Classical Chinese Medicine

CLASSICAL CHINESE MEDICINE

Liu Lihong

Translated by
Gabriel Weiss and **Henry Buchtel**
with **Sabine Wilms**

Edited by
Heiner Fruehauf

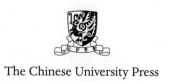

The Chinese University Press

Classical Chinese Medicine
  By Liu Lihong
  Translated by Gabriel Weiss and Henry Buchtel with Sabine Wilms
  Edited and introduced by Heiner Fruehauf

© The Chinese University of Hong Kong 2019

First edition 2019
Second printing 2019

ISBN: 978-988-237-057-9

The Chinese University of Hong Kong Press
The Chinese University of Hong Kong
Sha Tin, N.T., Hong Kong
Fax: +852 2603 7355
Email: cup@cuhk.edu.hk
Website: cup.cuhk.edu.hk

Printed in Hong Kong

CONTENTS

CHAPTER TWO
The Significance of Cold Damage

CHAPTER THREE
The Functioning of Yin and Yang

FOREWORD

The author of this book stood out from the many students I have taught. What made him remarkable was the extraordinarily heartfelt interest and curiosity with which he pursued his study of Chinese Medicine and its pertinent classical texts. It is highly commendable that he placed such importance on the classics, especially given their deteriorating status and the popular disregard for the great writings of the ancients. In a time when these important medical classics have been gradually downgraded to elective courses in prominent medical universities, it is this passionate pursuit of his studies that I find most gratifying.

The author's ardent study of the classics has brought him close to the limits of the current understanding of Chinese Medicine classics, and this is amply evidenced in the pages of this manuscript. I am convinced that, having read this book, the reader will have a similar impression. Just as the author of this book says, the study of the classics serves as the foundation of the study of Chinese Medicine, and there is still nothing that can adequately substitute for this foundation. For this reason, if one desires to learn Chinese Medicine well, if one desires to attain the utmost heights of what this branch of learning has to offer, then one must emphasize the classical texts, its very foundation. "If you want to cross the sea to a distant shore, only a boat can take you there." This is something both ancient and modern masters alike have recognized as a necessity. There is no other way.

What sort of book is the *Shanghanlun* (Treatise on Cold Damage[1])? It is

---

1   For better readability, classical Chinese texts in later occurrences are referred to by their translations in italics (*Treatise on Cold Damage* in this case). Where the translation of a classical Chinese text is long, an abbreviated translation, also in italics, will be employed for later mentions of the work.

a monumental medical work that serves as a link between the past and the future; it is almost universally esteemed by the most eminent physicians as a most important piece of classical writing; it is "an axe that can fell a mountain"; it is a springboard into the Dao; and it is, most importantly in my estimation, a treatise that expounds upon the many difficult and complicated pathological conditions one may encounter as a physician. The importance of the *Treatise on Cold Damage* to Chinese Medicine is beyond doubt.

The *Treatise on Cold Damage*'s unique significance in this branch of knowledge has led it to become, at all times and in all places, a focus of attention for Chinese Medicine physicians. As far as the textual merits of the *Treatise on Cold Damage* go, members of Chinese Medicine circles still sigh with admiration and say that it is good beyond comparison. And yet, this author has produced a rare piece of writing in which profound meanings from the classics are handled in a simple, straightforward, and absorbing manner that is both unassuming and pleasant. Confucius said, "Youths are to be regarded with respect—who knows whether they might exceed their forebears?" These words are worth keeping in mind as we read this book.

October 2001
Chen Yiren
Nanjing University of Chinese Medicine
Nanjing, China

Introduction

It is with much excitement and gratitude that I am announcing the English edition of Liu Lihong's milestone work, which represents a much-needed beacon for the profession of Chinese Medicine in the twenty-first century. *Classical Chinese Medicine* delivers a straightforward critique of the severe predicament that the "integration" of the traditional healing arts with Western science has spawned during the last 60 years, as well as a fervent call for the preservation of classical Chinese medical wisdom. Professor Liu's open and pointed style of presentation has made this book a best-seller that is read not only by medical students and doctors in China, but by multiple strata of the general population who long for a state of health and well-being founded in a deeper sense of cultural identity. Most importantly, Professor Liu's ardent appeal to regard Chinese Medicine as a science in its own right has inspired a mainland grassroots movement that is beginning to draw talented students to a field that was long regarded as a bleak second rate destination for professional development.

Eighteen years after its initial publication, it is more than time to bring this seminal work to Western readers. Oriental medicine education has made great strides since the 1970s in North America, Europe, and Australasia, but clear guidelines regarding the "traditional" nature of Traditional Chinese Medicine (TCM) remain murky and undefined. *Classical Chinese Medicine* not only delineates the educational and clinical problems the profession faces today in both East and West (despite quantitative "upgrades" such as doctoral-level status, extensive licensure, and the accreditation of ampler and larger schools), but also transmits concrete and inspiring guidance on how to effectively engage with ancient texts and designs in the postmodern age.

While Professor Liu's published voice represents one of the earliest objections to the direction that the standardized form of Chinese Medicine has taken since the foundation of the People's Republic of China (PRC) in 1949, it must be seen as the culmination of a cultural movement that first reacted to the sustained influx of Western science and medical modalities into China more than one and a half centuries ago. To cite an example, the medical philosopher Meng Jin wrote provocatively in *Yi yi yi* (Prescriptions for Healing the Present State of Medicine) in 1902:

> Most of today's Chinese Medicine doctors are utterly ill-advised—tens of thousands of miles removed from the advanced craftsmanship of the ancient sages. . . . As a result, the time-honored wisdom tradition of Chinese Medicine that once studied the microcosm of the body before the sophisticated backdrop of all macrocosmic sciences has now become an escapist haven for the ignorant and apathetic.[1]

Meng Jin goes on to lament the change from a medicine that was intrinsically founded upon functional and holistic parameters to an institution dominated by the presumptions of Western science—defined by the material eyes of anatomy and a diagnostic perspective based exclusively on structural changes in the body. Clinical outcomes, he declared exactly 100 years before Professor Liu published his book, were noticeably deteriorating.

Classical Chinese Medicine articulates the essence of this long-standing intellectual movement aiming to preserve the unique theories and techniques behind the clinical efficacy of Chinese Medicine. After other scholars in contemporary China realized that it was politically acceptable to share their genuine opinions about the government-issued doctrine of "modernizing," "integrating" and "unfeudalizing" Chinese Medicine, the dam broke and a flood of articles and books on the subject emerged. A pertinent example of the passionate tone adopted in the wake of Professor Liu's pioneering publication is provided by Mao Jialing, editor of the China Agency for Chinese Medicine and Pharmacology News. In 2005, he wrote

---

1   Meng Jin, *Yi yi yi* (Prescriptions for Healing the Present State of Medicine), in *Miben yixue congshu* (A Collection of Esoteric Medical Texts), edited by Qiu Qing-yuan, reprinted by Shanghai Shudian (Shanghai, 1988), vol. 5, p. 5.

in the preface to his influential essay collection *Zheyan kan Zhongyi* (Chinese Medicine in the Eye of Philosophy):

> If the field of Chinese Medicine continues to develop according to the fashionable directive of "glorious surface, collapsed interior," it won't be long before the chain of genuine knowledge transmission will be broken, before the market share of Chinese Medicine will dwindle down to zero, and until no more but an empty shell will remain of the profession of Chinese Medicine. In slightly more pessimistic and maybe exaggerated terms, one could say that the age-old profession of Chinese Medicine is presently facing a quiet death. Thousands of years of accumulated experiential knowledge gone in a flash—by finally having become "one with the rest of the world," by having become "scientific." The price: the sacrifice of its unique flavor and clinical benefits. Is this now a "revolution" that gives us reason to rejoice, or is it a "tragedy" or even a "sin"? However way we look at it, the development of Chinese Medicine has reached a state of extreme crisis! These may sound like empty words, overblown perhaps, but I believe that history will be the true judge of this statement. . . .[2]

We live at a most interesting point in history when pioneering scholars are actively exploring a more unbiased look at "the Other," arguably a prerequisite for all endeavors of true science and informed integration. It is one of the unfortunate characteristics of humanity that we all too easily become limited and determined by habitual patterns. After two centuries of donning the lenses of scientific materialism, mainstream views of reality have come to disregard the subtle domains of process and function, dynamic energy transformation, spirit, and the invisible threads that bind us to our ancestors in the transmission of knowledge—in essence, the core elements of classical Chinese Medicine. While these lenses have brought the gifts of logic, order and precision, they have also come with the qualities of arrogance, prejudice and, in a better scenario, esoteric amusement. We have become largely ignorant of the enormous potential that the ancient wisdom traditions offer for the task of healing the complex maladies of our time.

---

2   Excerpt from the preface to Chen Guiting and Mao Jialing, eds., *Zheyan kan Zhongyi* (Chinese Medicine in the Eye of Philosophy), Beijing Keji (Beijing, 2005), p. 1.

During the twentieth century, therefore, modern science all too often became an instrument that confirmed what we wished to see. When the first Egyptologists explored the treasures and mysteries of the pyramids, the Great Sphinx and the Valley of the Pharaohs, most of them described what their modern identity longed to corroborate: that these edifices, despite being built close to five millennia ago with engineering methods that mechanized building modes could not achieve until the 1980s, reflect nothing more than the fantastic belief system of stone-age barbarians. With a slightly different twist, late-nineteenth-century explorers of East Asia described what they longed to see: Japan was a land of geishas and *ukiyo-e* prints, mirroring the aesthetic preference of European authors such as the exoticist Pierre Loti. In turn, when Chinese artists went to the West during the 1920s, they tended to depict a two-dimensional landscape replete with flower-filled alcoves, blond women and romantic love, as in the work of the Japanese painter Tsuguharu Foujita (1886–1968) or the Chinese poet Li Jinfa (1900–1976).

A more productive and integrative approach to the Other was modeled by the symbolist authors R. A. Schwaller de Lubicz (1887–1961) and René Guénon (1886–1951), who independently coined the term "sacred science" during the 1920s. The concept of sacred science is based on the premise that ancient civilizations and their cultural legacy are containers of ageless wisdom, sorely needed at a time when all higher knowledge and the promise of enlightenment were assumed to lie exclusively in the future. The premise: in order to access and extract the acumen of these ancient traditions, we must first adopt an attitude of deep respect. When the labyrinth of seemingly nonsensical code—snakes and water lilies and scarab beetles; wood, fire, earth, metal, and water; *taiyang, yangming, shaoyang, taiyin, shaoyin, jueyin*; the hexagrams of the *Yijing* (Classic of Changes)—bewilder us, we should assume that this sentiment reflects our own ignorance on the subject matter, not that of its creators. As Liu Lihong points out, this vital piece of advice for the research of all ancient subject matter had been issued by China's primordial classic itself: "When you approach this book with the eyes of wisdom and compassion, all it will mirror back to you is wisdom and compassion," states one of the major commentaries of the *Yijing*.[3]

---

3   See the *Xici zhuan* (Tradition of the Appended Statements) commentary to the *Yijing*, chapter 1.5.

The implied meaning for modern readers: "When you approach this repository of ancient wisdom with the eyes of ignorance, you will most likely see nothing but senseless scribbles created by superstitious barbarians"—hardly a constructive attitude for the effective study of Chinese Medicine.

Once we have fully immersed ourselves in the symbol language of the ancient world and come to understand its concepts from within (as Schwaller attempted during his twelve-year studies of the hieroglyphs and the structural design of the Temple of Luxor in Egypt), true transmission of knowledge can take place and we begin to recognize its timeless meaning and modern significance. This is, perhaps, the most essential recommendation that *Classical Chinese Medicine* proposes for the study and practice of Chinese Medicine in the modern age. Liu Lihong employed this method himself when writing his doctoral dissertation on the *Shanghanlun* (Treatise on Cold Damage)—he meditated on the lines of the classic over and over again, and thus allowed the inner meaning to reveal itself, without consulting a single academic work on the subject.

In the epistemology of Western science, it took until the end of the twentieth century before this type of deeper integrative approach to the study of foreign or ancient Other made inroads into the realm of academic credibility. A throng of scholars from various fields spent their careers arguing vigorously against the limited view of human cognition that the materialist worldview of the Scientific Enlightenment had cast over most professional fields, including the domain of Chinese Medicine. Such scholars include the biologist and neuroscientist Francisco Varela, the authority on ancient mysticism Frits Staal, the physicist Fritjof Capra, the philosopher and cultural ecologist David Abram, the consciousness researcher B. Allan Wallace, the Daoism and Contemplative Studies expert Harold D. Roth, and many others. Liu Lihong's *Classical Chinese Medicine* echoes the multidisciplinary voices of these pioneering thought leaders. It exposes the scientist viewpoint as an obstacle rather than a liberating condition for the effective clinical practice of Chinese Medicine.

The term "integrative" has become a fashionable buzzword that has come to be used liberally in the brochures of both allopathic and alternative medicine colleges in East and West. Liu Lihong reminds us that true bridges of integration can only be built when both bridgeheads stand solidly grounded in their own foundation. As Chinese Medicine practitioners enter into the doctoral age, his challenge posits, it is vital for the integrity of the profession that we deepen our insights about the unplumbed depths of the past rather than the familiar minutiae of Western Medicine.

In order to understand the historical background upon which Liu Lihong's effort was conceived, it is important that we first understand the monolithic influence that the PRC brand of Chinese Medicine has exerted on the field during the last six decades. The following represents a synthesis of the development of TCM, the medical system that has monopolized the practice of Oriental medicine in mainland China, and that has come to serve as the primary mold for the evolving profession of Oriental medicine around the globe. It exposes a system that has been conditioned by a distinctly political agenda, and reveals its logo "TCM" as a grave misnomer— designating a medicine that is not at all aiming to preserve the traditional characteristics of Chinese Medicine, but, on the contrary, to expurgate, reform, and control the classical and folkloric texture of the traditional record in the name of progress.[4]

First Impact: The Modernization of China During the Late Nineteenth and Early Twentieth Century

At the beginning of the nineteenth century, the profession of Chinese Medicine was in peak season. Although many aspects of Chinese society were entering into a state of collapse and disarray by 1841, the culture of traditional medicine was alive with the multihued color and texture of a 2,500-year-old art. There was the stimulating discourse between the newly founded fever school and the school of the neo-classicists, there were numerous scholar physicians publishing influential discourses, and there was the arcane realm of esoteric discipleship, alchemical experimentation, and the kaleidoscopic facets of folk wisdom that always characterized the sensuous heart of the profession. The advent of Western Medicine

---

4   This historical synthesis was first published in shorter form in the October 1999 issue of the *Journal of Chinese Medicine*. I owe the inspiration for the original essay, as well as much of the detail information contained in it, to my mentor Professor Deng Zhongjia, Dean of the College of Medical Theory at Chengdu University of TCM.

presented the traditional healing system its first major challenge, from which it never completely recovered. It lost its rank as the one and only "medicine" (*yixue*) and became "Chinese Medicine" (*Zhongyi*), defined in contrast to "Western Medicine" (*Xiyi*). Immediately, however, there developed an early brand of progressive physicians who did not lament this situation, but attempted to integrate some of the paraphernalia of modern medicine into the traditional system. These pioneers are now collectively referred to as the Chinese-Western Integration School (*zhong xi huitong pai*). Main representatives are Wang Qingren (1768–1831), Tang Zonghai (1851–1908), Zhang Xichun (1860–1933), and Zhang Shouyi (1873–1934). It is important to note that these initial "integrators," often cited by TCM administrators as early visionaries of their own system of integrated medicine, were not proponents of the hierarchical superiority of Western Medicine, but rather tried to embody the traditional ideal of the broadly educated master physician. It was their erudite skill level in the art, philosophy, and science of the traditional thought process that allowed them to break new ground by, for instance, categorizing Western drugs in energetic terms, or by relating the Triple Warmer to certain anatomical tissues described by Western Medicine. Although it was their declared goal to incorporate some of the useful mechanics (*yong*) of Western Medicine into the traditional mother body (*ti*) of Chinese Medicine, their parameters remained clearly "traditional at the core"—as the programmatic title of Zhang Xichun's collected writings announces in 1933, *Yixue zhongzhong canxi lu* (Chinese at Heart But Western Where Appropriate: Essays Investigating an Integrated Form of Medicine).

The period during which curious Chinese physicians could explore the phenomenon of Western Medicine from an equal footing was soon eclipsed by a (still extant) period in which the Western scientific worldview dominates. During the first half of the twentieth century, a variety of events politicized Chinese Medicine as the despicable symbol of everything old and backward. It became a pawn that reformers from all political camps sought to abolish. When this endeavor failed due to vehement public protest, the new stewards of the Chinese Republic settled for banishing the unruly gargoyle of Chinese Medicine into a controlled existence that was subject to not only a rigorous purge of diagnostic methods and therapeutic modalities, but—most damaging to its integrity as a system in its own right—the gradual replacement of its essential standards with the "correct" parameters of modern science.

The political voice of Sun Yat-sen, the leader of the Republican revolution that toppled the dynastic system in 1911, was shaped by his Western science education, and reflected a deep suspicion of the old system of medicine. Later on, Kuomintang public health officials took this personal bias into the legislative arena and presented the radical proposal, *Feizhi jiuyi yi saochu yishi weisheng zhi zhang'ai an* (A Case for the Abolishment of Old Medicine to Thoroughly Eliminate Public Health Obstacles).[5] Authored by Yu Ai and Wang Qizhang, the proposition aggressively inferred that "the theories of yin and yang, the five elemental phases, the six atmospheric influences, the *zang-fu* systems, and the acupuncture channels are all illusions that have no basis in reality," and warns that "old medicine is still conning the people with its charlatan, shamanic, and geomancing ways."[6] The proposal, containing three major clauses (severely restrict the practice of Chinese Medicine; prohibit Chinese Medicine advertisements; bar the establishment of Chinese Medicine schools), passed the first legislative session of the Central Ministry of Public Health on February 26, 1929.[7] Although the proposition was not implemented due to thousands of protesting doctors and patients who took their passionate disapproval to the streets, the production of anti-traditional sentiment in an official document had a tremendous impact on the general mood of Chinese Medicine practice during the 1930s and 1940s.

Around the same time, the outlawed "communist bandit" Mao Zedong promulgated thoughts that were very similar to those of his nationalist adversaries. In 1942, he instructed his guerilla government to uproot all shamanic beliefs and superstitions in the Yan'an area and establish model public health villages.[8] Around the same time, he wrote that "old doctors, circus entertainers, snake oil salesmen, and street hawkers are all of the

---

5   Wa Zhiya, ed., *Zhongguo yixue shi* (A History of Chinese Medicine), Jiangxi Kexue Jishu (Nanchang, 1987), p. 278.
6   Wa Zhiya, ed., *Zhongguo yixue shi* (A History of Chinese Medicine), Renmin Weisheng (Beijing, 1991), p. 488.
7   Ibid., p. 489.
8   Wa Zhiya (1987), p. 288.

same sort."[9] This terse statement would have a truly devastating impact twenty-five years later when Mao's works became the one and only source for the country's definition of political truth. It was quoted in millions of copies of red "Mao Bibles" (*Mao Zhuxi yulu*), serving as the Red Guard's main license for the uncompromising persecution of the rich culture of traditional medicine and its unique modes of practice, education, and theoretical discourse.

Chinese Communism and the Conception of TCM, 1953–1976

The years 1953–1959 witnessed what appears like a remarkable reversal of Mao's earlier views on Chinese Medicine. Having graduated from the task of creating national respect for the "rural outlaw" who now donned the emperor's robes, he began to gradually advance his private ambition of asserting leadership over the legion of budding communist countries around the world. This objective required the conception of a socialist model that distinguished itself from the Russian paradigm of Marxist-Leninism by incorporating the regional attributes of third-world countries. Chinese Medicine fit well into this general scheme, since it embodied a medicine that was "self-reliant," "among the people," "native," and "patriotic"—all slogans that had been used to promote Mao's unique brand of communism. Mao sensed, furthermore, that China was beginning to become overly dependent on the influx of Soviet goods and expertise, especially in the areas of modern medical equipment and pharmaceutics. The catastrophic famines and the far-reaching collapse of infrastructure that followed the Russian walkout in 1961 were to dramatically confirm his premonitions.

It was for primarily political reasons, therefore, that Mao began to publicly embrace Chinese Medicine during the mid-1950s. This was the time when he issued the famous calligraphy that graces the front pages of so many TCM publications: "*Zhongguo yiyao xue shi yige weida baoku, yingdang nuli fajue, jiayi tigao*" (Chinese Medicine is a grand cache of knowledge that we should actively bring to light and further evolve). In the wake

---

9   *Mao Zhuxi yulu* (Sayings by Chairman Mao), no editor, no publisher, p. 54.

of this apparently new direction, two ministers of health, Wang Bing and He Cheng, had to resign due to their exclusive loyalty to the Western medical system that had made them trustworthy candidates for the position in the first place. In 1956, premier Zhou Enlai signed papers that authorized the immediate establishment of the first four colleges of Chinese Medicine, namely Chengdu College of TCM, Beijing College of TCM, Shanghai College of TCM, and Guangzhou College of TCM, followed by Nanjing College of TCM the following year. At the same time, a group that was to become the influential voice of the first generation of institutional TCM teachers— all of them still trained under the pre-institutional model of discipleship education—assembled in Beijing. They are generally referred to as the "five elders" (*wulao*), including Qin Bowei from Shanghai, Cheng Shenwu from Beijing, and Ren Yingqiu, Li Chongren, and Yu Daoji from Sichuan.

As if to set a good example for the new course that he had outlined, Mao publicly ingested the traditional remedy Yin Qiao San (Lonicera and Forsythia Powder) when he fell ill during the historic announcement of the Great Leap Forward at the Chengdu Conference in 1957. He restrained his one-time prejudice against "snake oil salesmen" and allowed Li Shizhi and Peng Lüxiang, both first-generation elders of Chengdu College of TCM, to be present at his bedside for an entire night.

In 1958, the political motives of Mao's actions fully revealed themselves when he issued his decreeing vision about the concept of "Chinese-Western Medicine integration" (*Zhong xi yi jiehe*).[10] The integration movement, in essence, mandated the establishment of "TCM"—a medical system which restrains the "wildness" and the "feudal elements" of the traditional art by taking it out of the hands of its lineage holders and assigning it to the control of modern science, one of the most trusted tools of Marxist-materialist ideology. Mao announced a nationwide search for "2,000 first-rate Western Medicine physicians who are to assist in the evolvement of Chinese Medicine." Special Seminars for the Study of Chinese Medicine by

---

10 See a series of articles published in 1958 in China's official newspaper, *Renmin ribao* (The People's Daily), i.e. "Dali kaizhan Xiyi xuexi Zhongyi yundong" (Let Us Give Strong Momentum to the Western Doctors Studying Chinese Medicine Movement). See Yu Zhenchu, *Zhongguo yixue jianshi* (A Brief History of Chinese Medical Science), Fujian Kexue Jishu (Fuzhou, 1983), p. 446.

Western Medicine Physicians On Leave (*Xiyi lizhi xuexi Zhongyi ban*) were established, administering pieces of a highly standardized extract of traditional knowledge over a period of one to two years. Qualifying participants were required to hold or exceed the "physician in chief" rank within the Western medical system. Of 2,000 doctors who initially entered into the program, only about 10 percent graduated. This low success rate may in part be due to the fact that the study of Chinese Medicine, even in abridged form, involves the memorization of scientific detail which all participants, including the successful graduates, had previously been conditioned to condemn as the nefarious byproduct of a social system riddled with feudalist superstition. Nevertheless, these Western doctors who participated in the "traditional medicine reform" efforts of the years 1959–1962 came to provide the main pool for TCM administrative positions in later years. Most top-level TCM administrators of the 1980s and 1990s were, in fact, Western Medicine graduates of the reform/integration seminars.

This situation is the primary reason for the plight of Chinese Medicine under the TCM system. Traditional medicine in mainland China continues to be managed by individuals who for the most part, and often openly, entertain deep-seated suspicions against the field that they are supposed to represent. In a radical sense, the history of TCM can be described as the history of implementing anti-traditional sentiments into the general atmosphere of Chinese Medicine education and practice. I personally know of very few TCM administrators who resort to traditional modalities when they fall ill themselves. TCM students and faculty, moreover, regularly take antibiotics when contracting a cold—"because it is more convenient and works faster and better." One of the personal memories I associate with this topic is a conversation with the grandson of Li Shizhi (the founding elder of Chengdu College of TCM who once prescribed Yin Qiao San to Mao Zedong)—himself a TCM doctor, scholar, and administrator at the College that is generally regarded as the "most traditional" among TCM institutions in China—in which he expressed concern about my enthusiasm for traditional herbology. He flatly admonished me to curb my faith in the efficacy of Chinese Medicine. In light of this situation, all of my more classically oriented teachers thus cautiously asserted that the "integration" project marked the beginning of a process that ruined the true nature of traditional medicine.

On the surface, however, this course of events caused a boost to the status of Chinese Medicine. The government had encouraged individuals of high scientific regard to immerse themselves in the subject of indigenous medicine and foster the betterment of the field. Furthermore, for the first time, TCM departments were established in many city hospitals. The actual result, though, was the genesis of a situation in which the old, clinically experienced Chinese Medicine practitioners were barred from participating in the domain of major league TCM. All of the doctors in charge were "Western doctors with Chinese knowledge" (*Xi xue Zhong*)—experts who styled their diagnosis entirely in Western terms, but sporadically included some cookbook-style Chinese Medicine modalities in their approach. Distinguished "folk" physicians, unable to practice privately under the communist system, were accessible only in outpatient departments, or occasionally summoned for a second opinion. Many observers of this practice bitterly remark that if a remedy prescribed by one of these elders resulted in a cure, it was most likely that all the credit was given to the Western modalities— even though it was their ineffectiveness that had initiated the traditional consultation. Chinese Medicine, after all, was not recognized anymore as a clinical science in its own right, and the traditional diagnostic approach of *bianzheng* (diagnosis by synthesis of pulse, tongue, and symptom profile) was progressively becoming eclipsed by the standardized procedure of *bian-bing* (diagnosis by Western disease name).

In the aftermath of these events, the status of Western Medicine became dramatically elevated with regard to institutionalized TCM education. Planned in 1961 and executed in 1962, all TCM colleges adopted a curriculum that required incoming students to first study Western Medicine for two and a half years, then Chinese Medicine for two and a half years, until finally entering into an "integrated" clinical internship for one year. The five elders immediately realized that this educational setup was responsible for an increasing loss of respect for the fundamental principles of Chinese Medicine, and composed a letter to the central government that summarized their concerns. Their protest led to an abolishment of the new curriculum and ushered in a brief revival of classical values—spawning a college program that started out with three years of exclusive Chinese Medicine training, including the reading and memorization of all major classics in their entirety, as well as palpation of 10,000 pulses and inspection of 2,000

tongues. However, the exigencies of the political sphere were soon to interfere in a most severe manner again.

In 1966, Mao Zedong found himself locked in an internal power struggle and unleashed the "Great Cultural Revolution" to neutralize his antago-
nists. For ten years, all forms of higher education came to a screeching halt.
In the field of Chinese Medicine, only the entering class of 1963 was able to
complete a TCM curriculum that for the first time truly deserved the label
"traditional." Since it was the main rallying cry of the Cultural Revolution
to eradicate every trace of feudalist influence, all of the old master practitioners of Chinese Medicine, including the Five Elders, became subject
to criticism, ridicule, and in some instances, public humiliation. As many
physicians frantically burned their stitch-bound volumes and other old-
fashioned belongings to avoid persecution, and as others died from grief or
physical abuse, much of the physical legacy of Chinese Medicine perished
irretrievably.

In this vacuum, Western Medicine reasserted its defining influence on
TCM, while it had to adapt to a political environment that despised erudite
learning of any kind itself. Already during the previous year, in a speech
given to healthcare professionals in Beijing on June 26, 1965, Mao had set
the stage for the anti-intellectual direction of the new medicine to come:
"Medical education needs to be reformed—it is completely unnecessary to
engage in so much studying. How many years of formal education, after all,
did Hua Tuo have? And how many Li Shizhen? There is no need to restrict
medical education to people with high school diplomas; middle school
and elementary school pupils will do. The real learning will happen during actual practice. If this type of lowly educated doctor is then sent to the
countryside, he will always be able to do a better job than the charlatan sha-
mans; and the peasants, moreover, will be able to afford such care. Studying is a stupid endeavor for a doctor."[11]

During the years 1966–1971, therefore, no new students were admitted by educational institutions, including schools of Chinese Medicine. In
1972, so-called Colleges for Workers, Peasants, and Soldiers (*gong nong bing*

11 Mao Zedong, "Dui weishengbu gongzuo de zhishi" (Instructions Regarding the
    Work of the Ministry of Public Health), in *Ziliao xuanbian* (A Collection of Mate-
    rials), no editor, no publisher (1967), p. 312.

xueyuan) were established, offering three-year vocational programs under the maxim of "open door schooling." This meant that there were no entry exams; the admission of students was entirely based on their political status as well as the social background of their parents. Textbooks were filled with quotes from *Mao Zedong's Collected Works*. The doctors produced by this system received a very rudimentary training in both Chinese and Western modalities, and provided the human resource for the well-known Barefoot Doctor Movement (*chijiao yisheng yundong*). The barefoot doctors, naturally, were never introduced to the essential concept of differential diagnostics. Meanwhile, the generation of Chinese Medicine elders was either dead or locked up as "bovine demons and snake-like goblins" (*niugui sheshen*) in so-called "ox stalls" (*niupeng*). Of the five elders, only Ren Yingqiu was still alive. He was banished to Qinghai province, China's equivalent to Siberia—allowed to bring only one cherished book, Li Shizhen's *Bencao gangmu* (Outline of the Materia Medica).

In the Name of Progress: The Introduction of "Superior Methodology," "Scientific Standards," and "Research Axioms" During the 1980s and 1990s

Another blow to the integrity of the traditional system, or what was left of it, occurred during the period of 1980–1985. At this time, the concept of "Chinese Medicine improvement by methodology research" (*Zhongyi fangfa lun yanjiu*) was introduced. The political leaders of TCM institutions, i.e. the communist party secretaries who are generally more influential than the college presidents, selected several fashionable theories of Western science and applied them to the domain of Chinese Medicine—once again motivated by the resolve to "further evolve" the field. These endeavors were generally characterized by the attempt to sanctify the "scientific character" of selected aspects of Chinese Medicine, and consequently, by denying scientific validity (and the ensuing right to be preserved and transmitted) to others. During the period in question, the theories elected for this purpose were cybernetics (*kongzhi lun*), system science (*xitong lun*), and information theory (*xinxi lun*).

The result of this "assistance" was the affirmation of the TCM system on theoretical grounds. The methodologists concluded that Chinese Medicine classics such as the *Huangdi neijing* (Yellow Emperor's Classic of

Medicine) already contain evidence of these progressive theories in embryonic form, apparently recommending an affirmative stance toward the tradition of Chinese Medicine. On the other hand, this position implied that the classics were to be viewed like dinosaurs—interesting to look at in a museum, but, in terms of their pragmatic value in a contemporary environment, vastly inferior to the eloquent treatises of information theory, cybernetics, and other domains of modern science. As a result, many TCM colleges actually established museums, and many publishers dared again to issue reprint editions of classical texts. The original regard for the classics as the primary source of clinical information, however, dwindled as the presence of original texts in the curriculum became minimized. Again, it was a situation where a group of individuals with no traditional medical background attempted to "reform" Chinese Medicine—motivated by ideological rather than clinical considerations.

The 1990s, in the opinion of my more classically oriented teachers and myself, have seen the most severe erosion of traditional core values. I will cite the following reasons for this assessment:

(a) Due to market-driven priorities, none of the numerous TCM journals made efforts to cover the philosophical foundations of Chinese Medicine. The government, furthermore, provided no money for the traditional category of textual research (which had been a possible area of specialization for graduate students until 1988), and no graduate research projects involving only Chinese Medicine theory were permissible.

(b) The new market economy obliged TCM hospitals to be profitable. The subject of profitability was and still is intimately tied to a standardized fee structure based on an official ranking system—which, in turn, is defined by Western Medicine values, such as the quantity of modern diagnostic equipment and the amount of available beds. The hospitals thus devote a tremendous amount of effort to the acquisition and application of paraphernalia that will boost both their quality ranking and their diagnostic income. As one TCM physician put it: "little money is to be made by just feeling the pulse." This tendency is echoed in private street clinics, where doctors are encouraged, even required, by the herbal pharmacies that employ them to prescribe large amounts of preferably expensive herbs to maximize profits.

(c) In 1994–1995, the Ministry of Health published a host of official guidelines aimed at standardizing the mandatory process of researching the effect of new patent remedies.[12] Along with the establishment of a Chinese FDA, it was decreed that the research of Chinese Medicine patents must be conducted according to the standards of Western pharmaceutical research. Most consequentially, this meant that the traditional system of differential diagnosis (*bianzheng*) had to be completely replaced by allopathic diagnostics (*bianbing*). According to these guidelines, research on the constitutional multipurpose remedy Four Frigid Extremities Powder (Sini San), for instance, must be conducted and marketed in the context of only one diagnostic category, i.e. "cholecystitis." Theoretical background research into the traditional rationale of a remedy is confined to 10 percent of the proposal, while disease-oriented research has to account for 70 percent. Another point that mirrors the research protocol of Western Medicine is the obligatory focus on laboratory animal research. This development has started to turn the broadly defined clinical science of Chinese Medicine into a discipline that is dominated by the narrowly defined and, most importantly, completely disparate parameters of modern pharmacology. It finalizes the process of "evolution by integration" that Mao had originally prescribed for Chinese Medicine 60 years ago—a process that involves eviscerating the indigenous art of its spirit and essence, and subsequently appropriating its material hull (i.e. herbs and techniques) into the realm of an integrated medicine that declares itself scientifically superior.

(d) A new class of graduate students began to develop who cannot diagnose in differential terms anymore, and who instead are

---

12 See the authoritative work in two volumes published by the Chinese Ministry of Health in 1994–1995, *Zhongyao xinyao linchuang yanjiu zhidao yuanze* (Guidelines for Clinical Research Pertaining to New TCM Remedies).

steeped in allopathic terminology and diagnosis. Virtually all of the doctoral theses presently produced in China fall into the field of Chinese-Western integration research, or laboratory animal research related to the ratification of new patent remedies. Integrated standards for students of Chinese and Western Medicine, moreover, have produced a situation where Chinese Medicine researchers are required to utilize unwarranted equipment such as electron microscopes to achieve doctoral-level approbation. In addition to the conceptual crisis outlined in this article, the system of state-sponsored TCM is also facing a grave financial crisis. Most institutions simply cannot keep up with the rising cost of the narrowly defined type of research prescribed by the system.

(e) Of an impressive-sounding five years in the TCM bachelor curriculum, much was (and still is) taken up by classes in foreign language, physical education, political studies, and computer training. By far, the most extensive classes are dedicated to Western Medicine contents such as anatomy, physiology, immunology, parasitology, and other topics that are unrelated to the diagnostic and therapeutic procedures of classical Chinese Medicine. From both a quantitative and a qualitative perspective, therefore, it would not be entirely inappropriate to state that the Chinese Medicine portion in the contemporary TCM curriculum has been reduced to the status of a peripheral supplement—approximately 40 percent or less of the total amount of hours. This issue is compounded by the ongoing division of students into Western-style areas of specialization, such as acupuncture or bone disorders. None of the specialty students, including acupuncture department graduates, are required anymore to familiarize themselves with the realm of original teachings, not even in the radically abridged form of classical quotations that still serve to bestow an air of legitimacy on most official TCM textbooks.

Voices of Dissent:
The Call for a Renaissance of Classical Chinese Medicine

Similar to earlier waves of elder physician protest, the increasingly declining depth of teaching and practice modes during the 1990s brought about polarization and internal dissent. While policy makers were interested in the appearance of a united front, a group of concerned scholars and administrators wrote letters to government leaders and editors of TCM journals, and circulated critical memorandums at scholarly meetings. In a communiqué entitled "A Call to Correct the Developmental Direction of Chinese Medicine and to Preserve and Cultivate the Unique Characteristics of Our Field," Lü Bingkui, former director of the TCM section of the PRC Ministry of Health, wrote in 1991:

> In recent years, the unique characteristics of Chinese Medicine, its advantages over Western Medicine, and its standards of academic excellence have not been developed according to the wishes of the people, but have rather been tossed into a state of severe crisis and chaotic actions. Underneath the bright and cheap glitter at the surface, the essence and the characteristics of Chinese Medicine are being metamorphosed and annihilated at a most perturbing rate. The primary expression of this crisis is the Westernization of all guiding principles and methodologies of Chinese Medicine.[13]

Other notable members of this critical group were Cui Yueli (Ministry of Health), Fang Yaozhong (Chinese TCM Research Academy), Deng Tietao (Guangzhou University of TCM), Fu Jinghua (Chinese TCM Research Academy), Li Zhichong (Chinese TCM Association), and Zhu Guoben (National Ministry of TCM).

In 1997, the topic of the erosion of Chinese Medicine integrity had become prevalent enough for a major publisher to bring these dissenting voices from the obscurity of back door communications to the fore by publishing them in a two-volume set, entitled *Zhongyi chensi lu* (Pondering Core Issues of Chinese Medicine). Scholars of lower administrative rank, however, remained cautious of voicing their opinions in public. While consulting with

---

13 Cui Yueli, ed., *Zhongyi chensi lu* (Pondering Core Issues of Chinese Medicine), 2 vols., Zhongyi Guji (Beijing, 1997), vol. 1, p. 25.

me about the details of a similar essay for the *Journal of Chinese Medicine* in 1999, for instance, one of my Chinese mentors encouraged me to publish the facts of the century-long "TCM Crisis" abroad, while choosing to circulate the Chinese translation of the article among students and colleagues at his institutions only in unpublished form.

In 2002, the critical examination of the TCM model reached a level of unprecedented openness in China. From the safe haven of a Hong Kong teaching position and backed by the preface of Deng Tietao, by now the most prominent sponsor of the classical essence movement, scholar Li Zhichong published a volume of essay collections entitled *Zhongyi fuxing lun* (Advocating for a Renaissance of Chinese Medicine). Featuring highly provocative section headings such as "Liberating Ourselves From the Century-Old Straightjacket of Delusion in Chinese Medicine" or "Westernization—The Mortal Wound of Chinese Medicine," these essays distinguish themselves not only by way of candor, but also by delineating clear guidelines for a revival of the science of classical Chinese Medicine. Here is a sample of the new tone introduced by Li's book:

> It is sad to see that because of several decades of wasted efforts and misguided energy, the core essence of Chinese Medicine has virtually been lost by the ignorant people who, from the top of their lungs, have been chanting the mantra of "modernization." Even though the outer shell of Chinese Medicine education is still there—the tall buildings, the books and the students and the instructors, and the herbs that fill the markets in abundance—the real science of our medicine, especially the true essence of our theoretical foundations has been lost almost in its entirety, or has become little more than an empty slogan. As an old Chinese saying goes: "When seeking the longevity of a tree, one must safeguard its roots"—this "root," that is the theoretical foundation of our field. A "flourishing" without root . . . is like an empty shell without *hun* or *po*.[14]

It was at this opportune time that Liu Lihong issued his passionate and comprehensive plea for a return to the medical values delineated in the classics. Since the publication of *Classical Chinese Medicine*, Professor Liu

---

14   Li Zhichong, *Zhongyi fuxing lun* (Advocating for a Renaissance of Chinese Medicine), Zhongguo Yiyao Keji (Beijing, 2002), p. 344.

has emerged as China's leading voice expressing the sense of cultural loss surrounding the knowledge system of Chinese Medicine as well as other time-honored arts and sciences. While the publisher was originally doubtful that he could move the 2,000 copies of the first edition, the Chinese version of this book has since sold more than one million copies and become one of the best-selling non-fiction books in modern China. In addition, several Chinese Medicine universities in China and the United States, including Guangzhou University of TCM and the College of Classical Chinese Medicine at National University of Natural Medicine in Portland, Oregon, have integrated the principles delineated in *Classical Chinese Medicine* into their core curriculum.

Professor Liu's thoughtful and forthright approach promptly elicited official leadership support in his home province of Guangxi. In the fall of 2004, he received permission to establish a state-funded educational research institute with the goal of inviting exceptional Chinese Medicine elders who had been ignored by the institutionalized TCM system to transmit their clinical knowledge to motivated disciples, many of them experienced physicians, doctoral-level students, and practitioners returning from abroad. The first "resident elder" of the Institute for the Clinical Research of Classical Chinese Medicine was Dr. Li Ke, a physician known for his successful track record of treating acute stages of heart attack, stroke, kidney failure, and other emergency disorders with Chinese herbs (administered through nasal tubes).[15] Since then, Liu Lihong has developed the Institute into an influential platform that has reintroduced multiple classical lineages to contemporary scholarly discourse, most notably the Fire Spirit School of Sichuan herbalism (*huoshen pai*), the traditional system of emotional healing synthesized by the Confucian educator Wang Fengyi (1864–1937), and classical five-element-style acupuncture. Each one of these efforts has had a considerable impact on the grassroots momentum of Chinese Medicine education in China.

---

15 See *Li Ke lao Zhongyi jiwei zhongzheng yinan bing jingyan zhuanji* (A Collection of Case Histories of Chinese Medicine Elder Dr. Li Ke's Treatments of Acute Emergency Disorders and Recalcitrant Diseases), Shanxi Kexue Jishu (Taiyuan, 2002).

Perspectives On "TCM" and
Classical Chinese Medicine—A Comparative Outlook

In addition to underscoring the immense significance of this book, it is a declared purpose of my introduction to make "TCM" transparent as a historically and politically conditioned system that is fundamentally different from the multifaceted traditions that constitute traditional Chinese Medicine. In this process, I am attempting to establish a defining line that helps individual Oriental medicine practitioners, schools, and agencies to clarify their own philosophical position. It is, however, not my point to denounce the phenomenon of "TCM." The standardization procedures of "TCM" are perhaps the main reason that Chinese Medicine is still a thriving profession today, after a prolonged period during which China and the rest of the modernizing world were willing to forsake their own traditions in exchange for the power of Western Medicine. The TCM barefoot doctor approach, moreover, did save many lives when expert healthcare was not available in the Chinese countryside. It is my intention, however, to expose the common practice of advertising the education and clinical practice of "TCM" under traditional insignia that suggest the transmission and application of an ancient Eastern healthcare system based entirely on holistic principles.

The general discourse on Oriental medicine in the West appears to have reached the realm of the 10,000 details (i.e. "what points work best for diabetes," "how to treat headaches with Chinese herbs"), while leaving the basic parameters of its scientific approach unexplored. To help stimulate a broader discussion on Chinese Medicine methodology, I have created a table (see Table 1) that contrasts the characteristics of "TCM" with those of traditional Chinese Medicine—here labeled "classical Chinese Medicine" in order to distinguish it more clearly from its modern cousin—as Liu Lihong and my own teachers have described it. This table is meant to be a starting point, a tool that may help Oriental medicine practitioners and institutions assess their inner mode of teaching and practice. It may be incomplete and, due to the nature of the black-and-white table format, overstate some of the differences that set the two systems apart.

Table 1 Some characteristics of classical Chinese Medicine and "TCM"

CLASSICAL CHINESE MEDICINE	"TCM"
Based on naturalist philosophy (Daoism, Confucianism)	Based on pragmatist philosophy (scientific materialism, communism)
Alchemical (synthetic) approach: scientific endeavor defined as acknowledgement and exploration of the complexity and multi-dimensionality of nature and the body	Analytical approach: scientific endeavor defined as elimination of complicating factors and unpredictable occurrences
Based on traditional parameters of Daoist and Confucian science (yin yang, *wuxing, bagua, wuyun liuqi, jing-qi-shen*, etc.)	Primarily based on parameters of modern science (virus, inflammation, blood pressure, etc.)
Views medicine as a branch of the Daoist and Confucian mother sciences (Huang Lao, *zhouyi, fengshui*, etc.)	Views medicine as a branch of modern science
Source-oriented: reliance on tradition (experience)	Branch-oriented: reliance on progress (experiments)
Requires broad base of knowledge due to intimate relationship to other traditional arts and sciences	Technical and highly specialized trade
Body is treated as a microcosm that follows macrocosmic laws and is continually informed by macrocosmic influences (totality of cosmic/calendric/seasonal patterns created by conjunctions of sun, moon, and stars)	Body is treated as an independent entity
Based on experience of human "subject" in environment of geocentric universe	Based on "objectivist" heliocentric worldview
Based on dualistic cosmology of becoming (process-oriented worldview observing the continuous change of physical phenomena, symbolized by the changing pattern of the moon)	Based on cosmology of being (concept of singular, metaphysical truth, symbolized by fixed position of the sun)
Impartial view of reality as continuous interplay between heaven and earth, light and shadow, "demons" (*gui*: lunar influences) and "spirits" (*shen*: solar influences), birth and death, male and female, yin and yang	Materialist method of dividing heavenly and earthly spheres and "rectifying the names" (*zheng ming*: convert the binary symbols of lunar mythology into the immutable and one-sided terminology of the solar perspective, and dignify an absolute position as "right/good/correct")
Communicates through symbols which contain and correlate multiple layers of meaning	Communicates through words and terms which refer to narrowly defined contents
Preserves the lunar element of complexity and "obscuring" mystery that defies exacting definition (*wuwei* maxim: "do not define categorically")	Demystifies and demythologizes the traditional record by "illuminating" aspects of lunar ambivalence, and by creating "clear and simple" textbook definitions (*youwei* maxim: "define as firmly and precisely as possible")

(Cont'd Table 1)

CLASSICAL CHINESE MEDICINE	"TCM"
Views body as field (traditional *zang-xiang* theory: *zang-fu* are primarily viewed as functional systems)	Views body as material entity (influence of modern anatomy: *zang-fu* are primarily viewed as structural organs)
Body—mind—spirit medicine	Body—(mind) medicine
Physician is intermediary to the sacred, cultivating the dual roles of the Daoist shaman (master of intuited knowledge) and the Confucian sage (master of scholarly knowledge), connecting above and below, inside and outside, energy and matter	Physician is skilled technician who rectifies imbalances between bodily humors and calibrates the structural composition of the body (eliminate viruses, etc.)
Physician aspires to the Dao of medicine, a process which requires the actualization of his/her individual path by working to become a self-realized being (*zhenren*)	Physician is part of a legally defined profession with standardized ethical standards
Major tools: *qigong* meditation, music, calligraphy, painting, poetry, ritual journeys	Major tools: standardized courses/tests on legal responsibility and liability issues
Highly individualized discipleship-based training	Highly standardized institutionalized training
Teachers are individual "master" figures who emphasize the creation of a lineage inspired atmosphere/culture	Teachers are assigned to standardized curriculum items, and thus in principle exchangeable
Transmission of "understanding" (may include *qi* transmission from master to disciple)	Transmission of data through "words" and "terms"
Multidirectional memorization:	Mono-directional memorization:
Memorization of classical texts that are interpreted situationally according to individual circumstances	Use of standardized textbooks that prepare for testing of knowledge in multiple choice format; classics are placed in museum
Health is defined as the active process of refining body essences and cultivating vital forces: concept of "nourishing life" (maximizing physiological functions)	Health is defined as the absence of pathology
Clinical diagnosis is primarily based on "subjective" experience of the senses	Clinical diagnosis is primarily informed by "objective" instrumental data (as provided by prior Western Medicine diagnosis)
Clinical outcome is primarily based on patient's subjective feeling of well-being and physician's collation of sensory information (tongue, pulse, etc.)	Clinical outcome is primarily monitored through instrumental data (reduction of viral load in blood, disappearance of lump on x-ray, etc.)
Highly individualized diagnosis: emphasizes *bianzheng* (diagnosis by symptom pattern)	Standardized diagnosis: emphasizes *bianbing* (diagnosis by disease name)

(Cont'd Table 1)

CLASSICAL CHINESE MEDICINE	"TCM"
Highly individualized treatment: favors flexible therapeutic approach which freely chooses from a wide variety of modalities, and within them, favors a flexible usage of prescription items	Standardized treatment: favors fixed modalities (herbs or acupuncture), and within them, promotes fixed herb regimens (patent medicines) and fixed-point prescriptions
Use of wide range of clinical modalities, including the external application of herbs to acupuncture points, umbilical therapy, *qigong* exercises, *waiqi* emission, five-phase emotional therapy, alchemical dietetics, *ziwu liuzhu* acupuncture, etc.	Selective ratification of certain modalities that have a measurable effect on the physical body and that can be explained from the perspective of modern science, such as the internal administration of anti-bacterial herbs and *ashixue* acupuncture
All-inclusive scope of practice (includes emergency medicine, bone fractures, serious diseases such as cancer, etc.)	Selective scope of practice (chosen areas in which modern studies have shown an advantage of TCM over Western Medicine, such as chronic pain or allergies)
All-encompassing training (may lead to clinical specialization in a traditional field, such as external medicine, if inspired by the clinical expertise of a specific teacher)	Progressive clinical specialization according to the model of Western Medicine (acupuncture, internal medicine, external medicine, gynecology, pediatrics, tumors, cardiovascular diseases, digestive diseases, etc.)
Combination of Western and traditional modalities, if employed, is performed according to Chinese Medicine criteria (i.e. Zhang Xichun's method of energetically classifying aspirin and integrating it as an alchemical ingredient into traditional formulas)	Combination of Western and traditional modalities is recommended in most cases; combination follows Western Medicine criteria (i.e. abdominal surgery plus post-operative administration of herbs with anti-adhesive effect such as magnolia bark)

With regard to the positions outlined in Table 1, most of us will find that our own convictions and modes of practice follow propositions that can be found on both sides of the dividing line. In particular, it is my experience that Oriental medicine practitioners in the West often proclaim to embrace the principles stated on the left, while their modus operandi in terms of diagnosis and treatment is much more closely aligned with the attitudes outlined on the right—much like Chinese officials used to aspire to the image of the philosopher-poet in their private life, while adhering to pragmatist values when acting in public. Others, after surveying this table, might find that although they were not aware of a "TCM issue" in the past, they certainly like the premises of "TCM" better than the mystifying conjectures of the classical path.

It is, therefore, not my goal to dignify the classical Dao of Oriental medicine and malign "TCM," although it has become clear in the course of this presentation what the nature of my own bias is. Neither do I suggest that any deviation from pre-twentieth-century ways of diagnosis and treatment automatically establishes the practice of "TCM." The use of modern equipment to measure the electric resistance of acupuncture points, for instance, thoroughly adheres to traditional *zang-xiang* theory ("examine the surface to determine the hidden factors inside"). In accordance with the principles outlined in Liu Lihong's book, I believe that the term "classical" does not imply that we should turn the clock back to the times of Zhang Zhongjing or Sun Simiao, but rather that we should utilize the timeless principles of the art and science of Chinese Medicine to assess, appreciate, and potentially incorporate new information from all branches of knowledge.

In conclusion, *Classical Chinese Medicine* represents a fervent call for respecting the art of Chinese Medicine as a science in its own right.[16] It is one of the most visible problems of twentieth-century Oriental medicine that the profession feels compelled to scour for legitimacy by conducting tests and experiments that conform to the parameters of Western Medicine. To illustrate the kind of absurdity that can potentially spring from this situation, I would like to relate an incident that I witnessed at the teaching hospital of the Chengdu College of Traditional Chinese Medicine in 1990. A respected doctor at the hospital was widely known for prescribing an herbal remedy that appeared to be highly effective in bringing about the speedy and painless delivery of babies by first-time mothers. Expecting mothers sometimes came to the hospital from as far as 50 miles away to obtain a prescription. After two decades of consistently positive feedback, a local pharmaceutical company decided to produce his formula as a patent. Before "modernization"

16　The issue of respect for the Chinese scientific tradition as a stand-alone body of science—and its demise at the hands of PRC administrators—was first introduced by the prolific work of Joseph Needham, and more recently, specified for the field of Chinese Medicine by Manfred Porkert, Leon Hammer, and Bob Flaws. See Leon I. Hammer, "Duelling Needles: Reflections on the Politics of Medical Models," *American Journal of Acupuncture* (AJA), 19.3 (1991); Bob Flaws, "Thoughts on Acupuncture, Internal Medicine, and TCM in the West," *Journal of Chinese Medicine*, 38 (1992); and Manfred Porkert, *Chinese Medicine Debased*, Phainon, 1997.

had become an issue, the positive testimonies of hundreds of patients would have sufficed to get the project started, but new codes demanded that direct action of the herbal solution on the uterus must first be verified in a laboratory setting. The lab director went through great pains to exclude factors that could potentially affect the outcome of the experiment. He put a female rabbit in a sterile incubator, stabilized the temperature and light exposure, surgically isolated the uterus and placed it outside of the rabbit's abdomen, and finally injected the herbal solution directly into the carefully extrapolated organ. To the researcher's surprise, nothing happened, even when he repeated the experiment with a number of other animals. In a second series of experiments, he injected a variety of other substances into rabbit uteri and, after observing that some of them induced contractions, proclaimed that they were more suitable for mass production. However, when the newly "discovered" herbs, which in traditional pharmacopoeias are not at all related to uterine effects, were tested on eager mothers by the old obstetrician, they failed to produce any clinical results. Thoroughly confused, the managers of the company decided to withdraw from the project.

This incident exemplifies how the elaborate procedures of reductionist science can project a highly distorted picture of the reality of the human body, producing results that are essentially non-scientific. The traditional doctor and most of his colleagues seemed undisturbed by the outcome of the experiment, since they adhered to a set of principles demanding verification in non-sedated, intact people who deliver babies in an uncontrolled real-life environment. According to their reasoning: (a) rabbits are different from humans; (b) human beings usually do not give birth in controlled conditions with their uterus hanging from their bellies; and (c) the remedy in question is designed to work via the digestive process of metabolic transformation rather than through direct injection into an isolated part of the organism.

Does not the prolific depth of Chinese Medicine present a scientific approach that bears the power and the promise to work the other way round? Do we always have to wait for a related discovery in Western Medicine before we sanctify *qigong* or other aspects of Chinese Medicine that were previously deemed "unscientific"? Could we not utilize so far inexplicable *Neijing* concepts such as *wuyun liuqi* (cosmic cycles) and *ziwu liuzhu* (chrono-acupuncture) to actively inspire the nature and direction of modern scientific experiments? As the profession of Oriental medicine is stepping into a greater stage of maturity in both China and the West, it greatly needs solid respect for its own wisdom traditions, which no gloss of doctoral-level ratification or other marks of progress can deliver from the outside. As Mao Jialing stated pertinently in 2005:

> "We need to revitalize Chinese Medicine! We need to bring about a renaissance of Chinese Medicine! We need to save Chinese Medicine!" For how many decades have we been shouting these slogans now, and how many administrative measures have been passed to support, to protect, and to develop the field of Chinese Medicine, but here we are years later, still talking about the exact same issues. The decade-old problems are still problems, trapped in a vicious circle that loops back and forth in a maze of never-changing questions: "What is science?" "Is Chinese Medicine a science?" "If Chinese Medicine is a science, what type of science is it?" "If Chinese Medicine is not a science, then what is it?" . . . We can only answer this slew of questions appropriately if we advance to a deeper and more fundamental level of discourse, by understanding the scientific significance of Chinese Medicine, and by seeking out the philosophical foundations that qualify Chinese Medicine as a scientific discipline in its own right. Only then can we generate a set of appropriate administrative measures and directives that can do justice to the unique nature and inherent advantages of Chinese Medicine, and only then can the persistent inequity between the two systems of medicine be resolved. Only in this type of environment can the genuine article prosper again.[17]

These, precisely, are the questions that *Classical Chinese Medicine* explores, and the task it has set for itself: to outline a timeless working model for the profession of Oriental medicine—a system that is intellectually satisfying in both its study and its practice, and that delivers consistent clinical results.

April 5, 2016
Heiner Fruehauf, PhD, *LAc*
Founding Professor, College of Classical Chinese Medicine
National University of Natural Medicine
Portland, Oregon

---

17   See the conclusion of Mao Jialing's preface to Chen Guiting and Mao Jialing, eds., *Zheyan kan Zhongyi*, p. 3.

Translator's Note

I first met Dr. Liu Lihong in the mountains of western Sichuan province while traveling with Dr. Fruehauf and a group of fellow Chinese Medicine students one summer. I was immediately struck by his serious and contemplative nature, which he tempered with a fiery passion for traditional Chinese culture and an uncanny ability to form warm rapports with both students and patients alike. At that time, I was only barely familiar with his book, primarily from references Dr. Fruehauf—or "Heiner," as we all call him—made in the course of his lectures.

After our return to Oregon, I made my first tentative forays into translating *Classical Chinese Medicine* under Heiner's close supervision and direction. It gradually became a weekly ritual to join Heiner and his family for dinner and then, after the table was cleared, to sit in the kitchen with dictionaries on hand, going through line after line. The way in which Dr. Liu deftly wove careful interpretation of passages from the classics together with his own insights and clinical anecdotes from his own experience and that of his mentors impressed me deeply.

As a translator and student of the Chinese language, the constant alternation between the syntax and distinct character meanings of classical medical Chinese to that of modern literary Chinese and finally to the colloquial infusions of Dr. Liu's unmistakable voice was dizzying and delightful. I felt that I had before me a sort of Rosetta Stone, one that allows the reader to collate the ancient with the contemporary and finally with the personal experience of a unique and gifted practitioner of classical Chinese Medicine.

Translating this book provided both joy and challenges. I am honored to have had my work joined with the skill and expertise of two other, perhaps better qualified, translators, Henry Buchtel and Sabine Wilms. It is my hope that our work, combined with Dr. Fruehauf's oversight, provides the reader with a book that is a pleasure for the student of Chinese Medicine to read and one that remains true to the complexity and variation of the original text.

Gabriel Weiss, ND, MSOM
Shanghai, June 2016

CHAPTER ONE

A Few Words about Studying and Researching Chinese Medicine

Taiji, the Great Unity,
is nothing but the laws of nature.

I. Establishing a Correct Understanding

I.1. The Importance of Understanding Theory

Chinese Medicine is as dear to me as my own skin. I feel duty-bound to study and practice Chinese Medicine, and the writing of this book derives from that same sense of duty and responsibility to Chinese Medicine. I dearly hope that this book will resolve certain problems or questions regarding Chinese Medicine. In particular, I hope that this discourse provides the reader with a sound foundation for a correct understanding of Chinese Medicine.

The thoughts in this book have undergone nearly ten years of fermentation, a degree of preparation most would agree to be adequate. However, despite my preparation, when it came to putting the pen to the paper, I was not sure where to start. It always seems as if the problems facing Chinese Medicine are too complex and interwoven. Which issues are more important? Which are more crucial, more pivotal?

From the layperson's perspective, Chinese Medicine is a medical modality best suited to the treatment of chronic illnesses, or as it is commonly expressed in Chinese: "*Xiyi zhi biao, Zhongyi zhi ben*" (西醫治標，中醫治本), meaning that Western Medicine treats superficial symptoms of the disease, while Chinese Medicine treats the root cause. But what does it actually mean to say that Chinese Medicine treats the root of disease? In current medical practice, this equates to Western Medicine being employed to treat emergent, dangerous, and serious diseases during their critical period, while afterward Chinese Medicine is permitted to help wrap up the case and provide further care. Chinese Medicine is looked upon as a modality that is only capable of treating non-fatal diseases.

To some people, Chinese Medicine is thus like the rooster crowing before the dawn. If the rooster crows, the sun rises; if the rooster does not crow, the sun still rises. That is the attitude of many, but is it really so? I consider this fundamental issue of understanding, perception, and recognition to be of critical importance.

I.1.a. The Current State of Chinese Medicine

The aforementioned attitude toward Chinese Medicine is not coincidental, nor is it without basis. In the past, there had been a number of graduating students who enjoyed coming to me to discuss their thoughts and observations. Many of them experienced the same thing: During their four years of Chinese Medicine study at the university, they were passionate about Chinese Medicine and had confidence in its capacity to cure disease. These students also hoped to have an opportunity to show something of their ability in the final year before their graduation. But by the end of their year as clinical interns, they had almost completely given up this hope and their passion toward Chinese Medicine had practically expired. Why?

One reason was that the Chinese Medicine they saw being put into practice was not at all the sort of Chinese Medicine they had previously imagined. Regardless of whether they were in a Chinese Medicine hospital or in the Chinese Medicine ward of a Western medical hospital, what they witnessed was Chinese Medicine used as a sort of decoration. To top it off, the Chinese Medicine practitioners they shadowed had little confidence in their profession. The instant they encountered any sort of difficulty, they would frantically resort to Western medications. Or they would add a bit of Chinese medicine to the Western medical protocol, going through the motions. Those who dared to practice Chinese Medicine in a manner true to their own high esteem for the medicine became easy targets of criticism and censure. Practicing in such a way, they found themselves outside the protection of the conventional guidelines for treatment established by the institutions in which they worked.

I can remember when, just after graduation, I practiced in a Chinese Medicine hospital as a clinician. That particular hospital had a well-emphasized rule: if Chinese medicine was used to treat a febrile illness and the fever did not abate within the space of three days, then the patient must be treated with Western medicine. To this day, I still cannot fathom how a Chinese Medicine hospital could make such a rule. Why shouldn't a Chinese Medicine hospital have the opposite rule—if the fever of a patient being treated with Western medicine does not come down within a period of three days, they must be treated with Chinese medicine? Demoted to such a lowly position, how can we expect confidence in the clinical efficacy of Chinese Medicine?

Yesterday, a woman who was nearing her date of delivery came to me, to thank me in person. During the seventh month of her pregnancy, for reasons related to overwork and fatigue, she began to have abdominal pain and vaginal bleeding, suggesting the possibility of a miscarriage. She received a round of Western medical treatment but did not improve. She was especially fearful because she had experienced previous miscarriages. A mutual friend introduced her to me for treatment.

After examining her tongue and taking her pulse, I prescribed Huangqi Jianzhong Tang. After the first dose of medicine, her bleeding decreased. After the third dose, her abdominal pain and vaginal bleeding stopped entirely and her appetite increased considerably. Following this improvement, she phoned her mother who lived in a northern province of China. After explaining what had happened, the first sentence out of her mother's mouth was: "Chinese Medicine really worked?" This mother's doubt reveals a mentality shared by the ordinary Chinese people toward Chinese Medicine.

This past May, I was invited to participate in a symposium on Chinese Medicine study and give a lecture titled "A Brief Discussion of Learning and Research in Chinese Medicine." After giving the lecture, a gentleman with a PhD approached me to chat. He commended me on the one hand for my passionate study and promotion of Chinese Medicine classics in this day and age, but at the same time he was also genuinely puzzled by this behavior. Among the throng of Chinese Medicine PhDs attending the symposium, there were only a few that had actually studied the classics. If one of them had a copy of the *Huangdi neijing* (*Yellow Emperor's Classic of Internal Medicine*, abbreviated below as *Yellow Emperor's Classic*) on his or her desk, it would invite ridicule. What books adorn these doctors' desktops? Invariably, we find texts related to molecular biology and modern biochemistry.

In their field, doctoral-level Chinese Medicine practitioners form an elite class. It will be their duty to modernize Chinese Medicine. For them to read books on molecular biology and biochemistry is simply good form. But why are they not interested in reading any Chinese Medicine texts, especially the medical classics? I think there is a simple answer. In their view, Chinese Medicine is nothing more than it appears to be at first glance and the classics are nothing more than what they appear to be at first glance. As far as they are concerned, it is unlikely that there is anything worthwhile to gain from reading the medical classics. There are many challenges confronting Chinese Medicine, but this disregard for the Chinese Medicine classics is the highest hurdle. These elite Chinese Medicine doctors have a bright future.

It is they who will become the leaders and policy makers of our profession. By the time these people have assumed their positions of authority, what will have become of Chinese Medicine? It is not hard to imagine.

At this juncture, it is important to raise these questions: Is the Chinese Medicine that we witness today and with which we in China are so familiar an accurate representation of what *real* Chinese Medicine has to offer? The standards of practice that we see exhibited in every facet of Chinese Medicine by these doctors, are they the true standards to which we must adhere? Where can we find the true standards of Chinese Medicine? Should we look for them in the present or in antiquity? There are various answers to these questions and from their variety, disparate attitudes toward Chinese Medicine become apparent. If Chinese Medicine is nothing more than what we witness practiced today, does it really merit such a great amount of time devoted to its study? Does it merit the energy a graduate student spends scrutinizing, scrupulously researching, and practicing it? Let me be the first to answer that last question—No, it certainly does not! Why should we be trapped in such a blind alley as that? Why should we expend such energy merely to play a secondary, and perhaps decorative, role? I am raising the question of "how to establish a correct understanding" in the hope that no one be confused by the current state of Chinese Medicine, and thereby lose confidence in what Chinese Medicine has to offer.

I.1.b. Does Chinese Medicine Theory Lag Behind Clinical Practice?

In the past ten years or more, many people have raised the following question: Is Chinese Medicine not up to the task of tackling problems encountered in the clinical setting? In any field of science, theory leads practice, and practice plods along, following the footsteps of theory. Later in this book, I discuss the relationship between theory and practice at greater length. In recent decades, why is it that Chinese Medicine has had no breakthroughs in this particular area? Why has the clinical efficacy of Chinese Medicine not improved in all this time? Whenever a patient has a high, persistent fever, the patient ultimately receives antibiotics. Why and how has this scenario become so prevalent? Chinese Medicine theory was established over 2,000 years ago. During the intervening time, there have apparently been no great breakthroughs and no great changes. Does this reflect the fact that Chinese Medicine theory is antiquated and backward, and thus unable to furnish useful guidance for the clinical practice of this medicine in modern times?

The question of whether or not Chinese Medicine theory has fallen behind what is necessary for clinical efficacy is an inevitable one. Does the relatively deficient clinical usefulness of Chinese Medicine as it is practiced today and the low expectations clinicians hold for it, point to a core theoretical deficit? My own view is entirely contrary to this or any low estimation of Chinese Medicine. On the contrary, I believe that Chinese Medicine theory is not at all backward or lagging. It is actually far ahead of its time. It shares this quality with a number of other traditional arts. The famous philosopher of modern times Liang Shuming said that China's traditional culture, such as Confucianism, Daoism, and Buddhism, could be classified as anthropologically precocious cultural constructs. I believe that Chinese Medicine is equally precocious, and that it matured to such a degree as to make it advanced even in present times. Within the system of Chinese Medicine theory, the problem of lagging behind the requirements of clinical practice is absolutely non-existent. If one says that Chinese Medicine theory lags behind clinical practice or that Chinese Medicine theory cannot offer guidance in the clinical setting, then I would ask: Does one really have a firm grasp of Chinese Medicine theory? Regarding Chinese Medicine theory in the *Yellow Emperor's Classic*, exactly how much of it have you comprehended? Do you understand it 100 percent? If you do not understand it 100 percent, how about 20 or 30 percent? If you have not grasped even 20 or 30 percent of the content of the *Yellow Emperor's Classic* (and there are those who have practiced Chinese Medicine their entire life and still are unable to distinguish yin from yang), how then can you declare that Chinese Medicine theory is deficient? A superficial and overly simplistic understanding of Chinese Medicine theory predominates in the modern world. Chinese Medicine is regarded the way a peasant from the mountains is regarded by the sophisticated Chinese urbanite. What is wrong with simplicity though? Simplicity is the highest accomplishment. Only by returning to simplicity can we return to authenticity. If you have yet to truly understand Chinese Medicine theory, or at the very least to have attained what resembles an understanding of Chinese Medicine theory, what basis do you have to determine whether it is primitive or advanced?

The previous question is a serious one, for if it goes unanswered, we cannot understand how the present crisis of Chinese Medicine has come about. What has brought about the low standards to which we hold Chinese Medicine in the clinical setting? If we mistakenly see these low standards as evidence of deficiency within the theoretical framework, and seek to find problems within the theory itself, then we will indeed lag behind!

I remember when, shortly after completing my undergraduate study, I was doing a clinical internship in a teaching hospital of my university. We received a female patient with pneumonia. The patient was 60 years old, and at the time she entered the hospital, her temperature was 103 degrees Fahrenheit. Her white blood cell count was near 20,000, with 98 percent neutrophilia. X-rays revealed a large shadow over her right lung. From a Western medical perspective, this patient was, almost without doubt, suffering from a serious case of pneumonia. It is dangerous when an elderly person suffers from serious pneumonia. However, since I was so green, and since the inexperienced often do not shy from adversity, I was eager to try the curative abilities of Chinese Medicine and chose to treat this patient with Chinese herbs. I diagnosed her situation as a case of lung heat. And so I prescribed a Chinese herbal formula intended to clear her lungs of heat pathogens. However, to my dismay, two hours after ingesting the medicine, the patient experienced a bout of diarrhea. Subsequent doses of the formula caused diarrhea at closer and closer intervals, until the patient had loose bowel movements within ten minutes of ingesting the herbal decoction. What came out of her looked just like the medicine she had drunk. Three days after being admitted to the hospital, her fever had not decreased one bit, and her other symptoms were not ameliorated.

According to hospital regulations, if her fever did not abate by the following day, we would have to begin administering Western pharmaceuticals. At this point, I may have been even more worried than the patient. I hurried off to the office of my mentor to beg for advice. After introducing the case to him, he pronounced that this was a case in which Taiyin and Yangming syndromes were intertwined. Yangming was hot and Taiyin cold, and so Yangming heat must be cooled, but the cold Taiyin could not handle the cold nature of the decoction and so the formula caused the patient to have diarrhea. The Taiyin and Yangming of this patient must be treated separately, yet without neutralizing each other. The original formula to cool Yangming should be continued and administered orally, while Lizhong

Tang plus Sharen should be ground into a powder, mixed with liquor, and applied with heat to the acupoint at the patient's navel to warm Taiyin. I hurriedly set about following his advice. At around nine that evening, I applied the topical medicine to the patient's navel. About an hour later, I had the patient again take the decoction I had previously prescribed to her. To my surprise, there was no diarrhea this time. The next day on morning rounds, I found her temperature had returned to normal, and she reported that during the night before her other symptoms had improved dramatically. To treat this illness, not a single Western Medicine drug had been used. In the course of the following week, the fluid in the patient's lung had been completely reabsorbed and she left the hospital.

This experience left a lasting impression on me, such that in the next ten years, whenever a patient did not respond as I had hoped to a particular prescription, I never suspected Chinese Medicine or Chinese Medicine theory to be the culprit. It is worth rethinking the contemporary understanding or perception that Chinese Medicine theory lags behind clinical practice. Once our doubts are dispelled, we will be prepared for the theoretical propositions set out in this book. In the future, when our prescriptions fail, we can seek the shortcoming in our own clumsy understanding rather than blame Chinese Medicine theory. In my own experience and that which I have observed, the vast majority of problems do not stem from theoretical shortcomings but from failures in our own understanding.

I.1.c. An Excursion into Twentieth-Century Physics

An irrefutable relationship exists between theory and practice, and likewise a clear relationship between theory and clinical application. This point is well illustrated by the role that physics played in the technological development of the twentieth century. At the conclusion of the nineteenth century, classical physics had already produced incredible intellectual achievements. Many believed that classical physics constituted the ultimate, and most comprehensive, theoretical explanation of reality. Physics's honeymoon with cosmology was rudely interrupted at the beginning of the twentieth century with the establishment of the special theory of relativity in 1905 and the subsequent general theory of relativity, and with the discovery of quantum mechanics shortly thereafter. There were fundamental changes in our knowledge of the universe at every level. This retooling of our perception of how the universe is structured and behaves led to a revolution in the development of technological applications, ranging from space travel to atomic energy to microelectronics. These changes affected all of us in an undeniable way and are all directly related to changes in theory. Within the framework of the classical physics of the nineteenth century, space travel, atomic bombs, and even modern communication devices would have been inconceivable.

Looking back on the technological advances of the past century, the importance of theory and how it governs the application and development of technology is obvious. Can the contrast between the technological advances of the last century and the lack of clinical efficacy of Chinese Medicine as it is currently practiced be the grounds on which we can suppose that Chinese Medicine theory is backward?

We arrive at the crucial question: Just how inclusive is classical Chinese Medicine theory? How far do its theoretical framework and precocious nature extend? Does it still have anything to offer in terms of guidance to the present-day clinician? This is what is important, not the fact that it was created some 2,000 years ago. If we can determine that this theory is definitely backward and that it is indeed unsuitable to the modern age, then we should destroy it without any hesitation, and establish in its place a something equivalent to the "theory of relativity." If this theory is not backward, and if within the framework there is already a "theory of relativity" as well as "quantum mechanics," why should we get rid of it?

At present in Chinese Medicine circles, there is a strange and even frightening phenomenon: a steady weakening of the teaching of the Chinese Medicine classics. Nowadays, the vast majority of Chinese Medicine schools have converted courses on the Chinese Medicine classics into electives. Venerable institutions in Chengdu and Nanjing that formerly stressed the importance of studying the classics are equally guilty of conforming to this trend. Is this progress? I doubt it. What is being substituted for classical Chinese Medicine theory? Have some fatal flaws been discovered in the theories that have served Chinese Medicine practitioners for decades? The classics remain the nucleus of Chinese Medicine, its very foundation. As such, the classics must remain an absolutely obligatory subject of study. How is it that we can turn the study of the most essential and fundamental facet of our discipline into an elective? Is there anyone who would contest the fact that a modern text such as *Fundamentals of Chinese Medicine* (Zhongyi jichu lilun) is anything more than a shadow of the *Yellow Emperor's Classic*? In present times, popular opinion favors such modern textbooks over the classics and deems them adequate replacements for their ancient predecessors, when in fact *Fundamentals of Chinese Medicine* and the *Yellow Emperor's Classic* are on completely different levels. They are so far apart in terms of quality that they should not even be mentioned in the same sentence!

Theory requires practice in order to be fleshed out and fully realized. This is the appropriate relationship between theory and practice, regardless of whether we are talking about physics or medicine. In modern science, the value of theory is obvious. Enrico Fermi's work on quantum theory is an excellent example. The average person cannot understand quantum theory or the theory of relativity. In the history of Chinese Medicine, there have been a number of brilliantly successful practitioners of classical Chinese Medicine theory, such as Zhang Zhongjing and Bian Que. Bian Que used the theory found in the classics to become a physician able to bring those past the brink of death to life again. Zhang Zhongjing's intensive study of the classics eventually led him to become a sort of medical sage. We can appreciate the real value of classical Chinese Medicine theory from the accomplishments of Zhang Zhongjing and other famous physicians of history, just as we gain a true appreciation for modern physics from famous physicists such as Enrico Fermi.

I.2. Chinese Culture As Recognized by Professor Yang Zhenning

On December 3, 1999, renowned physicist and Nobel Prize winner Yang Zhenning accepted an invitation from The Chinese University of Hong Kong to participate in a series of lectures on the "Culture and Science of China" held by New Asia College. During this lecture series, Professor Yang used sets of Chinese couplets to illustrate the distinctive features of Chinese culture. Professor Yang is one of the great physicists of the twentieth century, and has a degree of accomplishment in classical studies as well. Yang Zhenning's understanding of traditional culture can be summarized along the following lines: First, traditional culture sought universal principles but modern science seeks natural laws. According to Yang Zhenning, traditional culture did not seek natural laws, but modern science does. "Traditional culture sought universal principles, not natural laws," and this is what underlies all the differences between the two. Well then, what is meant by these universal principles? Professor Yang described "universal principle" as a sort of "spirit" or "state of consciousness." Should this be taken to mean that these do not exist within modern science?

Secondly, Professor Yang believes that, within traditional culture we find only the inductive method, but no logical deduction. In science, there are two methods of obtaining knowledge: the inductive method and the deductive method. The inductive method collects a number of conclusions regarding observed phenomena and arrives at an "induction": a definition, a universal principle, or a general law from a number of particular instances. Although these two may at first glance appear dissimilar, they share commonalities. The inductive process proceeds from the external to the internal. Logical deduction is another important method. This process is extremely rigorous. For instance, from one we may proceed to two, from two to three, and so on. This process can only proceed in a careful, sequential way. Present-day science possesses the inductive method as well as the logical deductive method, but logical deduction is its identifying feature. According to Yang Zhenning, within traditional Chinese culture there is only the inductive method and no deductive method, and this is what divides the traditional from the modern.

The third point made by Professor Yang is that traditional Chinese culture lacked formal experiments and a natural philosophy. A great number of people believe that Chinese Medicine and its teachings constitute a type of natural science, or better put, a sort of natural philosophy. Professor Yang, on the other hand, in his lectures, takes traditional Chinese culture as an example of one that is lacking in a natural philosophy, directly disagreeing with the observations of many others.

In modern science, experiments are extremely important. Without experiments, modern science can hardly move an inch. Even if we extend our observations to scientific classification, we find that this is the case. At the time I was a doctoral student, there was an unwritten rule governing doctoral students: if one wished to obtain a doctoral degree, one would have to perform experiments in one's research. I owe my good fortune that I, as a doctoral candidate, never had to do any experiments to my supervisor. In Yang Zhenning's opinion in the history of Chinese Medicine, there are no experiments. We do not find the Yellow Emperor asking Qi Bo: "This yin yang theory of yours, how did you arrive at it? Did you experiment with any white mice to arrive at this theory?" Certainly not. So we can say that it is indeed true that in Chinese Medicine or in other traditional sciences, there are no experiments in the modern sense of the word. And that, on the whole, is Professor Yang's understanding of Chinese culture.

I.3. The Structure of Traditional Theory

I am mentioning Professor Yang's understanding because it is representative of how most people see our medicine and other aspects of traditional Chinese culture. Does it describe the deeper implications of traditional culture? Personally, I think not. Traditional Chinese culture has many facets, but Chinese Medicine is arguably the most representative branch. Below, I will therefore use Chinese Medicine as an example to make a series of points concerning my perspective on traditional culture in general.

I.3.a. What Are "Universal Principles"?

First of all, the question we must answer is: What are these "universal principles" of traditional Chinese culture? When traditional culture diligently sought these "universal principles," was it merely due to a certain "spirit" or "state of consciousness" or did it include the concepts of "spirit" and "state of consciousness"? We can first investigate the concept of "universal principles" from the perspective of the Chinese character used to convey this idea. The book *Explaining Writing and Analyzing Characters* (Shuowen jiezi), a Chinese language dictionary dating back to the early second century, defines the character for "universal principle" (*li* 理) as "that by which jade is carved."

After being mined and collected, each piece of jade was carved and polished, worked at meticulously, and slowly took the shape of what was desired, becoming a work of art. The original meaning of the character for "universal principle" referred to this sort of process. In the eyes of the ancients, what was the finest and densest material? It was jade. Why was jade so cold and clear, and so very fine and smooth? It was because the veins and grain of jade are so exquisitely fine. Everyone is familiar with the story of Butcher Ding from the *Zhuangzi* and the saying that goes with that story: "When Butcher Ding cut apart an ox, in his eyes the ox was already in pieces." Why was this the case? It was because he was extremely knowledgeable about the "grain" (*li*, also meaning "universal principle") of the ox. He was extremely familiar with the trends of each piece of flesh and he knew that if he went with these trends, this grain, the ox would fall apart quickly and without the least expenditure of effort. The grain of jade is of course much denser and finer than that of an ox. To carve jade, one must be doubly careful, and even more cognizant of the hidden grain of the material. Going with the grain of the jade made it possible to carve and polish the material and thereby produce the desired art object. Going against the grain when carving might damage the stone. The original meaning of the Chinese character for universal principle was tied to its alternate meaning, that of grain or texture.

By extension, this means that if you proceed in one particular direction, it will work, but if you proceed in another way, it will not. Why is this? This is because of the very function of "universal principle," of the grain of things. Let us ponder this for a moment: If this sort of "universal principle" is not synonymous with "natural law," then what is it? Natural laws, the rules governing phenomena, are rules that cannot be circumvented; any effort to go around the laws of nature will be unsuccessful. As the saying goes: "If one grasps the universal principles, one can go anywhere; without an apprehension of the universal principles, it is difficult to move an inch." The significance of the Chinese concept of "universal principle" is illustrated by this idea. If you go with the grain, your method will be successful. This is "universal principle." That is the case with the "universal principle" or "grain" of people, of the cosmos, and of nature. The "universal principle" of nature is the grain that we must go with in order to get along with nature; the "universal principle" of people is that which we must concord with in order to get along with people. The point is that the ancient Chinese concept of "universal principle" is something very real; it is something that can be perceived with one's eyes and touched with one's hands. If you act in this way, everything works; if you act in that way, you will be rebuffed. "Spirit," on the other hand, is a concept that is abstract and intangible, dimly discernible, and impossible to grasp in a concrete way.

In Chinese Medicine, we esteem these "universal principles," rules, or laws most highly. And what are these "universal principles," rules, and laws? Merely yin and yang and the four seasons! Thus, we find the following statement in the *Plain Questions* (Suwen) chapter titled "Great Treatise on the Four *Qi* and the Tuning of the Spirit" (Siqi tiaoshen dalun):

So it is that yin, yang, and the four seasons are the beginning and end of the myriad things, the root of life and death. If you go against them, you will bring about disaster. If you accord with them, no severe illness will ever arise. This is called achieving the Dao.

Why is the phrase "achieving the Dao" used at this point? This is a fascinating question. This phrase "achieving the Dao" is one that was often used by the ancients in their writings. If one "achieves the Dao," one can ascend to the heavens, and if one can ascend to the very heavens, what is beyond one's abilities? How is it that one achieves the Dao? One realizes these principles and acts in accord with them. If one does that, of course one will achieve the Dao and enter upon the level plane of the high road. How is it that modern-day spacecraft are able to fly out into the sky? Isn't it because we clearly understand the principles conveyed by the theory of relativity? Thus, this "universal principle," this "Dao," this "rationality," are words and expressions laden with meaning for both the ancients and for modern people.

I.3.b. Combining Inductive and Deductive Reasoning

Is it accurate to say that traditional Chinese culture relied only on the inductive method of reasoning? I disagree on this point as well. The *Plain Questions* chapter titled "Treatise on Heavenly Truth in Remote Antiquity" (Shanggu tianzhen lun) clearly points out:

> The people of remote antiquity were knowledgeable of the Dao, their method was comprised of yin and yang and harmonized with numerical calculation.

Here, knowing the Dao is identical with obtaining the Dao. Those who have obtained the Dao are of course enlightened regarding it. Here, knowledge of the "universal principle" or "grain" of the Dao has two facets: one is yin yang, and the other is numerical calculation. Therefore, we are confronted with two problems: what is expressed by yin and yang is induction, as illustrated in the chapter "The Great Treatise on the Correspondences of Yin and Yang" (Yinyang yingxiang dalun) from the *Plain Questions*:

> Yin and Yang comprise the Dao of the cosmos, the warp and weft of the myriad things, the father and mother of changes and transformations, the root of life and death, the container for the spirit light.

In this passage, by attributing heaven and earth and the myriad things, all of the transformations and changes of phenomena, and even death and life to the concept of yin and yang, we are clearly speaking from an inductive perspective. There is no method more complete and consummate than yin and yang theory as an inductive method. What of "numerical calculations," as mentioned in the above passage from the *Plain Questions?* What is meant by "numerical calculation," translated literally as the "technique of numbers," is of course the deductive aspect, the logical methods as expressed in traditional Chinese culture. When one speaks of deduction and logic, one must of course make reference to mathematics. Professor Yang believes that ancient China did not develop mathematics until the seed was planted from the West in the sixteenth or seventeenth centuries. In his understanding, mathematics, in the true sense of the word, did not appear in China until the twentieth century when it was standardized in the curriculum of the two leading universities in China. Did traditional Chinese culture exhibit evidence of possessing mathematics? It certainly did. "Numerical calculation" refers directly to mathematics. In the *General Catalogue for the Complete Encyclopedia in Four Branches* (Siku quanshu zongmu), we have an explanation of this concept of "numerical calculations" that includes the following lines:

> When phenomena emerge, there are images; when images emerge, there are numbers. When the multiplications and divisions of numbers are studied and explained, diligently investigating the source of creation, this is called "numbering."

This passage does not refer to the sort of system of logic or mathematics we see used today, but it belongs, without doubt, to the category of deductive methods. And so, if we want to fully understand the Dao, if we want to truly grasp traditional knowledge and understanding, then we must have a firm grasp of yin and yang as well as a clear understanding of "numerical calculations." Traditional Chinese culture did in fact combine inductive and deductive methods, and the two were mutually indispensable.

I.3.c. Rational Thinking and Internal Experimentation

When Professor Yang Zhenning stated that traditional Chinese culture did not have experiments, he was only half right. Certainly, in traditional

Chinese culture, we do not see modern experimental research like what we see today. When we speak of medical studies, the ancients did not have experiments subjecting humans, white rabbits, little white mice, or other animals to a series of tests. However, in traditional Chinese culture, there was a very subtle and profound process of *internal* experimentation. It is due to the combination of internal experimentation and rational thinking that traditional Chinese Medicine and Chinese Medicine theory came into being. Of course, internal experiments are fuzzy because no part of internal experimentation can be observed objectively. There are no white mice to be observed, nothing to be seen, nothing tangible. It is entirely a sort of ability that emerges within oneself from one's own practice. As soon as someone acquires this ability he or she can with ease conduct a host of experiments that are vastly different from those conducted outside the system of the human body. This issue is therefore difficult to talk about but avoiding the topic is not a solution either. If we continue to insist that traditional culture is devoid of experimentation, then there is only one road to go down, with the following of two outcomes: either Chinese Medicine does not possess a theoretical framework and is a purely empirical medical science, or Chinese Medicine is entirely the result of contemplation. Let's think for a moment: If we were relying on a theory born solely of contemplation, would we be able to put our trust in it completely? Could Chinese Medicine's many theories and observations hold up in practice if they were based solely on subjective thought? Take, for example, the acupuncture channels or the many acupuncture points, and other such elements of Chinese Medicine. Could they be discovered simply by theoretical speculation? Take, for example, the acupuncture points Fengfu (GV 16, "Wind Palace") and Fengchi (GB 20, "Wind Pool"). What sort of speculative process would you rely on to come up with these particular points and name them "Wind Palace" and "Wind Pool"? What sort of thought process would you rely on to be able to say that the Shaoyang channel circulates like this and the Taiyang channel circulates like that? I believe that no matter how intelligent you might be, these are not things you could come up with via reflection. If you do not believe me, try to think up such a thing and see for yourself. It is obvious that if profound internal experiments had not been conducted, it would have been impossible for such ideas to develop. We have every reason to believe that in the course of the development of its theories, traditional

Chinese culture, especially in fields such as Chinese Medicine, employed both contemplation and experimentation. The argument that traditional culture did not possess experimentation does not have a leg to stand on. We have cause to differentiate internal experimentation from external experimentation, but we certainly have no reason to negate internal experimentation. This point should be crystal clear.

Rational reflection and subtle experimentation are the foundation of traditional sciences, and for this reason we can have complete confidence in the theories developed from this foundation. The problem lies in the reason why so many people do not recognize that traditional Chinese culture possessed experiments. It is because we have a very difficult time imagining what internal experiments are. In the case of the channels, for instance, Li Shizhen once said that if we do not trace the path of the channel by turning our gaze inward and observing them internally, then we will have a difficult time even saying where they are. What does it mean "to turn one's gaze inward and observe internally"? To turn one's gaze inward and observe internally is the very model of internal experimentation. If you possess this internal capacity, the channels and points are all things that you can see, despite the fact that you cannot observe them with even the most advanced technology. Even should you use the most state-of-the-art equipment, it is difficult to discern the channels and points. What you cannot see externally, you will find difficult to believe. Therein lies the difficulty.

If you would like to conduct internal experiments such as we just mentioned, it is necessary to have a certain degree of education, practice, and talent. If you cannot enter into this requisite state of internal experimentation, you will not be able to sense such things as the channels. Albert Einstein, to a great degree, was a believer in intuition. Without intuition, science is missing a leg. In my opinion, there may be people among the general population who possess the capacity to observe the internal landscape just as the ancients could, or there may not. But do you believe that this is possible? Some people ask me what they need in order to study Chinese Medicine. My answer is always this: If you cannot perform such introspective, intuitive investigations yourself, do you or do you not believe that this way of seeing is possible? What is the nature of this kind of internal experimentation? Liang Qichao said it well in a single sentence: "The illumination of the heart-mind is Heaven's universal principles." Incidentally, this is the same sentence used by Yang Zhenning during the course of his symposium lecture. This "illumination of the heart-mind" is by no means an understanding through mental analysis, and to see, to really see, with an illuminated heart-mind is not easy. The illumination of the heart-mind referred to here is the state of perception already mentioned in reference to internal experimentation. The illumination of the heart-mind can look within; it can turn inside and observe what it finds there, and perceive the path of the channels in one glance. Why do we say these are internal experiments? It is because they are not conducted outside of the human body but rather within it.

In the preface to the *Treatise on Cold Damage*, Zhang Zhongjing referenced a book titled *Fontanel Record of Medicinals* (Tailu yao lu). As we know, in the past, there was a *Fontanel Classic* (Luxin jing) that was concerned with pediatric diseases. In the case of the former book, we are also using a word referring to a fetus, and therefore we naturally take the *Fontanel Record of Medicinals* to be a book about pediatric medicine. If we were to use modern language to translate this title, we might translate this work as "Comprehensive Volume of Pediatric Medicine." However, if we open the history books, it becomes clear that it is unlikely that a book devoted solely to pediatrics existed prior to the Eastern Han dynasty. The *Divine Farmer's Classic of Materia Medica* (Shennong bencao jing) is divided into upper, middle, and lower substances, and not organized into categories such as internal medicine, external medicine, gynecology, or pediatrics. Even up until the Ming Dynasty, the book *Compendium of Materia Medica* (Bencao gangmu) is divided into sections such as "trees," "herbs," "minerals," "beasts," etc. Knowing this, we must change our thinking regarding the probable content of the *Fontanel Record of Medicinals*. The character for "fetus" does not refer to an unborn child here, but instead to "fetal breath," which is a breathing method whereby one returns to the fetal breathing state. Once a person has entered into the fetal breathing state, the "illumination of the heart-mind" state naturally arises, and the person enters into a deeply introspective state. At this point, a laboratory for introspective experiments can be set up. At this time, one is able to sense the effects of medicinal substances concretely. After ingesting medicines, their *qi* and flavor, the channel into which they enter and into which they will move next, and consequently also their appropriate use, all become completely clear and obvious. Thus, when the ancients spoke of a medicine's *qi* and flavor, or of the channel that it entered, these were not determined solely through contemplation, but from true experimentation. The *Fontanel Record of Medicinals* was a record of the movement and function of medicinal substances resulting from the ability to enter into the introspective experimental state. So we see that traditional Chinese culture, and in particular the structure of Chinese Medicine theory, is entirely a joint product of rational thought and introspective experimentation. We cannot accept that there was only contemplation and not experimentation. We can only accept the premise that Chinese Medicine did not have external experiments such as those of the present day.

I.3.d. The Application of Theory

After establishing Chinese Medicine theory, how should it be put into practice? The application of theory presents a unique problem. Within the realm of modern science, we can delimit three distinct areas: basic science, technological science, and applied science. What is technological science? It is a bridge between the basic sciences and the applied sciences. Why is modern science often mentioned in one breath with the term "technology"? It is because these two influence each other so greatly. Sometimes science determines technology, and sometimes technology determines science. Take, for example, the current research into the basic composition of matter. Without theory, nothing can be accomplished in this field, but without a functioning superconducting supercollider, the theory cannot be furthered. Science and technology are, therefore, intertwined. Within traditional Chinese culture, we find a very strange phenomenon: between theory and practice, we do not have a technological field in the modern sense of the word. There is no mediator or bridge between the two. When we look at modern medical science, there is a massive technological bridge between theory and practical application. The entire disciplines of modern physics, chemistry, and biology serve as these mediators. These make the application of medical theory extremely convenient. Nowadays, physicians rarely rely on their own bodies and senses to examine, palpate, ask questions, and listen, which originally comprised the four basic methods of diagnosing disease in Chinese Medicine. These direct, corporeal modalities have been replaced with technology, used to probe and measure and look into the body. In the field of Chinese Medicine, there is no such mediating layer that offers technological tools. The application of theory, and the proof that this theory actually works, relies entirely on our own ability to make this knowledge our own and become enlightened to its subtle depths. Naturally, this situation makes the study of this medicine quite difficult.

It is this point that comprises the biggest difference between traditional Chinese cultural understanding and modern science. In modern science, there is a level of technological mediation between theory and practice that is crucial in the process of actualizing theory. In the case of traditional Chinese culture, especially in the case of Chinese Medicine, there is no such go-between. The application of theory depends almost solely on the subject feeling and subjectively perceiving the pulse. How adept is the physician at pulse diagnosis? This will depend on the practitioner's mastery of direct perception and their ability to interpret that perception. By contrast, a scientific elite produces the medical technology upon which the practitioners of Western Medicine depend. As soon as the new technology exists, it can be manufactured *en masse*. Then, any ordinary technician can put this technology to use.

Qian Xuesen worked on the development of guided missiles, but he himself did not need to get involved in building bombs. The inventors of the first computers, after completing their work, did not need to go and build each computer one motherboard at a time. Technology enabled them to complete the production process. Modern technology is a very convenient thing. It can help us to actualize any theory, no matter how advanced. Therefore, for modern science, the most essential element is reproducibility. However, in the traditional fields, this particular convenience is missing. This means that, no matter how good the theory, if you cannot grasp it yourself, it amounts to nothing. Just imagine that we get ahold of the secrets of the theory of general relativity—what would be able to do with this knowledge? What practical thing would you be able to produce with the details of general relativity at your command? It is not different from if we were to have a firm grasp of the theory of relativity. Armed with this knowledge, what sort of contraptions could we come up with? If a person had the entire theory of relativity clear as crystal in their mind, what sort of device would they design? Personally, I find it very difficult to conceive of the answers to such questions. Just because one cannot construct a tool or other elements of technology with a particular theory, does it mean that the theory is backward? Was Albert Einstein's work meaningless? This is the sort of problem that Chinese Medicine faces. If it has fallen behind, then it has fallen behind at this particular junction. One cannot say that the theory itself is backward or primitive. History has already produced a great number of highly successful practitioners of Chinese Medicine, who have brought forth their equivalents of the "atomic bomb" and the "computer."

Keeping this particular insight in mind, we should approach any questions surrounding classical Chinese Medicine theory with an extremely clear head and ask us whether in case of any perceived deficiencies the theory itself should be blamed, or whether the problem lies in surrounding circumstances. Therefore, I would like to invite you to establish the following understanding: the science of traditional Chinese Medicine does not suffer from impractical theories that have become unsuitable for the needs of modern clinical practice. I guarantee that the power of traditional theory, once acknowledged, will be palpable and immediately useable—no need to bring up the "backward" argument ever again. How come then, we may ask, that Chinese Medicine finds itself in a situation of low clinical effectiveness and low esteem? The only fingers that should be raised here should point in the direction of our own self. How deep, really, is our understanding of the classical principles governing our medicine? Do we really have a masterful grasp of the ways in which this knowledge should be applied to clinical practice? Where will the problems we encounter as Chinese Medicine practitioners emerge? Will they emerge in the arena of theory, or will they emerge elsewhere? As a discipline, Chinese Medicine does not suffer from a deficiency of theory. Its theory does not lag behind practice. This is not the problem. Once you begin to study Chinese Medicine theory, you may begin to perceive things and you may benefit from what you have learned. How can the theory be said to lag behind? Since its challenges do not arise from theoretical weaknesses, why is Chinese Medicine theory doubted at this particular juncture? We must look for the reason in our own shortcomings. How thorough is our current comprehension of Chinese Medicine theory? Have we truly grasped the clinical application of the theory?

I remember when my mentor treated a hemothorax patient in 1987. The patient had already undergone a round of conservative Western medical treatments but his condition did not improve. He still had a high fever, difficult breathing, and the left lung was reduced in size by two-thirds. In this sort of situation, the only option left to Western Medicine is surgery. But the patient and his family were not willing to give up hope on conservative treatment, and conversely sought help from my mentor. After diagnosing the patient, my mentor recognized that this was a Yangming disease, in which Yangming forces would not descend. In his mind, one had only to think of a way to induce Yangming to sink back down, and the hemothorax would resolve. He thereupon prescribed 120 grams each of Yuzhu, Chenpi, Baizhi, and Dazao—four different herbs in all. After taking the herbal decoction, the patient had a large bout of diarrhea, and thereafter improved rapidly. By the fourth day, his body temperature had returned to normal. By the end of the week, the hemothorax was completely resorbed, and the left lung had recovered.

What relationship is there between a hemothorax and Yangming? On the surface, this is a matter of intuitive insight and the individualized approach of this practitioner, not a question of a direct theoretical link. The theory found in the classics, therefore, is not only adequate to the task of resolving problems of the twentieth century, it is also up to the challenges of the twenty-first century.

II. The Transmission of Knowledge

Next, we will discuss the transmission of knowledge, specifically the transmission of Chinese Medicine knowledge. For this purpose, we are intentionally using the word "transmission," a somewhat antiquated term. When a particular body of knowledge is passed down through generations, what does this process depend on? It depends upon this "transmission." Therefore, the transmission of knowledge is an important matter. Let us examine the matter in two parts and discuss it.

II.1. Modern Chinese Medicine Education

Expressed in modern terms, transmission is simply education. Therefore, let us first take a look at modern Chinese Medicine education. What exactly is "modern Chinese Medicine education"? It formally began when the colleges and schools that currently teach it were established. These institutions started operating in 1956. When we look back on the past decades of teaching Chinese Medicine, pros and cons are evident. First of all, it needs to be said that the way in which we were taught did not differ from the manner in which Western Medicine was taught at other colleges and universities. Currently, all Chinese Medicine students still pursue two different courses of study: Chinese Medicine and Western Medicine. What are the formal differences in the way these vastly different disciplines are studied? There are none! Therefore, so-called modern Chinese Medicine education is, in actuality, an imitation of modern Western medical education. What are the distinguishing features of modern education in general? Naturally, each educational system is tied to a specific style of teaching most suitable for the discipline in question. In the previous part of this chapter, Professor Yang Zhenning proposed a particular difference between modern science and traditional Chinese culture: modern science possesses mathematical logic and a system of deductive reasoning, whereas traditional Chinese culture does not. This system of logic is very precise, and the rationality that pervades it is robust and transparent. Hence, when it is taught, it is very easily accepted. Another especially important difference lies in the fact that modern technology acts as a mediator for modern science. This technological mediator acts as a sort of stockpile as well as a replicator of scientific ideas. Human intelligence can be compressed into this technological medium, as in the case of the personal computer. Then we can turn around and use this intermediate technology to gather more knowledge about reality, improve reality, and thus serve humanity. For this reason, we might call modern science, with its emphasis on technological mediators, a "middleman" science. Once this middleman or mediator is at hand, we have the means to replicate it. After the first computer prototype is built, computers can be produced in large batches. This is mass production, where it is no longer necessary to build each unit one at a time. The replicability of modern technology is superb, which in turn greatly expands its scope and influence. The reason why modern education has such a broad influence in today's society corresponds directly to this characteristic of modern science. In addition, the branches of modern science are extremely specialized and this specialization is reflected in the highly compartmentalized way in which modern educational approaches are organized. This distinctive feature of the organization of modern science is amply reflected in many aspects of Western culture, for example, paintings. When we look at a Western oil painting in the classical European tradition, what sort of feeling does it give us? It gives us the impression that we are looking at something very real. For instance, in paintings of the human body, the body is completely uncovered. The entire body is laid bare before you and sometimes even every hair is clearly depicted. On the other hand, what do we experience when we look at a Chinese painting? Chinese paintings do not depict the human body. When you scroll open a typical Chinese landscape painting, you usually get the impression of a vaporous mist, blowing about indistinctly, reminiscent of the phrase from Laozi: "Unexpectedly! Suddenly! There is an image in its midst." To paraphrase insider language, Western painting emphasizes realism; Chinese painting emphasizes expressionism. In the former everything is clear at a single glance, while in the latter things are dimly veiled. This distinction constitutes the difference between Chinese and Western culture, and it is precisely this difference that impels us to ask: Should there not be a difference between the instruction of Chinese Medicine and Western Medicine? In modern Chinese Medicine education, we see a tendency for branches of the discipline to become increasingly specialized. Some of these branches attempt to create their own version of "Fundamentals of Chinese Medicine," developing distinct disciplines from each division. Even the study of moxibustion and acupuncture is divided into smaller branches, such as channel study, the study of transport points, and the study of acupuncture alone. Does this sort of divergence into more specialized branches really improve the quality and effectiveness of study? From a certain perspective, Chinese Medicine is entering into a period in which it has an unprecedented number of specialists, undergraduate students, and researchers. This is especially evident in the wave of Chinese Medicine hospitals that have upgraded their status to universities. Clearly, the scale of Chinese Medicine institutions has been greatly expanded, but does this mean that the quality of education has been expanded as well?

In recent years, I have been asked many times by senior students at the four major universities of Chinese Medicine to come and lecture for them. What do they want me to lecture on? They want me to lecture on the topic "How Should We Best Study Chinese Medicine?" Why is this? It is because they are still perplexed by Chinese Medicine and still feel unclear about it. They do not know what method they should use to tackle clinical problems. Four years is not a short time at all, yet many masters of the past only studied for three years, as in the case of the famous twentieth-century physician

Pu Fuzhou. He started to apprentice with his grandfather at age 15 and after three years was able to open his own clinic. Nowadays, however, we appear to be still confused after four years—where might the problem lie? Could it be in the current method of education? Naturally, we assume this is the cause. Previously we mentioned that the nature of a science determines the model of education employed to teach it. Have we pondered this question carefully enough?

II.2. "Beyond Form" and "Form"

In the following passage, we will examine the implications of the previous topic, the appropriate way in which Chinese Medicine should be taught. Modern culture divides the world into two basic categories: the material universe and the spiritual world. Modern science limits the scope of its research to the physical world and barely touches on spiritual things. Therefore, materialism and positivism are primary, and spiritual matters are secondary. To what category of things does the material universe belong? We may temporarily set this particular point aside, and instead first examine how the ancients categorized the world. In ancient times, this kind of a division did exist between the physical and the metaphysical. As a commentary to the *Classic of Changes* states: "What is beyond form is called Dao; what is form is called 'vessel.'" Please take notice: here there is a division into metaphysical and physical, between the Dao and a tool. What is this so-called "vessel"? A vessel is something possessing physical form, something possessing structure, therefore it belongs to the realm of form. Obviously, the physical world into which modern science delves is this physical world of material tools. The category of things that modern science investigates is this physical category. What is the realm "beyond form"? "Beyond form" refers to things that are beyond or above having tangibility or form. Of course, this refers to something formless or intangible. This formless, "beyond form" thing is simply called the Dao. Is then the realm of the Dao synonymous with mind and spirit? We will have to think about this question a while longer, but we can say already that the two of them have certain similarities.

The crux of the dichotomy discussed in the preceding passage lies in the concept of "form." In the *Plain Questions*, there is a very specific description of "form": "*Qi* joins together and there is form," or translated differently: "*Qi* gathers together and becomes form." How is form constituted?

Qi gathers together and there is form; *qi* joins together and there is form. After *qi* gathers and joins together, we have a thing with an objectifiable form, a phenomenon, a thing belonging to the world of objects or tools. And in the case that *qi* has not yet gathered and joined together? What state are we concerned with in that case? Obviously, it is the state of formlessness, of being "beyond form." According to this manner of classification, the area with which modern science is concerned is the area in which *qi* has already joined and gathered together. For instance, physics investigates the structure and composition of matter and, consequently, we have the concept of elementary particles. What is matter composed of? It is composed of molecules, the molecules of atoms, and the atoms, in turn, of a nucleus and an electron. The nuclei consist of neutrons and protons as well as mesons. And what constitutes the mesons? Quarks! Quarks are the smallest components of matter known to modern science. Although they are exceedingly tiny, they still belong to the realm of form. The name "quark" was arrived at in a humorous way. Its origin reflects the attitude with which scientists pursue the most basic constituents of the material world. The word "quark" originated from a fantastic bird of Western mythology. This bird's call resembled the sound made by the word "quark." This bird did not call easily. Whenever the bird did make its call, the sun fell behind the mountains, darkness blanketed the earth, and nothing could be seen. Entrusting the name "quark" to the smallest known particle, it appears that scientists are unwilling to seek further for still smaller particles. Should they do so, what might happen? The sun will fall behind the mountains, the sky will darken, and nothing will be seen.

Considering this particular model of the physical world, when will we discover the ultimate constituents of matter? By all appearances not within the foreseeable future! Until that time, it is difficult to rely on any conclusions. The ancients did not hold their breath. They simply said, "As for that with form, it emerges from the formless," and did not go hunting after the ultimate foundation of matter, the material basis for form. Laozi said, "Under heaven, the myriad things are born from being, and being emerges from non-being." When we say that modern science is primarily concerned with the physical realm, we are saying that its scope is primarily that of the realm of "being." What is the scope of Chinese Medicine? Obviously, its scope is composed of both physical and metaphysical components. It is a field of study in which Dao and "vessels" are combined. Laozi and the *Yellow Emperor's Classic* emphasize the need for both form and spirit, for combining form and *qi*. Form and spirit are equally necessary. Chinese Medicine explores both that which precedes quarks and that which proceeds from quarks. There are a great many examples, too many to enumerate, that testify to Chinese Medicine being a study of both the physical and the metaphysical. Let us take the "five viscera" of Chinese Medicine anatomy and physiology as an example. When we look at the Chinese characters for the five viscera of Chinese Medicine physiology, we realize very easily that one of them stands out: the character for heart (*xin* 心) is the only one that does not possess the "flesh" radical on its left side. Flesh, of course, designates material objects. The ancients were very certain of the primacy of the liver, kidneys, spleen, and lungs within the human body. These organs belong to the "physical" category, the category of form and vessels. The heart, however, is different. The character for "heart" does not possess the flesh radical; in other words, it does not possess this "form-vessel" aspect. The heart is metaphysical, it is beyond the realm of form. The heart's classification as a spiritual or metaphysical organ is neither a simple nor a casual one. The heart's unique classification permeates Chinese Medicine as well as the whole of traditional Chinese culture. We can better understand the heart's special position by familiarizing ourselves with Chinese five-element theory. In this theory, the elements of metal, wood, water, and earth are all things with form. As material entities, each of these has a tendency to descend. They have mass and weight and are acted upon by the force of gravity. All belong to the scope of tools. But fire? Fire is difficult to describe in physical terms. Unlike the other four elements, it has a tendency to rise. Does it not have weight? Is it not subject to the force of gravity? Fire represents precisely this metaphysical realm, that which is called "beyond form," the Dao.

If Chinese Medicine were to discuss only the liver, kidneys, spleen, and lungs, would it be sufficient? Of course not—the heart must also be understood. Chinese Medicine is a discipline that explores not only physical phenomena, but also the metaphysical realm. Is there a difference in the relative importance of the two categories? The answer to this question is obvious. In Chapter 8 of the *Plain Questions*, titled the "Treatise on the Spiritual Orchid Secret Canon" (Linglan midian lun), we read: "The heart holds the office of the sovereign and ruler; spirit brightness originates from it." What does the phrase "sovereign and ruler" signify? I believe that every-one must be very clear about this. Another passage of this same chapter explains:

> As for these twelve offices, they must never lose contact with each other. If the ruler is bright and clear, there is peace below. To nourish life on the basis of this results in longevity. There will be no risk of failure till the end of all generations. To rule the world in this way results in great abundance.

> If the ruler is not bright and clear, the twelve offices are all imperiled. The Dao will be closed off and obstructed, and the physical form will be greatly harmed. To nourish life on the basis of this results in disaster. To rule the world in this way will greatly endanger the ancestral temple. Beware! Beware!

From both a "five-element" and a "twelve-office" perspective, we can see that in traditional Chinese culture, although there is an emphasis on the interdependence of form and *qi* as well as the spirit and body being merged into one entity, particular stress is laid upon the eminence of Dao, spirit, and *qi*.

The study of Chinese Medicine is a discipline that puts Dao before matter, regards spirit as primary to and superior to form, and esteems the metaphysical more than the physical. To illustrate this point with a more concrete example, we have the example of the way in which classes of physicians are ranked. The *Yellow Emperor's Classic* divides physicians into two classes: the upper-level physicians and the lower-level physicians. The higher level represents the exceedingly brilliant physicians. The lower level doubtlessly refers to very ordinary, average doctors. Can we perhaps differentiate between the upper level and the lower level in a more esoteric way? The *Spiritual Pivot* (Lingshu) section of the *Yellow Emperor's Classic* provides us with a very specific indicator of the true nature of this dichotomy: "The upper-level physician protects the spirit while the lower-level physician guards the form." What is the spirit? The spirit is a thing without a form; it belongs to the same category as the Dao and the metaphysical. The higher-level physician works to protect this aspect. That is to say, if someone is able to preserve this aspect of reality and is capable of understanding and curing disease from its metaphysical aspect, then we might consider them a "higher-level" physician. Conversely, if a physician deals with what has already taken on a form, and understands and treats disease from a physical, material level, then he or she is merely a lower-level physician. The second chapter of the *Plain Questions*, the "Great Treatise on the Four *Qi* and the Tuning of the Spirit," states:

> Thus, the sages do not treat what is already diseased but what is not yet diseased. They do not seek to regulate what is already chaotic but instead regulate before chaos ensues. As for treating disease with medicine after it has matured, or attempting to regulate chaos after it has fully developed, this is like digging a well after one is already thirsty, or forging weapons during a battle—far too late!

Preserving the spirit means treating disease before it has emerged, in other words, treating it before it has taken form. If you treat disease before it has taken form, it is a far simpler problem to solve! If you wait until the disease has assumed physical form, it is essentially indestructible. If you wish to get rid of it at this point, it will not be easy! You will be facing a difficult and thankless job. Every disease proceeds from a state prior to disease to a state of already being a disease. In accordance with Western medical interpretation, the pathological process of any disease begins in a prior stage where structural changes have yet to develop. During the pre-pathological phase, cure is relatively easy, but once one enters into a state of pathology that involves structural or biochemical changes, cure is far more difficult. For this reason, physicians must not only be adept at treating pathology, but also at recognizing the early signs of pathological change. When the disease is still in its pre-pathological phase, before it has assumed any physical form, can you discover it? Can you intercept and seize it, and make it disappear back into the formlessness from which it sprang? Such treatment would be like when Bian Que looked at the complexion of the Marquis of Qi. His disease was only at the depth of his skin when Bian Que noticed it. When disease is apprehended at this superficial layer, it requires very little to prevent it from going deeper. Zhang Zhongjing, moreover, is known to have diagnosed the royal advisor Wang Zhongxuan twenty years before the outbreak of his disease, giving him a prescription that could prevent his ailment from advancing. This is the ability to see what is coming from one small clue. How meaningful is it to wait until the patient has late-stage cancer? Currently, modern medical technology, on the whole, is only able to recognize diseases that have already taken form. Even if the current technology were to become even more advanced, it would still only be able to detect existing disease processes. Current technology is powerless to perceive diseases before they have blossomed into full-blown structural pathology. Genetic testing, examining the genes of an infant or a fetus, for example, can detect diseases before they manifest. In this sense, we can say that modern Western science is progressing in the direction of ancient Chinese Medicine.

The great majority of those who are interested in Chinese Medicine are familiar with it only from the perspective of structural pathology and diseases that have already formed. Familiar only with this aspect of Chinese Medicine, they find it markedly inferior to Western Medicine. I often use the following analogy to make this point: To which hospital would you take a patient having a heart attack? A Chinese Medicine hospital or a Western Medicine hospital? I think if you asked a hundred people, all of them would send an acute heart attack patient to a Western-style hospital. If Zhang Zhongjing himself were alive and well today, it is possible that even he would suggest such a patient go to a Western Medicine hospital, rather than send him to a Chinese Medicine hospital. Based on this example alone, every practitioner of Western Medicine will square their shoulders and raise their head, beaming with pride. Every Chinese Medicine practitioner will hang their head dejectedly, feeling they have entered into the wrong profession. If this is the sole basis of comparison, we practitioners of Chinese Medicine must admit defeat and say that Chinese Medicine is simply not that great.

If, however, we compare the desirability of providing preventative treatment to this patient so that his coronary artery disease never blossomed into a myocardial infarction, with the need to try to rescue him after he has already suffered a heart attack, the desirability of treating disease before its final outcome is immanent seems greatly preferable. It is better for society as a whole, better for the country, the family, and the patient himself. I think if you asked a hundred people whether prevention or treatment is preferable, they would all endorse prevention. If we compare Chinese with Western Medicine from this perspective, then perhaps we will place more stock in Chinese Medicine. Chinese Medicine specifically treats diseases before they have come into being, as Zhang Zhongjing stated in his preface to the *Essentials from the Golden Cabinet* (Jingui yaolüe): "The higher-level physician does not treat manifested disease but rather unmanifested disease." The ability to treat unmanifested disease, to dig a well before one is thirsty and forge weapons before the battle has ensued, is a valid starting point for the evaluation of any medicine. However, at present, the contest between Chinese Medicine and Western Medicine seems to revolve around their ability to treat diseases that have already manifested, that have progressed to the point of blatant, even potentially fatal, pathology. When such a comparison is made in reference to an emergent medical condition such as a heart attack or stroke, Chinese Medicine finds itself holding the short end of the stick. If we are talking about digging a well after one is already thirsty, or forging weapons in the heat of battle, how can we compare ancient methods to the speed of modern technology?

This issue is really the crux of the matter. Chinese Medicine is a science that primarily concerns itself with the realm of the metaphysical, and how this governs the realm of the physical. It is a medicine that treats pathology by focusing on the not-yet-manifested. However, at present, we view this science entirely through a materialist lens, and treat it exclusively as a field of knowledge that is mired in the realm of the material, as a type of medicine that treats structural diseases. We encourage scientific research and the modernization of Chinese Medicine education over all else. In this process, we use a sieve that only catches the physical, material aspects of Chinese Medicine understanding to filter its content, mistakenly thinking we are distilling its essence. In fact, we are merely collecting its dregs and gathering its dross. Let us contemplate what passes through this sieve and is lost. The metaphysical, immaterial portion of Chinese Medicine is lost. If we clearly consider the implications of this with regard to the current mode of Chinese Medicine education, it is obvious that the educational method adopted by Chinese Medicine schools is the path by which the lower class of physician, not the higher class, is cultivated. Perhaps you disagree with me and consider my point of view too extreme. We must, however, examine why students taught in the modern way lack confidence in the efficacy of Chinese Medicine. Why do Chinese Medicine clinicians who run into difficulties not attempt to discover a solution using Chinese Medicine and instead urgently switch to Western pharmaceuticals? Chinese Medicine offers a multitude of therapeutic methods. Its curative potential is not exhausted by trying out a few doses of a particular decoction.

Besides the current era's fixation on objective variables, how can we explain the current inferior status of Chinese Medicine? I think there are only two possible reasons: one lies in the way in which knowledge is passed on in the current educational method, and the other lies within Chinese Medicine itself. However, if we turn our heads to examine the accomplished physicians of Chinese Medicine in the past, we quickly discover that the problem is not with Chinese Medicine itself.

II.3. Reciprocity between Teacher and Disciple

Given that traditional Chinese Medicine involves this kind of learning, there must be many aspects where it differs greatly from modern science. Yet we continue to indiscriminately imitate the teaching methods of modern science, and hence many essential aspects of our medicine get lost. What we lose in this process might just be the most important aspect of Chinese Medicine. This leads us to contemplate what teaching model is best suited to Chinese Medicine.

II.3.a. Visiting Dr. Yu Lu

With its extensive 2,000 years of history, Chinese Medicine is rich with experience, much of which is worthy of our attention. One example is the emphasis laid on the teacher–apprentice relationship. I personally think this sort of pedagogical model is especially beneficial to the study of Chinese Medicine. In this context, I would like to share a story with you. In the first half of 1998, I went to Beijing for a conference. While there, I asked a friend if he knew of a Chinese Medicine "master." Of course, I was not looking for a master so that I could cross swords with him, but rather to find an opportunity to receive further instruction. Because I often feel that my own level of clinical maturity is still deficient, and because my own beloved mentor passed away in 1991, whenever I come to a new place I tend to seek out eminent physicians for guidance. My frame of mind when seeking out such individuals is much like that of a character in one of Jin Yong's Kungfu novels. My friend introduced me to a Dr. Yu Lu of Peking University of Traditional Chinese Medicine. Dr. Yu is known as an expert in the Warm-Disease (*wenbing*) School of Chinese Medicine and his teachers include many of the celebrated experienced physicians of our time. One of his teachers was a truly outstanding old physician, with a father, grandfather, and great-grandfather who were all physicians at the imperial court so that his family was thus deeply steeped in medical knowledge. Dr. Yu Lu himself has great natural talent and is able to express himself exceedingly well. He apprenticed with this master for three years and obtained most of his secrets. However, due to outside circumstances, their relationship fell into disharmony. Sadly, it eventually got to the point where they would not even greet each other in passing. When I visited Dr. Yu Lu, we discussed a great number of scholarly topics, and I asked many questions. When he bid me goodbye, Dr. Yu spoke with great sincerity straight from his heart: "Dr. Liu, to learn Chinese Medicine well, you need to know only two words: 'Teacher transmission.'" Saying it as he did, just at the moment of my departure, these two words made a deep impression on me. What is this "teacher transmission"? Teacher transmission is a traditional phrase denoting the transmission of knowledge directly from master to disciple. Considering the scope and scale of the current model of education, can we say that it features "teacher transmission"? We can safely say that it does not. The present system employs teachers who are technical experts but does not feature "masters" in the traditional sense of the word. Although his relationship with his own master was highly problematic, Dr. Yu had still sent me off with these words, revealing the depth of the impression his master had made on him. I believe this single phrase, repeated to me by Dr. Yu Lu, is a crucial link for the study and transmission of Chinese Medicine knowledge.

II.3.b. Teachers: The Greatest Treasure in Life

Now I would like to discuss my experience with my own master. At present, my mentor is the reason why I am able to discuss these impressions with you, and also why I have studied Chinese Medicine continuously and without interruption and continue to do so. From the time that I graduated from university, it has been twenty years now at the time of writing. During this time, I have pursued my studies tirelessly, never stopping or turning back, never breaking my stride. Despite the many obstacles I have encountered—tempting waves of business and high rank in the establishment, as well as the overbearing influence of Western Medicine—I have not wavered in my beliefs and pursuit of this medicine. I owe this fact to my master, my *shifu*. After graduating from college in 1983, on the eighth day of the first lunar month in 1984, I became a disciple to my *shifu*. My teacher's name was Li Yangbo, and he passed away over ten years ago. I followed my *shifu* for a total of eight years. During the first two years of my discipleship, we ate food from the same wok, slept in the same bed, and sometimes stayed up all night discussing scholarly matters. Eight years of life with my master opened to me the world of Chinese Medicine, and it was my *shifu* who initiated me. As the saying goes: "The master leads one through the door, but the practicing and perfecting of the art lies with the individual." This remark sums up the educational experience of adepts in all times. A *shifu* is needed in order to pass through the door. Unless you go through the door, you will forever remain strolling around outside. This point is extremely important. Why is it that some people strive their entire lives and never grasp the essence of our medicine? Why is it that some people fail to keep going on the path of learning? It is very probable that it is because they lack this one crucial link. As I now recount the process I underwent with my master, I must say that I received so much from him. Everyone loves pleasure more than suffering and difficulty. There is a Chinese saying regarding scholarship and study: "The sea of learning has no shore, and suffering is the boat." This saying has frightened many people who are, so to speak, yet to "enter through the door." As a matter of fact, once one has gone through that door, not only is the sensation not entirely one of suffering, but suffering and pleasure exist in equal parts. I would go so far as to say that the pleasure exceeds the sensation of suffering. Thus the opening line of the *Analects* (Lunyu) of Confucius states: "To learn and to review what has been learned at times, is this not a pleasure?" It does not say: "To learn and to review what has been learned at times, is this not suffering?"

Another common saying is that "the poor study and the rich engage in business." Those who engage in scholarly work are necessarily impoverished, and only those who trade become wealthy. Why is it then that so many people still pursue a life of study? Precisely because of the truth observed by Confucius, namely that the pursuit of real knowledge is pleasurable. Scholars are rich in terms of their inner life, and merchants are rich in terms of material possessions. Which is capable of truly bringing about peace and happiness—a rich inner life or material wealth? Nevertheless, the joy derived from study is not easily obtained. I believe that master–disciple transmission plays an important role here. One's *shifu* can point the way to discovering this pleasure, this happiness. Furthermore, in other fields of traditional Chinese culture, the significance of master–disciple transmission is even more pronounced. This is a process that, within the sciences embedded in traditional Chinese culture, specifically in the field of Chinese Medicine, I personally underwent. I am offering my own experience with this process as food for thought to the reader.

Whether we are talking about formal education or the passing down of information within a traditional lineage system, there are three levels of significance. The first is the teaching of the knowledge. The second is the application of what has been taught. And the last facet involves creation and innovation, bringing forth new ideas. We speak of knowledge when we are talking about things that as a culture we already know. We study those things that are already known and have been experienced. Old things tend to make us feel bored. People generally enjoy new experiences and grow tired of the old. Every student must make it through that phase of boredom and rejection of old things. If you do not study the knowledge of our forebears, how will you be able to use the old to bring forth the new? Those who pursue scholarship must be able to "enjoy the new and not be bored by the old." The *Analects* mentions a prerequisite to being a teacher, which is "to breathe life into the ancient and know the present . . . breathing life into the ancient and knowing the new, only then can you be a teacher." Whether or not you are a worthy teacher depends on whether or not you possess this special skill. Whether or not your scholarship will be transmitted down the line also depends on this.

What is this special skill? It is merely the joy that studying produces! If you experience joy in study, the path of scholarship will be renewed each day. Day after day it will be made fresh, and you will be able to deepen your study and persist as you continue. If you do not possess this, studying will be dull and dry. If that is the case, you might as well change professions and seek material wealth, trade study for commerce, and enter the market and chase money. Where does the joy of learning come from? From one's teacher! Those who are teachers are able to "breathe life into the ancient and know the present." They are able to instill in you the ability to know the present from the ancient. This is like a form of replication, of cloning. And the inheritance of scholarship and learning is a sort of cloning that is even more worthwhile!

II.3.c. An Unexpected Gift by Lake Lugu

My late teacher was an amazing man. In the past, he made believers of a number of Western Medicine doctors who had previously slandered Chinese Medicine. He relied on his clinical ability to do this. After I began following my teacher, the focus of his work shifted. He attempted to achieve in traditional Chinese Medicine what Einstein tried to accomplish in physics, namely to create a sort of "unified theory." His focus moved from clinical practice to the establishment of theory. Therefore, I received a great deal of influence regarding theory from my mentorship with him. I feel that the clinical instruction I received was relatively deficient. After my teacher passed away, I explored theory even more deeply. But in terms of my clinical ability, I could not find a clear way forward, I was without a definite plan, and my results were inconsistent. Sometimes I heard people say: "Liu Lihong is brilliant! If a stubborn case falls into his hands, he can cure it with just a few decoctions." At other times, however, I heard people discussing me, saying: "Liu's theory is pretty good but he's nothing special when it comes to clinical practice." In my own heart, I am very clear about this situation. It is especially difficult when patients come from far distant places and put all of their hopes into my ability to help them but I find myself unable to do much for them. At these times I feel especially perplexed and uncomfortable. All of these feelings are signs that I have reached another level, fraught with new obstacles that require the guiding hand of a master to cross over. Earlier I mentioned that there was a reason why in the past, whenever I came to a new place, I asked around for "experts," did I not? It was, in fact, because I wanted to resolve this particular problem.

In August 1999, at the invitation of Professor Heiner Fruehauf, the head of the School of Classical Chinese Medicine at the National College of Natural Medicine in Portland, Oregon, I conducted a series of lectures on the *Treatise on Cold Damage* by the shore of Lake Lugu, which lies at the boundary between the provinces of Yunnan and Sichuan. Heiner Fruehauf is a German sinologist who, among other places, studied Chinese literature at Fudan University in Shanghai. After completing his doctoral degree in the United States, Harvard University invited him to teach there. Due to a severe illness, however, he fell in love with Chinese Medicine and declined the professorship that had been offered to him. One can imagine what it means to receive a professorship from a university of this caliber. Yet Dr. Fruehauf forewent this position and became a student once again. This story should move those of us who have studied Chinese Medicine from the very start of our academic careers. Most of us were forced into the profession of Chinese Medicine and have studied it without much joy rather than feeling blessed to have had this opportunity. The motivation to become a Chinese Medicine physician could not be more different. At Lake Lugu, I lectured for ten days. Among the people listening to the lectures were people with multiple doctoral degrees, master degrees, undergraduates, as well as poets and painters, none of whom had ever before come into contact with Chinese Medicine. For the first few days, we only had lectures in the morning, and students made their own arrangements to fill their afternoons. After three days, the participants began to feel that only having lectures in the mornings was not sufficient and requested that we continue our studies in the afternoon. At the end of the ten days of lecturing, none could bear to part. They all gave me the thumbs-up and said I was a "great man." The praise that I received from this group renewed my sense of the greatness of the ancient wisdom. It also instilled in me the feeling that the interaction of Chinese and Western culture could overcome the barriers of culture and language if provided with an appropriate method.

Dr. Fruehauf was also deeply affected and, in addition to conveying his gratitude, felt compelled to share his personal life story with me, including his introduction to his teacher Zeng Rongxiu, an old Chinese Medicine doctor. Dr. Zeng had studied Chinese Medicine the old way, outside the regular university system. After initially teaching himself, he had had the extraordinarily good fortune during the Chinese Cultural Revolution to apprentice with the famous physician from Chengdu, Tian "Bawei" (田八味)—Dr. Tian "Who Never Uses More Than Eight Herbs." Anyone who hears this name feels a sort of thrill, as if confronted with a character from one of Jin Yong's martial arts novels. Master Tian, however, a real-life master physician, was known for his exclusive application of classical remedies and stringent use of just a few important herbs. Dr. Tian was a master of pulse diagnosis since his patients were many and in the course of a day he would have to diagnose three to four hundred patients and often had no time to ask them questions, having to rely exclusively on pulse diagnosis alone. Due to his great degree of accuracy in matching specific pulse patterns to specific herbal formulas, his clinical success rates were very high. After studying under Master Tian, Dr. Zeng eventually understood the importance of pulse diagnosis and, over time, added his own clinical experience to the transmission he had received. Thus, he developed a unique understanding of the many pulse patterns present in the *Treatise on Cold Damage*, and practiced according to the principle that when patients exhibit a particular pulse, they receive the corresponding formula. This method produced overall better results in comparison with other doctors. Dr. Fruehauf's account excited me. Although I had studied the *Treatise on Cold Damage* for many years and had formed a sense of its theory, I still felt uneasy when prescribing classical formulas in the clinical setting. To have studied the *Treatise on Cold Damage* and to still be unable to use any of its prescriptions, how can one be said to be an expert on Cold Damage diseases? I felt that Dr. Zeng possessed precisely what I most needed at that time and entreated Dr. Fruehauf to introduce me to his mentor. And so it was that after we returned to Chengdu from Lake Lugu, Dr. Fruehauf took me to see his teacher. After meeting Dr. Zeng, I expressed my sincere desire to become his disciple. Dr. Zeng turned out to be a straightforward person. We were almost immediately on close terms with one another. I had Heiner Fruehauf's recommendation, so he gladly accepted me as his student. In November 2000, I took Dr. Zeng with me to Guangxi province and spent a week transcribing his prescriptions. This week of study helped me immensely. With the help of Dr. Zeng, I finally found the agility to leap across the pit of difficulties I had encountered in the clinical arena. This experience once again instilled in me the feeling that if one wishes to study Chinese Medicine, the importance of having a teacher cannot be overestimated. When Dr. Yu Lu had sent me off with a reminder of that importance, the words had come straight from the bottom of his heart.

After apprenticing with Dr. Zeng, I still cannot employ classical formulas with his high level of proficiency, but my practice goes much more smoothly than before, and thus my clinical results are improving. Several days ago, I was treating a colleague of mine. The patient's left cheek was red, swollen, itchy, and painful. He had already used Western antibiotics with inadequate results. From a conventional Chinese Medicine perspective, we might think that because the symptom picture involved redness, swelling, and itching, we should clear heat, resolve toxicity, dispel wind, and stop the itching. In the past, this is how my diagnostic train of thought would have developed. However, when I felt this patient's pulse, I could tell it was floating, but it was also choppy, lacking its usual smoothness. What sort of pathology does this sort of pulse indicate? These are clear signs of a Taiyang syndrome, caused by disease in the exterior with inadequate sweating and a resultant stagnation of yang *qi*. The forty-eighth line of the *Treatise on Cold Damage* focuses on this problem, and the recommended treatment principle is to "induce more sweating to cure it." In accordance with this line, I prepared Mahuang Guizhi Ge Ban Tang. After one dose, the redness, swelling, pain, and itching were reduced by more than half. After the second dose, the inflammation subsided. Both Mahuang Tang and Guizhi Tang are originally used as formulas to treat disorders of the common cold variety. Why did I use them here to treat a red, swollen cheek? My colleague was most astonished. In the past, I may have been surprised myself and thought: "The left cheek belongs to the liver, and redness with swelling is a sign of heat—this calls for purging heat from the liver." I might have used Longdan Xiegan Tang, but I could not possibly have thought of using Mahuang Guizhi Ge Ban Tang. Personally, I consider this sort of progress in my thinking to be inseparable from Dr. Zeng's tutelage. This example may once again demonstrate the importance of teacher transmission. Why? It was entirely inspired by the nature of lineage transmission I received from Dr. Zeng.

This sort of lineage-based knowledge is much less transparent than most elements of Western science. There is no technological mediator here, only one's own subjective application of human faculties. This sort of educational process relies on teaching by personal example and verbal instruction. We must consider whether this personalized teaching is possible without the essential one-on-one mentorship of the traditional model. Since Chinese Medicine is a science that combines the material and the immaterial realms, its transmission must necessarily revolve around both of these aspects. We have already discussed how the pedagogical model selected by the current educational system is solely adapted to the scientific and materialistic aspect of knowledge. So what of the metaphysical, immaterial aspect of Chinese Medicine? This element is purely dependent on a transmission from teacher to disciple in the genuine sense. It depends on an ancient model of give and take epitomized by the master–disciple relationship. Therefore, the Chinese Medicine educational model must include both educational modes.

Generally speaking, we should applaud the establishment of graduate studies in Chinese Medicine as a positive event, for the role of academic advisor does bear some resemblance to a traditional mentor. Unfortunately, we can already see that this system has failed, since it has remained stuck in the regular material level of education. To compound the issue, those supervisors with personal experience of teacher transmission are retiring, one after another. The old masters are gradually passing from this world, and their successors are university graduates who have no experience and sense of true teacher–disciple transmission and therefore do not know how to find and teach suitable disciples themselves. Almost all graduate students, regardless of whether they are at the master's or the doctorate level, refer to their advisor as their boss. Why? This is not an incidental distinction; there is good reason for it. There is no comparison between a boss and the type of mentor Dr. Zeng was to me.

III. Seeking a Method That Works—Relying on the Classics

After issues of belief have been resolved, confidence naturally emerges. If in addition, one receives the requisite transmission from a teacher, then there is only one thing left, and I think that is the pursuit of still more effective methods. If one desires to truly rise to the level demanded by the study of Chinese Medicine and truly grasp its inherent value, apart from the technical aspects of this medicine, one should be deeply interested in Chinese Medicine as a science, as a philosophy, and as an art. One cannot accomplish this without heavy reliance on the classics. It may seem anachronistic to say that one must study the classics to master Chinese Medicine, since most Chinese Medicine colleges have turned the study of the classics into elective courses. Reduced from core curriculum to electives, the position of the classics has fallen considerably. This demotion signals that the classics are unnecessary to the study of Chinese Medicine. How did this development come about? The Chinese Medicine classics are 2,000 years old. Times are changing, everything is advancing, so why should we cling to the classics? Furthermore, one could argue that more recent textbooks like *Fundamentals of Chinese Medicine, Formula Studies, Diagnostic Techniques,* and those pertaining to each of the clinical departments are, after all, derived from the classics and include modern observations as well. Why should we hold on to the classics when we have books like these? And lastly, there is the collection of survey statistics by government departments. These surveys reveal that many practitioners regard the classics as having little significance. In the opinion of most people who are surveyed, little is lost by not studying the classics. It is because of a combination of these three reasons that the fate of Chinese Medicine classics has been relegated to its current position. My own experience is directly opposite to this assessment. I believe that the importance of the classics should not be weakened, but rather strengthened. Below, I will discuss the reasons why I think that reliance on the classics is necessary in our field.

III.1. The Experience of History

Are the classics ultimately relevant or not to the study and comprehension of Chinese Medicine? Should they be an obligatory part of the curriculum or not? The answer is clear when we look at it from a historical perspective. When we examine history, we see that from the time of Zhang Zhongjing clear up until the Qing dynasty, in over a thousand years of history, the vast majority of preeminent physicians emerged from a foundation of serious study of the classics, and again a great number of these individuals relied on the classics to produce their most highly regarded accomplishments. Chinese Medicine, as a unique historical phenomenon, cannot but compel us to wonder why the classics have cast such a powerful spell over its most distinguished adherents. Ever since the Eastern Han dynasty, there have been countless books by Chinese doctors. In this vast sea of medical texts, there is not a single one that does not profess to be a direct product of the classics. However, in terms of significance, they cannot replace the classics and certainly do not surpass them. There are even times when they may actually hinder our understanding of the meaning inherent in the classics's text itself. It was for this reason that, as late as the Qing dynasty, the great physicians Chen Xiuyuan and Xu Dachun called for the incineration of these later medical texts. Of course, the point of view held by Chen and Xu is a bit too extreme, but their overweening passion should not prevent us from recognizing the importance of the Chinese Medicine classics from a more moderate perspective.

From the historical facts alone, we can see that since ancient times physicians have emerged from the foundation of the classics. This was the experience of the ancients, but how about the experience of doctors who are closer to our own time? We need only glance at Zhou Fengwu's *The Path of Venerable Chinese Medicine Doctors* (Minglao Zhongyi zhi lu) to find a very similar sentiment. Let us take Pu Fuzhou, with whom we are perhaps most familiar, as an example. When Master Pu was just beginning his medical career, he already saw a great number of patients, some of whom he treated effectively and some not. On account of this, Master Pu suddenly closed his doors and stopped his practice for three years in order to study more deeply. He read the medical classics repeatedly, pondered their essence, and contemplated them over and over. After three years behind closed doors, he resumed seeing patients and found that his clinical proficiency was now much more adequate. The final result of this concentrated study was that after the founding of the People's Republic of China, he topped the list of the country's most eminent physicians. Regarding this unusual episode of cloistered study, Master Pu had this to say: "At the time there were many people who did not understand my state of mind. They thought that I had closed my doors and stopped treating disease as a means of raising my social status, when in fact it was simply that I did not understand the merits of the classics." It was not by coincidence that another famous physician, Master Qin Bowei, also emphasized that every Chinese Medicine practitioner needs to take at least three months each year to review the classics. The experiences and advice of these two master physicians deserve our serious attention.

The late Professor Lin Peixiang was a teacher who I greatly respected. Master Lin was not only an expert of Chinese Medicine theory, but also an accomplished clinician. Besides internal medicine, he specialized in gynecology, pediatrics, and ear, nose, and throat issues. But Professor Lin never read specialized texts for internal medicine, external medicine, gynecology, pediatrics, or texts devoted to the diseases of the five senses. He relied solely on his single copy of the *Yellow Emperor's Classic* to cure disease. During one of his lecture courses, he is quoted as having said: "As for the content of the *Yellow Emperor's Classic*, if you fully understand even one sentence, you will be able to receive nourishment from that for your entire life." In other words, if one is able to fully grasp even one of the problems presented in the *Yellow Emperor's Classic*, if you can make a single sentence completely comprehensible, then you will be able to benefit from it for the rest of your life. These are words of wisdom, words from the bottom of the heart! Think about this. Isn't this the magical power of the classics that we spoke about earlier? If one single sentence can provide that much inspiration, then what about two sentences, or three sentences, or even the entirety of the *Yellow Emperor's Classic*? If you decipher all of it, how many lifetimes of use will you gain from it? From the example of Master Lin's life, we can see that the longevity and the continued importance of the classics are inestimably great. They are truly manifestations of the utmost maturity of ancient wisdom and a perennial source of creativity.

III.2. Clearing Away Obstructions to Understanding the Classics

It is not easy to persuade people to take a fresh look at the classics, a topic that has gradually been getting discarded and turned into elective courses, and ascribe new importance to them. Almost everyone is accustomed to using modern scientific thinking to consider medical problems. Along the same lines, we tend to think that anything new surpasses the old. How can we possibly believe that the classics are able to transcend time and space, cross over many eras, and even surpass later generations? It is difficult to believe, but this is indeed what has happened in many traditional disciplines.

If we wish to clear away any ideological resistance that we may have to this argument, we must yet again return to the topic of theory. Earlier we spoke of how the Chinese Medicine classics do not solely rely on a rational structure; they also contain knowledge that was discovered and validated by internal experimentation. The classics represent a perfect merging of these two cognitive methodologies. It is precisely this sort of perfect integration that Liang Shuming referred to as the "precocious cultural product that has the ability to spawn future civilizations." But the span between this future and this precocity is extraordinarily great. This is true to such an extent that even now we have no means whereby to fully understand the deep meaning contained in the classics. For instance, the non-material aspects of ancient theory have barely been touched upon by modern science. As yet, there are no substantive means by which many of the elements contained in the classics can be explained, and as a result, they tend to be ascribed to superstition and pseudoscience. This accusation cannot hold—many aspects of classical theory have simply superseded the level of the material world of "vessels" and material things. In order to understand them, we must employ calipers not confined to the physical world of "vessels." If we solely use a material lens to look upon the more ephemeral aspects of the classics, we will have great difficulty perceiving them. To produce this different sort of thinking, we must rely on the method of internal experimentation, not external experimentation.

We already discussed how internal experimentation potentially presents problems that are difficult to discuss. At this juncture, however, we cannot proceed without talking about genuine internal exploration as part of Chinese Medicine. This experimentation does not rely on how much equipment you buy, or how technically advanced your apparatus is. It does not involve at a concrete laboratory that you can see or touch. It arises purely from a process of serious cultivation and intense training and has the potential to pierce the veil of the material realm. This ability is, on some level, related to talent. Several days ago, I was browsing through a copy of *Discovering Our Mother* (Faxian muqin) by Wang Donghua. This book contains a wealth of information. One of its chapters is concerned with the problem of individual talent and uses plants as examples: identical seeds raised in different conditions with different stimuli emerge as very different plants. Take for instance a tomato. Those who have spent time in the countryside will surely have some experience with this. How many tomatoes can one tomato plant produce? According to what I have personally seen in rural areas, I assumed that a tomato plant can produce at the most ten to a hundred tomatoes and, if given a lot of extra care and nourishment, perhaps a few hundred tomatoes. However, a group of Japanese breeders succeeded in cultivating a tomato plant that was able to produce more than 13,000 tomatoes! It is hard not to twist one's tongue repeating this number. At the time, this specially cultivated tomato caused quite a sensation in Japan and set a new record. This example reveals the breadth of latent potential. The same seed receiving different cultivation results in a very different product. From the latent potential contained in the seed of a plant, we can infer how great the latent potential of a person is. What is the hidden potential of the brain? Difficult to quantify indeed.

Rationally, we are therefore completely capable of deducing the existence of this internal experimentation. Once a sort of special "cultivation" process is undergone, the conditions for this type of experimentation can be achieved. And once these conditions are there, all kinds of experiments that serve the process of verifying the classics can be conducted. In this manner, the linear data stream and the more invisible part of Chinese Medicine that requires internal experimentation can be combined, and the deeper meaning of the classics can become apparent. In the post-classical period, however, we tend to only study the theoretical data and do away with the core of internal cultivation and experimentation. As time goes by, we lose the ability to conduct these experiments altogether, and in the very end doubt that they are even possible. In the time of Zhang Zhongjing, there was no such suspicion toward internal experimentation. In the preface to the *Treatise on Cold Damage*, Zhang Zhongjing wrote: "I have always esteemed the formulas and methods. Please allow me to serve with these words here." The fact that the formulas and methods Zhang Zhongjing refers to here are the sort of internal experiments we have been speaking about and not just herbal formulas, has been extensively researched by historians. When we consult the biographies of "masters of formulas" in the *Book of the Han* (Hanshu) and the *Book of the Later Han* (Houhanshu) we can see that "formulas," meaning medicinal formulas but also any other treatment method, was a phenomenon that 2,000 years ago primarily referred to the art of internal alchemy.

As time has passed, people have become more and more distant from this system of internally verified experimentation. Why was it that during the Song and Ming dynasties, the Confucian schools of rationalist philosophy emerged? The answer is very obvious: by this time people were already unclear about the knowledge obtained through internal verification, so they employed rationality and mental deliberation to figure things out. Was the advent of this rationalist philosophy actually the result of losing internal verification? We can form a judgment about what people in the Song and Ming dynasties thought on this point by examining the four-character phrase: "investigate things to perfect knowledge" (*gewu zhizhi*). At this point, we are not ready to fully understand the meaning of the phrase "to investigate things to perfect knowledge." We must first clarify some fundamental principles. Originally, the word *zhi* ("to know") did not represent the sort of general knowledge obtained through study or in-depth analysis. The meaning here is "to perceive or feel" and is identical with the "illumination of the heart-mind" state discussed above. It is this "illumination of the heart-mind," this perceiving, that is required in order to enter into the state of internal verification, and only then can one engage in internal experimentation. How does this state arise? It arises through "investigation," but this "investigation" is not like the thorough probing into the laws of nature as the Song and Ming–dynasty rationalists deemed it. This "investigation" means to distance oneself from worldly desires. It is a sort of mental or spiritual outlook. It is only once one has obtained this state that one can carry out internal experimentation.

This kind of outlook toward the world is contained in the wisdom teachings of Confucianism, Buddhism, and Daoism. The saying by Confucius "The gentleman eats without seeking satiety, and rests without seeking quiet" is actually referring to this state. The *Great Learning* states: "After one knows when to stop, one can have certainty; after there is certainty, one can have quietude; after there is quietude, one can have peace; after one has attained peace, one is able to strategize contemplatively; once one can strategize contemplatively, there is achievement." This "stopping," this "certainty," this "quietude," this "peace," this "strategic contemplation," if this is not "investigation," what is it? If you do not "eat without seeking satiety, and rest without seeking peace," all day long your desires will overflow; you will be thinking about the price of this stock rising and the price of that stock falling. If that is the case, will you be capable of "stopping," "certainty," "quietude," and "peace"? And if you are not, how will you obtain what you seek? How will you acquire knowledge? In Daoist philosophy, Laozi said, "Engage in study and gain something each day, practice the Dao and lose something each day; lose and lose until you arrive at non-action (*wuwei*). What is lost? The material world is lost, and this loss is later understood as an external probing into material things. The "investigation of things" in Buddhism is clearly related to the process of detachment. Confucianism, Buddhism, and Daoism all make reference to this process in their own way. The details vary in each school of thought, but the main point is the same. This understanding of "investigating things" is obviously completely different from the understanding held by Song and Ming–dynasty rationalism. If one wishes to obtain the ability to see internally, this "distancing from the material world" is one of the most fundamental requirements. If this prerequisite is not met, or if it is maligned, then there is nothing to speak of as far as internal experimentation goes. The scholars of the Song and Ming dynasties analyzed this concept of "investigating things" in minute detail. Although they debated the concept exhaustively, they never realized true internal verification and never conducted any of the experiments made possible by this ability.

It is easy to see why certain problems in Chinese Medicine are difficult to understand and why we are perpetually confused about the value of the classics. Why is it that we constantly harbor suspicion toward so many aspects of Chinese Medicine? It is because we lack the discerning eye of internal verification. This is a crucial factor in the obstruction of our comprehension of the classics. If we wish to comprehend Chinese Medicine, and especially the Chinese Medicine classics, we must sweep away this hindrance in our thinking.

III.3. Three Types of Culture

Earlier, we emphasized the significance of understanding theory. Why should we emphasize this issue? In the past, many famous physicians practicing Chinese Medicine did not require a rational system before beginning their undertaking. They began directly with their pursuit of perceptual knowledge. This kind of knowledge is a strange thing—very powerful. Once the power of intuition is tapped, all other problems are resolved. The ancients, for the most part, studied Chinese Medicine primarily through perception and intuition. This is exemplified by Zhang Zhongjing in his preface where he writes: "I was deeply moved by the loss of my family's former glory and the loss of so many lives and thus sought the guidance of the ancients, collecting a multitude of formulas." It is also exemplified by the author of *The Basic Canon of Acupuncture and Moxibustion*, Huangfu Mi, as well as other doctors who threw themselves headlong into the pursuit of Chinese Medicine knowledge after being moved by a particular event.

Please, now, take a good look at your own motivation for studying this medicine. From my perspective, most practitioners do not possess this burning flame inside them, and even if they do, it tends to be confused. Ask yourself, therefore, the question of how you came to this profession. In China, the honest answer to this question is that the entrance examination scores of most Chinese Medicine students were not high enough to enter Tsinghua University or Peking University; they were not even high enough to enter average polytechnic institutions, and so the choice was made to enter Chinese Medicine colleges instead. Are there any students in our field who could have attended Tsinghua or Peking University? I think not! If students are entering their education in this sort of psychological state, without a strong positive motivation toward their discipline, how will they be able to study Chinese Medicine well?

My mentor often stressed that Chinese Medicine cannot be learned by the average person, and that it required the same caliber of student as those found at Tsinghua University in order to learn Chinese Medicine well. Modern science requires great talent, and so does Chinese Medicine. The Song dynasty physicians Lin Yi and Gao Baoheng also held this view. In the preface to the *Unabridged and Annotated Plain Questions of the Yellow Emperor's Classic* (Chongguang buzhu Huangdi neijing suwen), they write: "If an utterly sophisticated and subtle Dao is transmitted to an utterly base and shallow person and that person does not just give up and discard it, how fortunate is that!" And so we have the current situation in China: highly talented people disdain to consider a career in Chinese Medicine, while those with little talent from the very beginning fail to learn Chinese Medicine well. So it is indeed fortunate that they do not just give up! If this sort of situation is not corrected from the very foundation, how can the legacy of Chinese Medicine be transmitted? How can it blossom and thrive?

Why, now, do the gifted, at least in modern-day China, look down on Chinese Medicine? This has much to do with their environment. At present, everyone is surrounded with the informational buzz of modern culture. We are therefore accustomed to using a certain cultural perspective to ponder any question that comes before us. In this sort of intellectual environment, it is extremely difficult to be deeply moved from a place of direct perception that urges us to preserve the wisdom of traditional culture, including Chinese Medicine. I hope to be able to provide some rational reasons that may help to develop a more intimate relationship with our tradition, and Chinese Medicine in particular, and a motivation to study them.

In fact, culture is multifaceted and not limited to one paradigm. It is simply the case that everyone is already accustomed to this one paradigm, and they use the constructs of this one paradigm to understand their world. This constraint produces a unilateral and highly limited perspective. The culture to which everyone has become so accustomed is, of course, the culture of modern science, or to abbreviate the term, the culture of science. This culture has a distinguishing feature that it meets the needs of its time. This culture progresses in step with its era. We can describe this culture as something that renews itself each day. Take a moment to ask yourself: Is this daily change something you can relate to in your life? Compare the previous decade with this decade: Are there differences? The differences are huge. All of us clearly perceive this tidal change and it naturally causes us to think that all culture is like this. "Each wave of the Yangzi River pushes the wave before it"—each new generation surpasses the old. Times are advancing, all culture is progressing, the new culture is always stronger than the old, ancient things lag behind the culture of today: it is inevitable. Coming from this sort of understanding, how could one possibly be satisfied with Chinese Medicine? How could one attach importance to the classics?

When we say that culture is multifaceted, we also mean that it cannot be confined to the model described above. The phase of scientific culture causes us to feel that as time progresses, so too will the culture of science. Are there any other cultures that possess this characteristic? For instance, is it the case that as time progresses, artistic culture also progresses? We do not need to do a lot of research in art history to answer this question. A brief look at the development of art in- and outside of China confirms that progression over time is not at all what has happened. We can take poetry as an example. In the Tang dynasty, Chinese poetry was highly refined and stylized. During the centuries of the Tang, a sublime form of literature known as Tang poetry was explored exhaustively. Is it the case that when we come to the Song dynasty, this poetry improved still further, and progressed in some way? On the contrary, this is not the case. Our forebears knew that Tang Poetry represented a climax in the art of literature and could not possibly be further improved upon. Knowing this, the poets of the Song dynasty did not go rooting around in the dregs of the Tang to try to create something better. Instead, they went in a different direction and created the highly distinct form of Song dynasty lyrics. The verses of the Yuan dynasty underwent a similar process. How about music? Or painting? Their circumstances are more or less the same. Every New Year in Vienna, there is a musical concert to commemorate the passing year. What music is played at these concerts? It is almost exclusively the works of Johann Strauss and Johann Strauss Jr., not just to commemorate them but because nobody after them has been able to surpass the standard they set. The standard has been set by musical geniuses such as these, geniuses of the same caliber as Tchaikovsky and Beethoven. Has this music been produced in the previous year? In the case of music, is it the case that after some decades or centuries, we can expect music to exceed that of these great composers of the past? Those who study music are in agreement: no such development is on the horizon. The fields of music, painting, and poetry can be considered examples, but they are different from the field of science. They are not, after all, fields that progress in an entirely linear fashion. In these disciplines, once a summit is reached, another cultural apex may be reached in a matter of years or centuries, but that second peak may or may not exceed the first. Science is linear, but these artistic disciplines are not. Science progresses steadily forward and these other disciplines meander back and forth in curved paths. Clearly, then, these aspects and paradigms of culture differ greatly.

Besides the two expressions of culture described above, there is yet another special category of culture formed in antiquity, such as Buddhism. Buddhist culture originated more than 3,500 years ago with Prince Siddhartha Gautama, also known as the Shakyamuni Buddha. In contrast to other cultural models, especially that of science, Shakyamuni did not predict that Buddhist culture would develop endlessly. In contrast, he predicted that Buddhist teaching would experience three distinct phases, the Three Ages of Buddhism: the Age of the Right Law, the Age of the Apparent Law, and the Age of the Conclusion of the Law. At the moment, we will not analyze this problem with regard to the question of why the Buddhist tradition has chosen a path that appears to diverge from the norms we are accustomed to. For now, let us simply take note of this phenomenon and not discuss it further. In addition, Daoism and Confucianism followed similar paths. After these expressions of culture were established, they experienced a period of prosperity and then gradually diminished until now, when they exist in name only.

So we see that culture is highly variable and is not restricted to one particular pattern or mode. Looking at everything through the lens of "progress" simply does not match reality. Among the cultural categories that we have just described, where do we place Chinese Medicine? Or is it the case that Chinese Medicine belongs to all three categories at once? Let us ponder this question. In my opinion, Chinese Medicine, at the very least, is not solely restricted to the same category as that of science. To regard and research Chinese Medicine solely from this perspective is bound to produce problems. Regarding Chinese Medicine, sometimes we must look to what lies behind us and sometimes we must look to what lies ahead of us.

I often say, that if we wish to determine what type of culture Chinese Medicine belongs to, we should examine ourselves to find the answer. What level of mastery of this medicine do we find when we look at ourselves? Better than the past or worse? If you are a graduate of a TCM college, or even a master's or doctoral-level practitioner, and if your Chinese Medicine skill is indeed excellent and in both theory and practice you have no trouble, and if you are unhindered in your understanding of the classics, then maybe, in your case, Chinese Medicine has experienced a linear sort of development. If the situation is the opposite of this and your skill in Chinese Medicine is as mediocre as your understanding of its underlying theory, you are unable to resolve clinical quandaries, and you are completely clueless regarding the classics, then Chinese Medicine has experienced problems in your case and regressed instead. Being absolutely clear where we stand ourselves before answering this question is imperative.

Another important consideration is one's familiarity with the classics. An appraisal of the classics must be based on the extent to which we have benefited from their study. If we have not reaped any benefit from these treasures, then our appraisal of them is simply empty talk. So I strongly advise those who wish to criticize the classics to think twice before speaking. Otherwise, your perspective will reveal your ignorance. Confucius said it best in his *Great Commentary* (Xici) of the *Classic of Changes*:

> When benevolent people see it, they call it benevolence; when wise people see it, they call it wisdom. Common folk use it every day and do not know what it is. Thus the Dao of the noble person is ever so rare!

The content of the classics is indeed regarded by the benevolent as benevolence and by the wise as wisdom. There is one more thing that needs to be said here, but the reader may ponder it carefully. Why is it that courses in the classics have become optional? It is of course because certain people have come to regard the classics as increasingly unnecessary. Another reason for relegating the classics to the status of elective study is evidenced by a statistical survey of popular opinion. Hundreds or even thousands of questionnaires were given out and recipients were asked to approve or disapprove a list of topics. A great number of people who completed the survey marked the topic labeled "Classics" as irrelevant. The results of this study validated making a study of the classics optional, since many people considered the classics as having little significance. However, if we are to apply Confucius's standards, this sort of statistical investigation does not have the slightest significance, since this is a matter of the benevolent seeing benevolence, the wise seeing wisdom, and the mediocre finding mediocrity. If you are seeking wisdom but do not possess any yourself, how will you find any "benevolence" or "wisdom" in the classics? You will, of course, say that the classics are devoid of sense, and may not even want them to be taught as electives. Previously, we discussed how one must be perceptive and receptive to study the classics. If this sensitivity has not yet been kindled, you will most certainly be unable to say a single good word about the classics. An accurate assessment of the classics cannot be had from just anyone.

Let me give you an example. There are four great classic works of Chinese literature: *The Romance of the Three Kingdoms* (Sanguo), *Journey to the West* (Xiyouji), *Outlaws of the Water Margin* (Shuihuzhuan), and *Dream of the Red Chamber* (Hongloumeng). The first three of these I have read more than once. As for the *Dream of the Red Chamber*, I really want to read it and have seen it praised by many notable scholars. Mao Zedong especially loved this book. But when I read it, I get through a few chapters, twenty at the most, and then I cannot read anymore, though I do not know why. So up to this day, I have not read this great classic through even once. I only know its famous idiom, the Chinese equivalent of "For we bring nothing into the world and it is certain we can taking nothing out." Imagine if someone were to ask my opinion about this particular book—I would look like a fool. The renowned physician I spoke of earlier, Professor Lin Peixiang, could easily forgo reading modern Chinese Medicine books on internal medicine, gynecology, or pediatrics, but he considered reading the *Yellow Emperor's Classic* to be indispensable. Professor Lin did not bother with modern expositions on special topics, he relied solely on the *Yellow Emperor's Classic*. Despite this, he did a beautiful job treating all sorts of diseases, including gynecological and pediatric conditions. If Professor Lin were given a survey, you can bet how he would respond. And so, regarding the difference of attitude toward the classics, it is not the case that because so many people consider them useless, they are useless. It is simply the case that those who have not benefited from the classics have failed to comprehend their usefulness. If someone goes into the stock market to become a millionaire but instead ends up losing money, they will certainly say the market is no good.

III.4. The Importance of Studying the Classics

III.4.a. It Is Not "Holding On to the Old"

Previously, we discussed the classics from a cultural perspective. The purpose of this discussion was to demonstrate that despite the age of the classics, they are not by definition out of date or backward, so we should not simply refute or abandon them because they are old. At the same time, when we emphasize learning from classics from 2,000 years ago, people are bound to be a bit nervous that this might be too conservative an approach, which might lead to a rejection of new ideas. To gain perspective on this, we must consider the concept of new and old on many levels. Zhang Zhongjing states in his preface to the *Treatise on Cold Damage*:

> In the ancient past there were the Divine Farmer, the Yellow Emperor, Qi Bo, Bo Gao, Lei Gong, Shao Yu, Shao Shi, and Zhong Wen. In mid-antiquity there were Chang Sang and Bian Que. During the Han dynasty, there were Gongsheng Yang Qing and Cang Gong. After these, we have not heard of anybody.

Zhang Zhongjing uses this passage to remind us of a particular conundrum: Why is it that at the time the classics were created, the most famous masters of Chinese Medicine were so numerous? And why is it that all of a sudden "we have not heard of" any more great masters since? Let us consider this phenomenon for a moment. Stressing the importance of the classics is done for no other reason than to stress that the distance from the time when the classics were created grows ever farther. However, if we study correctly, is it possible that we can come closer to them? Coming closer to the classics, we find ourselves closer to the great masters of antiquity. After we have studied the classics thoroughly, we become more like Lei Gong, Shao Yu, and Shao Shi. What's wrong with that? I believe that this is the most fundamental significance of studying the classics.

In a later passage of the preface, Zhang Zhongjing touches on this point:

When I look at today's doctors, they do not study and ponder the meaning of the classics in order to advance what they know. Each has inherited his family's skills and from beginning to end merely follows along in the old ways.

In this passage, written 1,700 years ago, Zhang Zhongjing explains the difference between being conservative and innovative. The physicians of that time conserved the tidbits of experiential knowledge gleaned by their families, which is what is called "holding on to the old." This is contrasted with those who "study and ponder the meaning of the classics in order to advance what they know." This sort of sincere study of the classics is innovation. When we study the classics, such as the *Yellow Emperor's Classic* or the *Treatise on Cold Damage*, we are "advancing our knowledge." What does it mean to advance our knowledge? To "advance" means to further deduce, to enlarge, to develop, to continue. Serious study of the classics is able to stretch the limits of our understanding, to broaden our perspective. We are always saying that Chinese Medicine needs to innovate in order to blossom, but what do we rely on in order to innovate? This point requires personal experience to be fully understood. Only when you yourself have studied the classics earnestly can you truly understand them and put them into clinical practice. Talk is not enough.

I frequently mention that to be a scholar, you must "delight in the new and not grow weary of the old." This was, of course, Confucius's thinking. Confucius made a crucial point for scholars when he said: "To study without thinking results in confusion. To think without studying is dangerous." Regardless of the topic you study, whether it be Western or Chinese Medicine, this idea is valid.

To study, what does it mean to study? It means to study what has come before, what has preceded the present moment, things that are, to varying degrees, all "old." Is it enough to simply study what is presently available? This sort of study—study for the sake of studying—was considered by Confucius to lead to confusion. Simply acquiring information, even to the point of becoming a sort of walking lexicon, is not enough. In that case, you might have knowledge but you are not necessarily a scholar. This understanding of the ancients is very reasonable. Thus, Confucius said that when we study, we must also think. What does it mean to "think"? Thinking or contemplation is the process by which different pieces of information are brought together and combined in new ways. Various ideas and thoughts collide, exchange parts, and become something new. This process is one of innovation. To "delight in the new" is something everyone does. But the new cannot spring out of nothingness. The new comes from the old, so "to think without studying is dangerous." If we do not have building materials, how can we build anything? Studying the classics is like this. If we wish to harvest what they have to offer, we must act accordingly. If one simply studies without thinking, how can one hope to gain anything? One is simply laboring and confused! I hear many people say that the *Yellow Emperor's Classic* and the *Treatise on Cold Damage* do not matter, and so they either toss them aside or even leave them to collect dust on a high shelf. It is hard for me to stomach. To see such precious objects regarded as meaningless is painful to witness! Therefore, to study the classics, we must contemplate and study, study and contemplate.

III.4.b. All Change Is Encompassed by the Classics

We have said that the importance of the classics cannot be overestimated, and this is the truth. I would like to tell a couple of stories about my own experiences.

In the first half of 1998, as luck would have it, I came to know an old Chinese Medicine practitioner of Binyang County near Nanning. His name was Liao Bingzhen. I like to refer him as Old Liao. Old Liao had been practicing Chinese Medicine for some decades and had his own unique experiences in treating certain diseases. But what most impressed me was his medical ethics and character, and it was these that made it so delightful to visit him. The difference in age did not prevent us from being friends, and he never hesitated to share the knowledge he had gained from long study. One time, Old Liao was telling me of remedies for snakebites. Prior to the founding of the People's Republic of China, there were some quack doctors who possessed methods for treating snakebites but who would always hold back a trick or two when it came to curing patients. This step or two was ingenious—no one could guess it. When these charlatans would cure a snakebite, they would first treat the bite so that the patient was out of death's way and many of the associated symptoms were removed. But the wound would never quite heal, and after a time it would begin to fester so that the patient would have to return to the doctor to buy some more medicine that needed to be taken for two or three months. And so it would drag on for a year and a half or more. Among these unscrupulous practitioners of the medical arts, this practice of curing the patient incompletely to prolong the course of the recovery was referred to as "the quack hooking the patient, and the patient supporting the quack." The crucial trick for treating snakebites, not revealed by these impostors, was passed on to Old Liao from his father's side after he inquired about it. The trick was simply to avoid salt. If the patient did not eat salt for several days while taking several doses of the medicine, the wound would heal quickly and would not fester. The secret was this simple, but not knowing it meant that the patient would suffer terribly.

After hearing Old Liao's story, I wondered if this connection between festering wounds and salt derived from the *Yellow Emperor's Classic*. According the *Plain Questions* chapter "Treatise on True Words in the Golden Cabinet" (Jingui zhenyan lun):

> The north is associated with the color black. Entering the body, it communicates with the kidneys, the orifices it connects with are the anus and the urethra and it stores essence in the kidneys. Therefore its disease is in ravines, its flavor is salty, its overarching category is that of water, and the domesticated animal associated with it is the pig. The type of grain belonging to it are legumes. In its correspondence with the four seasons, in the sky it is the planet Mercury. Therefore we know that its disease is in the bones. Its sound is *yu*, its number is six, and its odor is rotten.

The smell related to the kidney is rotten and so it stands to reason that the pathological processes resulting in a rotten smell are connected to the kidney. Those suffering from disease related to the kidney should avoid salt as instructed by the *Yellow Emperor's Classic*: "Eating too much salt damages the kidneys." This is also common sense to most people. Wounds from snakebites turn rotten. By avoiding salt for a few days and taking some ordinary Chinese Medicine, the wound heals. This is so mysterious and at the same time so simple! The contents of the classics are just like this. Before one has uncovered them, they are extremely mysterious. Afterward, they seem very simple. This reflects the saying "Once you have reached the Dao, it is uncomplicated." This sort of knowledge is used every day by ordinary people, and yet they are unconscious of it. It is certainly unknown to these quacks that the step they are omitting originated in the *Yellow Emperor's Classic*. The classics are precisely this above-mentioned "*Dao* of the noble person."

Old Liao also related his experience of treating bone cancer. Among cancers, bone cancer is one of the most intensely painful. This pain is also very difficult to treat. Even the use of strong anesthetics may not help much. Old Liao had a trump card when treating this sort of pain. Although bone cancer often turns out to be incurable, he could get rid of the pain very quickly, and this went a long way toward relieving the patient's suffering. What medicine did he use? He would add a special ingredient to some medicinal herbs and then the patient would bathe the affected part repeatedly in the resulting decoction until the pain gradually disappeared. This particular ingredient was very efficacious. If added, the pain would stop quickly. Without it, the decoction did nothing. And what was the special ingredient? It was plant material that had grown out of soil from beneath a buried decomposed coffin. In the past, when a person died in China, their body was put in a wooden coffin and buried. The body slowly began to rot, and the rotten remains oozed into the wooden bottom of the coffin. This putrid material joined with the very fiber of the wood, and, after a time, from this special wood at the bottom of the coffin, this special ingredient began to grow. One can imagine the quintessential putrescence this wood contained after receiving the sluggish infusion of a corpse's decomposition. In accordance with the above passage from the *Yellow Emperor's Classic*, one must realize that whatever grows in such a rotting and festering material would have a strong affinity with the kidneys, and by extension with the bones of the body, since the bones are understood in Chinese Medicine to pertain to the kidneys. This explains, from a classical Chinese Medicine perspective, why such an organism would contain the medicinal properties that allow it to assist in treating bone cancer. At one point, I asked Old Liao who had taught him this method. Old Liao did not go into all the whys and wherefores. The method was not inherited from anyone else, nor was it adopted from a strict theoretical framework. His thinking was that bone cancer is a remarkably insidious and strange disease, and so a strange and unique medicine was called for. In this, he employed the method of curing like with like. He never dreamed that the effect would be as dramatic as it turned out to be. When I showed Old Liao the passage from the *Yellow Emperor's Classic* in which the connection between the kidneys and the rotten smells are described, he suddenly realized that his selection of remedies was in accord with the classics.

Despite being rather unusual, these two examples could both be explained by the teachings in the *Yellow Emperor's Classic*. Of course, the role of the *Yellow Emperor's Classic* in these cases was passive, in that it was after events had already occurred that we went searching for evidence. However, through this kind of passive guidance, we can discover the inner meaning of the classics as well as their latent capacity to guide our understanding toward solutions. If we regard every sentence in the classics as having merit, and underestimate no part of it, then we can change passive to active, and actively use the teachings of the classics to contemplate the world in front of us, resolving many difficult problems. It is my belief that even a cure for AIDS can be found within the pages of the *Yellow Emperor's Classic*. A number of years ago, two particular books caused quite a sensation in China. *The Learning Revolution* by the American Gordon Dryden, and *A Great Revolution in the Brain World* by the Japanese author Shigeo Haruyama. It was this latter book in particular, drawing upon research on the brain, that caused an uproar. One focal point of *A Great Revolution in the Brain World* is the exploration of how to improve the efficiency of the brain and awaken the vast potential of each brain cell. Furthermore, this discussion was concentrated on how to evoke alpha waves in the brain and how to bring about the secretion of endorphins in the brain. In his discourse concerning increasing endorphin secretion and alpha wave activity in the brain, Dr. Haruyama wrote about a variety of effective techniques including exercise methods, dietary regulations, and mind-body techniques. In terms of nutrition, Shigeo Haruyama's research revealed that one particular food stood out from other Japanese foods in terms of its ability to increase the release of endorphins. This food, miso, is much beloved by the Japanese and is similar to Chinese fermented soybeans. Miso is a food eaten by nearly all Japanese, especially beloved at breakfast. Why does miso improve brain function to such a remarkable degree? If we take a look in the *Nejing*, the answer can be found.

From the *Fundamentals of Chinese Medicine* textbook, we understand clearly that the brain and nervous system are most closely associated with the kidneys. It is said that "the kidneys rule the bones and give rise to the marrow; the marrow is closely connected with the brain." Therefore, if one contemplates how to improve brain function from a Chinese Medicine perspective, one must proceed from the kidneys as a starting point. This is a basic principle. Having oriented oneself toward the problem in this way, it becomes easy to address. As we read in a passage from the *Plain Questions* in the chapter called "Treatise on True Words in the Golden Cabinet," the type of grain associated with the kidney is the legume, and its odor is rotten. It is fitting that beans are associated with the kidney. Anyone who compares the shape and form of the bean to the physical appearance of the kidney would agree that the similarity is striking. Beans do look like miniature kidneys. Beans have a special relationship with the kidneys. After the beans are fermented, this relationship with the kidneys becomes even closer. Fermentation is essentially a rotting process. Beans that have been fermented have a very strong affinity for the kidneys. Their affinity for the kidneys gives them an affinity for the brain. This affirms the assertion of Shigeo Haruyama's research from a classical perspective.

We have used this short passage from the *Yellow Emperor's Classic* to elucidate three separate medical matters. We could keep going. Through this process, we begin to fathom the mystery of the classics. Regardless how complicated the matter is, or how sophisticated the pathological process, it never strays from the wisdom of the classics. This is why it is said that "all change is encompassed by the classics."

III.4.c. Studying the Classics Awakens Wisdom

I strongly feel that studying the classics engenders wisdom, not merely knowledge. If one mistakenly considers the classics to be simply a means of acquiring certain information, then the significance of the classics is not very great.

Possessing a lot of knowledge is not equivalent to being wise, nor is it equivalent to possessing deep scholarship. Studying the classics, however, most definitely increases wisdom and deepens scholarship. I often say that scholarship begins with reading the classics. Many people agree on this point.

In the modern understanding of the brain, the left side of the brain is the logical brain. It rules spoken and written language and logical thinking. For most people, this left side is the dominant hemisphere. The right hemisphere is associated with intuition. Most of the time, this hemisphere is relatively inactive. This inactivity is of course related to the emphasis placed on logic by modern science. In recent years, scientific researchers have started aiming their investigation at the virgin territory of the right brain. In his book, Shigeo Haruyama also discusses this topic at some length. When the brain is in a state of high alpha wave activity, this reflects a state of awakening and activation of the right hemisphere.

I would like to use a different concept to describe and define the right and left hemispheres of the brain. The left brain, which we often refer to as the logical brain, I would like to call the "modern" brain. The right brain, the one we refer to as the intuitive brain, might be defined as the "traditional" brain. Therefore, the relationship between the left and right hemispheres is analogous to the relationship between modernity and antiquity.

In concrete terms, what is this contemporary brain that we are talking about here? By implication, this modern brain is the brain of this age. All of the information you have collected since birth is stockpiled in this modern brain. How much information can be collected and stored in the left hemisphere? That is directly proportionate to each person's experience. The amount of experience is dependent upon the person's age, and the matters in which each person has experience are dependent upon the particular course of their life. In any case, each person's experience can be measured in decades, at most a hundred years. The traditional brain, the right brain, is different. The traditional brain has a much greater store of information. It could be said that all of the experiences of humankind throughout history might create connections within the right brain. It can be said that the information stored in the right brain, or rather the integrative connections that occur in the right brain, are not limited to the information that can be collected in the span of mere decades or even a century. The connections formed here might span time periods of hundreds of years, thousands of years, tens of thousands of years, perhaps up to a hundred million years. Furthermore, this information is not individualized, but rather can be shared by the whole of humanity (in this sense, it resembles Richard Dawkins's concept of "memes"). If we borrow a term from Tibetan Buddhism, the right brain might be thought of as the "hidden treasure" mind. What is the "hidden treasure" mind? It is the collective experience derived since time immemorial and buried in the right hemisphere of the brain. When we compare and contrast the right and left brains in this way, we know that their differences are so vast that it is difficult to even compare the two. It is regrettable that nowadays most people do not recognize this point. They only know the brain of modernity, and do not understand the ancient brain, and do not seek methods by which to access it and develop its capabilities.

Please contemplate the following—when we recognize the right brain and begin to develop its capacities, we are standing atop the shoulder of a colossus. When one proceeds from atop such a lofty foundation, how could the experience of several decades possibly compete? The significance of the recognition and investigation into the left and right hemispheres of the brain is inestimable. To consider this phenomenon to be of little value or to think it as mere fiction would be a grave mistake. It is not fiction! In *A Great Revolution in the Brain World*, we are introduced to this interesting trend. Of still greater interest are the recent conclusions of the Russian biologist Alexander Kaminski, who proposed that besides the memory stored in our own nervous systems, we also possess hereditary memory, as well as immune memory. He refers to our hereditary memory as "nature's reserve fund." This shares strong similarities to the "hidden treasure mind" we just discussed.

In the brain, there is a structure that connects and coordinates the two hemispheres called the corpus callosum. The existence of the corpus callosum demonstrates that connections between the left and right hemispheres of the brain are inevitable. The information amassed in the right hemisphere can be transmitted to the left hemisphere and used there. By extension, this physiological evidence shows that the integration of the traditional or ancient and modern modes of thinking is also inevitable. The title of the present subsection is "Studying the Classics Awakens Wisdom." How is it that studying the classics brings about wisdom? Diligently reading the classics, researching the classics, can help us to unearth the "hidden treasure" brain and, from there, the collective knowledge of humanity, which can then continue to flow into each individual. If this process is realized, wisdom and scholarship are attained. If you read the classics with this approach in mind, you will find the classics rife with meaning and easy to comprehend. This process is what is meant by "the never-ending flow from the source"!

Of course, there are many people who will not only refrain from praising this point of view, but who may also snort in contempt when presented with it. They like to present traditional and modern knowledge as being in opposition to one another, and believe that the traditional texts of antiquity are actually a hindrance to modern advances in our understanding and should be cast aside altogether. In reality, this sort of thinking demonstrates a lack of understanding of tradition and of antiquity in general. To discuss tradition without even a basic knowledge of it, or to be afraid of it while lacking any real familiarity with it, is no way to act. Professor Wang Caigui of Taichung Normal University expresses this sentiment perfectly: "Those who regard tradition as a burden are not simply feeble-minded, they are good-for-nothings!" I hope for a day when we have no feeble-minded people or good-for-nothings. Who could possibly regard tradition as a burden? It is our capital! After making a suitable "investment," it can lead to the development and growth of our enterprises.

III.5. Understanding the Classics and Modernity

In the following pages, we discuss the classics from a different perspective. We can divide this discussion into three aspects.

III.5.a. The Question of Conservatism

Whenever we mention the classics or tradition, it is unavoidable that the issue of conservatism is raised. It is assumed that modern culture is open-minded and liberal and that traditional culture must be conservative. Why has China fallen behind? Why has China not produced a modern-day science of its own? Why has no Chinese scientist ever received a Nobel Prize? The answer to all of these questions would seem to lie within our very culture. They would seem to be the product of intrinsically conservative factors inherent in our culture. Hence, traditional practices are regarded as hindrances. However, we must ask ourselves whether this is really the case. I believe that holding this point of view demonstrates a lack of understanding of Chinese culture.

In 1998, yet another overseas Chinese scientist from Hong Kong was honored with a Nobel Prize. Dr. Yang Zhenning was inspired by this fact to present a talk at a symposium on the subject of why no scientist from mainland China has yet received the Nobel Prize. He proposed that the conservatism of Confucian culture was a major factor. At this point, I want to take up this issue of the conservatism of Confucian culture and consider Professor Yang's opinion.

Professor Yang's opinion that Confucian culture is conservative is representative of the opinion of many. If you were to ask ten people whether they agreed with this assessment, I bet that nine of them would. But is Confucian culture really conservative? If it is conservative, there should be proof of it. Likewise, if it is not conservative, we should be able to find evidence to the contrary. If we are to seek such proof, we should look for it in Confucius and in the orthodox teachings of Confucian culture. The *Analects* is arguably the most important classic of Confucianism. If we examine the *Analects*, where do we find evidence of this so-called "conservative Confucian culture" in the text? We can find no such conservatism. On the contrary, we discover a different quality in the text, namely open-mindedness.

The first chapter of the *Analects* is titled "Studying." In order to evaluate whether or not a particular school of thought is truly conservative, whether it is complacent and insulated, it is important that we take a close look at their understanding of "studying." This first chapter of the *Analects*, "Studying," opens with these lines:

> To study and at times to review what one has learned, is this not a joy? To
> have friends visit from far away, is this not delightful? To be unknown to
> others and yet to remain undisturbed, is this not being a gentleman?

In this opening passage, Confucius outlines three important keys to proper study. The first key is contained within the line: "To study and at times to review what one has learned, is this not a joy?" This sentence is not merely an admonishment to regularly review what one has studied. What is emphasized here is the enjoyment that comes from studying and then reviewing or putting into practice one's achievements. There is a unique sort of pleasure that arises from study and practice. If one becomes attuned to this joy, study and practice are delightful. Most of our experience tells us that studying is suffering. There is the old Chinese saying: "The sea of learning is boundless, and suffering is one's boat." This attitude explains why so few persist in their studies. If study is perceived as drudgery, it becomes something worth avoiding. It is only drudgery if the "joy" is missed. The first line of the *Analects* points to this joy. In recent years, many scholars in China have turned away from academia and entered into business. The reason for this is simple. A life of books is perceived as menial. The acquisition of wealth is deemed fun. How many people actually witness the beauty and luxury that lies within books, the jade maidens, the golden chambers? Whether or not a person can devote their life to learning depends upon whether they can perceive this "joy of studying." It lies in Confucius's little question: "Is it not a joy?"

Among Chinese scholars, this joy is referred to as "joy of studying," while Buddhists call it "pleasure of the dharma" and aim to be full of this pleasure. Why do we refer to a Buddhist monk at the very beginning of his studies as a "monk practicing suffering"? Because this stage is extremely difficult and devoid of any pleasures. He must rely on faith and the commandments of religious doctrine to restrain him and see him through this period, or he will not prevail. Once he has studied to the point of applying what he has learned, he discovers the pleasure of his practice, the "pleasure of the dharma." This brings about a dramatic shift from pain to pleasure. When this shift happens, the monk no longer worries whether his faith is sufficient to sustain him or the religious edicts strong enough to restrain him. He no longer needs to seek anything external to compel him to continue on his path. When the "pleasure of the dharma" is discovered, he naturally and effortlessly conforms to the path of the Bodhisattva. In the Chinese understanding, this is referred to as working without the effort entailed by diligence. Without "the joy of studying," without "the pleasure of the dharma," neither the path of study nor that of Buddhist practice would be bearable. In the very first line of the *Analects*, Confucius tells us that if we are able to find this kind of joy in learning, our scholarship is guaranteed. In education, especially where young children are concerned, it is essential to have an interest in the subject; this is also related to our topic.

The second key is found in the next line: "To have friends visit from far away, is this not delightful?" Confucius is not referring to fair-weather friends or acquaintances seeking some advantage. These are friends engaged in the same pursuit of scholarship, those who can help the student to further his or her study. The ancients said: "One's fellow disciples are friends and those of like mind are companions." "Fellow disciples" should be understood in a broad sense, as all those whose hearts and minds are set upon study and scholarship. These are your friends and suitable companions. During Confucius's lifetime, China was divided into a number of entirely separate states or kingdoms, each with its own ruler and system of government. When Confucius speaks of friends coming from afar, he is not simply referring to a neighboring county or the next city over. They may even be coming from another kingdom: the kingdom of Qin, Zhao, Chu, or Yan, for instance. They might even come from a state that is at war with his own. These scholars from far-away kingdoms would of course bring with them different cultures and scholarship. An exchange with a person from afar infuses the host with fresh ideas and insights. Little wonder that such meetings would deserve special mention and be worthy of celebration. When we consider today's geographical and cultural situation, such a friend from afar might be one who comes from the West, from the United States, perhaps. This second key emphasizes Confucius's promotion of the open exchange of ideas and perspectives among scholars—hardly a conservative attitude. In another passage of the *Analects*, Confucius clarifies the issue further by saying that "those who study alone but do not have companions are ignorant and oblivious."

"To be unknown to others and yet to remain undisturbed, is this not being a gentleman?" This line holds the third key. A scholar must possess the capacity for solitude. This capacity is crucial to traditional scholarship, especially in a field such as Chinese Medicine. If one wishes to study Chinese Medicine but is impatient and hopes to make a name for oneself in two or three years, if that person cannot sit still and study, then I strongly recommend a change of course. A career in finance or computers might be more suitable. One must be able to sink down into one's studies to learn Chinese Medicine well. If, after ten or twenty years, you are still unknown to the world but remain undisturbed by this, you may stand a chance of studying Chinese Medicine adequately. To become a scholar, you must first take interest in your study. You need to discover the joy of studying. This is the first requirement for in-depth study. Secondly, you have to be open to the ideas of your contemporaries and allow for the exchange of ideas. You cannot be isolated and complacent, ignorant or oblivious. Third, in order to study deeply, in order to become a scholar in the true sense of the word, you must be capable of profound solitude. Not one of these three requirements can be overlooked. When we consider these three key points, it is no longer possible to consider Confucianism to be conservative.

Just now, we have discussed the issue from the theoretical angle. Let us go over some relevant historical facts. There are three main schools of thought in Chinese culture: Confucianism, Buddhism, and Daoism. Of these, Confucianism and Daoism are native to China while Buddhism came from another part of the world. Of these three, Confucianism is the dominant cultural influence. When speaking of these three cultural influences, we should ask ourselves: How was it that Buddhism entered into Chinese culture?

Confucius was born in 551 BCE and the founder of Buddhism, Siddhartha Gautama, was born around the same time, approximately 565 BCE. The earliest record of Buddhism entering China was in 2 BCE, during the Western Han dynasty and hundreds of years after the time of Confucius. This interim period between the founding of Confucianism and the introduction of Buddhism into China was a period in which Confucianism flourished. During this time, Confucianism became the dominant cultural influence and the source of mainstream culture, and the emperor used Confucianism to regulate the people under his rule. It might be said that during this period, Confucian culture permeated every aspect of thinking and culture. This poses an interesting question: If Confucianism is truly a conservative, insular culture, how could Buddhism possibly have entered Chinese culture and taken hold? The answer is obvious—it could not have. On the basis of this fact alone, we can say that Confucianism is a very open and accepting culture, not the least bit conservative. When we say that Confucian culture is conservative, it is clear that we are speaking of a culture that is distinct from the school of thought established by Confucius. We are referring to a culture that has been distorted by later generations, his disciples and their followers. These distortions are not Confucianism. If we wish to evaluate Confucianism, it is only right that we look first at Confucius's teachings. Only in this way can we arrive at a correct and orthodox understanding. Likewise, if we wish to study Chinese Medicine correctly, we must begin with the classics. That is the only way we can avoid piling error upon error.

III.5.b. Classical Music and Popular Music

If we wish to compare the classics with works of the present day, we can draw upon an apt parallel to illustrate their differences: a comparison between classical music and modern popular music. Let us look at the very different situations in which we find classical and popular music at present.

If we were to undertake a survey to determine how many people prefer to listen to classical music and how many prefer modern, popular music, I bet we would find that the vast majority prefer popular music, and that very few prefer classical music. Just look at music stars from Hong Kong, Taiwan, or China and the sort of turnout they get at their concerts. As soon as they get on stage and shut their eyes before a sea of fans, a wave of excitement spreads and the fans go wild. Compare that picture with a classical music performance. It is quite a different scene. The concert hall is completely quiet and the audience much smaller. At most, there is some applause after each piece of music ends. The contrast is striking.

Why do modern people prefer popular music to classical music? The explanation is simple. It is a reflection of the person's inner world. To penetrate into the reason for this phenomenon, we might pose a number of questions. In China's past, popular music was referred to as "songs of the rustic poor" and was regarded as a simple and superficial sort of music. For instance, if it was a love song, everything was laid bare. If the topic of the song was the pining of the lover for the beloved, the mad desire of love, with one quick listen you would know that you were listening to a love song, regardless of your mental or emotional state at the time you listened to it. Classical music is a different story. Take for instance Beethoven's *Moonlight Sonata*. If you do not settle in and commune with the piece, then you will not have any idea what the theme is.

Music and song are means of expressing one's inner state, of giving a voice to powerful emotion. Although popular music is very straightforward and blunt in its expression, it is as the ancients said: "Written books do not fully express spoken words, and spoken words do not fully express what is in the heart and mind." When it comes to a profound state of mind or complicated emotions, these sorts of simplistic melodies fall short of expression. Why then do people prefer popular music? We can deduce from this preference the restless psyche of the modern person, and the desire for quick gratification. When they listen to music, they want to feel something immediately. The prospect of stilling their minds and entering into the sort of receptive state where classical music could be appreciated worries them.

We can draw strong parallels between this phenomenon in music and the steady decline of the classical texts in the world of Chinese Medicine. Classical music is like the Chinese Medicine classics and pop music is analogous to modern Chinese Medicine texts, including modern textbooks. The content of the classics is different from that contained within modern textbooks. The classics require that you intuit their meaning. They demand of you that you come to certain realizations by adopting a patient and receptive state, just as you would when listening to classical music. Appreciating classical music may not be easy at first, but once this ability is attained, the deeper mystery and vitality of music is revealed, just as the essence of Chinese Medicine can be found in the classics.

Everyone has tasted both tea and cola. What is the difference between the two? To drink a cola, you just open one up and drink it. You can taste it immediately. It exemplifies convenience. Tea is not so convenient. To prepare tea properly, it must be correctly infused. A great number of variables affect its flavor: the temperature of the water used to infuse it, the amount of time it has been allowed to steep. This is especially true in the case of the *gongfu* ritual of tea preparation, where small teapots with relatively large amounts of tea leaves are used to slowly uncover the layers of flavor in the tea. This method of preparing tea takes considerable skill and attention to detail in order to perform properly. Many people do not possess this patience and simply drink a cola. But the effect of cola, both its aftertaste and its effect on the mind and body, cannot begin to compare with that of tea. The difference between reading the Chinese Medicine classics and reading books written in later ages is a bit like the difference between savoring tea and drinking soft drinks. If we listen to classical music in the same state that we listen to pop music, or if we drink tea with the same attitude that we would drink a cola, we will be disappointed at best. The subtle flavors of tea cannot be appreciated with a mouth expecting carbonated corn syrup.

III.5.c. Can Modern Chinese Medicine Texts Replace the Yellow Emperor's Classic?

In contemporary TCM universities in China, the study of Chinese Medicine classics has been relegated to elective coursework. There are many who might prefer to do away with studying the medical classics altogether. An important reason for this is that textbooks such as the *Fundamentals of Chinese Medicine* are regarded as superior substitutes to classical works such as the *Yellow Emperor's Classic*. People argue that these modern teaching materials are derived from the classical sources but are clearer and more comprehensible than the *Yellow Emperor's Classic*.

It is an undisputed fact that the *Fundamentals of Chinese Medicine* are derived from the *Yellow Emperor's Classic*, but it is ludicrous to say that such textbooks encompass the content of the *Yellow Emperor's Classic*. These new books are no substitute for the classics. Let us look at a couple of examples to illustrate this point.

The first is the notion of the "disease mechanism" (*bingji*), a key concept in Chinese Medicine. This concept derives from Chapter 44 of the *Plain Questions*, "The Great Treatise on the Essentials of Ultimate Truth." If we search the entire *Neijing*, it is only in this chapter that this particular concept is discussed. That this concept is put forward in a chapter dealing with "ultimate truth" only highlights its importance. In the *Fundamentals of Chinese Medicine*, there is also a section devoted to these "disease mechanisms," and the chapters in this section are filled with quite a bit of content. But when you have finished reading this section of the book, it might make you think of the Chinese saying "hanging up a sheep's head to sell dog meat." Why? Because although they use the term "disease mechanism," there is absolutely no discussion of the wealth of information on this topic in the *Yellow Emperor's Classic*. To title a chapter "disease mechanism" and then completely ignore the *Yellow Emperor's Classic* in a book about the "Fundamentals of Chinese Medicine" is almost too much to believe.

Besides this, there is also the issue of how "disease mechanism" is defined in the *Fundamentals of Chinese Medicine*. To quote from the text: "Disease mechanism refers to the mechanistic principle by which diseases arise, develop, and change." Can we thus regard the notion of "disease mechanism" as identical to the "mechanistic principle" of disease? Let us investigate this passage from a purely linguistic angle. Is the character used for the concept of "disease mechanism" in the *Yellow Emperor's Classic* really identical to the modern notion of the "mechanistic principle"? If we consult the ancient dictionary *Explaining Writing and Analyzing Characters* or the *Kangxi Dictionary*, there is no support for this interpretation. We can derive the actual meaning of the ancient character *ji* (機) from *Explaining Writing and Analyzing Characters*: "That which governs the release of something is referred to as *ji*." When the arrow is notched to the bowstring of the crossbow and ready to be released, this trigger (*ji*) must be pulled for the arrow to be released. All phenomena are like this. All have a particular trigger that will set certain events in motion if pulled, and, if not triggered, even if all the other requisite conditions for its effect are in place, will prevent the phenomenon from occurring. This term *ji* therefore is the factor most crucial to a particular phenomenon transpiring. The *ji* is a concrete point, not a large area. But if you touch this tiny point, this special spot, the entire face of the object changes. To translate the term *bingji* from the *Yellow Emperor's Classic* as "disease mechanism" is somewhat misleading. We might do better to refer to it as "disease trigger." When we think of it in this way, we see that the "trigger" is very different from the "mechanism" or "mechanistic principle" of the disease process. The *bingji* is the most crucial factor in the emergence, development, and transformation of the disease, but it is obviously distinct from the mechanism of disease. This allows us to see a difference between *Fundamentals of Chinese Medicine* and the *Yellow Emperor's Classic*. At times, it is difficult for the former to explain the latter.

My second example concerns the line from the *Yellow Emperor's Classic*: "The lungs are in charge of *qi*; the lungs are in charge of *zhijie*." In the standard modern textbook *Fundamentals of Chinese Medicine*, the *qi* in the phrase "The lungs are in charge of *qi*" is interpreted as the *qi* of the entire body as well as the *qi* that is derived from respiration. But do the lungs actually govern the *qi* of the entire body as well as the *qi* of the breath? As we know, the meaning of the statement "The lungs are in charge of *qi*" is explained in the *Plain Questions* in Chapter 9, "Treatise on the Six Nodes and Visceral Manifestations" (Liujie zangxiang lun): "The lungs are the root of *qi*." Before discussing this important function of the lungs, this chapter explores the concept of *qi*. Let us examine this particular dialogue between the Yellow Emperor and Qi Bo:

> The Yellow Emperor said: I want to know what is meant by *qi*. Please clear away my confusion and remove my doubts concerning this concept.
>
> Qi Bo answered: This is a secret from the Emperors on high. What I know has been passed down from previous teachers.
>
> Huangdi said: Please let me hear it.
>
> Qi Bo said: Five days are called a *hou*, three *hou* comprise a *qi*, six *qi* make up a season, and four seasons are called a year. Each follows that which is responsible for governing it.

This conversation between the Yellow Emperor and Qi Bo is a crucial one, but is not lacking in humor! The Yellow Emperor asks to have the concept of *qi* explained to him, and requests that Qi Bo clear away his doubts and confusion. However, this question puts Qi Bo in a difficult spot, as the answer to this question is not the sort of stuff that he ought to speak of openly. It is a secret that originated with the ancient rulers, and one that has been passed down from individual to individual for many generations. In spite of his reservations, in such an audience with the Yellow Emperor he is compelled to answer, and answer honestly he does. Each year is divided into four seasons consisting of 90 days, which in turn are divided into six *qi* of fifteen days each. Thus, in the 360-day period comprising one year, there are twenty-four *qi*. What, then, is a *qi*? It is a "node *qi*" (*jieqi*), also translated as "solar term." Elementary school children in China memorize a song that details the twenty-four *qi*, or solar terms, of the year. If we flip through a Chinese calendar, we can see for ourselves. The fourth day of the second month heralds the *Lichun* (Beginning of Spring), fifteen days later is the period called *Yushui* (Rain Water), and then the next fifteen-day period is called *Jingzhe* (Awakening Insects). This simple division of the Chinese calendar into twenty-four periods is well known in China, and pervades the lunisolar calendars of East Asia. Imagine, however, the power this knowledge would imbue to the person who knew of it at the time when the *Yellow Emperor's Classic* was written. Knowing this sequence of *qi*, one knew the secrets of the annual procession of natural changes, the very rhythm and pace of nature. The question posed by the Yellow Emperor is no small matter.

One distinguishing feature of Chinese Medicine is holism, the concept that humans and nature form an organic whole, behave as one, and are interwoven on virtually every level. How are humans and nature woven into one? Put simply, as heaven and earth change and transform in the course of the seasons, people must change accordingly. Human beings need to keep pace with the rhythms of nature. From this concept of *qi*, we know that the basic rhythm of nature is *qi*, and that it is a rhythm consisting of fifteen-day divisions. As long as people change in accord with this rhythm, people and nature are one. Within the human body, the internal organ that is responsible for keeping us in time with nature's rhythms are the lungs. When the *Yellow Emperor's Classic* says that "The lungs are the root of *qi*," it is talking about this phenomenon. This *qi* actually has very little connection with the *qi* of the breath or the *qi* of the physical body.

The second issue is the way in which the phrase "the lungs are in charge of *zhijie*" is understood in the *Fundamentals of Chinese Medicine*. In that modern textbook, the two characters for *zhijie* are explained as meaning "governing and harmonizing." This would seem to be an even greater confusion than the last example. What does *zhijie* actually refer to? This concept emerges in Chapter 8 of the *Plain Questions*, "Treatise on the Spiritual Orchid Secret Canon." The concept of *qi* as we have just discussed it, as a fifteen-day period marking a change in the seasonal expression of nature, is actually a general term. A more precise way of referring to this is to say that a month consists of two *qi*, one of which is called the *jieqi* ("node *qi*") and the other the *zhongqi* ("central *qi*"). Together, these are known as the twenty-four *jieqi*. With this in mind, we can see that *jie* and *qi* are extremely similar concepts. The term *zhijie* (literally "governing the nodes") therefore refers to this regulation of the *jieqi*. How has this been distorted to mean "governing" and "harmonizing"? Even if it did mean "harmonizing," then what was being harmonized?

There is another way we can understand how the lungs govern the twenty-four *qi*. The lungs are in the chest and are encased by the ribs. If we count the ribs, there are twelve on each side, twenty-four in all. Is this simply a coincidence? Which came first: Were twenty-four divisions of the year correlated with the ribcage, or were the ribs counted and the number of that rhythmically expanding and contracting portion of the skeleton imposed upon a cyclical natural rhythm?

Also, these "nodes" (*jie*) also have a relationship with the *guanjie*, the joints of the body. If we look at the large joints of the four limbs, there are twelve in all, three per limb. Each joint has two articular surfaces, so that there are twenty-four articular surfaces in all. One of these surfaces corresponds to the "central *qi*" (*zhongqi*) and the other to the "node *qi*" (*jieqi*). Each of the four limbs has six large articular surfaces, and if each of the limbs corresponds to a season, then we have a nice parallel between human anatomy and the cosmology of "six *qi* make up a season." It is common knowledge that the joints of the body relate to seasonal changes in weather. If we were to ask elderly people, especially those with joint problems, we would find that the sensitivity of their joints to changes in weather is sometimes more accurate than the instruments used by meteorologists. The weather forecast may call for rain, but based on the feedback from their ailing joints they will disagree with this, and in the end they are right. How is it they are so confident about their ability to predict the weather? Because their joints respond to changes in the weather such as impending rain, and when no rain is on the way, their joints make no complaint. We can think of the joints of the body as weather sensors. These weather sensors are managed by the lungs.

Now that we have clarified the connection between the lungs and the "node *qi*," a fundamental change in the meaning of "lungs" has occurred. The correspondence between humans and the natural world is in a large part derived from this concept of "the lungs are in charge of *qi*" and "the lungs are in charge of governing the nodes (*zhijie*)." If this aspect of the classical text does not get discussed and if instead we rush to replace the *Yellow Emperor's Classic* with the *Fundamentals of Chinese Medicine*, this crucial point gets lost entirely.

III.6. How to Study the Classics Well

III.6.a. Intuition and the Importance of Reference Tools

To study the classics, we must have a method. One of the most basic methods is to thoroughly understand the importance of reference books. At the latest, the classics were written before the Eastern Han Dynasty. Partly because of the limitations of their historical context, they employed very concise language to express their far-ranging and profound content. How do we comprehend this deep content in our study of the classics? There simply is no other way than to start with the language, with the characters. And to understand the characters, you need reference tools. A modern dictionary like the *Xinhua Dictionary* is simply not adequate for the task of studying the classics of Chinese Medicine.

The ancients said that "written language is used to convey the Dao." If we wish to understand the Dao, we must first know and understand Chinese characters. The *Kangxi Dictionary* should be our most indispensable reference, a constant feature on our desktop. If you spend time with this outstanding lexicon, you will gain an appreciation for the many advantages inherent in the Chinese language and will develop affection for it. The Chinese written language uses pictographs as the basis for characters and emphasizes the relationship between form and meaning. When we look at a character, we need to do more than just look it up in a reference text. We need to analyze its construction. This means not only discerning the "radical" or "signific" part of the character (i.e. the semantic part, the component of the character that indicates its range of meanings), but also the phonetic part, as both are highly significant for its overall meaning.

We can take the character *wei* (味), meaning "flavor" or "taste," as an example. Flavors pertain to the mouth, and we see this reflected in the meaning portion: *kou* (口), the "mouth" radical, on the left. The phonetic portion is the character *wei* (未). The meaning of a character is related not only to the semantic component. In this particular instance, it would seem to be even more closely connected to the meaning of the phonetic component. On its own, the phonetic part represents one of the twelve earthly branches. It is positioned in the southwest, and among the five elements the southwestern direction belongs to earth and late summer. Among the postnatal hexagrams, it is made up of six yin lines and called *kun* (Responding). Among the five viscera, it is associated with the spleen. By examining the implicit meaning of this phonetic component, we are thus able to understand why it is used to construct the character *wei* (taste). It is clearly not simply a phonetic marker.

If we have studied the *Fundamentals of Chinese Medicine*, we know that the spleen is associated with the mouth as its orifice and it is only through the spleen and the mouth that can discern flavors. This is to say that the spleen governs the sense of taste, the spleen belongs to the earth element, the earth element is in the southwest, and the earthly branch that occupies this position, *wei*, just so happens to be the phonetic component of the faculty governed by the spleen, namely our sense of taste. Thus, by using the phonetic *wei*, the meaning of the character already includes the physiological role of the spleen in tasting and the faculty of taste.

Secondly, the meaning of "taste" or "flavor" in ancient texts was very broad. In the *Yellow Emperor's Classic* there are five flavors, but in a broader sense all ingested materials, as a class, belong to the category of "flavors," including medicinal substances. Let us consider for a moment at what time of year most food crops, especially grains, the chief staple of human diets around the world, ripen. They ripen in late summer. Thus we can say that the flavors ripen in late summer, narrowing the association between flavors and the phonetic part *wei*. The position of this earthly branch is the southwest, and in China the Southwest is where we find Sichuan province, nicknamed the "Storehouse of Heaven." It has this nickname because the agricultural products of Sichuan are so abundant and because the flavors of the foods that come from there are so plentiful. From a classical cosmological perspective, the crops and flavors of Sichuan are so abundant because it is in the southwest, its earthly branch is *wei*, its element is earth, and the myriad things emerge from the earth. Through an analysis of the creation and construction of a character, we get some sense of its profound meaning. The depth of meaning conveyed by the character *wei*, for example, derives not only from its pictographic component, but also by what might otherwise be disregarded as a mere phonetic marker. An understanding of its entire structure allows us to glimpse its significance. Of course, analysis of character composition is not always as fruitful as it was in this example.

Understanding Chinese characters is one of the keys by which we can unlock the hidden significance of the classics. To fully understand Chinese characters, we must of course rely on secondary resources, as well as on an intuition about the inherent structure of the character. Both of these are indispensable.

III.6.b. Zeng Guofan: The Art of Reading the Classics

When reading the classics, it is extremely important to read them over and over again until one is completely familiar with them. The ancients said: "Read a book a hundred times and its meaning will be self-evident." This saying is especially pertinent to the study of the classics. As far as books from later ages that merely discuss the classics go, it is not necessary to read them a hundred times. More often than not, once will suffice. But when it comes to the great classics, such as the *Treatise on Cold Damage*, it is absolutely essential that you read them at least a hundred times.

Some people read the classics once or twice and feel that it is enough. Having read them once or twice, they cannot come to any sort of realizations. They will end up putting the book aside, mistakenly believing it to be of no value. How can this be regarded as having truly read the classics? One might as well confuse a rare oolong tea with soda pop. If you treat a piece by Bach the same way you would one by Lady Gaga, I doubt you will ever appreciate Bach's music.

We can draw useful instruction from a passage in a letter that Zeng Guofan, a noted scholar, philosopher, and political and military leader, wrote to his disciples during the early part of the nineteenth century:

> When studying a classic, you must concentrate on that one classic alone and not skip around to other books. When reading the classics, you should view comprehending their meaning as most important, and examination of the words as a secondary consideration. The meaning is like the taproot and the words used to signify this meaning are like leaves in the upper canopy of the tree. There is a saying that describes the patient endurance needed to read the classics properly: "If a sentence does not make sense, do not read the next sentence; if today it is not clear, read it again tomorrow; if it makes no sense this year, read it again the next." This is the sort of patience that is required to study the classics adequately.

Zeng Guofan's formula for "patient endurance" is a remarkable technique for deep study of the classics. Of course, we may not necessarily forgo reading the next sentence when the sentence we have just read is not entirely comprehensible to us, but his advice that we should read the classics again tomorrow if we cannot understand them today, and read them again next year if we cannot make sense of them this year, should definitely be heeded. In one word, reading the classics is not the sort of undertaking that is completed in only a few years, much less a few months, or a semester. Studying the classics is a lifelong endeavor. The classics should not only adorn our desk, but also constantly occupy our hearts and minds. Reading the classics is a compulsory and lifelong endeavor. If you truly want to study Chinese Medicine and the classics properly, you should plan on this.

III.6.c. Basic Requirements

In order to study the classics well, we must pay attention to yet another issue: we must fulfill a basic requirement, namely to approach them with an attitude of receptive trust and reverence. These days, most people read the classics with a critical eye. They presume that the classics are not scientific and were written at a time when people were ignorant of science. They regard themselves as intellectually superior to the authors of these works. This sort of contrarian attitude prevents the reader from gaining much from the medical classics. The attitude you have when reading the classics is crucial. You should have absolute confidence in the validity of the work, accept everything that is written as truth, and then afterward contemplate how to realize the thoughts and ideas you have found in them. This is the only way that you will truly access the information contained in the classics and the only way you will get anything out of them. The classics have endured extremely long and thorough testing, and so many revered physicians have depended upon them. What do you have to worry about? For this reason, you can absolutely have an attitude of complete trust and reverence toward the classics.

Why do I mention this requirement and attitude here? Because it is that important! If you lack this attitude, studying the classics will simply become an obstacle. I remember once when I was reading the *Compendium of Materia Medica*, in one passage that discusses the medicinal Baizhu, the author Li Shizhen quotes a precedent from Zhang Rui's *Emergency Prescriptions from Rooster Peak* (Jifeng beijifang):

> If you observe a person's teeth growing by the day to the point where they gradually have difficulty eating, this is called marrow-spilling disease. Simmer Baizhu to prepare a decoction and have the patient gargle with this. This will cure the disease.

What is the first thing you feel when you read this example? I bet many will be skeptical. The teeth grow to a certain length and then stop. How could they possibly keep on growing to the point that eating becomes difficult? Implausible. Supposing one did suffer from marrow-spilling disease, the teeth are so hard—how could simply gargling with Baizhu cause them to recede? It's simply too unscientific an explanation. But I do not think like that. When I read this passage, I start out by simply believing it. Then I think about what it might mean.

First of all, the name of this disease is intriguing. The teeth are regarded as the surplus of the bones, and they are governed by the kidneys. The kidneys rule the bones and produce the marrow. The bones and the kidneys are, in a way, different names for the same thing. If the teeth are growing a little longer every day, it gives the appearance that the marrow is spilling over and pushing the teeth outward, hence the disease name. Then we must contemplate why the teeth would be getting longer every day and why the marrow would be spilling over and pushing the teeth outward. This is obviously a problem with the system that normally restrains and contains the growth of the bones and marrow. The bones and marrow are governed by the kidneys, and the kidneys are the internal organ that is related to the water element. If the bones and marrow belong to water, it is obvious that they would be restrained by the earth system, since in the five-element cycle earth controls water. If there is a problem with the earth element, and the earth is deficient, then of course there will be a problem with water spilling over, and as a result, with spilling marrow. If the marrow is excessive, the teeth will naturally grow longer day after day. Once we understand this reasoning, the use of Baizhu to tonify the earth in order to control water and thereby control the excessive marrow makes perfect sense. This was my thinking process with regard to "marrow-spilling disease" and its method of cure.

In 1991, I saw a patient with bone spurs on both her heels that were so painful she could not put her heels down when she walked and instead needed to walk on her toes. This made her life very difficult. In accordance with common practice, I used kidney-tonifying, blood-invigorating, pain-stopping, and *bi*-eliminating methods. None of these helped her case in any notable way. Just as I started to feel in a quandary, I thought of the line we just discussed from Zhang Rui's writings. Bone spurs are also referred to as osteophytes. They result from the calcium leaching out of the bone and depositing on its surface. When this happens, it looks like something is growing on the surface of the bone. When the calcium of the bone leaches out from within and looks like the bone is growing, how is this any different than Zhang Rui's "marrow-spilling" disease? It must be the same. I set about following Zhang Rui's advice: I made a decoction with Baizhu and then had the patient soak her heels in the decoction two to three times a day for twenty minutes at a time. To my amazement, after just a few days, her pain diminished to the point that she was able to place her heels on the ground. This improvement continued for a month until her condition resolved completely.

This example affected me very deeply. How did it affect me? It instilled in me exactly the above-mentioned attitude of "trust and receptive reverence." Because I believed Zhang Rui's advice, I took the time to contemplate it. If I had not, there is no way it would have occurred to me to treat this patient's bone spurs with a decoction of Baizhu. Confidence is the first requirement. Only if you have confidence in the content of the classics is there any possibility that your research will bear fruit. If, from the beginning, you are skeptical, then you will be reluctant to engage in the sort of contemplation that might later allow you to put into practice what you have learned. The sort of trust and reverence that we have been discussing in this section is absolutely necessary to the successful study of Chinese Medicine.

In this chapter, we discussed certain fundamental issues for studying and researching Chinese Medicine from a universal perspective, from a rational perspective, and from the perspective of certain attitudes. Only when these fundamental issues are fully resolved can the study of Chinese Medicine and the study of the classics proceed without hindrance.

CHAPTER TWO

THE SIGNIFICANCE OF COLD DAMAGE

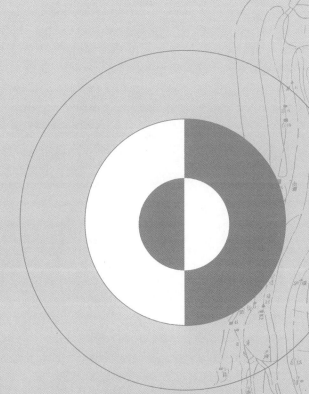

Yin and yang
are the Dao of heaven and earth,
the warp and weft of the myriad things,
the father and mother of all change,
the root of birth and death,
and the palace of the spirit light.

I. The Content of the *Treatise on Cold Damage*

The following paragraphs discuss various topics from the *Treatise on Cold Damage and Miscellaneous Diseases* (Shanghan zabing lun). Before we delve into these issues, let us examine both the title and the basic premise of this text, and thereby gain a sense of what sort of book we are dealing with.

I.1. The Meaning of "Cold Damage"

Cold damage is the central focus of this book that we are currently discussing, and in order to understand the book, we thus need to be very clear about the implied meaning of this concept. The concept of "cold damage" (*shanghan*) is explicitly defined in the *Plain Questions* chapter titled "Treatise on Heat": "As for heat diseases, they all belong to the category of cold damage." This definition illustrates a striking characteristic of cold damage: heat effusion. All illness that manifests with fever, or to put it another way, all illness that is characterized by heat effusion belongs to the category of cold damage. The *Yellow Emperor's Classic* defines cold damage disease according to its most basic aspect, but when we expand upon this one aspect, the definition becomes very inclusive and is not so easy to grasp. It is not until we look in the *Classic of Difficulties* (Nanjing) that we find a more concrete definition. The "Fifty-eighth Difficulty" of the *Classic of Difficulties* explains: "There are five types of cold damage: wind-strike, cold damage, damp warmth, heat disease, and warm disease." Those of us with sufficient clinical experience would say that the definition of cold damage given in the *Classic of Difficulties* is very specific, and that most of the illnesses that present with fever in clinic do in fact belong to one of these five categories. Therefore, if you wish to research cold damage disease, you must pay special attention to these five types.

The other issue that we must pay attention to is the fact that the *Classic of Difficulties* discusses cold damage in two different senses. The first type of cold damage is cold damage in the general sense. This sense of cold damage is the broad category of diseases described in the "Treatise on Heat" in the *Plain Questions* cited above. Modern textbooks now refer to this category as the "cold damage in the broad sense." There is also a more specific pathological picture referred to by the term "cold damage," and this is what we refer to as "cold damage in the narrow sense." In the present section of this book, where we are discussing the Chinese title of this book, we are most certainly talking about cold damage in the first sense. There must be no confusion on this point. Having understood this, we know that Zhang Zhongjing is not simply talking about cold but is also discussing damp warmth, heat disease, and warm disease.

傷寒論卷第一　仲景全書第一

漢　張仲景述
晉　王叔和撰次
宋　林億校正
明　趙開美校刻
沈琳仝校

辨脈法第一
平脈法第二

辨脈法第一

問曰。脈有陰陽。何謂也。答曰。凡脈大浮數動滑。此名陽也。脈沈濇弱弦微。此名陰也。凡陰病見陽脈者生。陽病見陰脈者死。

I.2. The Meaning of "Miscellaneous Diseases"

The primary theme of the *Treatise on Cold Damage*, or the *Treatise on Cold Damage and Miscellaneous Diseases*, is cold damage. But there is an important secondary theme, namely that of "miscellaneous diseases." When we compare "miscellaneous diseases" with cold damage diseases, what specifically does this term mean? Let me begin by telling you a story from the Chinese Cultural Revolution.

During the Cultural Revolution, Wang Hongwen was appointed as Vice Chairman of both the Communist Party and of the Military Commission of the party's Central Committee—two very important positions. However, everyone knew that this former low-level flunky was not especially talented. At one time, then Vice Premier Deng Xiaoping asked Wang Hongwen to tell him how many latrines there were in China. When Vice Chairman Wang heard this question, he was dumb-struck and at a loss on how to answer. He thought to himself: "I haven't really done any survey to determine that number . . . and hadn't Chairman Mao famously said that 'those who have not examined [a problem] do not have the right to speak'?" Seeing Wang Hongwen's awkwardness, the Premier attempted to help him out of his predicament. He explained that there was no need to conduct a survey to answer this question, as in China there were only two latrines: a men's latrine and a women's latrine.

Although this is just a joke, it actually illustrates a profound philosophical point that we can relate to the concepts of "cold damage" and "miscellaneous diseases." If we categorize all disease in relation to fever, there are diseases that exhibit fever and those that do not. That is obvious. Since the category of cold damage includes all conditions that involve heat effusion, any condition that does not manifest with a fever can be categorized as "miscellaneous diseases" or a febrile disease. Thus, when we speak of "cold damage and miscellaneous diseases," we are thereby speaking of all diseases that could ever arise. This is the true implication of the title *Treatise on Cold Damage and Miscellaneous Diseases*.

A clear understanding of this implied meaning resolves many of the possible reservations we might have toward the book. Prior to this understanding, we might have worried that only studying one category of disease, namely cold damage, might be too limiting. We might worry that those who study cold damage can only treat diseases caused by external factors and cannot treat internal disorders, or that we can only treat cold damage, and not warm disease, or that it only provides us with tools for treating patients in the internal medicine department and that we cannot treat diseases from other departments such as dermatology, gynecology, and pediatrics. Now that we understand the thesis of this classic, we understand the broad scope of the *Treatise on Cold Damage and Miscellaneous Diseases*, and we know that our worries are unfounded. This is why, when reading ancient books, comprehending the meaning of their titles is very important.

I.3. The Meaning of "Treatise"

The last word in the Chinese title *Treatise on Cold Damage and Miscellaneous Diseases* is the character *lun*, translated here as "treatise." The concept of *lun* was an important one in Chinese antiquity and was complementary to that of *jing*, which we have translated as "classic." To understand the concept of *lun*, we first need to understand the concept of *jing*.

What does this term *jing* mean? *Jing* in the present context serves as an abbreviation of *jingdian* ("classical texts"). Chinese Medicine has its classics (*jingdian*), Daoism has its classics, and Buddhism has its classics. What is the significance of these "classics"? It often signifies the highest authority in a particular field of study. The time period in which the classics of a particular school of thought were written tends to represent the golden age of that particular discipline. This is a different model of development from that of modern science. This identifying characteristic of the Chinese classics determines that we must rely on them in order to study a particular field. We have already discussed this point at some length above. The authors of classics are always exceptional. For instance in Buddhism, the sum of all the Buddhist writings of authors after Sakyamuni does not amount to the value of Sakyamuni's teachings. In Confucianism, we find the same thing. The writings of Confucius and his commentaries on the *Classic of Poetry* (Shijing), the *Classic of Documents* (Shujing), the *Record of Rites* (Liji), and the *Classic of Changes* (Yijing) are the Confucian classics. The same cannot be said of any work by authors after him. The classics are invariably the writings of the founder of a particular school of thought, never the products of its followers. The founders of these schools are sages. In Confucianism, only Confucius is considered to be a sage. Thus, Confucius was called the "Supreme Sage and Ancestral Teacher of Great Accomplishment," but those after

Confucius did not rise to the position of sage. At best, the title of "lesser sage," as in the case of Mencius, was achieved. In other words, Mencius was less than the sage, a follower of the sage. After these sages left the world, their followers went into these classics and annotated them, expounded upon them, developed their ideas, and elaborated them. These direct elaborations are what are called "treatises" (*lun*). To say that the treatises are complementary to the classics makes sense when we consider that treatises cannot exist without the classics. If a book is referred to as a treatise, we know that it is an elaboration and annotation of the writings in the classics.

Now that we have examined the classics and the authors of these classics in other schools, it becomes clear that there is a very strange phenomenon in Chinese Medicine: Zhang Zhongjing, the author of the *Treatise on Cold Damage and Miscellaneous Diseases*, is considered a sage, but the Yellow Emperor and Qi Bo, the authors of the *Yellow Emperor's Classic*, the true classic of Chinese Medicine, were never elevated to the status of sages. This phenomenon has its reasons. In a way, Zhang Zhongjing rescued Chinese Medicine when it was endangered, and it was through his works that Chinese Medicine has managed to survive until the present day. His contributions must not go unrecognized. It is on account of these contributions that his followers considered him a sage and elevated him to the status of a sage. Zhang Zhongjing himself was very modest. He did not append the distinction of "classic" to his books, avoiding the mistake made by Huangfu Mi and Zhang Jiebin (two authors who included the word "classic" in the title of their writings).

We can use yet another approach to define the relationship between "classic" and "treatise": the difference between "substance" (*ti*) and "function" (*yong*), respectively. The classics constitute a linguistic system, the substance out of which the function, or apparent usefulness presented in the treatises, derives. Without the substance of the classics, nothing can be accomplished, just as our intellect would fail if it lacked a healthy body to support it. Thus the substance, the body, is the foundation. By the same token, the use of that body, the function of substance, is equally important. If we have a body but cannot use it, how will the use or purpose of the body ever come to light? If we have a strong and healthy body but never put it to any sort of use, it is meaningless, nothing more than a mound of flesh and bones.

The relationship between "classic" and "treatise" is thus as vital as the relationship between "substance" and "function," and between the body and its various actions. It is clear that in order to study Chinese Medicine well, we must read not only the classics but also their discourses, the "treatises." So where does the *Treatise on Cold Damage and Miscellaneous Diseases* stand in this schema? It is both a classic and a treatise; both a logical system and an explanation of how that system can be implemented. Being this kind of a masterpiece, is this not a book that must be read? Is this not a book that you should rely on?

II. Pursuing the Ultimate Principle by Comprehending Yin Yang

After we have gained clarity on our topic above, we have in effect "opened the door to look at the mountain." Now, let us attempt to answer three questions. First, the *Plain Questions* states: "As for heat diseases, they all belong to the disease category of cold damage." Clearly, heat disease is simply heat disease, so why is this disease category ascribed to the classification of cold damage? Cold and heat would seem to be exact opposites, so why are they being lumped together? The second question is related to the first one. Cold damage is cold damage, in the sense of being a specific type of disease in its own right, is it not? Why then does the *Classic of Difficulties* say that "there are five types of cold damage: wind-strike, cold damage, damp warmth, heat disease, and warm disease"? How can this one disease, cold damage, also include so many other types of diseases? A third question that requires an answer is why Zhang Zhongjing chose cold damage as the central thread of his work. Why did the writer Wang Shuhe, who revived Zhang Zhongjing's work after the original texts were lost, choose cold damage for the title of the book? Before we read the *Treatise on Cold Damage* we must first answer these three questions. Unless we are clear on these points, we will not understand the book.

How can we arrive at clarity on these points? Here, we can follow the course of action prescribed by the famous physician Zheng Qin'an of Sichuan from the late Qing dynasty: "If students are able to pursue the ultimate principle by comprehending yin and yang, they have the foundation necessary to enter through Zhang Zhongjing's door." In accordance with this advice, we must first explore yin and yang in order to prepare ourselves adequately for studying the *Treatise on Cold Damage*.

II.1. Comprehending Yin Yang

What is the most important element of Chinese Medicine? What is its most central theme, around which all other aspects revolve and which none can do without? The answer is yin and yang! The beginning of the "Great Treatise on the Correspondence of Yin and Yang" explains: "Yin and yang are the Dao of heaven and earth, the warp and weft of the myriad things, the father and mother of all change, the root of birth and death, the palace of the spirit light. To cure disease, we must seek the root!" This passage from the *Plain Questions* gets right to the heart of the matter. The passage is both dense in meaning and broad in scope. When one considers the breadth and depth spanned by yin and yang in Chinese cosmology, and their incredible importance—the very father and mother of all change, the root of life and death—their centrality in Chinese Medicine theory is undeniable. In any field of study, but especially in medicine, we cannot leave the realm of heaven and earth, and yin and yang are the path to that universe. The *Yellow Emperor's Classic* refers to yin and yang as the warp and weft, literally the systematic arrangement of a lead rope and the net that it is holding together. Yin and yang form the interconnecting pattern of the "myriad things"— shorthand for the multifarious phenomena of this world. In physics, we seek a unified theory to explain all phenomena. For the authors of the *Yellow Emperor's Classic*, and for the Chinese Medicine practitioner of any age, the unifying theory to explain all phenomena is yin yang theory. Yin and yang are the father and mother of all change. When we investigate phenomena, we undoubtedly investigate the way in which they change through time and space. And what guides these changes? Yin and yang. We come in contact with human society, and we come in contact with the natural world. Regardless of whether we are talking about something from the human or the natural world, whether it is plant or animal, organic or inorganic, the universe or the Milky Way, its entire process is no doubt a process in which it emerges into existence and then passes out of existence, is born and then dies. How is this process of birth and death brought into being? It is brought into being by yin and yang. Furthermore, "Yin and yang are the palace of the spirit light." Spirit light means consciousness and thought, so this line is particularly relevant to us as human beings. Consciousness is also related to yin and yang. The last point relates to the notion of curing the root cause of disease. In China, everybody likes to repeat the line: "Western Medicine treats the branches, Chinese Medicine treats the root." And yet, when asked, Chinese Medicine practitioners cannot say how it is that they treat the root, or by what means they are able to treat the root. In fact, the "root" is precisely this yin and yang, and to treat the root we must seek for it in yin and yang. If the ultimate origin of any aspect of any phenomenon, including disease, is sought, we eventually arrive back at yin and yang.

How well do we all understand yin and yang? Is our understanding on a par with that of the *Yellow Emperor's Classic*? As a professor, I enjoy posing this question to my undergraduate and graduate students. The answers I receive from my students are invariably derived from their *Fundamentals of Chinese Medicine* textbook. Their explanations of yin and yang consist of phrases such as "mutual restraint," "rooted in one another," "waxing and waning in equilibrium," "mutual transformation," and so on. If I ask more probing questions that demand deeper explanations, they have no answers. If you are studying yin yang and all you know are the stock concepts from the *Fundamentals of Chinese Medicine*, it is simply not enough. What sort of "opposition" are we talking about? What does it mean that they are "rooted in one another"? You should be able to answer these sorts of questions in concrete terms. You must be able to discern the yin or yang of the permutation of any phenomenon, to perceive and distinguish the yin and yang aspects of all phenomena as an action that is as simple and as ordinary as raising your hand or taking a single step. Only in this way will you be able to use yin and yang to resolve actual, concrete questions.

II.1.a. The Relationship between Yin and Yang

When we speak of yin and yang, we speak of the interaction between the two. The simple fact that there are two brings up the question of their relationship. In fact, this is the most important question in the study of yin and yang. This issue is addressed incisively in Chapter 5 of the *Plain Questions*, the "Great Treatise on the Correspondences of Yin and Yang": "Yang births and yin grows, yang kills and yin stores." This line deals with the essential interactions of yin and yang. If we understand this line, the relationship between yin and yang becomes clear.

"Yang births and yin grows, yang kills and yin stores." This line is primarily discussing the transformation of yin and yang through the course of a year as it affects all living things. "Yang births and yin grows" refers to the first half of the year, and the changes that pertain to spring and summer. Within this process, yang gradually gives birth and engenders, while yin gradually makes things grow, and the relationship between the two is very closely coordinated. In relation to the natural world, with the arrival of spring, periods of daylight grow progressively longer, the temperature gradually increases, and everywhere we have the sense that the yang *qi* increases unceasingly. Yang transforms the *qi*, and yin gives it form. As yang increases, the myriad living things, which belong to this yin category of form, follow the growth of yang and become more resplendent, flourishing and blossoming. This process illustrates a relationship as is described in the saying "the husband sings and the wife follows," of yang birthing and yin growing. The antagonism or opposition between yin and yang that we mentioned earlier would seem to be different from the harmonious process we are describing here. We are not looking at a process in which yang produces and generates and then the myriad living things, in contradiction, perish and disappear. This is not at all the case. We can use modern metaphors to describe this process. We can compare yang *qi* to energy or electricity and imagine that this energy is stored by nature in a sort of power station. During the spring and summer, the energy is in the process of being released from storage. After the energy is released from the power station and living things begin to receive it, they emerge, grow, and blossom. The growth and blossoming of living things is induced by the release of this energy. This is yang emerging and yin growing.

As for yang killing and yin storing, this relates to the changes of fall and winter. We should not regard "yang killing" to mean extermination. The word *sha*, which is translated as "to kill," can also mean to terminate, weaken, reduce, or abate. "Yang births" and "yang kills" are complementary concepts. The emerging yang of spring and summer refers to the release of yang, the release of energy. Can this release of energy continue endlessly without interruption? Probably not. It can be compared to boxing. When a boxer throws a punch, he has to bring his fist back before he can throw another. The yang *qi* of nature is like this: It cannot constantly induce growth, and cannot be unceasingly released into the world. Energy is released up to a point, and then the energy is retrieved and put back into storage. This is complementary to the concept of "yang emerging" and is what is meant by "yang abating" or "yang terminating." As yang abates and the energy begins to be stored, the myriad things no longer receive this supply of energy, their growth slows to a stop, they gradually wane and wither, and we have before us the image of autumn and winter. This sentiment of solemn desolation is described perfectly in this line from a poem: "The autumn winds blow the waters of the Wei river, the fallen leaves fill the city of Chang'an." This is a description of this phase of withering and dying and of retreating into storage.

This entire process forms a cycle that repeats over and over, like a ring without an end. Once the energy is retrieved to a certain degree, a new cycle of growth and release of energy is begun. This is in accord with the statement in the *Yellow Emperor's Classic*: "Utmost yang must become yin, utmost yin must become yang." Yang indicates the process of emerging and releasing, while yin indicates the process of receiving and storing. "Spring and summer stand for yang, fall and winter stand for yin" also indicates these processes.

It is especially fitting to use the *Plain Questions's* line, "Utmost yang must become yin, utmost yin must become yang," to illustrate this process. To understand it more thoroughly, we can include some information from the *Classic of Changes*. The *Classic of Changes* specifically discusses the transformations of yin and yang by using two-dimensional images for the purpose of illustration. This makes the transformations of yin and yang clearer and more perceptible. In order to describe the transformations of yin and yang throughout the year, it has twelve tidal hexagrams, combinations of six yin and yang lines: *fu* (Turning Back, ䷗), *lin* (Approaching, ䷒), *tai* (Advance, ䷊), *dazhuang* (Great Strength, ䷡), *guai* (Eliminating, ䷪), *qian* (Initiating, ䷀), *gou* (Encountering, ䷫), *dun* (Retreat, ䷠), *pi* (Hindrance, ䷋), *guan* (Watching, ䷓), *bo* (Falling Away, ䷖), and *kun* (Responding, ䷁). The hexagram *fu* corresponds to the eleventh month of the lunar year, *lin* to the twelfth month, *tai* to the first month, *dazhuang* to the second month, *guai* to the third, *qian* to the fourth, *gou* to the fifth, and *dun*, *pi*, *guan*, *bo*, and *kun* to the sixth, seventh, eighth, ninth, and tenth months, respectively.

These twelve hexagrams are referred to as the "differentiated" hexagrams in the system of the *Classic of Changes*. They are created by compounding two "classic" trigrams each. The trigrams create the system of eight trigrams or *bagua*, which through various combinations form the system of 64 hexagrams. We can see that, of these twelve tidal hexagrams, all are composed of a combination of both yin and yang lines, except for the hexagrams *qian* and *kun*. *Qian* and *kun* are different from the rest because they consist exclusively of yang or yin lines and are thus pure yang and pure yin. The hexagram *qian* is composed of two *Qian* Heaven trigrams one atop the other. For this reason, this hexagram is referred to as "double," "stacked," or "utmost" yang. In identical fashion, the *kun* hexagram consists of two *Kun* Water trigrams and is referred to as the "utmost" yin hexagram. As we proceed through the tidal hexagrams, we see that yang *qi* is steadily building and increasing until we reach the hexagram *qian*, consisting of six yang lines and representing the climax of yang release. Proceeding from here, we see an apt illustration of the phrase: "Utmost yang must turn to yin." In the following hexagrams, beginning with the hexagram *gou*, there is a gradual increase in yin.

The hexagram *gou* corresponds to the fifth month of the lunar calendar, and the onset of increasing yin coincides with the "apex of summer" (*xiazhi*) or summer solstice at this time. The character *zhi* ("apex") is often translated as "arriving at" or simply "reaching." Here, a different meaning is intended: the "utmost reach" or "furthest extent" of something. Summer is yang, and at the summer solstice we find the utmost extent of yang, the point at which yang can proceed no further and yin is born. As the hexagrams progress from this point, yin steadily increases and yang withers. This process continues until we arrive at the hexagram *kun* (Responding), the double or utmost yin hexagram that indicates the turning point back to yang. Thus, with the hexagram following *kun*, we have the hexagram *fu* (Turning Back) and a gradual increase in yang lines. At this point, a new cycle of "yang birthing and yin growing, yang killing and yin storing" is set in motion, hence the title of the hexagram.

With regard to the present discussion, it is important to keep in mind one more detail: the change when utmost yin must become yang, and the advent of the first yang line in *fu* does not occur at the beginning of spring, but rather in the dead of winter. Likewise, the hexagram *gou* is not positioned at the beginning of fall when yin begins to predominate, but rather at the summer solstice, at yin's inception in the cycle of the seasons. This corresponds to another characteristic of yin and yang: yang emerges from yin, yin emerges from yang; in the heart of yin there is yang, in the heart of yang there is yin.

The above example illustrates how discussions of yin and yang, and discussions of Chinese Medicine as well, become more convenient and clearer when conducted in conjunction with an examination of the *Classic of Changes* and a thorough investigation of implied significance of this classic. Throughout history, prominent physicians have pointed out the relationship between Chinese Medicine and the *Classic of Changes*. Most notably, the legendary physician Sun Simiao wrote: "If you have not studied the *Changes*, you cannot become a great physician." This is a point we should heed.

II.1.b. The Issue of Hierarchy

In the previous discussion, we saw how yin, following the emergence of yang, grows, and how yin, following the autumnal killing influence of yang, stores. This is an opportunity for us to shed light on the question of the two types of hierarchy in concrete terms. In the first type of hierarchy, we have a cooperative hierarchical relationship between yin and yang where neither is in opposition to or constraining the other. This is the relationship illustrated by the saying "the husband sings and the wife follows," which we already mentioned before. In real life, the most concrete example of yin and yang in this kind of a relationship can be seen in the relationship between man and woman, husband and wife, and the relationships of a family. Imagine if, in the course of marital life, both partners tried to dominate the other, with one facing south and the other facing north, as incompatible as fire and water; it would make life impossible to the point where they would not even be able to have a normal family life, much less careers. Therefore, in the relationships of the family, or of marriage, the relationship between yin and yang must be guided by cooperation.

In the second paradigm of hierarchy, yang is dominant over yin. In reality, this sort of hierarchy is already evident in the first type of hierarchy. In this explanation of the hierarchical relationship between yin and yang, the changes of yang give rise to a guiding action, a deciding function. The changes of yin are seen as subsequent to the changes that yang undergoes. We can see this relationship between yin and yang in many aspects of nature and society. The *Plain Questions's* line "yang births and yin grows, yang kills and yin stores" is in fact referring to the progression of birth, growth, harvesting, and storage. This cycle of emerging, increasing, gathering, and going into storage refers to the dominant themes of spring, summer, fall, and winter. But, as a matter of fact, it is the changes and transformations of yang through the course of the year that the line refers to in particular: the emergence of yang, its growth, its harvesting, and its storage. Through the changes of yang, the birth, growth, gathering, and storage of the myriad things are initiated. This point is made clear in Dong Zhongshu's *Luxuriant Dew of the Spring and Autumn Annals* (Chunqiu fanlu):

> Animals are born and die in accordance with yang; numbers heed yang as their beginning and end. . . . Yang is the lord of the lifespan, all of the insects of the world take notice of yang to determine their emergence and egress, all of the vegetation of the earth abides by yang to flourish or perish, the three sovereigns of this world defer to yang in order to establish governance.

Is it not the case that regardless of whether we are discussing vegetation, insects, plants, or animals, all must comply with the changes of spring, summer, fall and winter? How do spring, summer, fall, and winter come about? What determines the four seasons? They are determined by the angle of the sun. A single cycle of the sun along the path of the ecliptic is equivalent to the spring, summer, fall, and winter of a year. The four seasons correspond to the changes of time, but more importantly, they reflect the changing disposition of yang. Spring is, in fact, the period of time that is dictated by yang *qi* being in a state of emergence. Summer is a period of time dictated by yang *qi* being in a state of growth. Autumn is the period of time dictated by yang *qi* being inclined toward gathering and harvesting. And winter is the period when yang *qi* assumes a posture of storage. Spring, summer, autumn, and winter are generated by the changes of yang, and the changes and transformations of the "myriad things," of all living things, are in accordance with the seasons. From the perspective of society, the fact that the yang (male) clearly holds the position of leadership is even more obvious and does not need to be discussed at length.

Above, we used the twelve tidal hexagrams to illustrate the transformations of yin and yang. When we look at the changes in the hexagrams, it might be easy for everybody to look at yin and yang separately and in terms of their mutual antagonism. For instance, when we look at the changes in the progression of hexagrams from *fu* to *qian*, it is obvious that yang is increasing and yin decreasing. Yang wins and yin loses, yin dies and yang lives. The antagonism seems clear as the light of day. However, this perception is incorrect. When we say yang increases, we are speaking of its growth and its increasing outward release. When we say yin diminishes, we are not saying that as yang grows there is some independent thing that is slowly decreasing. If we understand yin and yang in this way, we will encounter a number of fundamental problems. If we watch the progression from the hexagram *fu*, where we see only one yang line at the base of the hexagram, to the hexagram *qian*, consisting of all yang lines, we do see a gradual decrease in the yin lines within the hexagrams, until, when we have reached the hexagram *qian*, there are no yin lines left whatsoever. But can we say that during the time governed by *qian*, there is absolutely no evidence of yin? If so, if there was no yin at all, then we would have solitary yang! The *Yellow Emperor's Classic* states that yang, when solitary, does not emerge and that yin, when solitary, does not grow. And yet, during the three months of summer, all living things flourish splendidly. It is clear that we cannot look at yin and yang in this way.

To understand these changes correctly, we should remember that yang is alternately released outward and then gathered back in; it is born and then dies. The metaphor of the movement of a boxer's fist is helpful. The boxer must first extend his fist and then recoil it. It would be impossible for a boxer to both deliver a punch and wind up at the same time. The extension and retraction of the fist are like the release and gathering of yang. Although we speak of waxing and waning, we are really discussing an issue of changes in yang *qi*.

Another common confusion regarding the twelve tidal hexagrams has to do with the progression of yin. Most people regard the progression of the hexagrams from *gou* to *kun* as an illustration of yin flourishing and yang withering. If we take a superficial view of things, this is precisely how it appears. If we stop and think about it, though, this point of view has obvious problems.

Why do I say that this view has problems? Beginning with the summer solstice, yang *qi* begins to gather inward after reaching the utmost extent of its outward release. It gradually gathers inward, entering a stored state. What is the purpose of this gathering and storage? It is as we previously described, like the fist retrieved by the boxer after he throws a punch. The purpose of cocking the fist is so the boxer can throw another. When the yang *qi* is retrieved, it is in order to release it. If the yang *qi* were to weaken after being gathered back, it could not then be released. The released state of yang *qi* may weaken and falter. The goal of retrieving, of gathering back in, is to compensate for this attenuation and weakening. From a quantitative perspective, the period of fall and winter when yang *qi* is gathered back in, represents the period in which "yin triumphs and yang becomes feeble." This attenuation of yang *qi* is in actuality the process by which it is restored and through which it increases. Only in this way can a new cycle of growth and release be set in motion. In relation to our own bodies, during the day when we work, yang *qi* is being released, and at night when we rest and recuperate, we are gathering and storing our yang *qi*. The purpose of resting in the evening is to ensure reinvigoration for the following morning. If, on the contrary, after resting, our yang *qi* were reduced and weakened, why would we feel refreshed? If that were the case, who would want to rest or sleep? If we consider the issue in this way, it is easy to understand.

Understanding yin and yang rests on our ability to see that the two are one and that the one is two. When regarded separately, it appears as if there were two separate, independent entities, one male and one female. When we observe their interactions with one another, we see that they constitute a single, solitary organism. If we can only consider questions of yin and yang while thinking of the two as entirely independent of one another, unable to see the two as one, it is indeed very difficult for us to comprehend key points. We encounter a similar difficulty when we seek to understand issues regarding cold and heat. If we think about them being like water and fire, two things that could never be combined, it is challenging to regard these two seemingly opposite and independent entities as one. However, if we examine them more deeply, we can see that they are in fact one, and that the question is once more a question of understanding the nature of yang *qi*.

Earlier, we talked about how yang *qi* can be compared to energy, or even thermal energy. Why is spring warm and summer hot? This is because yang *qi* is being released in these seasons and so we have the heat of yang. Why then is autumn cool? Why is the weather of winter frigid? Yang *qi* is being gathered back and stored, and with it the warmth and heat of yang. This causes the weather to turn cold. This is to say that cold and heat accompany the emergence, growth, gathering, and storage of yang *qi*. When yang *qi* is released, there is warmth; when it is retrieved, there is coolness.

When the weather turns cold, it is not because cold exists as an independent entity; cold is the absence of warmth.

When contemplating problems such as these, it is important to carefully distinguish between the manifestations and the substance of the dynamic at hand. If we contemplate these issues until they are absolutely clear, we can fundamentally resolve questions regarding yin and yang. The *Plain Questions* emphasizes this point:

> As for yin and yang, if we count ten variations, we can deduce a hundred. If we count a thousand, we can deduce myriad. If we count myriad, our deductions are beyond counting. In truth, there is only one essential factor.
>
> If we understand this crucial factor, we can discuss it and draw our conclusions. If we do not understand this crucial factor, our comprehension will be endlessly scattered.

In this passage, the "counting ten and deducing a hundred" refers to counting the multifarious possible manifestations of yin and yang. Manifestations are ultimately limitless in number, whereas the substance of these variations is singular. If we understand this essential element, we are finished. This is what is meant by the saying: "If you are able to understand the one, the myriad can be accomplished"; if we do not understand this crucial element, our efforts are scattered endlessly.

The transformations of yin and yang and the hierarchy that characterizes their relationship can be understood at their roots from an astronomical perspective. The *Arithmetic Classic of the Gnomon and the Circular Paths of Heaven* (Zhoubi suanjing) describes the earliest calculations of the sun's orbit and the method by which a year can be divided into twenty-four calendrical periods. When the sun is directly overhead at noon, a staff eight feet (*chi*) in length is held vertical and its shadow is measured. The length of this shadow indicates the position of the earth, in its orbit, relative to the sun, and by extension, which of the twenty-four calendrical periods is current. The *Arithmetic Classic of the Gnomon and the Circular Paths of Heaven* tells us that this shadow's maximum length is approximately thirteen and a half feet (more precisely, one *zhang*, three *chi*, and five *cun*) and its minimum length is sixteen inches (one *chi* and six *cun*). Which season corresponds to the longest shadow and which to the shortest? The longest shadow pertains to the winter solstice and the shortest to the summer solstice. The shadow cast by this staff is indicative of the yin shadow of the sun.

During the hot mid-summer months of China, anyone who goes outside prefers to be in the shade of a tree or hopes for the shadow of a cloud to come along. This shade blocks the rays of the sun and offers a bit of cool respite from the summer heat. The shadow cast by the staff acts as a measurement of the extent to which yang is gathering and storing. The shadow cast by this staff is longest at the winter solstice, because at this time the gathering and storing of the yang *qi* is strongest. After the winter solstice passes, this shadow grows gradually shorter, corresponding to a weakening or abatement of yang gathering and storage, and a concomitant strengthening of the sun's intensity. After the winter solstice, daylight grows longer each day and the dark of night shorter. These correspond to the alternation of gathering and storing with emergence and growth. This shadow gradually shortens until the summer solstice when it is twenty inches long. If we compare a shadow that is twenty inches long with one that is seven and a half feet long, there is really no comparison. At the summer solstice, the yang *qi* is at the zenith of its release and is almost completely unimpeded. Utmost yang must turn to yin, and so after the summer solstice this shadow grows longer each day. Accordingly, the daylight grows shorter and shorter and the nights longer and longer. After the yang *qi* is completely released, it gradually turns toward gathering and storage.

We can see that the expansion and contraction of the shadow cast by the staff at noon corresponds to the changes of the four seasons of the year and the transformations of the twenty-four calendrical periods. These changes are, in effect, the result of the alternation between the release and gathering of yang *qi*. Once we understand this guiding principle, every aspect of yin and yang's interrelations becomes evident.

II.1.c. The Relationship between Substance and Function

We can also discuss yin and yang from the perspective of substance and function, or put another way, theory and praxis, for the Chinese words *ti* and *yong* embody both of these concepts. The dichotomy of form and function represents an important concept in traditional culture. Form or theory refers to the theoretical basis. Function or praxis refers to the practical application, the utilization of theory. Without theory, there is no praxis.

Without praxis with which to put theory into use, theory is essentially meaningless. Substance and function follow one another. How do theory and praxis, substance and function, relate to yin and yang? More specifically, between yin and yang, which one corresponds to theory and which one to praxis? It is obvious that if we regard yin and yang as an organic whole, yang corresponds primarily to praxis and yin primarily to theory. In the *Fundamentals of Chinese Medicine*, the section on the liver includes a discussion of the notion that the liver's *ti* ("substance") is yin and its *yong* ("function") is yang. In fact, it is not only the liver that is like this; yin and yang correlate like this in everything else as well. If we look at the course of a year, spring and summer are yang and autumn and winter yin. During spring and summer yang is being applied or put into use. Spring and summer are characterized by sunlight, warmth, the flourishing of plants and animals, which all reflect the exuberant application, the praxis or function, of yang *qi*. Therefore, when we say that spring and summer are yang, this yang refers to the practical application of yang, its outward function. This concept is not too difficult to understand. Here, the function of yang corresponds to the state of yang release that we discussed earlier. The withered and cold aspect of fall and winter do not accord with the application of yang. This is because the praxis of yang, its exercise out in the world, is being gathered back in and stored. What you see is not the function of yang, but something else made visible by its absence. What becomes visible when the function is withdrawn is the substance, the body of yang, its *ti*. This "substance" refers to the foundation, the capital. The yin of fall and winter, its inherent gathering and storing, is essential precisely in order to foster and nurse this foundation, to conserve this capital. Once this foundation is solidified, this capital increased, the function of yang can be brought into full play. From this perspective, form and function and yin and yang are in correspondence with one another. The two complement each other and are mutually derived. Neither is dispensable.

The function of yang is easily perceived, but its prominence does not warrant that we ignore the significance of substance. As we should know, this substance does not stand in a relationship of opposition to the function of yang. It is not enough to speak only of the rights of men; we must also promote women's rights. Isn't there a popular saying: "Behind every successful man, there is a successful woman"? This saying is very true, and many situations are like this. Nowadays many men, once they gain success, discard the woman who helped them achieve it. This is not only immoral, but foolish, and may very well doom them to disaster.

Yang refers to function or implementation, and this function is reflected in many aspects. First of all, we have the way in which "yang births and yin grows," the *qi*-transforming yang that is able to bring about the birth and growth of the myriad things. Why is the appearance of spring and summer so fresh and luxurious? It is because of this transformative yang power. The second aspect of the function of yang is illustrated by yang as the foundation for longevity. The "Treatise on the Vital *Qi* Connecting to Heaven" (Shengqi tongtian lun) in the *Plain Questions* states: "The yang *qi* is like the sun in the sky. If it is lost, the lifespan is shortened and obscured." The connection between longevity and yang *qi* highlights the importance of yang. Whether a person lives to old age or dies young depends upon it. Those who live long have, by definition, adequate yang *qi*. If the yang *qi* declines, we can predict that the person's life will be shortened. Third, "Yang circulates on the exterior and acts to secure and consolidate the exterior of the body." This is also a very important aspect of yang function. The question of whether or not our bodies are firm and sturdy, whether we are able to ward off infection, depends on how well yang is defending the exterior. This particular aspect of the function of yang has a strong connection with our overall health. We consider the greatest problems facing the human body, excepting perhaps the challenges posed by our careers and economic situations, to be health and longevity. The function of yang is directly related to both of these.

Yin refers to substance or body (*ti*). How and where is this substance expressed? Let us take a family as an example. In particular, in a traditional Chinese family in the past, women had the sole function of bearing children and performing the domestic chores. So how did we gauge the usefulness or "function" of such women? We looked to see if the males in the family had good prospects. If the men did well in their work, this meant that "inside helpers" of the family were good. Why were the wives called "inside helpers"? Because they "helped" the yang. It is as if to say that the significance of yin is its ability to assist yang, to help yang obtain proper development and prospects. Yin acts as the basis of yang, yang acts as the utilization of yin. "Yang is on the outside, the envoy of yin; yin is on the inside, the keeper of yang." The relationship of these two can be understood by this line.

Yin acts as the foundation, and one of the most salient functions of yin is its ability to store essence (*jing*). In the "Treatise on the Vital *Qi* Connecting to Heaven" in the *Plain Questions*, we read: "Yin stores essence and is compounded into being, yang defends the exterior and acts to consolidate." In actuality, what is this "essence"? Essence is neither yin nor yang. Currently, many people are confused regarding this concept of essence in Chinese Medicine, and view it as purely yin, going so far as to consider yin synonymous with essence. If essence is the same as yin, then how can we talk of yin storing essence? How would it store itself? It would be logically impossible. Strictly speaking, essence is yang *qi* in its stored form, or in other words, the stored form of energy is called "essence." The more boisterous and vigorous a person's energy is, the better their energy stores. Of course, in both the *Yellow Emperor's Classic* and the *Fundamentals of Chinese Medicine*, essence has a number of other explanations. At this juncture, I am analyzing it only from its most basic theoretical perspective. Essence is yang *qi* in its congealed, gathered state, but not in its emitted, released state. The ability of yin to store essence reflects its role in assisting this gathering process. The ability of yang *qi* to gather together and shift from a released, emitted state to a stored state depends upon this function of yin. Where, specifically, is this *jing* stored? In "The Treatise on the Six Nodes and Visceral Manifestation" in the *Plain Questions*, we find the following statement: "The kidneys rule hibernation; they are the root of sealing and concealing, the dwelling place of essence." Hibernation refers to hiding and concealing. The kidneys rule storage and concealment, thus they are the root of sealing up and concealing. And what is it that is sealed up and concealed? They seal up and conceal the yang *qi*; they seal up and conceal the essence. This essence, this yang *qi* in condensed form, is sealed up and hidden in the domain of the kidneys. Thus, they are called the "location of the essence." Of the seasons of the year, the kidneys belong to winter, and winter governs storage. Among the five viscera, the kidneys belong to yin; they are the yin within yin. The kidneys correlate closely with the substantial aspect of yin, as well as its essence-storing capacity. Both substance (*ti*) as a whole and the process by which yang *qi* is stored depend in great part on the kidneys. The ability to seal up and store the essence, the ability to adequately store yang *qi*, to recuperate and rebuild, all depend on the proper functioning of the kidneys. Only if accumulation and storage are sufficient will the ability to release yang *qi* be adequate and the energy ample. If we wish to understand the condition of a person's overall strength and vigor, we must look at the kidneys.

Now that we are clear on how yin refers to "substance" and how the purpose of this corporeal form is to assist the yang function of the body, it is difficult to still regard the relationship between yin and yang as antagonistic. At this point, we can understand any opposition between yin and yang as emerging from a basic unity of the two, whereas before we might have seen it as a purely antagonistic opposition.

The relationship between yin and yang as form and function can be demonstrated by countless examples from everyday life. Taking rest as one example, previously we might have had a very general understanding of rest. Hence, we might have considered sitting down to be resting, or sleeping. If we look at the Chinese word for resting, we see that it consists of two characters (*xiuxi* 休息), which pertain to two different aspects of "resting." The general understanding of "resting" just mentioned actually refers to the first part of this word, the character *xiu* (休). *Xiu* refers to taking a pause from the activities of life, taking a short breather, or stopping. A *xiu*-type of rest might refer to simply taking a break during a busy day, or going to bed to sleep. This character derives from the character for person (人) on the left and the character for wood (木) on the right. It literally refers to a person lying down on a wooden bed. The goal of rest is to have more energy afterward. When we go to sleep at night, it is in order to restore vigor for the next day. Likewise, when we take an afternoon siesta, it is so that we have renewed energy in the second half of the day. Those who are accustomed to taking an afternoon nap become drowsy and muddled for the rest of the day if they happen to miss their little siesta. For this reason, the function of "rest" is described by the second character (*xi* 息). This character can be understood by examining its meaning in other contexts. Why do we put money in the bank? To earn "interest," which is one of the other meanings of the character. If ten years ago, we made a deposit of 10,000 dollars, and each year we earned 8 or 9 percent in interest, then we would have 10,900 dollars after a year. This "interest" is why people are willing to put their money into a bank account. The meaning of *xi* is "to increase." Our money increases when we put it in the bank, therefore interest is referred to as *xi*. So what exactly do we mean by *xiuxi*? Obviously, we mean that by taking a rest, we can renew, literally increase, the energy that has been lost through activity and work. Rest is the process by which we return to a state of renewed vigor and vitality, and the Chinese concept of *xiuxi* is comprised of two characters: one that relates to its substance, namely *xiu*, and one that relates to its function, namely *xi*.

Spring and summer are yang; fall and winter are yin. But in fact, what we are saying is that spring and summer are function, and fall and winter are substance. Whether the function is operating properly depends to a great extent on whether or not the substance is good. Therefore, to determine how spring and summer's function will be, we need to ascertain the state of fall and winter, but especially the state of substance as it relates to winter. The "Great Treatise on the Four *Qi* and the Tuning of the Spirit" chapter of the *Plain Questions* states: "The sages cultivated yang in the spring and summer and yin in the fall and winter, thereby abiding with the source." In the past, many people have misunderstood the concept entailed by this cultivation of yin and yang. They think that cultivating yang during spring and summer is like putting oil on a fire and cultivating yin during fall and winter is like putting frost on a snow bank. The *Chinese Medicine Journal* (Zhongyi zazhi) organized a public forum to discuss this very topic. Actually, when viewed from the perspective of substance and function, what is there left to discuss? Cultivating yang during spring and summer means to promote the development of function during this time. Cultivating yin during autumn and winter means we should nourish substance during this period of convalescence. This is how we discuss yin and yang from the perspective of substance and function. Of course, these ideas could be expanded upon endlessly and applied to any number of concepts and examples.

II.2. A Summary of Cold Damage

Above, we discussed two different aspects of yin and yang: one was their hierarchical relationship, and the other was their relationship in terms of substance and function. Now that we understand these aspects of yin and yang clearly, we can easily answer the three questions we posed prior to our investigation into yin and yang.

II.2.a. The Qi of Winter Is Cold

First of all, if we think about cold, it is the *qi* or weather of winter. We need look no further than the *Fundamentals of Chinese Medicine* to learn this much. Spring is warm, summer hot, fall cool, and winter cold. How is cold produced? This is a question we discussed earlier. The nature of yang belongs to the category of heat, and when yang *qi* is in its released state, heat emerges in the environment and the weather becomes warm. During spring, the degree to which yang *qi* has been released is relatively less than that of summer, so the weather of spring is not as hot as that of summer. When autumn comes, the yang *qi* is reined back in, and with it the heat of yang begins to close. The weather gradually turns cool and then cold. The gathering and storage of yang *qi* during autumn are not as intense as during winter, and so the weather of winter is significantly colder than that of autumn. This is an important aspect of winter. From this particular aspect, we can see that cold is the outward manifestation of the retrieved and stored state of yang *qi*. It is not only the *qi* of winter, however, it is also the *qi* of storage.

Let us shift our discussion from temporal changes to spatial considerations for a moment. In my country, China, it is clear that the Northwest is much cooler than the Southeast. During the winter, the weather reports always indicate a number of places in the north where the weather is ten or twenty degrees below zero Celsius, while the temperature in places in the south is greater than twenty degrees above zero. The contrast is huge. When a resident from Hainan province goes north on a business trip, he gets on the plane in little more than a shirt, but when he arrives at his destination, he has to put on a fur-lined jacket! Why is there such a difference? We can look to the *Yellow Emperor's Classic* for an answer. The "Great Treatise on the Correspondences of Yin and Yang" in the *Plain Questions* states: "The northwest is yin; the southeast is yang." Yang is function, the state of release. Yin is substance, the state of collection and storage. From a geographical perspective, the entire Northwest of China is governed by collection and storage, and the Southeast by release. This explains their vastly disparate climates. This example illustrates an important issue. In our study of Chinese Medicine, it is important to pay attention to spatial considerations as well as the temporal dimension. Time and space are the same in Chinese

Medicine—they are integrated. This notion must be anchored firmly in the mind.

Earlier, we delineated how it was not enough to rely on standardized textbook learning for the purpose of comprehending the concept of yin yang, but how we must also have a personal, subjective sense of this concept. We should cultivate the ability to understand all issues from the perspective of yin and yang. For instance, the people who live in Nanning, in the South of China, wear short-sleeved shirts and short pants right up until the Chinese New Year. Why is this? If the student of Chinese Medicine cannot answer this from a yin yang perspective and clarify his or her answer from the same angle, then that student will become insensitive and apathetic toward the most basic tenets of Chinese Medicine theory. That apathy and insensitivity will most certainly prevent such a student from learning Chinese Medicine well.

II.2.b. How to Nurture Storage

Once we understand the basic attributes of cold, its significance, and the type of weather that it represents, we realize that cold is in no way a bad thing. From the appearance and extent of the cold, we can deduce the degree to which the yang *qi* has been gathered and stored; we can see the state of the substance (*ti*).

Winter should be freezing cold, because the yang *qi* needs to be sealed up and stored during winter, and because substance must be conserved. To reinforce this point, the *Plain Questions* specifically discusses the issue of nurturing storage. During the three months of winter, storage is nurtured, while during the three months of autumn, gathering is nurtured. What this means here is obviously that in both fall and winter, yin is nurtured. The "Great Treatise on the Four *Qi* and the Tuning of the Spirit" contains a monograph regarding this point. Here we shall examine only the discussion of the three months of winter:

> The three months of winter are called the time of closing and storing. Water freezes and the ground is split with cracks. Do not disturb yang. One should go to bed early and rise late. One must wait for the light of the sun before getting up. The will should be as if hidden, as if one had private intentions, as if one's aims were already obtained. Get rid of cold and seek warmth. Avoid sweating and thereby disturbing the *qi* that is

now in a state of storage. These are the mandatory actions in winter, and these constitute the way to nurture storage. To go against these rules harms the kidneys, and then in spring there will be wilting and reversal, and little growth will be had.

This treatise from the *Plain Questions* discusses the "four *qi* and the tuning of the spirit." The four *qi* refer to the *qi* of spring, summer, fall, and winter, indicating the *qi* of emergence or birth, growth, harvesting (or killing), and storage. What does the "tuning of the spirit" refer to? This refers to the human factor. How do we accord with the emerging *qi* of the three months of spring, or the growth *qi* of summer, the harvesting *qi* of fall, or the storage *qi* of winter? We must cultivate and nourish emergence, growth, harvesting, and storage in each season respectively. Nowadays, people only talk about cultivating the generation or emergence of *qi*, in the popular ideal of *yangsheng* ("nurturing life"; the Chinese character for "life" used in the compound "nurturing life" is the same character as the one used for "generation" or "emergence" in the description of the four types of seasonal *qi*: *sheng* 生). They say nothing of its growth, harvesting, or storage. This is a very one-sided approach.

The passage quoted above focused on nurturing storage. During the three months of winter, how do we cultivate storage and how do we accord with the state of closing and concealing? The key point is to "not disturb yang" during this time. The three months of winter are yin, and the *Plain Questions* clearly indicates that we should "nourish yin in fall and winter." By emphasizing in the same passage that we should "not disturb yang," this statement demonstrates that we can regard the emergence, growth, retrieval, and storage of spring, summer, fall, and winter as revolving around yang as the dominant principle. The phrase "do not disturb yang" tells us that during the three months of winter, the yang *qi* is sealed up and enclosed. Because it is sealed off and stored away, it should not be disturbed. This is analogous to when we stay in a hotel and hang a "Do Not Disturb!" sign on the doorknob of our room. Everyone has experienced the particularly uncomfortable sensation of being rudely awakened from sound slumber. Now then, how do we manage to avoid disturbing the yang? The above passage discusses four aspects.

Firstly, we must be cautious in our daily routine. During the three months of winter, our daily routine should entail retiring early and rising late, waiting for the light of day before rising, as the *Plain Questions* tells us. Personally, I detest oversleeping, and I do not make a habit of wasting my morning lazing in bed. However, the *Yellow Emperor's Classic* suggests that we make an exception during the three months of winter. We are instructed to go to bed a little earlier and get up a bit later, after the light of day is upon us. I have always thought that Chinese Medicine schools should disregard daylight savings time and instead adopt a schedule in accord with the "Great Treatise on the Four *Qi* and the Tuning of the Spirit." Such a schedule would provide for a period of relative rest during the three winter months, and thereby accord with the principles of Chinese Medicine, harmonizing human activity with the four seasons. I believe that retiring early and rising late, waiting for the light of day before rising, would be welcome advice to most people. Who doesn't like to sleep in a bit during the winter? Maybe this bit of advice alone is enough to make you like the *Yellow Emperor's Classic* and Chinese Medicine.

Why should we retire early and wake up late during the winter? This is in order to nourish the storage of yang *qi*. Sleeping is a state in which we are storing up and recuperating, and since the three months of winter are the season of storage, we should naturally extend our sleep. During the winter, the days are short and the nights are long; the shadow of the staff at noon is over seven feet long in winter and less than a foot long in summer. The long shadows and long nights of winter reflect a state of storage and concealing in winter. Just as nature tucks things away, so it is only appropriate for us to also get into bed a little earlier and leave its warmth and comfort a little later than usual. In Chinese Medicine, it is often said that humans and nature should correspond to one another, but what kind of "correspondence" are we talking about? Nurturing storage in winter is one example of this sort of correlation; retiring early and rising late during the three months of winter is another.

If we want to understand mutual correspondence, we must realize that the temporal dimension is very important. During the winter months, heaven and earth are collecting and storing. When nature is collecting and storing, you too should collect and store. When nature is releasing and loosening, you should do the same. In concrete, practical terms, sleeping is collecting and storing, and working is releasing and emitting. In the present day and age, many people work at night and sleep during the day. This turns the natural organization of yin and yang upside down and is definitely harmful to the body. When a person is young, this harm may not be evident, but it will certainly be felt in old age. Students of Chinese Medicine must avoid this sort of inversion of yin and yang and instead seek to make their behavior reflect the temporal patterns of nature.

Secondly, this passage discusses the need to harmonize the emotions. The ideal emotional state during the three months of winter is described as: "The will should be as if hidden, as if one had private intentions, as if one's aims were already obtained." Here, the word "will" has two layers of meaning. One is willpower, or resolution, as defined in the *Kangxi Dictionary*: "The desires of the heart and mind are called the will." The second is what we might simply refer to as the "emotions." The *Commentary of Zuo* (Zuozhuan) contains a discussion of human emotions that summarizes them into the six "wills." Hence, this term can connote not only one's will or resolution, but also just the emotional state in general. During the winter months, we should keep our desires and emotions hidden below the surface. We should remain emotionally reserved during this time, and not be prone to emotional displays or overt expression. We tend to encourage others to be open and expressive about their emotions, but during this time we should tend toward introversion. "As if one had private intentions" means that we should keep our desires and intentions to ourselves and not tell others, concealing them inside our heart. "As if one's aims were already obtained" recommends that we assume an attitude of already having obtained what we desire and of not needing to seek it outside ourselves, so that we can remain peaceful. Put simply, our aims and resolutions, as well as our emotions, must be hidden instead of publicized; doing this is beneficial for storage.

Thirdly, it is fitting to ward off cold with warmth. During the three months of winter, we should "get rid of cold and seek warmth." This is an important point. Much of what we have already discussed depends upon this point. This point also presents us with a problem: we have said that cold is the *qi* of winter, and that cold is also the *qi* of storage. If we wish to nurture storage, it would seem, at first glance, that we should increase cold, not dispel it. Actually, there is no contradiction. In the summertime, we wear more than just our underwear. We also wear short-sleeved shirts and women wear skirts. In any case, whatever can be left bare is as exposed as possible. This manner of dressing is not simply a matter of staying cool; it has a cosmological correlation. At this time of year, heaven and earth are displayed. The days are especially long, and anything that can sprout from the earth is at the height of its growth. And so, our manner of dressing during this time accords with this sort of exhibition; this is a way of cultivating growth. During the winter, especially in the north, people wear thick fur coats, hats, gloves, and thick scarves. Wrapped up like this, their apparel parallels the winter theme of storage and concealment. This manner of dressing is also in complete accord with the dictum "Get rid of cold and seek warmth." By swathing the entire body so that it is almost completely hidden and shut off from the outside world, people in the winter accord with the mandate to nurture concealment and storage of their yang. Presently, of course, this manner of dressing is not considered fashionable. As a result, during even the coldest months here in China, we see women wearing short skirts and showing their skin. An understanding of Chinese Medicine causes us to disapprove of this style of winter dress. Among my friends are those who choose to wear skirts during the winter, and I find myself advising them against it. I tell them: "Right now you are young and you can take it, but once you have aged a bit, your joints are going to ache, you will develop bone spurs, and by then it will be too late." Of course, dispelling cold and increasing warmth includes a number of other methods for preserving heat and protecting against cold.

Fourthly, we should restrict our activity. During the three months of winter, we are admonished to "Avoid sweating and thereby disturbing the *qi* that is now in a state of storage." Naturally, we sweat when we engage in vigorous exercise, and this sweating causes a diminishment of *qi* and damage to the yang. The three months of winter are a time for sealing and storing, and during this time the skin should correspondingly be sealed off and closed up. Excessive sweating should be avoided. This statement prescribes the sort of exercise we should engage in during the winter months. The type of movement we engage in during the winter should be different from the other seasons of the year and have its own unique characteristics. Athletes who love vigorous exercise should pay particular attention to this advice. During the winter, athletes should avoid exercise that causes excessive sweating and engage in more meditative forms of training. In this way, they will act in accordance with the winter season. In this way, they will nourish storage.

II.2.c. Cold Damage Means Storage Damage

The four aspects we just discussed are in correspondence with winter and with nurturing storage. They all revolve around one basic principle—do not disturb the yang! In light of this fact, what about cold damage? Why is cold damage so significant? Its importance derives from this central theme, a violation of the above-mentioned basic principle of not disturbing the yang. Winter rules storage, and cold is the companion of this storage. Therefore, the cold of winter is extremely important. If the winter is not cold enough, what does this indicate? This indicates that the yang *qi* is still liberated and has not been collected and stored. That is why if a winter is warm rather than cold, farmers know that this does not bode well for next year's harvest. To use an idiom used by the ancients: "The rice will be expensive in Chang'an."

In my hometown in Hunan province, we have a saying: "When you hear thunder in winter, of ten cattle pens, nine will be empty." Thunder should not be heard until the spring. The third seasonal term after *Lichun* (Beginning of Spring) is called *Jingzhe* (Awakening of Insects), and it is during this period that thunder should begin to rumble. The thunder that sounds during the spring causes the myriad hibernating forms of life to awake and emerge from their deep sleep. The sound of thunder heralds the rousing and release of yang from storage. What does it mean when thunder occurs during the winter months? The sound of thunder signifies that the sealing and storage of yang are shattered. When the sealing and storage are broken in this way, the yang *qi* is released at the wrong time, disrupting the storage of yang, and causing the substance of yang to be deprived of its proper measure of nourishment. If the substance of yang is insufficient, what can the function of yang bring into play? Thus, in the coming year, the function of yang is debilitated. If the creatures of the earth do not receive the benefit of yang activity, the whole natural order of things becomes confused. This portends not just a natural disaster but calamity for the whole planet. Not only plants, but also animals are affected by this sort of imbalance, as is suggested by the warning that ". . . of ten cattle pens, nine will be empty."

There is another popular saying in China: "An early spring snow foretells a year of abundance." Why is this so? In modern understanding, the freezing temperatures with a snowstorm in early spring kill plant diseases and noxious insects, thereby improving the harvest in the coming year. Of course, this is just one aspect of the way in which an early spring snow benefits agriculture. More importantly, such an event indicates that yang *qi* is in an exemplary state of storage. If the yang *qi* has been well preserved, the substance of yang receives ample nourishment, ensuring that when it is released, it will be especially beneficial. If the myriad things are amply supplied, there will naturally be an abundance of the "five grains." Furthermore, this timely snow indicates that yin and yang are especially well balanced, and that the natural order is undisturbed. This greatly reduces the likelihood of a natural disaster, boding well for the coming harvest.

We can also shed light on this process from a classical perspective. The *Plain Questions* tells us that "To stay in good health, we must attend to storage," and that "those who attend to yin live long." When you read the statement that "those who attend to yin live long," you may feel that its meaning contradicts what we said previously about the functional aspect of yang. If yang reflects and dominates longevity, why doesn't the *Plain Questions* say "those who attend to yang live long," instead of "those who attend to yin live long"? In the present day and age, people seem only to know about *yangsheng*, about nurturing the "emergence" (*sheng*) associated with spring, and about ideas like "movement is life." But where does "emergence" or birth come from? "Emergence" arises out of storage. The reasoning behind the five-element understanding that the water element gives birth to the wood element is clear to almost everyone. If we look at the natural world, especially the animal kingdom, we see that those animals that are especially quiet and reposeful live a long time. For instance, tortoises, snakes, and cranes are all tranquil animals that live relatively long lives. On the contrary, those animals that are quick to move about tend to live short lives. Daoists speak of attaining a state of emptiness and preserving genuine stillness; Confucians speak of contemplative sitting and of knowing when to stop; Buddhists discuss tranquility and the concentration of Chan (zen) meditation. All of these emphasize quiet and storing. Therefore, people cannot simply know activity, but must embrace a combination of activity and quietude.

As soon as our understanding of these principles is unobstructed, we can return to the original question. The *qi* of winter is cold, and this cold is the result of the yang *qi* of heaven and earth being covered up and concealed. The human realm corresponds to heaven and earth, and so at this particular time, people must also store up their yang *qi*. However, if winter weather is cold, at this time yang *qi* must still be released to warm the body, must it not? Since winter is supposed to be the time for storage, how do we resolve this apparent contradiction? This depends upon how well we succeed in "getting rid of cold and seeking warmth." During this time, we need to cover our bodies with adequate clothing and, if necessary, turn the heater on. We need to rely upon the accoutrements of our man-made environment and allow our yang *qi* to rest and recuperate. After our yang *qi* has undergone this process of reaccumulation, then we can go about our usual implementation of its functional aspect. If we fail to practice "getting rid of cold and seek warmth" effectively, our body experience cold damage. When the yang *qi* is not permitted to sit quietly but is instead roused from its slumber, it of course immediately enters into a state of release. When the yang *qi* is disturbed in this way, the process of "nourishing yang" is disrupted, and the "substance" aspect of yang is spoiled. This of course has a thoroughly negative effect on the functional component of yang. From this perspective, it should be clear how significant the concept of cold damage really is. In reality, "cold damage" is the same as "storage damage." It destroys the entire process of nourishing yang. When the "substance" of yang *qi* is harmed and this fundamental element of human health is not secure, there is nothing for the functional aspect of yang to utilize or implement. If this functional aspect has nothing to utilize, it cannot act as the safeguard of longevity, and it cannot circulate on the exterior or consolidate. As a result, the organism suffers not only from wind-strike, cold damage, damp warmth, heat disease, and warm disease, but from any of the hundred diseases that may arise. There are more than just five types of cold damage; there can be ten, a hundred, a thousand, or even myriad.

When we contemplate cold damage from the perspective of it breaking either of the two relationships discussed above, namely cooperative hierarchy or the substance-function relation, we can easily see how important it is. Going back to the original discussion, and the three questions we asked at the outset, this understanding of cold damage explains why the *Yellow Emperor's Classic* says that heat disease belongs to the category of cold damage, why the *Classic of Difficulties* divides cold damage into five categories, and why Zhang Zhongjing used the term "cold damage" in the title of his book.

Having completed this introduction to the guiding theme of cold damage, a series of related questions emerge. This is our opening to the classics, and at the same time one method for studying the classics.

CHAPTER THREE

THE FUNCTIONING OF
YIN AND YANG

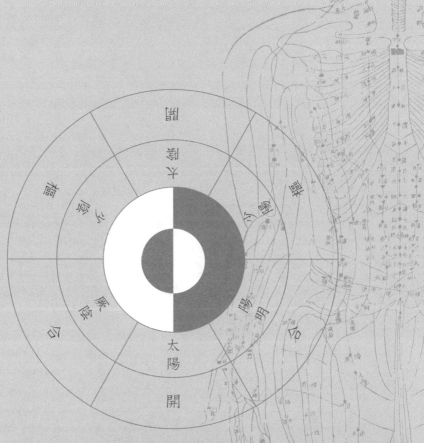

As for yin and yang,
if we count ten variations, we can deduce a hundred.
If we count a thousand, we can deduce myriad.
If we count myriad,
our deductions are beyond counting.
In truth, there is only one essential factor.

In the previous chapter, we discussed the significance of cold damage. Cold damage means impairment of the retrieval and storage of yang, impairment of the substance or body of yang. The consequences of this influence then create a ripple effect that touches all aspects of yin and yang. We already described the process of transformation between yin and yang above, but in broad terms that were not thorough enough for a process of such complexity. In this chapter, we will therefore look at this process in more specific detail.

I. The Dao Produces the One, the One Produces the Two, the Two Produce the Three, and the Three Produce the Myriad Things

I.1. Change Contains the Supreme Ultimate, Which Is What Produces the Two Polarities

We have already discussed yin yang above in quite some detail and made a number of observations. Now let us look at mechanism by which yin and yang operate. Once we have a clear understanding of this, many issues surrounding the *Treatise on Cold Damage* will be easily comprehended. Yin and yang constitute an organic whole with two aspects, one thing that is divisible into two. Its origin is closely related to the *Classic of Changes.*

Confucius in his *Great Commentary of the Classic of Changes* said: "Change contains the Supreme Ultimate (*taiji*), which is what produces the two polarities." What are these two polarities? They are yin and yang. Therefore, yin and yang come from the Supreme Ultimate. The Supreme Ultimate is an important concept in the system of the *Classic of Changes.* If this concept is not clearly understood, many Chinese Medicine concepts do not make sense. The character *tai* (太, "supreme") in *taiji* is quite commonly used in the Chinese language, and it can be translated into English as "extremely" or "excessively," but it also denotes seniority, respect, and grandness. The character *ji* (極, "ultimate") is a different story. The early dictionary *Explaining Writing and Analyzing Characters* defines *ji* as the ridgepole of a house, the highest point of the roof. The term *taiji* thus clearly refers to something that exceeds or is higher than this uppermost point. In this sense, it is an abstract term and might be thought of as "higher than the highest point." But does it have a more concrete definition? Regarding the concept of *ji*, we find a specific definition in the *Arithmetic Classic of the Gnomon and the Circular Paths of Heaven*:

> The way to calculate yin and yang is by the sun and moon. Nineteen years is called a *zhang*. Four *zhang* constitute a *bu*, equivalent to 76 years. Twenty *zhang* form a *sui*, equivalent to 1,520 years. Three *sui* form a *shou*, equivalent to 4,560 years. Seven *shou*, finally, form one *ji* ("Ultimate"), equivalent to 31,920 years. At the completion of this large cycle, the counting is concluded and all living creatures start over again. Heaven recommences its movements, and a new calendar is instituted.

The preceding passage discusses five important concepts, each a measure of time: *zhang* ("chapter"), *bu* ("shed"), *sui* ("succession"), *shou* ("chief"), and *ji* ("ultimate"). One *zhang* or "chapter" is nineteen years, and this unit of time would appear to be a sort of pervasive law. Why, for example, does the "Great Treatise on the Essentials of Ultimate Truth" in the *Plain Questions* speak of only nineteen disease triggers? Why isn't dryness, for example, added into the mix, as the renowned physician Liu Wansu did in the twelfth century? Here, it is a question of structural integrity: we cannot casually add to or subtract a condition from the nineteen that are listed. This structural pattern is strictly adhered to and absolutely unambiguous. Continuing on, we find that four "chapters" form a "shed," twenty "sheds" form a "succession," three "successions" form a "chief," and seven "chiefs" form an "ultimate." And how many years is an "ultimate"? No less than 31,920! That is to say, 31,920 years constitute an "Ultimate." After this period of time, there is an enormous transformation: "The counting is concluded and all living creatures start over again."

When this farthest point in time is reached, everything that can be counted ceases to be, and all life and the conditions that permit life end. Afterward, everything starts over, and all living things begin again in an ever-renewing cycle. Thus, the world and the universe proceed in a sort of rhythmic advance. At the beginning of every new "ultimate," astronomically speaking, a new era begins, and with it a new historical period.

This ancient information about "ultimate" periods should not be dismissed as nonsense. Consider modern science's understanding of the universe and its most basic cosmological underpinnings. From the perspective of a thermodynamic "heat death" of the universe, the big bang theory, and the law of entropy, the universe is born from a "big bang," and after this birth, continuously develops in accord with the law of entropy, until it reaches the point of maximum entropy. At this point, all the energy of the universe has been completely expended, everything becomes deathly still, and the universe faces an unavoidable death. This is equivalent to "the counting is concluded and all living creatures start over again," or in other words, the time when the end of a *ji* ("ultimate") cycle is at hand. Can it be that this state of "heat death," of maximal entropic exhaustion, persists indefinitely? If that were the case, how can we account for the universe prior to the big bang that set the current known universe in motion? How did our current civilization come into being from a state of seeming nothingness? This state of heat death cannot persist forever; it must change and transform, bring forth another big bang, and allow for a time when "all living creatures start over again." This process was referred to by the ancient Indian philosophers as successive stages of "becoming, remaining, decaying, and emptiness." After the universe takes shape, there is a long phase of "remaining" that takes place. But this "remaining," if we take into account the law of entropy, is a process of constantly increasing entropy. This entropy increases up to a point and then produces a state in which all energy is completely annihilated. At this point, entering into a state of complete emptiness is inevitable. This sequence of transformations forms one cycle, and when that cycle is complete, a new one begins, and another process of "becoming," "remaining," "decaying," and "emptiness" ensues.

From the information above, we can see that the *Arithmetic Classic of the Gnomon and the Circular Paths of Heaven*, the ancient Vedic texts, and modern science all agree in many respects, but that there is still a major discrepancy in terms of the overall length of the cosmological cycles. Of course, modern scientists have advanced technological devices that allow them to ascertain the true length of this process. The ancients did not have such technology and were therefore able to intuit the overall process and its immense scale but not its actual timeline. This alone should remind us that we cannot take the writings of the ancients lightly. If we pass over their writings as too simple and naïve, we will miss much that is profound.

In China, the ancients clearly delineated the cycle of coming into being, remaining, decaying, and fading back into nothingness as one that lasted 31,920 years and was called "Ultimate." At the end of each cycle, they wrote, massive changes take place, life and all phenomena cease, and everything is destroyed. Nevertheless, if everything is destroyed, how do the myriad living creatures come back into being? The ancients realized that in order for there to be a transition from one *ji* cycle to the next, there must be something higher than this cycle itself, something external to the Ultimate. Just as, when we find a child, we assume that there must be a mother, the ancients presumed there to be a superior accompaniment to this Ultimate. And this superior progenitor was what they called "Supreme Ultimate" (*taiji*). This is how the concept of Supreme Ultimate came into being. After the complete annihilation at the end of the cosmological cycle, it is the Supreme Ultimate that permits phenomena to come back into being, that allows for the resurgence of life and renewal of the cycle of becoming, being, decay, and oblivion.

So what sort of thing is this Supreme Ultimate? It is the mechanism whereby the cosmological cycle can be renewed instead of being broken, and life can come to an end and then return. The Supreme Ultimate is like a ring that has no end. If we look at the "Chart of the Supreme Ultimate" (*Taijitu*) map passed down by Zhou Dunyi of the Northern Song dynasty, we see that it consists of a completely empty circle. This sort of picture, of an unbroken circle, is the perfect representation of the meaning of *taiji*. It is regrettable that later many people adopted the black and white yin yang pattern that is so readily seen nowadays to represent the Supreme Ultimate. That symbol is a completely inaccurate representation. The yin yang symbol represents the two polarities of yin and yang, and might be considered a depiction of yin and yang. Of course, if the empty circle representing the Supreme Ultimate is depicted around the yin and yang symbol, then it might be referred to as a Supreme Ultimate yin yang symbol. That is acceptable. But to regard the yin yang symbol as a depiction of the Supreme Ultimate would be like regarding a picture of the child as depicting the mother. That is nothing short of ridiculous.

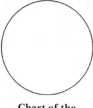

**Chart of the
Supreme Ultimate**

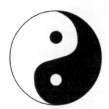

**Chart of the
Supreme Ultimate and yin yang**

In Confucius's Great Commentary of the *Classic of Changes*, he writes: "That which gives birth to creation is called change." He further states: "Change contains the Supreme Ultimate, which is what produces the two polarities. These two produce the four images, and the four images produce the eight trigrams. The eight trigrams determine good and bad fortune and our fortune determines our accomplishments." What is this "change"? Change is the material thing but also the principle that produces life. In this way, we can regard change as synonymous with the Supreme Ultimate. Several decades ago, when insulin was first synthesized, there was a trend of thought that emerged among scientists who believed that life could also be synthesized by science. They reasoned that if proteins could be created, and human beings are composed of proteins, we should also be able to create human beings. In the final analysis, can life be synthesized? Liang Shuming expressed a traditional perspective on this issue in his *The Human Mind and Human Life* (Renxin yu rensheng):

> In nature, the creation of life always begins with the differentiation and proliferation of cells, but the artificial creation of things by humans has always started from combining structures. I sincerely doubt that the current claim that we can synthesize life by combining structures is possible.

When life is created from a single cell, as it is in cloning technologies, the natural process of division and differentiation that nature employs to generate life is preserved. The growth of living things can only proceed through this sort of division of cells—how could it be otherwise? Life cannot be put together piece by piece. Only if the Supreme Ultimate creates the two yin and yang lines (literally the "two polarities"), and these produce the four images (i.e. combinations of two lines), and these in turn produce the eight trigrams, can life be created. This process cannot be reversed. Therefore, there is no basis for the possibility of synthesizing life, either in the world of modern science or in the ancient classics. On this point, we can see that both the traditional and the modern scientific views are in harmony. In my opinion, the deeper we go into the classics, the more profound the parallels between the understanding of the ancients and the discoveries of modern science. Of course, the opposite is also true. The more deeply we study science, the stronger of a foundation we have for an understanding of the ancient classics. Therefore, a robust dialogue between the ancient classics and modern science should be fostered. Only in this way can Eastern and Western cultures engage in a mutually meaningful and profitable exchange of what each has to offer. This dialogue must be balanced between the two perspectives if it is to be instructive. If one perspective dominates the other, a true exchange cannot be achieved.

When we consider our discussion regarding phrases such as "change is that which gives birth to creation," we realize that the classics should not be disregarded as irrelevant to a deeper understanding of modern science. The classics are pertinent not only to ordinary questions, but also to the most profound scientific problems. Life emerges from division and differentiation, not from synthesis. The Supreme Ultimate producing the two polarities is a process of division. The two polarities creating the four images is also a process of division. At the stage of the two polarities, yin and yang have just been established and life has not yet come into being. Only when we have the four "images" do we have a parallel with the cycle of emerging, growing, retrieving, and storing. At this point, very simple life forms such as microscopic plants can exist. At the stage of the four "images," there are four combinations of two lines: two yin, two yang, "greater yang and lesser yang," or "old yang and young yang." Further division brings us to the three yin and the three yang, and the advent of life as we know it. Therefore, if we wish to research life, especially human life, we must pay particular attention to the "three yin and three yang" phase of existence.

I.2. The Three Yin and Three Yang

In the system of the *Classic of Changes*, the levels of the two "polarities" and the four "images" are followed by the level of the eight trigrams (*bagua*). The eight trigrams also have three yin and three yang, but their meaning differs widely from what we mean by three yin and three yang in the context of Chinese Medicine. It should be mentioned here that the three yin and three yang of Chinese Medicine is a unique and almost independent sort of system. If we look at the *Plain Questions*, we find that the first few chapters talk only about two kinds of yin and two kinds of yang. This is especially true in Chapter 4 of the *Plain Questions*, "The Great Treatise on the Four *Qi* and the Tuning of the Spirit," where these two kinds of yin and two kinds of yang are referred to as Shaoyin, Taiyin, Taiyang, and Shaoyang. It is only once we get to Chapter 6, the "Treatise on the Separation and Union of Yin and Yang," that the three kinds of yin and three kinds of yang are clearly delineated. In addition to the two yin and two yang mentioned earlier, Jueyin and Yangming are added. The concept of yin and yang is found in almost every aspect of traditional Chinese culture, and every formal pursuit and profession makes use of yin and yang as part of their theoretical basis. Jueyin and Yangming are distinct in that they are found only in Chinese Medicine. No other field of traditional Chinese culture makes use of these concepts. This should lead us to the correct conclusion that Jueyin and Yangming are especially important in Chinese Medicine.

What is Yangming? What is Jueyin? The *Plain Questions* gives us a specific definition of these two concepts: the two yang, when they unite, become Yangming, and the two yin, when they exchange completely, become Jueyin. The other two yin and two yang are not specifically defined in the *Plain Questions*. This emphasizes the particular significance of Jueyin and Yangming to Chinese Medicine theory. There is a fundamental concept in Chinese Medicine, or, we might say, one of its most fundamental characteristics, which we have already discussed above: this is the holistic conception of the human body, in which the human being and the rest of the fabric of the cosmos are integral, where humanity and nature are one. This conception permeates Chinese culture just as yin and yang do. Confucianism, Daoism, every field of thought, has inherited this basic element. It might be said that this concept is the rock foundation on which the mansion of all traditional Chinese culture rests. In previous sections of the present book, we quoted from the "Great Treatise on the Four *Qi* and the Tuning of the Spirit." As a matter of fact, these above-mentioned passages were discussing this very concept.

As we have already discussed in previous chapters, why is it that we should nourish yang in spring and summer, and yin in fall and winter? Why should we nourish the emergence of life in spring and growth in summer? To stay in step with heaven and earth. When nature is in a state of bringing forth new life, so should you. Whatever the pattern of change and transformation assumed by heaven and earth, we should assume a like pattern. This is the mutual correspondence of humanity with the cosmos; this is the conception of the human being as an organic microcosm. This is precisely the Dao! Those who obtain the Dao will be greatly assisted, while those who lose sight of the Dao receive little support. This has been the gist of the traditional view of nature from the beginning. If we wish to keep pace with the changes of nature, we must first have a clear understanding of how heaven and earth change and transform. The most obvious unit, or layer into which the cycle of macrocosmic changes can be arranged, is the year. Every year, heaven and earth undergo a significant transformation. For instance, as of the writing of this book, the year 2000 is a *gengchen* year in the sexagenary cycle, while 2001 is a *xinsi* year in that cycle. *Gengchen* years are characterized by metal movement emerging early in a *taiguo* ("overstepping") pattern, with Taiyang cold water ruling heaven and Taiyin damp earth residing at the source. But in a *xinsi* year, the water movement emerges late in a *buji* ("falling behind") pattern, with Jueyin wind wood ruling heaven and Shaoyang ministerial fire residing at the source. One is characterized by the movement of metal, the other by the movement of water. In one case, this movement emerges early; in the other, it emerges late. Vast change thus occurs in just a single year. And within the framework of these large changes, there is a more fundamental, smaller unit of change, namely *qi*.

We have already discussed the concept of *qi* in Chapter One. It was originally one of Qi Bo's secrets but he was forced to explain it to the Yellow Emperor when asked. Thus, he told him that each year is divided into twenty-four *qi*, that within the framework of the year, a *qi* is the most basic unit of change, and that heaven and earth are constantly changing in accord with the succession of these units: from *Xiaoxue* (Minor Snow) to *Daxue* (Major Snow), from *Xiaohan* (Minor Cold) to *Dahan* (Major Cold). If humans wish to accord with the changes of the cosmos around them, they must do so in accord with these changes. When the cosmos shifts to the pattern of a new *qi*, we must follow in step. If we remain in the pattern of the previous *qi*, this is referred to as "falling behind." If heaven and earth have not yet shifted to a new pattern yet you stride ahead, this is called "overstepping." Whether you fall behind or overstep, you are still failing to correspond to the cosmos. What do we rely on to keep pace with the procession of *qi* without overstepping or falling behind? We must rely on the lungs. The *Plain Questions* chapters titled "Treatise on the Spiritual Orchid Secret Canon" and "Treatise on the Six Nodes and Visceral Manifestations" include the following two statements: "The lungs are in charge of governing the nodes," and "The lungs are the root of *qi*." These statements point out the particular capacity of the lungs. Concerning this question, which we already analyzed in detail in Chapter One, the lungs in the movement of *qi* and in the "Great Treatise on the Correspondences of Yin and Yang" are associated with Yangming. Yangming is the dry metal and rules the lungs and the large intestine. Therefore, in terms of the relative importance regarding the human correlation to nature, Yangming is exceptionally prominent.

If Yangming acts as the intermediary between heaven and earth with regard to *qi*, what does Jueyin do? Jueyin is associated with the wind and wood, and it rules the liver and gallbladder. In the *Plain Questions* chapter "Treatise on the Six Nodes and Visceral Manifestations," we learn that "The liver is the root of dismissal of the ultimate (*baji*) and the domain of the *hun* soul." What is the meaning of "dismissal of the ultimate"? In accord with many historical statements, including the position of the *Fundamentals of Chinese Medicine*, the general consensus is that this term *baji* refers to extreme exhaustion, but this interpretation seems somewhat illogical. Why is this? It is because the "Treatise on the Six Nodes and Visceral Manifestations" explores the normal physiological functions of the viscera and the bowels: the root of life, the root of storage, the root of *qi*, and the root of the granary, all of which touch upon the most important aspects of essential life processes. How then can we suddenly arrive at the "root of *baji*" and change the topic to fatigue and exhaustion? Suddenly, we find ourselves confronting a sort of reverse logic. What is this *baji* referring to exactly? Let's start with *ji*, which we have previously translated as "ultimate" in the term "Supreme Ultimate." In the previous description of the cycles of time, we learned that seven "chiefs" constitute one *ji* ("ultimate") and that one *ji* adds up to 31,920 years. Once that most distant point in time is reached, we arrive at the transformation described as follows: "At the completion of this large cycle, the counting is concluded and all living creatures start over again." Who will be able to witness this change? Who will live for a span of 31,920 years? Even the ancient Pengzu, famous for his longevity, only lived to be 800 years old. No one will survive long enough to witness this change. Luckily, this is irrelevant and does not prevent us from understanding it because we can use another concept from the arsenal of the *Yellow Emperor's Classic* to understand this idea: the concept of "images" (*xiang*). In the *Spiritual Pivot*, we find a chapter that focuses on this topic, titled "Division of the Proper Flow of *Qi* of One Day into Four Times" (Shunqi yiri fenwei sishi pian). Usually, the "four times" are the four seasons that take place over the course of a year. How then does this section in the *Spiritual Pivot* describe a day as consisting of spring, summer, fall, and winter? This is called "the principle of using the identical image." In terms of the "image," what is the most important aspect of spring, summer, fall, and winter? Spring, summer, fall, and winter are none other than the progression of birth, growth, gathering, and storage throughout the year. As we put it another way earlier, they can be described as "yang births and yin grows, yang kills and yin stores." These four aspects are clearly evident in the course of the year, but what of the far shorter cycle of a day? A day too exhibits birth, growth, gathering, and storage. So it is that Qi Bo said: "Morning is like spring, the middle of the day like summer, sundown like fall, and midnight like winter." Despite the significant difference in length, in symbolic terms and in terms of the transformations of yin and yang, there is really no difference between a day and a year. How can we say that "Morning is like spring, the middle of the day like summer, sundown like fall, and midnight like winter"? It is because in the morning the yang emerges, through the day yang grows, at sunset the yang is retrieved, and during the night yang is stored.

The lengths of the cycles may be different, but the changes and transformations of yin and yang are identical. This is what is referred to by "the principle of using the identical image." To take the season of spring as an example, it lasts for three months, while morning lasts for six hours or three of the twelve traditional Chinese two-hour periods into which the ancients divided the day. That is the only real difference.

Once we have recognized the relationship of "using the identical image," many difficulties are resolved. We know that vast cycles called *ji* are punctuated by a phase in which all life is extinguished and living things must be re-created. Is there a similar transformation at some point in the course of a year? We can compare the three months of winter with the three months of spring. The three months of winter are a period of closing and storing. This is particularly true in the north, where we see thousands of square miles frozen over, tens of thousands of square miles of snow in thick drifts. This is the perfect image of the myriad things withering and falling away, and the cessation of all birth and procreation. But when the harsh winter has passed and spring returns, the multitudes of living things surge back into life in all their glory. This transition from the absence of all life to the return of life's splendor, is this not more or less the same as the final phase of the *ji* period? We can see that the apparent changes that characterize the course of one year are analogous to those of a *ji*. The sequence from one year to the next is no different from the sequence from one *ji* cycle to the next, and operating from the same basic principle, the four seasons of the year can easily be discerned in the course of a single day. The mechanism by which we go from one year to the next is the same as that which allows one *ji*, when dismissed, to transition to the next *ji*. This brings us back to our discussion of the term *baji*. The meaning of this term is exactly as was just described: it impels one year to become the next, and drives the changes of the sexagenary cycle. It is the factor that drives the movement from one *ji* to the next. For instance, when a *gengchen* year shifts to a *xinsi* year and suddenly the pattern of excessive metal transport is replaced with one of insufficient water transport, we are faced with an abrupt and remarkable change.

As a human being, how do we make the transition from the energetic pattern of one year to the next, how do we handle the change and make the necessary shifts in our own bodies that ultimately will preserve us? We must rely on Jueyin for this, on the liver, on this "root of dismissal of the ultimate" (*baji zhi ben*). To connect with heaven and earth at the level of the transition from one year to the next, we must rely on the source or root of the "dismissal of the ultimate," on Jueyin. To connect and correspond with the cosmos during the transition from one of the twenty-four calendrical periods or node *qi* to the next, we must rely on the root of *qi*, on Yangming. This is similar to a radio. In order to listen to a particular radio program, the radio must be tuned to the same frequency as the one that the program is broadcast on. To do this, we turn the tuning knob. Often radios have two such knobs, one for fine-tuning and the other for making larger changes in the frequency received. Jueyin is the rough tuning knob, and Yangming the fine tuning knob. With these two, we can "attune" ourselves to whatever changes in "frequency" occur in the natural world. It is these exquisite mechanisms, of Jueyin and Yangming, that allow humans to accord with both the changes of the seasons and the changes of each year, thus preserving life. We can thus see that the structure of Chinese Medicine theory is not casually or randomly composed. It is very precise, concrete, and not to be underestimated.

II. The Mechanism of Yin and Yang Separating and Uniting

In the previous section, we discussed the significance of including Jueyin and Yangming to make the six-fold division of three yin and three yang. We also explained the importance of these two concepts and showed how some basic aspects of Chinese Medicine theory were determined after the three yin and three yang were established. Arriving at the sixth chapter of the *Plain Questions*, we see that it is called "Treatise on the Separation and Union of Yin and Yang." What is meant by this "separation and union" of yin and yang? To start with, when we speak of "union" (*he*), we are referring to a synthetic vision of yin and yang, viewing them as organic wholes. Here, yin and yang are discussed in the most general terms. At this level, there is one yin and one yang. From this unified or holistic perspective, in the system of the *Classic of Changes*, yin and yang might be referred to simply as the Dao. Therefore, the *Great Commentary of the Classic of Changes* states: "One yin, one yang, this is the Dao." When we earlier discussed how "Yang births and yin grows, yang kills and yin stores," we were talking at this unified, synthetic level. What then of the separated perspective? Here we are talking about yin and yang being differentiated into smaller fractions. The *Plain Questions* cites the infinite divisibility of yin and yang: "As for yin and yang, if we count ten variations, we can deduce a hundred. If we count a thousand, we can deduce myriad. If we count myriad, our deductions are beyond counting." If we divide it up in this way, how will we ever grasp its meaning? Therefore, when we speak of dividing yin and yang, we need not go so far. If we divide each into three parts, that will suffice. Dividing yin into three and yang into three, we have the three yin and the three yang. To use a Daoist saying: "A single *qi* contains three distinct creative potencies." Seen in this way, the phrase "separation and union of yin and yang" is talking about a sort of cooperation through a division of labor. This cooperation brings about what we discussed in the second chapter: the emergence, growth, expiration, and storage of yin and yang, or in other words, the release and retrieval of yang *qi*. In order to achieve such a process, we must have different mechanisms of action and engage in a division of labor. This issue is the key focus of the *Plain Questions* chapter "Treatise on the Separation and Union of Yin and Yang."

II.1. Introducing the Concept of a Hinged Door

When the "Treatise on the Separation and Union of Yin and Yang" in the *Plain Questions* discusses the separation and union of yin and yang in concrete terms, it states: "In the separation and union of the three yang, Taiyang opens, Yangming closes, and Shaoyang acts as the pivot. In the separation and union of the three yin, Taiyin opens, Jueyin closes, and Shaoyin acts as a pivot." One opens, one closes, and one acts as a pivot: What does this discussion refer to? Clearly, we are discussing a door. A door's function is clear to all. Open it and you can enter or exit through it. Close it, and you prevent entering or exiting. And what, exactly, allows a door to open and close? Its hinge. Therefore, if we differentiate the general concept of a door into its most basic elements, we find that there are three: open, close, and pivot. If a door does not close or open, it cannot even be considered a door, and in order for a door to open and close smoothly and with little effort, it must have some sort of pivot or hinge.

Earlier in this book, we discussed how the changes and transformations of heaven and earth are without exception changes that are characterized by rising and falling, exiting and entering. Therefore, the "Great Treatise on the Six Subtleties" (Liu weizhi dalun) of the *Plain Questions* explains: "Rising and falling, coming out and going in only pertain to vessels." And if something is marked by rising and falling, exiting and entering, then of course it also involves emerging, growing, gathering, and storing. What sort of "rising and falling, coming out and going in" are we talking about? The ancients contemplated this at length. Imagine if the concept of a door were not at hand, how would we be able to conceive of the sort of change that is characterized as exiting and entering in the *Plain Questions*? When do we exit, when do we enter, from where do we exit, and from where do we enter? An actual location is required. For this reason, the concept of the "door" came into being. Once we have this concept of a door, we can understand the rising and falling and entering and exiting changes of yin and yang far more easily.

In the "Great Treatise of the Four *Qi* and the Tuning of the Spirit" in the *Plain Questions*, we read:

> As for the four seasons and yin and yang, they are the root of the myriad things. Therefore in spring and summer the sages cultivate yang, and in

fall and winter they cultivate yin, following the essential course of each. Thus by following this root, they float and sink together with the myriad things at the door of birth and growth.

In this passage, the concept of the "door" is clearly taking shape within the intellectual framework of the *Yellow Emperor's Classic*. Here, "floating and sinking" entail exiting and entering as well as rising and falling. Sinking denotes entering, and floating exiting. On the one hand, we have "floating" at the "door of birth and growth." This process is none other than the emerging and rising of yang *qi*, which is in fact the same as the release of yang that we discussed earlier. On the other hand, we have "sinking" through the "door of birth and growth." This process refers to the entering of the yang *qi*, its descent, and is synonymous with the gathering and storage of yang. Why does this passage from the *Plain Questions* use the phrase "float and sink together with the myriad things"? Clearly, it is using the floating and sinking of the myriad things to represent the floating and sinking of yin and yang. The floating and sinking of the myriad things represent the varied physical manifestations that stem from the changes in yin and yang. Therefore, whenever we investigate any phenomenon, whenever we look, listen, ask, or feel the pulse, the goal is always to penetrate through this outer layer of physical manifestations and see to their root, the changes and transformations of yin and yang. The *Yellow Emperor's Classic* emphasizes this point when it states: "When diagnosing by observing the complexion or feeling the pulse, first you must distinguish yin and yang." Chairman Mao once wrote in a poem: "Ask the vast and boundless land, who rules floating and sinking?" If we borrow that question and answer it here in this discussion, it is certain that it is yin and yang that rule floating and sinking.

Now that we have established the concept of the door, we need some sort of working structure by which we can implement its function. This is the opening and closing pivot mechanism that we discussed earlier. In concrete terms, the three yang have their pivot for opening and closing, and the three yin their pivot for opening and closing. This means that we must have two separate doors: one yang door, dominated by the three yang, and one yin door, dominated by the three yin. The above-quoted passage from the *Plain Questions* only mentions one door for birth and growth. This is either an abbreviation or a deliberate omission, as there is also a door of gathering and storage. The yang door that is ruled by the three yang is the door of birth and growth, and the yin door ruled by the three yin is the door of gathering and storage. When the yang door is opened, that is to say, the door of birth and growth, the yang *qi* rises and is released. Following this release, the natural world displays the transformations of spring and summer, and the myriad things undergo a gradual process characterized by rising and floating. When the yin door of gathering and storage is opened, the yang *qi* enters and sinks downward, going into a state of storage. At this time, fall and winter begin, and the myriad things gradually sink back down.

Each door has its own separate function, but their action needs to be extremely well coordinated. This reflects the idea that they are separate but united. When the yang door opens, the yin door must gradually close at the same time. Otherwise, the yang *qi* will be exiting and entering at the same time, even to the point where more yang might be going in the yin door then what is exiting the yang door. Should this happen, the changes of spring, of birth and life, cannot come into being. Likewise, if the yin door opens but the yang door does not gradually close at the same time, the amount of yang exiting from the yang door may exceed that which is entering through the yin door, and the process of gathering and storage is thwarted. This process demonstrates the importance of yin and yang cooperating in coordination instead of being in opposition to each other. If the yang door opens and the yin door also opens, then the entire process of exiting and entering becomes chaotic. Again, according to "The Great Treatise on the Six Subtleties," "When exiting and entering are ruined, the transformation of the spirit trigger perishes; when rising and falling cease, the *qi* is orphaned and endangered." If the transformation of the spirit trigger perishes and the *qi* is orphaned and endangered, how can life be preserved? This is a matter of great concern!

When the *Treatise on Cold Damage* describes the six conformations in terms of three yin and three yang, in reality the book is talking about the two doors that we have just discussed above. These two doors must collaborate in close coordination, and the opening, closing, and pivoting of the three yin and three yang must be coordinated well. When this is the case, the rising and falling, exiting and entering of yin and yang cannot possibly malfunction, and as a result the spirit trigger and the coursing of the *qi* will not malfunction either. As the result, the person's life and health will be free of irregularities. With this understanding in mind, not only is the entire *Treatise on Cold Damage* clear, but also the rest of Chinese Medicine. Below, we discuss this matter more concretely.

II.2. The Opening, Closing, and Pivoting of Yin and Yang

II.2.a. The Opening, Closing, and Pivoting of the Three Yang

In the preceding discussion, we emphasized that close coordination of opening, closing, and pivoting is of the greatest significance for these doors. First, let us examine the "door" of the three yang. Among the three yang, Taiyang is responsible for opening. The expression "Taiyang opens" clearly denotes this responsibility. After Taiyang begins the process of opening the yang door, the yang *qi* gradually begins to rise as it is released and emerges from storage. In the natural world around us, this is clearly visible in the seasons of spring and summer, when nature displays her beautiful luxuriance. How does this luxuriance manifest in the human body? Every aspect of the function of yang *qi* aims at completely expressing its full potential. However, if Taiyang remains open too long and in a state of release for an extended period of time, it is like a person who works and works but never sleeps. It is unlikely that such a person will ultimately be successful. We have discussed this at some length in earlier passages and explored the shortfalls of constantly overextending ourselves. Taiyang opens up to a certain point, and then, by virtue of an innate mechanism, gradually begins to close again, causing the luxuriance of nature to recede and wither. The aspect that carries out this closing of the door of yang *qi* is Yangming, as pointed out in the *Plain Questions* line: "Yangming closes." Taiyang opens and Yangming closes. But how does one transition to the other? The transition between opening and closing depends on the pivoting function, and, as the *Plain Questions* points out, Shaoyang acts as this pivot.

II.2.b. The Opening, Closing, and Pivoting of the Three Yin

Now, let us examine the three categories of yin. Once the yang *qi* has risen and become released to a certain degree, the closing of the door by Yangming acts to cause a gradual attenuation of the yang *qi*. At this point, the yang *qi* changes its direction completely. Rising turns into falling, exiting into entering, and floating into sinking. At this time, the door of gathering and storage must start opening, so that the yang *qi* is not left outside. This process depends upon Taiyin, as the phrase "Taiyin opens" so aptly points out. Once Taiyin initiates the process of opening the door of gathering and storage, the yang *qi* enters into the state of gathering and storage in earnest. We have talked about what happens to the yang *qi* when left in a prolonged state of release. Would it be any better if it were perpetually left in storage? What sort of lazy good-for-nothing spends all his or her time sleeping in bed? Therefore, the yang *qi* is stored away up to a certain point, and then this storing action gradually diminishes. The door that has opened to commence the gathering and storage of yang *qi* slowly closes under the auspices of Jueyin. Taiyin opens, Jueyin closes, and Shaoyin acts as the pivot or hinge to facilitate the transition between opening and closing. This is the relationship of the three yin.

II.2.c. Collaborative Action

Regarding the two aspects we just discussed, we can see that close coordination between yin and yang is exceedingly important. Taiyang rules opening, and the opening mechanism and the release of yang *qi* begin. Once the yang *qi* is liberated to the appropriate degree, the release of yang *qi* ends, and it is Yangming that governs the closing of the opening mechanism. The timing between the functions governed by Taiyang and Yangming must be tuned precisely. As the release of yang *qi* diminishes, the trend must turn toward retrieval and storage. It is at this time that the yin door opens. If this fails to happen, and the release of yang *qi* diminishes without the beginning of gathering and storage, the rising and falling of yang *qi* goes awry. Therefore, the link between Yangming and Taiyin is especially important. One yin, one yang, one opening, one closing; in addition, there is a sort of tacit agreement between the two of them that allows for the smooth transition between release and storage of yang *qi*. On the other hand, once the act of storing has proceeded to a particular point, this process also slowly comes to a stop and the opening turns to closing under the guidance of Jueyin. Of course, just as with the transition from Yangming to Taiyin, the transition from Jueyin to Taiyang must be seamless and perfectly timed to avoid a blunder in the coordination of the rising and falling action of yin and yang. And so here too we have one yin, one yang, one opening, one closing, and a tacit agreement between Jueyin and Yangming that allows the transition from the sinking, entering process to the rising, exiting process.

During this process, yin and yang help one another. The opening of Taiyang requires the assistance of Jueyin. The opening of Taiyin requires the help of Yangming. The cooperation of Taiyang among the opening, closing, and hinging aspects of the three yang is very clear. The "Great Treatise on the Essentials of Ultimate Truth" in the *Plain Questions* states: "When attempting to cool a disease results in an increase of heat, approach it from the yin. When warming a cold disease paradoxically results in an increase of cold, approach it from the yang." We can take this idea presented in the *Plain Questions* and adjust it slightly to say: "When treating the yang, should it fail to recover, ask for assistance from yin. When treating the yin, should it fail to recover, ask for assistance from yang."

For instance, when we treat a disease that is clearly a Taiyang disease, but our efforts meet with no success, then we must remember that the opening of Taiyang is in part dependent upon the proper closing of Jueyin, and, applying the principle of "asking for assistance from yin" and try treating Jueyin. If we are confronted with a Taiyin disease, and there is no mistaking that it is Taiyin, but efforts to cure the illness using methods directed at restoring Taiyin are ineffective, then we should consider "asking for assistance from yang," and treating Taiyin by means of Yangming.

Here we have two methods, i.e. "When attempting to cool a disease results in an increase of heat, approach it from the yin. When warming a cold disease paradoxically results in an increase of cold, approach it from the yang"; and "When treating the yang, should it fail to recover, ask for assistance from yin. When treating the yin, should it fail to recover, ask for assistance from yang." To these two methods, we may also add the content of the following chapter in the section on the nineteen disease triggers, in which we discuss the method of treating each of the viscera through the five dominations. Once these methods are understood, they will allow us to treat many illnesses that are otherwise difficult to cure.

II.3. Pathological Changes of Opening, Closing, and Pivoting

We have discussed how loss of the normal functioning of the opening, closing, and hinging functions can result in pathological changes. Diseases of the six conformations, Taiyang, Shaoyang, Yangming, Taiyin, Shaoyin, and

Jueyin, are the result of imbalance between these three functions: pathology deriving from opening, closing, and pivoting.

II.3.a. Pathological Changes of Taiyang Opening

Taiyang governs opening, and is responsible for opening the yang door. In brief, the function of the opening mechanism of Taiyang is to assist the outward emergence of the yang *qi*, and to assist with the effective expression of the yang *qi*. Why does the function of Taiyang sometimes encounter problems? The cause can be internal or external or both simultaneously. External factors are typically more representative. We often see cold damage and wind-strike resulting from pernicious external influences attacking, hindering, or fettering the opening mechanism. This causes the yang *qi* to become constrained, and Taiyang illness ensues. Besides external factors, what internal factors induce Taiyang disease? If the yang *qi* is deficient, and the vitality of the person's body insufficient, then the opening of Taiyang can become problematic. Problems can also arise from water-rheum, accumulation of damp within the body, or other such variables that hinder the hinder the yang *qi* from emerging outward, and Taiyang's opening function may also encounter problems.

As we discussed earlier, the functions of the yang *qi* include outward dissemination, circulating and defending the exterior of the body, the transformation of *qi*, and so on. If the opening aspect of Taiyang encounters an obstruction, the various functions of the yang *qi* are influenced, and the advent of Taiyang diseases are directly related to this influence. The most common Taiyang disease is disease involving the exterior of the body, in which the attack of an external pathogen hinders the free circulation of *qi* on the exterior of the body. In addition, if the yang fails to transform the *qi*, fluid metabolism is disturbed, and we have diseases related to the accumulation of fluids and their subsequent interference with physiological processes.

If we examine the rubrics of Taiyang disorders—external syndromes, water *qi*, phlegm-rheum, and water amassment making up the vast majority—we can see that these all create pathology by interfering with the function of yang in the body, and all inhibit the opening of Taiyang. When we understand Taiyang disease as a failure of the opening mechanism of Taiyang, we have grasped its guiding principle.

II.3.b. Pathological Changes of Yangming Closing

The opening of Taiyang causes the yang *qi* to rise and be emitted outward. The closing Yangming causes the yang *qi* to be retrieved and to sink downward. After the yang *qi* is collected and descended, the weather turns dry, cool, and so Yangming corresponds to autumn. Now, if the closing mechanism of Yangming encounters a hindrance, that which should be collected by the yang *qi* is not collected, that which should descend does not descend, and circumstances characterized by heat and failure of the normal descending in the body result. Therefore, the two most salient features of Yangming disease are heat and a failure to descend. Heat manifests in the Yangming channel syndrome, while failure to descend appears in the Yangming bowel syndrome. Of course, heat, failure to descend, channel syndrome, and bowel syndrome can all mutually influence one another.

In the Yangming channel syndrome, Baihu Tang is used. This is very interesting. What is the "white tiger" (*baihu*)? The "white tiger" is the spirit of the western direction, and dominates the changes and transformations associated with that particular cardinal direction. What are those changes associated with the west? Principally, the collection and descent of the yang *qi*. When we use Baihu Tang to treat a Yangming disease, we are essentially saying that there is a problem in the collection and descent of the yang *qi*.

II.3.c. Shaoyang Pivoting Disease

Shaoyang governs the pivot, or hinge, and is responsible for regulating the opening and closing functions. If neither the opening nor the closing show any signs of trouble, it is unlikely that there are any problems with this hinge mechanism. If we look at the section of the *Treatise on Cold Damage* devoted to the three yang, there are 179 lines regarding Taiyang, and also a large number devoted to Yangming, but there are only ten or so lines devoted solely to Shaoyang. Is this because Shaoyang is unimportant? This is most certainly not the case. Shaoyang governs the hinge, whereby Taiyang and Yangming open and close. How could Shaoyang possibly be unimportant?

The relative scarcity of writing on the topic of Shaoyang is due to the fact that many of the pathological changes associated with Shaoyang are addressed in the lines devoted to Taiyang and Yangming. For instance, even though Xiao Chaihu Tang is universally recognized as a formula directed at diseases of Shaoyang, it is only mentioned once in Shaoyang section and appears multiple times in both Taiyang and Yangming sections of the *Treatise on Cold Damage*. The hinge mechanism rules opening and closing, so it is little wonder that the pathological changes associated with this hinge mechanism often center upon the functions of opening and closing. This is a key characteristic of pathology related to the pivot process.

In our previous discussion of cold damage and miscellaneous diseases, we discussed how we could categorize all diseases based on whether or not they involved fever. Disorders involving heat emission belong to the category of cold damage, and those that do not exhibit palpable heat production belong to the category of miscellaneous diseases. At this point, we can do something similar and categorize all diseases as opening or closing: diseases resulting from problems with opening, and diseases resulting from troubles with closing. Why can we say this? Because human physiology primarily relies upon rising and falling, exiting and entering. If the rising, falling, exiting, and entering of the body are normal, then the entire body will be normal. The instant the rising and falling, exiting and entering become irregular, all of the disease processes corresponding to that abnormality may arise. As we have already discussed, that which controls rising and falling, entering and exiting, are the opening and closing mechanisms. From this perspective, dividing all diseases into "closing" and "opening" categories is a theoretically valid approach. If we extend this concept a little further, we can see that the opening and closing functions are intimately linked with movement of the hinge or pivot. Hence, if we adjust the pivot, we are easily able to adjust the opening and closing. And the opening and closing allows us to adjust the rising and falling, exiting and entering. When we realize the relationship between the pivot mechanism and the rest of the organism, we also realize that by adjusting it, we can make countless adjustments in the rest of the human body.

Many of history's physicians gave preference to formulas containing Chaihu, an herb that has a special affinity with the pivot. One such formula is Xiao Chaihu Tang, which adjusts the yang pivot. Another is Sini Tang, which adjusts the yin pivot. Apt use of these Chaihu decoctions with the correct modification of other ingredients provides the physician with the tools to treat countless illnesses across the clinical spectrum. For instance, the late Chen Shenwu, an eminent physician of the Beijing Chinese Medicine

College, as well as Jiang Erxun, who lived in the medicinal herb producing mountains of Sichuan, both gave preference to formulas that featured Chaihu.

History often refers to the physicians who hold a preference for Chaihu formulas as members of the Chaihu school. The emergence of an entire school based on the use of a single formula is quite something, and this phenomenon merits serious contemplation. How is it that modified Chaihu formulas can cure so many different diseases? One reason for this is its particular action on the pivot. Therefore, instead of thinking that because Shaoyang section only has ten lines of writing it must be unimportant, we should consider the specificity of the pivot mechanism. If the pivot's influence alters the opening of the organism, then the pathological changes will manifest in Taiyang. If alterations in the pivot affect the closing aspect, then the disease will manifest in Yangming. And so it is that many diseases encountered in the clinic that have pathology related to either Taiyang or Yangming fail to respond when the treatment is directed at the particular conformation, but we find that these same diseases can often be readily resolved by addressing the pivot.

II.3.d. Pathological Changes of Taiyin Opening

Taiyin governs the opening of the yin door (the door of collecting and storing) through which the yang *qi* enters into storage. If Taiyin opening mechanism becomes disturbed, its effects will influence the passage of yang *qi* inward. This internalization of yang *qi* has two functions: it allows yang *qi* itself to rest and recuperate, and in addition the internalized yang *qi* warms and nourishes the internal organs. So when the internalization of the yang *qi* is hindered, the resulting disharmony has two facets: first, the yang *qi* cannot recuperate; second, the internal organs are not properly warmed and nourished. When the organs fail to receive warmth and nourishment, Taiyin disease can come about.

Therefore, the dominant themes of Taiyin disease are summed up in the first line of the outline on Taiyin:

> When Taiyin becomes diseased, there is abdominal fullness and vomiting, inability to eat, severe spontaneous diarrhea, intermittent spontaneous abdominal pain, and downward purging results in a hard bind below the chest.

All of these symptoms result from a loss of warmth and nourishment in the organs—or, put another way, cold exerting its influence upon the organs. This is just as it says in line 277: "Spontaneous diarrhea without thirst belongs to Taiyin. It is due to cold among the viscera, and it should be warmed. It is suitable to use a Sini formula." These two excerpts from the *Treatise on Cold Damage* make it clear that a loss of warmth in the internal organs is the dominant theme of Taiyin disease. If Taiyin opening mechanism is out of order, yang *qi* does not recuperate well, the person's vitality is not reinvigorated or restored and the yang *qi* is enfeebled. At this point, the situation can make a grave turn, and turn into Shaoyin disease. When treating Taiyin disease, we primarily use warming and nourishing approaches like a Sini type of decoction, which also serves to illustrate this point.

Taiyin belongs to spleen-earth, and the earth element in the body is in charge of fostering storage. Storage of what? Storage of the yang *qi*. The earth has the ability to bring forth and nourish the myriad things and relies upon this yang *qi* to do so. It is by means of this yang *qi* that the earth is able to bring forth every sort and color of living thing. The earth, and here we mean the soil and ground, not the planet, is in this sense inseparable from the "opening" and "storing" of the yang *qi*. If the opening mechanism encounters an obstacle, then the storage, and birthing and nourishing functions will be impeded.

II.3.e. Shaoyin Pivoting Disease

Shaoyin also governs the pivot or hinge, and its functioning, like that of Shaoyang, can influence either opening or closing functions. The importance of the Shaoyin pivot mechanism is somewhat greater than that of Shaoyang pivot, as Shaoyin guides the pivotal transition between water and fire. Shaoyin is the layer associated with both water and fire, and so its pivoting has an effect on the regulation of fire and water in the body. Water and fire are not incompatible with one another; in fact, they must mingle with one another, rely on one another, and harmonize each other.

If the Shaoyin pivot malfunctions, it will have an influence on the harmonization of water and fire in the body. This may manifest as excess water and cause cold, or it may manifest as an excess of fire, and give rise to heat. Thus, the nucleus of the Shaoyin section is centered on cold transformation and heat transformation.

Shaoyin is truly centered on the form of yang. We say that the three yin comprise the form and the three yang comprise the function. Yin is form and yang is function. The pathology of the three yang is characterized by a hindrance of yang function. When the function is impeded, it is not a very big problem. To use a modern medical term, we are still in the realm of "functional disease"—in other words, disease in which the symptoms cannot be directly related to any detectable lesion or structural derangement. Diseases of the three yang rarely kill anyone. When the disease process progresses to the three yin, the physical form is threatened. This is what is referred to as "organic disease," in which there is an appreciable physical damage to the organs or tissues.

Form and function: the first denotes the material substance and its quality, the second denotes its usefulness and efficacy. The Shaoyang pivot is crucial to the function, whereas the Shaoyin pivot is crucial to the form. The preservation of the form depends upon the function of the Shaoyin pivot, so its turning is extremely important. Why are there so many fatal syndromes that belong to Shaoyin disease? It is because if Shaoyin is disordered, the physical form of the yang cannot be maintained.

II.3.f. Pathological Changes of Jueyin Closing

We have already discussed how Jueyin is in charge of closing the door through which the yang *qi* is stored, and how once this closing process is set in motion, the process of storage is terminated, and the state of release ensues. As we have said before, Jueyin is the root of the *baji* (dismissal of the ultimate), and the *baji* is what brings about the transition from a state of storage to a state of rebirth. In fact, it reinitiates the entire cycle of birth, growth, harvesting, and storage. As described previously, Taiyin and Shaoyin are both harvesting and storing, and once we arrive at Jueyin, this process comes to an end and turns into a state of rising, emitting, and emerging. If this process is hindered, the result is that the yang *qi* cannot emerge when it ought to, and there is a buildup of heat. This heat is different from Yangming heat. Yangming heat is the result of yang *qi* that remains on the external part of the body, yang that should descend but fails to descend and thus produces heat. Jueyin heat is the result of yang *qi* trapped in the interior; it cannot escape and heat is generated. Based on this understanding, we can differentiate Yangming and Jueyin heat in the following way: the first is external heat, and the second is internal heat; the first is heat of the *qi*, and the second is heat of the blood.

The factor that most easily creates an obstruction to the closing mechanism of Jueyin, the influence that most readily prevents the transition from collection and storage to the emergence of the yang *qi*, the energy that is most antithetical to the process of emerging outward, is of course cold (*han*). Cold governs contracture and tautness, and so by definition, it most easily hinders the process of emergence and growth. This is further demonstrated by the fact that much of the section on Jueyin disease is concerned with heat and cold complex. Thus, the herbs that are discussed in this section are the very cold, very bitter Huanglian and Huangbai as well as the highly acrid and very hot Chuanjiao, Xixin, Fuzi, Guizhi, and Ganjiang. At first glance, this mix of hot and cold herbs seems contradictory, but in reality this is the very situation with Jueyin, namely that it is susceptible to heat and cold complex: the erroneous melding of cold and heat. In the past, many have found the section on Jueyin to be the most maddening part of the *Treatise on Cold Damage*. When analyzed from the perspective of its role as a closing mechanism, we discover that it is not so difficult to comprehend.

At this point, we have discussed the opening, closing, and pivot mechanisms with regard to the three yin and the three yang, as well as the six conformation diseases. Although our discourse so far constitutes only a rough outline of the topic, the basic order of the six conformation diseases is now revealed to us. On this basis alone, it should be acknowledged that this perspective provides an exceptionally expedient route to study the *Treatise on Cold Damage*.

II.4. Cold Damage Is Transmitted through the Legs, Not the Arms

In the "Treatise on the Separation and Union of Yin and Yang" in the *Plain Questions*, the three yin and three yang of the legs are mentioned, but the three yin and three yang of the arms are not. Furthermore, in the *Spiritual Pivot* chapter "Clinging Root," the issue of opening, closing, and the pivot are discussed in relation to the leg channels. When the channels of the arms are discussed, this topic is never brought up. In addition, in "Treatise on Heat" in the *Plain Questions*, the origin of the concept of cold damage (*shanghan*), the legs are discussed but not the arms. These examples caused later generations to mistakenly assume that cold damage was transmitted through the legs but not the arms, and that warm disease was transmitted through the arms, and not the legs.

An important concept of Chinese Medicine is the organic conception of the human body. If human beings and the cosmos are one unified, organic entity, and changes in the cosmos have an effect on the human body, how then could the arms and legs not have any effect on each other? How could there be no transmission between the two? However, when these issues were discussed in *Yellow Emperor's Classic* and *Treatise on Cold Damage*, there is no doubt that they laid particular stress on the legs. Why? If we wish to clarify this question, we must first ponder it from a few different perspectives.

First, in terms of our cultural significance, what are human beings? Human beings are the most favored of all creatures. It is no small thing for us to have been given this life, so we really ought to do something good, something that is of benefit to oneself and to other people. There are some types of work that benefit one's self, without necessarily benefiting one's country or other members of society. The practice of medicine, however, only requires that you make up your mind not to do evil, and you will almost invariably bring benefit both to yourself and to others.

In the *Plain Questions*, it often says: "People are born from the *qi* of heaven and earth." Therefore, to observe and study human beings, we must place them within the framework of heaven and earth. The ancients often spoke of heaven and earth in terms of *jing* and *wei*, referring to the lengthwise and side-to-side threads used in weaving. In the *Romance of the Three Kingdoms*, we often come across the phrase "heaven *jing* and earth *wei*." *Jing* was used to refer to heaven and *wei* to earth. *Jing* connects north and south, above and below; and *wei* connects east and west, right and left. This conception of *jing* and *wei* is seemingly simple, but can we use this simple concept to contemplate some deeper issues in Chinese Medicine? Let us consider for a moment why we are the most favored among the myriad things. Among animals, with the exception of humans, all crawl on four legs, with its body horizontal. Humans are the only animals that stand upright. From this perspective, humans are the only creatures that walk aligned with *jing*; all the other animals walk aligned with *wei*. In terms of the amount of *qi* that we receive, humans receive the greatest amount of celestial *qi*, and the rest of the creatures receive relatively little. This is an important factor influencing how humans became the most favored of all creatures.

Second, most readers will be familiar with the "heavenly stems" and "earthly branches" of Chinese astrology. However, has anyone ever asked why we do not refer to the stems as earthly and the branches as heavenly? It is because the stem is vertical, and the branch horizontal. Therefore, the stem corresponds to heaven and the branch corresponds to earth. Although all living things grow upon the earth, if these creatures wish to grow well, then they cannot do without the heavens and cannot go without the sun. During the Cultural Revolution, we often sang a communist song that expressed this idea. It went like this: "Sailing the great sea we rely on the helmsman, all living creatures depend on the sun." Although the flowers, leaves, and fruit grow on the branches, they depend upon the stem or trunk to receive nourishment. The concept of stems and branches reflects the significance of heaven and earth, of *jing* and *wei*, and of the difference between humans and other animals.

Third, whether the animal walks upright like a human or crawls on all fours, from the perspective of image (*xiang*), the head corresponds to heaven and the feet to earth. Hence, it says in the *Plain Questions*: "The sages used the image of the heavens to nourish their heads and the image of the earth to nourish their feet." What does it mean to nourish one's head? The sages were very clear about this: it means to contemplate the heavens. This activity was able to nourish their heads and develop their brainpower. Of course, this is a postnatal activity, and there is no way to change prenatal characteristics, which are already fixed.

Human beings walk aligned with *jing*, the axis of heaven. We are endowed with the greatest amount of celestial *qi*, and the head corresponds with the heavens. Why do humans have such a well-developed intellect? Why is it that only humans have a capacity for intellectual thought? Why are humans the only creature that possesses our sort of intelligence and wisdom? Why are we so different from all other animals? The essential reason lies with our endowment of celestial *qi*. What about the other creatures of the earth? They walk in line with the *wei*, and in terms of their prenatal endowment, they receive the greatest amount of terrestrial *qi*, which corresponds with the legs. The legs of an animal are incomparably stronger than those of a person. Who can outrun a horse, a tiger, or a monkey? We cannot even outrun a cat or a dog, or, for that matter, a chicken. Even China's great runner Ma Jiajun could not accomplish this feat! Why? Animals are imbued with a full store of terrestrial *qi*, and humans possess far less. Of course, we could argue that we are faster on our feet than some animals, such as ants or tortoises. However, if we consider speed relative to size, or compare endurance, then there is still no comparison.

Fourth, let us consider the posture humans assume in sleep. There are those who might ask, considering our connection with *jing*, why do we lie horizontally to sleep? This is a good question. Of all animals, only the sleeping posture of humans is different from the one assumed when awake. Do the postures of other animals change when they sleep? Besides a change in the overall height of their posture, their horizontality does not change. When we are awake, we are erect, vertical. When we sleep we lie level. When we are upright, we receive the celestial *qi* and when prostrate, the terrestrial *qi*. Why does it say in the *Plain Questions* that people are born of the *qi* of both heaven and earth, and that both our celestial and terrestrial *qi* are complete? The answer is reflected in the change of posture between waking and sleeping. Human beings receive not only celestial *qi*, but also terrestrial *qi*. Our "brains are not simple, and our four limbs are also developed." Of course, in terms of relative amounts, our share of terrestrial *qi* cannot compare with that of animals.

The strength in Ma Jiajun's legs is excellent, she can run ten kilometers in no time at all because her coach Ma Junren knew how to train the strength and endurance of his team members. However, I believe that if Coach Ma did some research into Chinese Medicine, and discovered a method whereby his runners could maximize their quotient of terrestrial *qi*, his team would be able to win even more Olympic gold medals.

Fifth, with regard to the factors that we have just discussed and which contribute to humans being the most favored creatures on earth, the crucial factor lies with the fact that humans are born of the *qi* of both heaven and earth, of *jing* and *wei*, and of these two it is the heaven *jing* that we are predisposed to. It is this aspect that is key in defining what makes humans unique. It is this aspect of *jing* gathering together *wei* that defines humans and their role in the world.

This also leads us to think about why it is that in Chinese Medicine the acupuncture channels are referred to as the twelve *jing* rather than the twelve *wei*! And why it is that the writings of the sages are referred to as *jingdian* (classics)! Once we have made sense of a few of these theoretical underpinnings, we can begin to unravel some of the puzzles introduced at the beginning of this section. Let us apply our new understanding to the question of cold damage being transmitted through the legs.

Among the twelve channels of the body, which channels truly traverse the north and south of the body, and link the upper with the lower? The channels of the arms only traverse half the body, and in that sense, they are not really *jing*, as they do not truly represent that which makes us uniquely human. Only the channels of the legs connect north with south in a truly longitudinal fashion. They travel from the head to the feet, from heaven to earth, traversing the entire human body. Therefore, the leg channels truly represent the concept of *jing*.

In the *Yellow Emperor's Classic* and the *Treatise on Cold Damage*, when it comes to discussing important questions, they only mention the leg channels. The reason these are used as representatives is because they are *jing* in the true sense of the word. In reality, the leg channels connote the arm channels as well, since the channels of the arms are gathered together or embraced by the leg channels, in the way that the side-to-side threads in a piece of cloth are held together by the lengthwise threads. And so when these texts mention the leg channels, they are not speaking of the leg channels solely, nor are they talking about a situation in which a pathogen traverses the leg channels without continuing to the arm channels. The preceding discussion should make this point more clear.

Sixth, now that we have discussed the above issues, we can discuss six conformation syndrome differentiation and how it is different from other methods of syndrome differentiation. Of course, those practitioners who are from Warm Disease schools of thought emphasize differentiating the four levels (defense, *qi*, construction, and blood) and the three burners (*sanjiao*), while those who study the viscera and bowels may say that only organ syndrome differentiation and eight-principle syndrome differentiation are needed. So when those of us who focus on cold damage emphasize the six conformation differentiation of syndromes, aren't we just another seller hawking our own wares in the marketplace?

I do not believe this is simply a case of different sellers all hawking their own wares. There has to be a good reason for choosing one diagnostic method over another, and for me, it is not simply a matter of personal pref-erence or emotional attachment. So why is six conformation differentiation superior? For the very reasons we just discussed: it is a longitudinal method of differentiating syndromes, it traverses both heaven and earth, and it is truly is a *jing* method of differentiation in all the senses of the word. For these reasons, this particular method of differentiation is best matched to the essential nature of human beings, it is most capable of reflecting that which makes humans human, and therefore it is best able to reveal the essence of disease.

In the *Plain Questions*, it says: "To treat disease, we must seek the root." We might say that this model of syndrome differentiation is the simplest method to arrive at the source of disease. Little wonder then that later gen-erations referred to six conformation differentiation as the model able to "indicate the hundred diseases." Other models of differentiating disease, such as defensive *qi*, *qi*, nutritive, and blood; triple burner; and even viscera and bowel differentiation, emphasize horizontal, latitudinal, terrestrial, *wei* differentiation. As a result, these methods of differentiation are all limited in their own way, while six conformation differentiation—or put another way, yin yang differentiation—is unlimited.

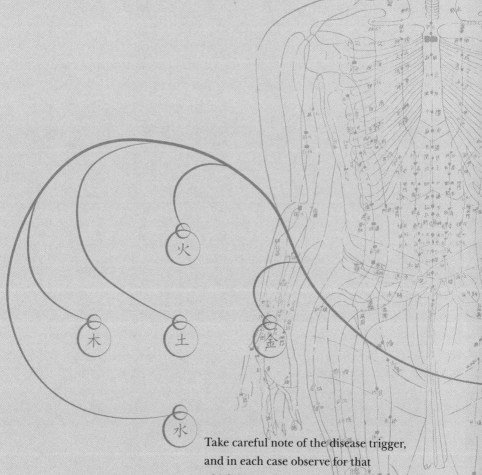

CHAPTER FOUR

THE ESSENTIALS OF TREATING DISEASE

Take careful note of the disease trigger,
and in each case observe for that
which is associated with it.
Seek presence and absence,
probe abundance and deficiency.

Before we enter into a formal discussion of Taiyang, we will discuss the essentials of treating disease. Only if we make this issue clear and grasp it completely will we, as physicians, have something solid to lean upon.

I. Two Ranks of Physicians

In 1936, the eminent physician and scholar Chen Cunren compiled and edited a collection of famous Japanese medical texts called the *Imperial Han Medical Series* (Huanghan yixue congshu). In this book, there is a chapter called "Ten Maxims for Physicians," which constitute ten issues that physicians should pay close attention to. Among these ten maxims, there is one in particular that has left a deep impression on me, one that my master told me more than ten years ago. My master explained many things that I have already forgotten, but this particular exhortation remains fresh in my memory, and for the last ten years I have been reciting this injunction and using it to keep myself in line, spur myself on, and motivate myself.

I am relying upon memory to reiterate the maxim here:

> In medicine there are higher physicians, and there are lower physicians. To see only the obvious and desire a quick cure is the way of the lower physician. To observe the syndrome, investigate its trigger, and harmonize with medicinals is the way of the higher physician. It may seem circuitous to investigate and harmonize, but it is in fact quite direct. This is understood by the wise, and lost on the foolish.

We can see that this maxim classifies physicians as high or low. The higher class described here are those we would today characterize as brilliant healers, and the lower class as inferior physicians, as quacks.

When we read this admonishment, as students of medicine we must make a choice. I would say that most people hope to be in the higher rank of physician. If not, there is no sense in studying medicine. If not, at the end of one's life, one would be no more than a physician of the lower class, a charlatan. Now that would be disappointing. There is no middle road for a physician to take, as one is either rescuing people or harming them. When you prescribe a formula, it will have an effect, and if that effect is not therapeutic, then it is injurious. There really is not much middle ground here. Therefore, those who choose the path of the physician must tread cautiously. In the words of the great Qing dynasty physician Xu Dachun: "If you are to be a physician, there are only two paths to take: either become a great physician to the common people, or a great robber of life."

I.1. The Rank of Lower Physician

What is a higher physician? What is a lower physician? What is the basis for judging one or the other? The maxim given to me by my master clarifies this for us: "To see only the obvious and desire a quick cure is the way of the lower physician." What exactly does this mean?

A few days ago, I was teaching a class of undergraduate medical students. After class during break time, a student asked me: "In my hometown, a friend of mine has an enlarged thyroid. Professor, what formula should he take?" Another student chimed in: "Professor, lately I have been having insomnia, what formula should I take?" At this point, let us forget about the questions with which we opened this section of the book and address another question. Chinese and Western physicians are similar in many ways. When a Western physician treats an enlarged thyroid gland, does she immediately reach for a scalpel to cut it out, or administer medicine to reduce the swelling? Not at all. First, she would attempt to diagnose the disease methodically. An enlarged thyroid gland or goiter is, after all, only a sign of disease, a relatively superficial manifestation of the underlying pathology, not a diagnosis. The diagnosis that the Western physician seeks is one that considers the factors causing the goiter. What caused the thyroid to swell? Is it due to an iodine deficiency? Is the thyroid hyperactive? Is it a tumor of some kind? Could it be cancer? Each of these diagnoses requires their own corresponding tests, perhaps administration of iodine-131, or a biopsy, or some other imaging, or blood tests. Once the cause of the goiter is determined, the physician can devise a strategy to treat it. It is common in our field for people to say that Western physicians "only treat symptoms." I disagree with this statement. The process of diagnosis and treatment in biomedicine is also a process of "treating the root" as we say in Chinese Medicine, the only difference being the level at which this root is found.

When this particular student told me about her friend with the goiter and asked me to prescribe a formula, a great number of steps were being skipped. Chinese and Western Medicine are the same in this respect. Whether we are speaking of a goiter or insomnia, these are only symptoms of disease. A distinguishing feature of Chinese Medicine is its emphasis on diagnosis based on an overall analysis of the patient's condition. Once this analysis is complete, we can determine the cause of the disease and then an appropriate method of cure can be undertaken in accord with this cause. In Chinese Medicine, this is called "differentiating syndromes to determine the cause, and determining treatment in accordance with the cause."

If you simply say "goiter" or "insomnia" without undertaking a process of diagnosis based on an analysis of the overall picture of the disease, without any diagnosis whatsoever, how can we possibly prescribe a formula? There is no way to prescribe a formula. On the basis of this understanding, we may find we not agree with the many irrational aspects of the post-classical Chinese Medicine field of "internal medicine." In Western Medicine, tuberculosis, for example, is both a disease name and a diagnosis, and this diagnosis includes an understanding of the cause of the disease. Even in the case of diseases like rheumatoid arthritis or systemic lupus erythematosus for which the etiology is not yet very clear, the names of these diseases include an understanding of the disease causes.

But in current Chinese internal medicine textbooks, when it says "cough" or "stomachache" or "diarrhea," these are all diseases. What is a "cough" or a "stomachache"? These are merely symptoms! There is absolutely no etiology entailed by the names of these symptoms. And so, if Western medical physicians should like to laugh at us Chinese Medicine practitioners, I think they have good reason to do so. If we are going to imitate a certain aspect of Western Medicine, then it ought to be done after a great deal of careful consideration. The results of blind imitation are often an unhappy mish-mash undeserving of respect.

Of course, the diagnostic methods of Chinese and Western Medicine are vastly different. Western Medicine has modern techniques upon which it relies for diagnostic data, and these become more advanced every day. Chinese Medicine has no such tools. One can only rely upon one's self. In this respect, the study of Chinese Medicine is more difficult than that of Western Medicine. The student of Western Medicine is assisted by the whole world of science and technology: physics, chemistry, biology; all of these are at their disposal.

The student of Chinese Medicine finds herself in a very different camp. Not only must she rely solely upon her own faculties as diagnostic tools, but she is surrounded by those who find fault with her faith in a "backward" medicine and make the endeavor still more difficult. Therefore, if you wish to study Chinese Medicine well, especially in this day and age, it is very difficult. If you wish to study Chinese Medicine, you should consider this problem with a clear mind, and fortify your faith in the validity of your undertaking.

The two students who separately asked for a prescription for insomnia and goiter are perfect examples of what is meant by "To see only the obvious and desire a quick cure is the way of the lower physician." There are many who study Chinese Medicine their whole lives and are still like this. As soon as they hear the word "goiter," they reach for a goiter formula, and if in addition the patient says they have a stomachache, then they put a couple of herbs into the formula that are used to relieve stomach pain. And if the patient says that they have lower back pain to boot, well then they add a couple of herbs for the lower back pain. At present, there are many Chinese Medicine practitioners who treat patients in this way.

Some of my students have told me that in Chinese Medicine hospitals, at present, real Chinese Medicine is nowhere to be seen. If someone has a myocardial infarction, then they are immediately given a set formula to boost the *qi* and nourish the yin, invigorate the blood and transform blood stasis; this has already become standard practice. Of course, some patients with myocardial infarction may actually benefit from boosting *qi* and nourishing yin, but the thinking behind the prescription is misguided.

A myocardial infarct is entirely a Western diagnosis. It points to a particular etiology: the obstruction of coronary arteries and subsequent ischemia in the cardiac tissue. So how does Chinese Medicine understand this particular malady? A Chinese Medicine doctor would not necessarily attribute this directly to the heart itself. The Chinese Medicine practitioner would "observe the complexion and feel the pulse, and first differentiate yin and yang." How can these would-be Chinese Medicine practitioners simplistically administer a formula that boosts *qi*, nourishes the yin, invigorates the blood, and transforms stasis? How are they any different from those who "see only the obvious and desire a quick cure"? This is absolutely the lower practice of medicine. We must devise a way to completely avoid this type of practice, to walk a different path.

I.2. The Rank of Higher Physician

This higher path is to "observe the syndrome, investigate its trigger, and harmonize with medicinals." What is the trigger? This is the *bingji*, the disease trigger. When one observes a syndrome, the first thing one must do is determine the disease trigger. Only then should one prescribe a formula. The formula should conform to the trigger of the disease as perfectly as possible. In this way, one is on the path toward becoming a "higher" physician.

"To observe the syndrome, investigate its trigger, and harmonize with medicinals is the way of the higher physician. It may seem circuitous to investigate and harmonize, but it is in fact quite direct." Is this method circuitous and roundabout? Well, it certainly appears so to some! "Investigate the trigger" . . . who wants to go to such trouble? Here is a myocardial infarction, and here is your *qi*-boosting, yin-nourishing, blood-invigorating, stasis-transforming formula. That was fast, wasn't it? "Investigate the trigger" . . . why bother? However . . . what about the result? I am afraid the outcome of such a treatment plan would be disappointing. This is what is meant by "It may seem circuitous to investigate and harmonize, but it is in fact quite direct"! Here is a patient with a sore throat, and here are your heat-clearing throat-disinhibiting medicinals: Xuanshen, Maidong, Jiegeng, Gancao . . . how does that sound? This certainly seems to be a direct solution to the problem, and anything but roundabout, but what about the actual result? I am guessing that most of you have had your own experiences with such a methodology.

Some days ago, I saw a patient with a painfully sore throat and generalized fatigue and weakness. She had lost her voice and used a pen and paper to communicate with me. What formula should be used? Based on this information alone, you cannot create a formula. If you were to hurriedly prescribe Shandougen and Niubangzi, then you are nothing more than a "lower" physician, because you "see only the obvious and desire a quick cure." Instead of hurriedly administering Shandougen, you should remember to "observe the syndrome [and] investigate its trigger."

In the case of this patient, I felt her pulse and found that both of the *chi* positions were floating and tight. Tightness in the pulse denotes cold, and floating indicates that the syndrome is on the exterior. From this tight and floating pulse, I realized that this was cold on the exterior of the body, a classic case of Taiyang cold damage syndrome. When there is Taiyang cold damage, we should of course use Mahuang Tang. I also looked at her tongue and saw that it was covered with a white, greasy coat, indicating that she was also afflicted by dampness. This damp pathogen was responsible for the feeling of weakness that she felt throughout her entire body. Therefore, I gave her Mahuang Tang with Cangzhu.

The patient's initial visit was in the evening, after having already taken antibiotics for several days with no results. She decocted the formula I prescribed later that same evening. The next morning, she called me on the phone to tell me her sore throat was 70 to 80 percent better and she had regained her voice. After the second dose, all her symptoms were relieved. Think for a moment about this particular case. When I used a tongue depressor to look in her throat, I could see that the mucosa was congested with blood and her tonsils were very swollen. Based on this picture, one might think that it would be best to clear heat, disinhibit the throat, and reduce swelling. So why did I instead "pour more oil on the fire" with the pungent and warming herb Mahuang? Because her tongue and pulse revealed that this was without a doubt an exterior cold syndrome, so it was necessary to use Mahuang Tang to warm and disperse the cold on the exterior of her body. As soon as she ingested the warming, dispersing medicine, her throat no longer hurt. This is what is meant by "observe the syndrome, investigate its trigger, and harmonize with medicinals." This is the process of clinical diagnosis. As the ancients said: "You must put aside that which normally governs and search for the origin of the disease."

I recently saw a different female student who also had a sore throat. The swelling and pain was so bad that she had been given penicillin by IV drip for the last three days and nights. In spite of this, she was still so sensitive that even the slightest of provocations, like walking past an apartment where someone was frying food, her throat would immediately swell up and begin to suppurate. Now she is fine. Not only can she smell food like that, but she also enjoys eating it!

A sore throat is simply a symptom, not a diagnosis, and it is not a justification in and of itself to prescribe Shandougen and Jiegeng. You must obtain a diagnosis. Your treatment must be directed at your clinical diagnosis, not at the symptoms your patient complains of.

The Chinese character for the biomedical concept of inflammation consists of two "fire" radicals arranged one on top of the other (炎), and it is tempting to equate inflammation with the Chinese Medicine concept of heat, or fire. If the patient's symptoms are truly the result of a fire pathogen, then using medicinals like Xuanshen, Maidong, Gancao, and Jiegeng is definitely a good idea. Fire has a very distinctive appearance. It is bright and brilliant, red in color, and burning hot. When the human body is afflicted by a fire pathogen, it also has a very distinctive manifestation, with clear indicators as to its presence. However, when I saw this student in the clinic, her face had a greenish cast, her tongue and lips were pale, her hands were freezing, and her pulse was deep and thin. There were no signs of fire at all! According to her tongue and pulse picture, according to the four methods of Chinese diagnosis (looking, listening/smelling, questioning, and taking the pulse), this patient was not afflicted by pathogenic fire. Despite this, the treatments she had received in the past consisted of approaches like Niuhuang Jiedu Pian, Xuan Mai Gan Jie Tang, etc., to clear heat and disinhibit her throat. If you saw this patient, you would quickly realize why it is that Chinese Medicine is often so ineffective. In the case of this patient, my treatment from the beginning consisted of supporting yang. At first I used Gui Qi Jianzhong Tang, and then Fuzi Lizhong Tang. Now, not only does her throat no longer hurt, but her entire constitution has improved.

This case reiterates the difference between the path of the "lower" physician and that of the "higher." The path of "observing the syndrome and investigating its trigger" may seem circuitous and meandering, but in the end, it gets much faster and better results. This is precisely what is "understood by the wise, and lost on the foolish." If one were to immediately prescribe herbs that clear heat and benefit the throat, or look through a materia medica for herbs that help with throat pain or herbs that have an antibiotic and anti-inflammatory effect, it might seem to be a faster, more direct route. But is it really? This girl had already taken that route, and years had gone by and she had seen no improvement. From senior-middle school to college, she constantly took antibiotics and expensive medicinals like Niuhuang Jiedu Pian. In this case, she needed only take the proper prescriptions for a month to resolve her symptoms, and furthermore to improve her overall constitution. Which way is faster?

The wise have merit precisely because they follow this method, and the foolish are foolish because they are ignorant of the importance of "observing the syndrome and investigating its trigger." It is my hope that from here on, anyone reading this will endeavor to be wise and not foolish. All that is required is a careful investigation, analysis, and diagnosis of the illness with the aim of finding its underlying cause. From here on, every patient should be treated with this requirement in mind. At the beginning, one's analysis may not be correct every time, but there is no shame in that. The important thing is that the physician be pointed in the correct direction and move forward.

At first, the novice is bound to be inaccurate, but with time, a ten-percent success rate will turn to twenty, then thirty, and so on. Eventually, the rate of success will be more like 80 or 90 percent. If the physician is able to help eight or nine patients out of ten in this way, then that physician might well be considered a "higher" physician. The novice must have confidence that the method is correct, and that the only obstacle is time and lack of experience.

II. Observing the Syndrome and Investigating the Trigger

The *Imperial Han Medical Series* advises us that the way of the higher physician is to "observe the syndrome, investigate its trigger, and harmonize with medicinals." This line might be reduced down to "investigate the trigger and harmonize with medicinals." The "trigger" refers to *bingji*, the disease trigger, a concept we discussed in Chapter One: a trigger (*ji*) is the key factor, the crucial element that causes something to occur. The disease trigger, therefore, is the most crucial factor in the development of a particular disease. This is a vastly different concept from that of pathomechanism, which refers to the pathological changes that come about in the course of a disease. The disease trigger is similar to the finger on the button that launches an atomic warhead. It is absolutely crucial to the sequence of events that follow it, but it is not identical to those changes.

II.1. How to Investigate the Trigger

The concept of the "disease trigger" is derived from the "Great Treatise on the Essentials of Ultimate Truth" in the *Plain Questions*. This chapter, in accordance with its title, contains the most authentic and substantial discussion in the *Plain Questions*. The fact that the concept of the disease trigger originates here in this chapter indicates to us that it is very crucial. Before the "Great Treatise on the Essentials of Ultimate Truth" discusses the concept of the disease trigger, Huangdi provides an introduction:

> As for the advent of the hundred diseases, they all emerge from wind, cold, summer heat, damp, dryness, and fire, and from these they change and transform. The classics say to drain the abundant, and supplement the deficient. I have given this knowledge to alchemists, but their use of it to treat is imperfect. I wish to pass on this essential method, such that it produces immediate effects like a drum produces sound when struck, and that it can be used to make a clear and immediate difference, just like removing a thorn or cleaning away filth. May I hear of these therapeutic methods employed by simple practitioners, skilled physicians, spirit-like physicians, and sage-like physicians?

In this opening passage, Huangdi discusses with his advisor Qi Bo how the hundred diseases are inseparable from wind, cold, summer heat, damp, dryness, and fire. These pathogenic influences then bring about other changes in the body.

Although, when we see a patient, we may clearly see the disease that was wrought by these changes, it may not be obvious that the original pathogenic influence, wind, cold, damp, etc., still affects the body. However, the original pathogen must not be forgotten; we must be clear on this point. This is why Huangdi's statement is so unequivocal. After making this point, Huangdi continues by saying that "The classics say to drain the abundant, and supplement the deficient." However, when he teaches this method to physicians and they try to apply it clinically, their results are imperfect and dissatisfying, and their ability to cure with this method is not absolute. Huangdi tells Qi Bo that he wants to pass down the most authentic and essential medical method so that physicians can quickly grasp it and use it to cure disease, just like removing a thorn or cleaning away filth.

Can clinical treatment of disease possibly be as simple as removing a thorn? When you strike a drum, it responds immediately; when you stand a pole under the sun, you immediately see its shadow. Could curing illness be the same? Is there really such a method? Qi Bo's answer is a resounding "Yes!" "Carefully investigate the disease trigger, and do not miss the appropriate *qi*, this is it!" This single sentence reveals the importance of the disease trigger. Carefully observe the disease, apprehend its origin, and then curing disease is as simple as removing a thorn, or cleaning away filth. But if the origin of the disease is not apprehended, then this sort of cure cannot be brought about, and the clinical results will never be perfect. How then do we carefully observe, and thereby apprehend, the disease trigger, the crucial element? One key to carefully observing the disease trigger is "not miss the appropriate *qi*." The "appropriate *qi*" (*qiyi*) is mentioned twice in the "Great Treatise on the Essentials of Ultimate Truth." The second time it is worded slightly differently: "Carefully attend to the appropriate *qi*, and do not miss the disease trigger." These two lines clearly parallel one another, and the reversal of the "appropriate *qi*" and the "disease trigger" indicates that the two are essentially interchangeable. The disease trigger is the appropriate *qi*, the appropriate *qi* is the disease trigger; these two are one and the same thing.

So what is the "appropriate *qi*" (*qiyi*)? It is what we just spoke of: wind, cold, summer heat, damp, dryness, and fire, and the factors related to the six *qi*. It is the orderly state of heavenly circulation and related weather patterns in nature. We are told to carefully observe the disease trigger so as not to miss the appropriate *qi*. How then do we ascertain the appropriate *qi*? For instance, let us say that right now the sky has turned yin and overcast, and it is about to rain. In this case, we know that the predominant *qi* is damp. We can directly sense the effect of this kind of *qi*, and we can predict the sort of pathological change that will ensue from the effects of this *qi*.

If the person were to become ill when this *qi* is dominant, regardless of what illness they have contracted, their malady is related to this dominant *qi*. If you thoroughly grasp this point, if as Qi Bo said you "do not miss" this point, then you have grasped the concept of the "disease trigger." If suddenly the weather turns cold with the arrival of the north wind, the "appropriate *qi*" is cold. The type of *qiyi* is called an "external" *qiyi*, or "manifest" *qiyi*. Of course, there is also a different type that is not so easily detected. Not surprisingly, this type is called "internal" or "hidden" *qiyi*. This appropriate *qi* can be discerned from examining the tongue and feeling the pulse.

In addition to these methods, is there an even easier way to determine the *qiyi*? As a matter of fact, all seven of the "Great Treatises" of the *Plain Questions* discuss this question.

Here we need to touch upon the specialized field of the study of the five movements and six *qi* (*wuyun liuqi*), the study of the cyclical transformation of universal *qi*. In the ninth chapter of the *Plain Questions*, "Treatise on the Six Nodes and Visceral Manifestations," we find this line: "If you do not know what each year contributes, the abundance and weakness of the *qi*, and how deficiency and excess arise, then you cannot be a practitioner." This is a serious statement. Right now, how many Chinese Medicine practitioners are there who know how to count the years in terms of their astrological influence? I assure you there are few to speak of. Despite this lack of ability, these same practitioners still practice Chinese Medicine. This is just the state of affairs in the present-day world of Chinese Medicine.

The year's contribution, the abundance and weakness of the *qi*, the rise of deficiency and excess—all of these are referring to matters of *yunqi* (movement and *qi*, an abbreviation for the five movements and six *qi*). As I write this during the year 2000, it is a *gengchen* year in the sexagenary cycle, so what does this year contribute to our state of health? The *geng* heavenly stem belongs to the metal element, and the heavenly stem refers to transformation and unification (*hua he*). The heavenly stems *yi* and *geng* transform metal, so this year is characterized by metal movement.

After determining the year's movement (*yun*), we must determine the earthly branch to deduce the *qi* of the year. This year *chen* is the earthly branch. *Chen* indicates that Taiyang cold water rules the heavens, and Taiyin damp earth resides at the source. In this year, metal movement emerges early in a *taiguo* ("overstepping") pattern, cold water rules the heavens, and damp earth resides at the source; this constitutes the overall framework of the appropriate *qi* that is characteristic for this year. If we are to examine the appropriate *qi* in greater detail, then we must look at the "host-guest" relationships: the host-guest relationship of the *qi* as well as that of the *yun*. The *qi* is divided into six steps, and the *yun* into five steps. This is the general principle of the five *yun* and six *qi* system. In the clinic, when we investigate the appropriate *qi*, our investigation must proceed in large part from this angle.

For instance, right now, we have already stepped into the two-week segment of the year called *Xiaoxue* (Minor Snow). This period is the last among the six *qi*, as well as the last among the five *yun*. The host *qi* of this time period is Taiyang cold water, and the guest *qi* of this period is Taiyin damp earth. All maladies that occur during this particular period, regardless of the disease, are related to this particular synthesis of appropriate *qi*. We must consider these factors when investigating the disease trigger, and when treating the disease. Furthermore, these factors can result in both externally contracted disease and internal injuries. With that in mind, we should seek out the appropriate *qi* (*qiyi*) whether the disease is externally contracted or arises from internal conditions.

If you understand the *qiyi*, if you understand the combined effects of the *qiyi* as we just discussed, and you understand "what each year contributes, the abundance and weakness of the *qi*, and how deficiency and excess arise," then you have become a practitioner in the classical sense. It is this understanding that allows the path of the physician to open up wide before you, as boundless as the sea and the sky. The study of *yunqi* is very important!

There is a famous physician in Nanning called Ceng Yongsheng who is also a teacher of mine. He spends his entire day studying the "what each year contributes, and how deficiency and excess arise." Some years ago, he operated an outpatient service. Each day he would see 100 to 200 patients, some days up to 300 patients, with half the visit numbers reserved for patients from the countryside.

How could one person see so many patients? It was because he understood the "what each year contributes, the abundance and weakness of the *qi*, and how deficiency and excess arise." When the appropriate *qi* is clear, and it is correlated with observation of the patient, then the disease trigger is easily understood. Once the disease trigger that is responsible for the emergence of the disease is worked out, determining the correct medicinal formula is a simple matter. In this way, he was able to diagnose diseases both quickly and accurately. The crux of understanding the disease trigger lies in ascertaining the appropriate *qi*, the *qiyi*; and if one wishes to grasp the *qiyi*, then one must know what each year contributes!

II.2. The Nineteen Disease Triggers

After learning of the relationship between the disease trigger and the appropriate *qi* (*qiyi*), Huangdi follows up with a request: "I wish to hear about the disease triggers (*bingji*)." Qi Bo replies, "All wind with swaying and dizziness belongs to the liver. All cold with contraction and pulling in belongs to the kidney. . . ." Qi Bo responds with a total of nineteen such lines, and these constitute the famous nineteen disease triggers of the *Yellow Emperor's Classic*. Although I personally have not studied the nineteen disease triggers very deeply, I have gained an appreciation of their importance.

It is a fact that very few people these days study these triggers seriously. For instance, in the chapter about "disease mechanisms" (as *bingji* is often understood to mean in post-classical Chinese Medicine) in the modern standardized textbook *Fundamentals of Chinese Medicine*, these nineteen disease triggers, which ought to form the nucleus of the discussion, are hardly mentioned. This is a direct reflection of a lack of recognition of their importance, and those who disregard them most probably think that pathology is so complex and intricate that nineteen lines would never be able to summarize it all. But can the nineteen disease triggers summarize all pathology? The answer is a resounding "Yes!" Qi Bo's use of the word "all" at the outset of each phrase in this particular passage indicates his certainty.

All "wind," all "swaying and dizziness," has a connection with the liver. If you begin your investigations with the liver, then you will, without doubt, discover the disease trigger, the crucial factor that led to the advent of the disease. On this point, Qi Bo has given you his guarantee. In the same way, "All pain with itch and sores belongs to the heart." We know that all symptoms like pain, itching, and sores belong to the heart, so we must seek out the instigating factor in relation to the heart. Below, we will discuss how to do this.

In this passage in the *Plain Questions*, after listing each of the nineteen disease triggers, Qi Bo probably realized that Huangdi might be experiencing the same doubts that we expressed above. In order to dispel any remaining uncertainty, Qi Bo quotes a passage from a lost classical work abbreviated as the *Great Essential* (Dayao):

> Take careful note of the disease trigger, and in each case observe for that which is associated with it. Seek presence and absence, probe abundance and deficiency. First attend to the five dominations, then open the flow of blood and *qi* so it is regulated and far-reaching. This will bring about harmony.

The disease trigger should be carefully noted, and known with absolute certainty. We must be quite clear on this point. Wind with swaying and dizziness, regardless of what sort of wind, swaying, or dizziness, all must be sought out in the liver. How do we seek them out? This takes us to this principle: "Seek presence and absence, probe abundance and deficiency. First attend to the five dominations."

For instance, with regard to the wind with swaying and dizziness that we just mentioned, if we see a disease characterized by swaying and dizziness, or vertigo, there is no question that this is ascribed to the liver. When we observe the patient, we compare the patient's presentation with that which we expect from someone with a disease centered around the liver. If his face has a greenish cast, and his pulse is wiry, then both the color associated with the liver and the characteristic liver pulse are obvious. This is what is meant by "presence" in the above passage. Seeking the presence of correlative signs is relatively easy, because it is so straightforward.

What if the vertigo patient presents with no correlative signs? What if his complexion has no greenish hue and his pulse is not in the least bit wiry? In that case, neither his color nor his pulse indicates that his disease belongs to the category of the liver. This situation is what is meant by seeking "absence" in the above passage. Absence must be sought out as diligently as presence. In any case, the disease at hand is related to the liver and there is no doubting that. So how do we understand this disease's relationship to the liver? This has to do with the instruction to "attend to the five dominations."

What is meant by "the five dominations"? This refers to the relationships between the five elements. In the case of the vertigo patient, the illness clearly belongs to the liver, why then is the color of the liver absent from the complexion and the pulse not wiry? This is a question that the student of Chinese Medicine could contemplate: What can account for this "absence"? The method is simple. We take the liver as the focus, and then use the five-element principles of generation and control to investigate the possible etiology. In the above example, if we find no liver signs and instead find signs of marked kidney deficiency, then you will of course presume that because the kidneys are deficient, this patient has a case of kidney water failing to engender liver wood. This pattern is generically referred to as the "mother failing to engender the child." In such a case, the treatment method entails tonifying the mother so that the child can flourish. In other words, if we tonify the kidneys, the vertigo patient will recover nicely.

If there are no signs of kidney deficiency, then keep looking. Is there a problem with the lungs? If there is, then you must determine whether that problem is the result of deficiency or excess. If lung is exuberant, if metal is excessive, then the liver wood is being overly controlled. In such a case, we should reduce the excess lung metal so that the wood is not disadvantaged. The patient will then be able to recover.

What if the lungs are deficient and the metal is insufficient? In that case, we should assist the metal to balance the wood. If the lungs are not in any trouble, then look elsewhere. How is the heart? How is the spleen? If the heart is deficient, then we have a case of "the child stealing the mother's *qi*." If the heart is exuberant, then fire is dominating metal, and metal is therefore unable to control wood. In this instance, if we drain heart fire, the disease will disappear. Sometimes, it may be that the earth element is at fault. When earth is deficient, it cannot nourish metal.

From the process we just illustrated, we can see that the search for the disease trigger becomes far easier once the focus of the disease is determined. Once the center point for the disease is determined using the nineteen disease triggers, then the principles of the five dominations and engendering and controlling can be used to determine the etiology and subsequent method of treatment. Imagine if this focal point were not provided! The physician would be more or less lost in a sea of possibilities. The guidelines provided by the *Plain Questions* are just amazing. They provide the disease trigger, the most crucial piece of information regarding the disease!

These lines tell us that the most relevant factor producing wind with swaying and dizziness is the liver. Consider for a moment what this must have meant to the physicians of antiquity. To them, this was the secret of success, the decisive technique: a treasure! We, on the other hand, for the most part anyhow, do not regard it as such. We mistake a golden vase for a chamber pot. Small wonder that the ancients said that one should not transmit your knowledge to those who would only spill the celestial treasures. At present, very few people delve into this invaluable process of differentiating syndromes. Personally, I intend to research it diligently, and I hope that the reader of this book will do the same.

In the Qing dynasty, the renowned physician Wang Xugao developed the "Thirty-Six Methods for Treating the Liver." How were these thirty-six methods developed? They were developed from the process we just explained, that of the five dominations. Each of the possible relationships between the five viscera was explored separately, such that diseases that clearly belonged to the liver could be treated by addressing a different viscera. He used ordinary medicines, and though he hardly uses any herbs specific to the liver, his methods cure diseases that are centered upon the liver.

Imagine that you use every ounce of your ability in an attempt to directly calm the liver and sedate wind, perhaps with a hefty dose of Lingyang Gouteng Tang, or Longdan Xiegan Tang, but it is of no use. Why is this? If you have not thoroughly investigated the pathology, and all you do is "see only the obvious and desire a quick cure," if all you know is "all wind with swaying and dizziness belongs to the liver" and are ignorant of how to "seek presence and absence, probe abundance and deficiency," and if you further do not understand the principle of "first attend to the five dominations," and you do not know "the liver transmits its disharmony to the spleen; first fortify the spleen," then like all lower physicians, you can only sit foolishly waiting for an unlikely windfall.

The potential permutations of a single disease trigger are countless, but they will never completely depart from the original trigger. If we use the principles provided by the *Great Essential*, and use the appropriate focal point while investigating the etiology of the disease, we will be able to determine the crux of the illness. Here, I have only provided only a general outline of the process required to properly diagnose and treat diseases using Chinese Medicine. I hope that the reader will use this outline as the basis of further research and, moreover, will put it to use in the clinical setting.

In the preceding passage, we discussed the nineteen disease triggers, and also introduced the general concept of the five movements and six *qi* (*wuyun liuqi*). I hope that this discussion has made a deep impression on you, the reader. As I write this, we have just passed through the *Xiaoxue* (Minor Snow) node *qi*. What sort of appropriate *qi* (*qiyi*) do we feel? It is very moist and damp, people feel foggy and drowsy, and many people suffer from colds. However, the cold that is going around now is different from that which circulated earlier in the year. If one does not know the year's contribution, and is not clear about *yunqi*, then curing this sort of cold is far more difficult.

At present, cold and damp prevail, with an emphasis on dampness. This moist dampness rivals that of spring. Several days ago, I saw three different patients: one had a malignant tumor in his upper palate, one suffered from sciatica, and one had stomach pain. I used the same formula with all three of the patients, Wuji San, from the *Official Prescriptions of the Harmonious Pharmacy* (He Ji Ju Fang). The cancer patient could not take the formula due to extenuating circumstances, but it had a good effect on the other two patients.

When one treats three different diseases in the same way, as I did here, this is what is meant by the Chinese Medicine saying "different illnesses, same treatment." In reality, the treatment is the same because the crucial factor underlying each of these different illnesses is identical. This underlying factor is the *qiyi*. If the *qiyi* is well understood, then it is easy to ascertain the disease trigger. When the disease trigger is clear, developing a treatment strategy is easy. In the clinical setting, this is a very efficient method.

The patient with the malignant tumor in his palate is only 26 years old. Observing his color and his *qi*, there is clearly something wrong. He himself does not feel much discomfort. He has a bit of a heavy feeling in his head, and a slight cough, due to the metastasis in his lung. His pulse on the right side was wiry and slippery, and the second position was rough. On the left side, his pulse was deep and fine, and when I applied pressure with my fingers, it disappeared. His tongue was dusky, and the tongue coat was white, wet, and slippery.

How do we assess such a patient? When I looked at what medicines he had taken previously, I saw that they consisted mostly of large doses of Banzhilian and Baihuasheshecao. The first thing I did was propose to him that he discontinue using these herbs. Banzhilian and Baihuasheshecao are both herbs that clear heat. If the patient's tumor was formed from an accumulation of heat-toxin, then these herbs would be indicated and would indeed have an anti-carcinogetic effect. But if the patient were suffering from a tumor wrought by cold and damp, as this one was, then using cooling herbs such as these would only add insult to injury.

If you encounter a cancer patient and the first thing you want to do is give him or her Banzhilian because of its purported anti-carcinogetic effect, then you definitely fit with the "lower" physician who "sees only the obvious and desires a quick cure." If that is your attitude, you are a Western physician, not a practitioner of Chinese Medicine. In Chinese Medicine, without a syndrome, there is no formula.

The *Yellow Emperor's Classic* laid down the following principle: cool that which is hot and heat that which is cold. This basic principle must be followed. If the disease is characterized by cold, then you must use medicines that warm, regardless of whether the patient is suffering from cancer or some other disease.

This patient's condition began in 1994. 1994 was a *jiaxu* year. The *jia* heavenly stem indicates that the earth movement was emerging early in a *taiguo* ("overstepping") pattern. The *xu* earthly branch indicates that Taiyang cold water is ruling heaven, and Taiyin damp earth is residing at the source.

It is very difficult in the case of a cancer patient such as this to clearly determine which day his illness began. It is very different from a common cold, where the exact day of onset can be determined. Therefore, it is the pattern of the year in which he first noticed his illness that is most important. We know the year's contribution in the year 1994, and the abundance and weakness of the *qi*. The main factor was that year's abundance of cold damp, especially dampness. Why didn't his disease appear in 1993? It is possible that the cancer was already gestating in 1993. Why did it choose to emerge in 1994?

We can be certain that the year's movement of 1994, the particular changes in the six *qi*, were especially conducive to the flare-up of this particular cancer. That is why this particular case of cancer became perceptible in this particular year. When we look at the year in which I am writing this book, we find ourselves in a *gengchen* year. Just as in 1994, cold water rules the heavens and damp earth resides at the source. This only serves to remind us that this particular illness is related to cold damp. This explains why cold and damp are detrimental to this patient's internal environment, counter to his immune system, but beneficial to the cancer that is afflicting him. Knowing each year's contribution is very useful, is it not? If we correlate this information with the patient's tongue and pulse, then we find that they agree with the contribution of the year in which his cancer first became obvious and confirm the nature of the disease trigger. Therefore, you can disregard the name of the disease and treat the patient according to the cold and damp aspect of the disease trigger. If you can eradicate the factors that benefit the cancer and damage the health of the patient, even if the patient does not recover from his illness, at the very least you will not be an accomplice to evil.

Regarding the beginning of a disease, Huangdi made a similar point: "As for the advent of the hundred diseases, they all emerge from wind, cold, summer heat, damp, dryness, and fire, and from these they change and transform." Here, Huangdi's use of the term "hundred diseases" means that all potential illnesses are affected by these factors. He does not name tumors as an exception. Tumors, like all other diseases, are influenced by the larger environment, and are influenced by these six pathogenic *qi*. All you need to do is clearly determine which pathogenic factor is at play and then devise methods to interfere with or change this factor, and you will have a beneficial effect on the course of the illness.

From this perspective, a formula such as Wuji San can combat cancer. However, we should not take this as a justification to do a study or create a research experiment, as such a research study may not show any positive results. As a result of this fact, there are many people that might be discouraged by Chinese Medicine. They might think that Chinese Medicine is unscientific, that it not universally applicable, that the results of its methods are not reproducible. Practically speaking, it is not that Chinese Medicine is not universal or lacks reproducibility. It is just that the particular process that the Chinese physician engages in to diagnose each illness cannot be reliably reproduced in a clinical study.

Wuji San counters the pathogenic factors of cold and damp. If it is used to combat cold and damp, then the results of using this formula are very consistent. If, however, you try to use this formula to treat other pathogenic factors, how can you expect any consistency or reproducibility? It is no different from the universality of antibiotics in the treatment of bacterial infections. If you attempted to test its efficacy on viral infections, would you expect consistent results? However, this is the very state of affairs in Chinese Medicine research at the present time. Their experiments are equivalent to administering antibiotics to patients with viral infection, and blaming the antibiotics when the treatment is ineffective. Since when is it principled to blame one's own mistakes on others?

I regularly see articles in journals touting the use of a particular formula or herb to treat a particular sort of illness. In this type of research, it is of course important to have enough subjects with that particular disease, as if the number is too low, the result will not have statistical significance. Now, let's be realistic: In actual clinical practice, is it ever possible to find a high enough number of subjects with the same disease and same disease-causing factor? Of course not. So what happens? All sorts of other totally unrelated patients are enrolled as subjects as well. This way of doing Chinese Medicine research, this type of attitude, is truly worrisome. On top of this, the policies set down by our regulatory departments, as well as the policies of these Chinese Medicine research journals, only add fuel to the flames.

The disease trigger (*bingji*) is a central focus of the clinical practice of Chinese Medicine. Previously, we said a few words about the line "All wind with swaying and dizziness belongs to the liver." What about "All pain with itch and sores belongs to the heart," "All dampness with swelling and fullness belongs to the spleen," "All sudden rigidity belongs to wind"? These lines are equally significant, and we could use a like method to analyze them one by one. Without exception, these nineteen lines provide you with a sort of compass.

If you take the information in these nineteen lines at face value, and take the crucial disease factor listed in each according to the disease before you to be the center of your investigation, and then conduct your inquiry as outlined in the previous pages of this book, then you will be able to determine the pattern of the pathology before you and treat it successfully. Once you become thoroughly familiar with these nineteen lines and the subsequent investigative method, you will be skilled at your job, and will find that "the hand accomplishes what the heart wishes."

II.3. Apprehending the Primary Symptoms and Recognizing the Disease Trigger

The previous discussion regarding how to investigate the trigger is extremely important, and should be considered to be classic teachings. A secondary facet of this discussion is "apprehending the primary symptoms," a method proposed by Professor Liu Duzhou. Professor Liu is an authority in the world of Cold Damage study. Regarding this subject, in China there is a saying: "Northern Liu, Southern Chen." The "Liu" in this saying is Liu Duzhou, and the "Chen" is my doctorate advisor, Professor Chen Yiren.

Liu Duzhou has a book called *Fourteen Lectures on Cold Damage* (Shang

Han Lun Shisi Jiang). Although this book is not very long, it is filled with Professor Liu's personal experiences and therefore very useful. The last lecture in this book addresses the issue of obtaining the all-important syndrome diagnosis by apprehending the primary, or governing, symptoms (*zhu zheng*). Professor Liu believed that apprehending the primary symptoms corresponds with the highest level of syndrome differentiation. Therefore, whether or not one understands the primary symptoms is a crucial question in clinical diagnosis.

Why is it so important? In my understanding, there are two important reasons. First, it is most often the key symptoms that best reflect the essential trigger that results in disease, and only the symptoms that completely reflect the disease trigger can be called "primary symptoms." Secondly, the primary symptoms are the best indicator of the appropriate path by which the pathology can be eliminated from the body. It tells you whether to induce sweating, or to purge, or to induce vomiting, or to use a different method. Ascertaining the dominant symptom is like the last step of "painting eyes on a dragon to bring it to life"; it brings the whole analysis of the disease to life and provides the physician with an organic overview that determines how she will commence treatment. The primary symptoms must convey these two basic characteristics.

Why did Professor Liu raise this issue in his *Fourteen Lectures on Cold Damage*? For the obvious reason that in every one of Zhang Zhongjing's passages, many of the symptoms he describes are in fact primary symptoms. If you look at the *Treatise on Cold Damage*, many of them are extremely simple, such as line 155: "If there is a sensation of a lump below the heart, and aversion to cold and sweating are seen again, Fuzi Xiexin Tang governs it." Or line 301: "Shaoyin disease: if at the time one contracts it, one contrarily has heat effusion, and the pulse is deep, Mahuang Xixin Fuzi Tang governs it." It might be said that the text of the *Treatise on Cold Damage* is permeated with the descriptions of the primary, or governing, symptoms.

I would like to provide an example. Three or four years ago, a female worker from a radio factory came to see me. Her Western Medicine diagnosis was of a kidney stone and subsequent hydronephrosis, and her condition was relatively serious. She had seen both Chinese Medicine and Western Medicine physicians but without any real improvement, and was introduced to me by an old patient of mine. The conventional approach for treating kidney stones is to use herbs that pass stones and free urination, but I did not spend much time contemplating these methods. Instead, I quietly listened to the patient's description of her illness. I listened and contemplated what she said. She spoke of how for the past month she had suffered from diarrhea, her heart was agitated, and she could not sleep well. In that instant, I apprehended her dominant syndrome.

I gave her Zhuling Tang, without any additions or subtractions, and without adding any stone-passing herbs. Why did I give her Zhuling Tang? Line 319 says very clearly: "For Shaoyin disease with six or seven days of diarrhea, cough and retching accompanied by thirst, vexation and inability to sleep, Zhuling Tang governs it." In this line, the *Treatise on Cold Damage* clearly states that diarrhea as well as vexation and insomnia can be treated with Zhuling Tang. This patient exhibited these symptoms at the same time, which quickly led me to this formula.

Regardless of whether the patient suffers from kidney stones or edema, the ideal treatment for her syndrome is Zhuling Tang, so that is what I used. The patient left after I gave her the prescription and she did not return, and about six months later, she introduced another patient to me. From this patient, I learned that after taking the formula, her symptoms quickly disappeared, and two weeks later she was examined and found to be free of kidney stones. Her hydronephrosis also went away. This particular case made a deep impression on me. I became ever so faintly aware of what Professor Liu meant by "apprehending the primary symptoms."

Those with clinical experience know that there are patients with very complicated conditions. This is especially true in the elderly. Some of my older patients could talk all day about the particulars of their illness. By the time they get to the end of their story, it is hard to remember the beginning. With these sorts of patients, it is even more essential that you apprehend their primary symptoms. They speak at length, but there is inevitably a sentence, or a symptom, or a pulse that arouses your attention, and it is this that will lead you to the primary symptoms.

A few days ago, I saw a student's mother in the clinic. Her chief complaint was a common cold with fever, which had come and gone for some ten days and still had not resolved. From a cold damage perspective, a common cold with fever should be regarded as a Taiyang disease, and in Taiyang disease, regardless of how the cause, the pulse, as a rule, is floating.

This patient's pulse, on the contrary, was very deep. An exterior syndrome with a deep pulse: this is unusual, this is a crucial point, this is a primary symptom.

This exterior syndrome with a deep pulse revealed that the external contraction spanned both the Taiyang and the Shaoyin conformations. The use of an ordinary common-cold formula would not do the job. I prescribed her two doses of Mahuang Xixin Fuzi Tang, and after taking the decoction, her fever quickly abated. In order to affect a clinical cure, you need only grasp the primary symptoms, and in the end you will produce results just as striking a drum produces sound.

How then do we accurately apprehend the primary symptoms? This depends in part upon experience and in part upon paying attention to three points. First, understand the theoretical principle. For instance, if the patient starts to get a Shaoyin disease, but contrary to expectation, she is feverish and her pulse is deep, why would a situation like this come about? In such a situation, why use Mahuang Xixin Fuzi Tang? You must understand the answers to these questions in order to draw inferences and use this information in other situations. Only then will you be able to use these formulas flexibly.

Second, learn by heart. Why do we stress the importance of reciting the *Treatise on Cold Damage* when we study it? If you wish to become a good Chinese Medicine practitioner, you must commit some things to memory. Even if you cannot remember every single word perfectly, you must be able to commit the general meaning to memory. You must be very familiar with each line, and especially those lines that contain formulas along with their primary symptoms. At any time, you should be able to summon from memory the gist of these lines. Only if you achieve this level of familiarity will you be able to put the *Treatise on Cold Damage* to good use. If you are not familiar with the lines, how will you grasp the primary symptoms? If you do not grasp the primary symptoms, then your use of classical formulas will not be efficacious.

Third, use what you have learned. Study with the aim of applying what you have learnt. After we study the chapter on Taiyang disease, we should practice our observation skills on each other to see if we have any signs of Taiyang disease. Hiding alone in your study will not give you the practical skill you need to become a good doctor. If you get a cold, you should determine whether you have a Taiyang cold or a Shaoyang cold, or a combination of Taiyang and Shaoyang disease.

If somebody who studies Chinese Medicine, especially someone who has studied the *Treatise on Cold Damage*, runs into someone with a cold and reaches for a pre-packaged herbal cold product and vitamin C, they have been wasting their time studying. I fear such students will only ever be "lower" physicians. Keep in mind: regardless of what disease you encounter, you must rely upon the pulse diagnosis and differentiation of syndromes. Only if you see a certain pulse-syndrome should you use the formula corresponding to that syndrome. You should have a definite target in mind before you release an arrow.

I wish to transmit to you these essential methods of curing disease. The reader should constantly keep in mind the difference between the higher physician and the lower physician, and what each of these entails. Although we cannot instantly become higher physicians, we must keep this goal firmly in our mind. We must constantly cultivate the habits of the higher physician, and avoid the behavior of the lower physician. If a cancer patient comes to you, do not let your head swim with desire to give him Banzhilian or Baihuasheshecao in order to combat the cancer. This is not Chinese Medicine. At best, it is the sort of Chinese Medicine practiced by a dabbler in the art.

Since you are practicing Chinese Medicine, you should also think Chinese Medicine. You should carefully observe the symptoms and seek the disease trigger. Only in this way will you gain understanding and a feeling for Chinese Medicine. Otherwise, even if you manage to cure the patient, you will not know why they improved. And if you fail to cure them, you also will not know why you failed. You will spend your entire life bumbling about. What a pity! There is really no point in practicing Chinese Medicine this way.

I hope that the reader of this book can become a higher physician, or at least be ready to become one. I believe that if the physician truly understands and behaves in accord with the procedures I have already described, then that physician will already be a higher physician in spirit. Before we enter into a formal discussion of the Taiyang section of the *Treatise on Cold Damage*, a clear comprehension of this guiding process is absolutely necessary.

CHAPTER FIVE

The Essentials of Taiyang Disease

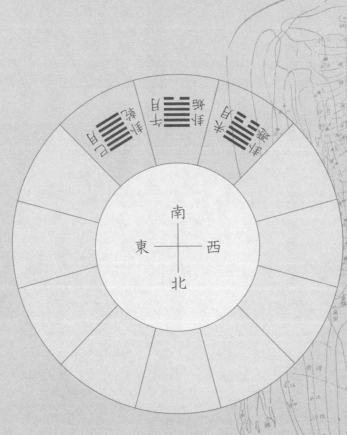

Taiyang disease tends to
resolve in the time from *si* to *wei*.

I. An Explanation of the Chapter Title

Before we read the Taiyang section, we must first take a look at the title of this section, just as we would read the title of a book before opening its cover. This is a habit that the student of Chinese Medicine must foster in his or her studies. It is especially true with regard to the Chinese Medicine classics, where the meaning of each and every word is indispensable. When reading the classics, we have to clarify three levels of meaning: the meaning of each character, the meaning of the sentence, and the overall meaning. If you are able to understand all three levels of meaning, then will be no classic that you cannot read.

Let us first examine the global meaning of the title of this section: "Differentiate Taiyang: disease, pulse, syndrome, and treatment." What does this title mean? It indicates that this section of the book will discuss the differentiation and determination of the disease name, disease trigger, pulse, and syndrome related to Taiyang, as well as the relevant treatment methods. By thoroughly analyzing each and every one of the topics mentioned in the title, we will get a firm grasp of certain important characteristics of Chinese Medicine.

In modern times, many people think that Chinese Medicine only discusses syndrome differentiation and does not concern itself with determining the name of the disease. Or they believe that Chinese Medicine is very detailed in its determination of the syndrome, but foggy about determining the exact disease. This is why, when integrating with Western Medicine, the Western Medicine disease is diagnosed first, and then the Chinese Medicine syndrome is differentiated next. With regard to these people, I often say that they clearly have not read the *Treatise on Cold Damage*, and their talk is not that of a Chinese Medicine practitioner. If you have read the *Treatise on Cold Damage*, then you know that it is nonsense to say that Chinese Medicine does not differentiate individual diseases. In fact, in Chinese Medicine we first determine the disease, and then we determine the syndrome. If in the first place you do not determine that you are dealing with a Taiyang disease, how will you take the next step to affirm whether it is the result of a wind-strike or the result of cold damage? Therefore, to say that Chinese Medicine does not differentiate between diseases and only analyzes the syndrome is a gross misunderstanding.

I.1. Explaining Differentiation

First, let us explain the character *bian* (辨). This character is a relatively simple one to explain. *Explaining Writing and Analyzing Characters* (Shuowen jiezi) says this character means "to judge." *Extensive Rhymes* (Guangyun) says it means "to differentiate." Taking these definitions together, the character *bian* means to judge or to differentiate. The *Kangxi Dictionary* (Kangxi zidian) cites that, in the *Record of the Study of Rites* (Lixueji) it says: "*Bian* means to examine orally to make a clear determination"; and that in the *Official Documents of the Rites of Zhou* (Zhouli tianguan shu) it is written: "*Bian* means to analyze a subject and make it clear to the point that no confusion remains."

If we gather all the above definitions into a comprehensive definition of *bian*, it would be: to take all the data received by various channels, and subject this information to thoughtful analysis and evaluation and thereby produce a definite and very clear conclusion. In Chinese Medicine, this process of differentiation might be described as taking all the information gleaned from the four diagnostic methods, subjecting this data to contemplative synthesis and analysis, and thereby achieving a clear diagnosis.

I.2. Explaining Taiyang

I.2.a. The Meaning of Taiyang

What are some meanings of Taiyang? Originally, Taiyang referred to the sun, and even in modern Chinese, the word *taiyang* (太陽) is interchangeable with sun. Its second meaning is brought up in *Spiritual Pivot*, "Nine Needles and Twelve Sources" (Jiuzhen shieryuan) where it says: "Taiyang among all yang is the heart." Why is the heart used as an analogy for Taiyang? Zhang Jiebin says, "The heart is the yang among yang, therefore it is called Taiyang." With regard to its implied meanings, Taiyang means "grand" or "magnificent" yang. Therefore Wang Bing says, "The yang *qi*, where magnificent, we call Taiyang."

I.2.b. The Meaning of the Taiyang Channels

In the past, those who have researched the *Treatise on Cold Damage* have held differing opinions regarding the meaning of the *liujing* (the six channels or conformations). Some have thought that the *liujing* referred to the channels of the body; some have thought that besides the channels, this term also referred to the internal organs; and some have taken the *liujing* to refer to six planes or surfaces. This informs us that the concept of the *liujing* is rich and multifaceted.

Here we will look at the significance of Taiyang from the angle of the channels of the body. There are the Taiyang channels of the arms and of the feet, and those of the feet are especially important, as we discussed in some detail earlier in this book. What are the distinguishing features of the leg Taiyang channels? The leg Taiyang channel begins at the inner canthus of the eye with the point Jingming, then proceeds upward to the top of the head and continues over and down the nape of the neck and back, on either side of the spine. It continues down the back to the back of the legs, before ending at Zhiyin (BL 67) at the end of the little toe.

If we compare the twelve regular channels, the leg Taiyang is the longest channel. The areas of the body into which its divergent channels branch are the longest and broadest of all the channels. It is especially significant that these channels and its divergent branches infiltrate the entire posterior aspect of the human body. When the wind blows in your face, you probably do not think much of it. But when it blows on your back, and this is especially true for those who are sensitive to wind, you find yourself suddenly uncomfortable. This is because "it is easy to parry a spear thrust in the open, but difficult to dodge an arrow shot from hiding." The *Yellow Emperor's Classic* time and again emphasizes that "the sages avoided wind as they would arrows or thrown stones." Wind should not be underestimated.

In the era in which the *Yellow Emperor's Classic* was written, what were the things that could injure a person from a distance and without any warning? Arrows and stones. Even so, if someone shoots an arrow or throws a rock at you from somewhere in front of you, you have a fighting chance of dodging it, but if an arrow comes flying at you from behind you some distance, evasion is almost impossible. In Chinese Kungfu novellas, there are characters who manage to evade such attacks, but outside the world of fiction it is very difficult indeed.

By comparing wind with dangerous projectiles, the message is clear: wind has the potential to cause great harm. When the wind blows in our face, we have some possibility of warding it off, but the wind that blows from behind is far more difficult to defend against. The wind that blows from behind us, sneakily, is called a "thief wind" (*zeifeng*) in Chinese Medicine.

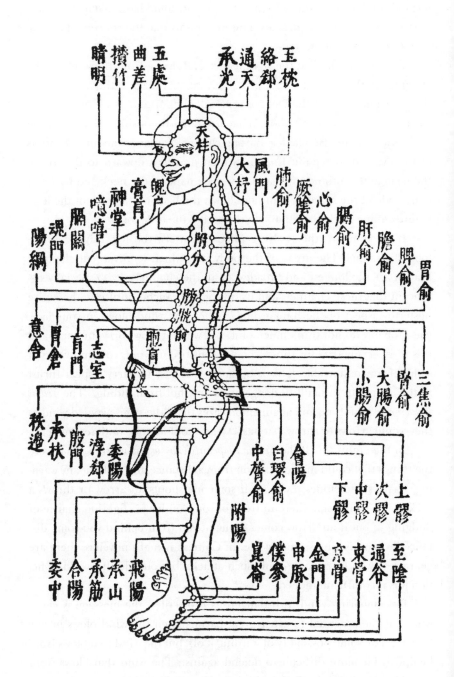

The human body relies upon Taiyang to defend against these "thief winds" that attack from behind. This is why Taiyang preponderates on the posterior of the body. Our ancestors compared Taiyang to a defensive border in the body. However, Taiyang's role as a defensive line should not be taken as an indication of its low status. The part of the body traversed by a particular channel is an important indicator of that channel's function. We should take careful note of this aspect of the channel, as it plays an important role in the differentiation of syndromes from a six channel perspective.

If a patient complains of leg pain, or pain in any other part of the body, you need to ask very specifically where the pain is located. Do not just dismiss it as leg pain. Ask if the pain is on the anterior or posterior, lateral or medial aspect. If the pain is in the popliteal fossa behind the knee, then you know with certainty that it is related to Taiyang. You must devise a treatment strategy that will address Taiyang, and this necessity will naturally draw you into six channel syndrome differentiation. It is clear then that if you wish to study the *Treatise on Cold Damage*, then a clear understanding of the channels is of great importance.

I.2.c. The Meaning of the Taiyang Bowels

The leg Taiyang channel corresponds to the urinary bladder and the Taiyang channel of the arm corresponds to the small intestine, both of which are hollow bowel-type organs. "The urinary bladder holds the office of regional rectifier. The body liquids are stored in it, and when *qi* is transformed, then body liquids can originate from it." Therefore, the bladder is the storehouse of the bodily fluids, the storehouse of water. Why would the storehouse of water be associated with Taiyang? This connection demonstrates the intimate relationship between *qi* transformation and water. Much of the content of the Taiyang chapter in the *Treatise on Cold Damage* is related to this relationship between water and the transformation of *qi*.

The small intestine is not as prominent as the bladder in the Taiyang section, but nevertheless its significance is indicated by the following passage from the "The Treatise on the Spiritual Orchid Secret Canon": "The small intestine holds the office of accepting. The transformation of things originates from it." With regard to *shou sheng*, translated here as "accepting" to match Wang Bing's interpretation, he further comments that:

In compliance with the demands of the stomach, the small intestine receives dregs from the stomach. It receives them, and in turn transforms them. Then, it conducts what has been transformed to the large intestine. Therefore, it is called the "official of accepting, the transformation of material emerges."

And Zhang Jiebin writes:

The small intestine resides below the stomach, it receives the water and grain from the stomach and separates it into clear and turbid. From here the watery fluids proceed to the front and the dregs fall back. That which the spleen *qi* transforms rises, and that which the small intestine transforms descends. Therefore it is said that "the transformation of matter emerges."

Both Wang Bing and Zhang Jiebin take the phrase *"shou sheng"* to be a compound word meaning "accept" or "receive." This reading is not necessarily appropriate. Because *shou* by itself carries the meaning to "receive" or to "accept," it already contains the above interpretations. What then is meant by the character *sheng*?

Explaining Writing and Analyzing Characters says that *sheng* is "the millet that has been placed in the utensil and is ready for sacrifice to the spirits." The character *sheng* originally referred to sacrificial grain! How ironic then that Wang Bing understood *sheng* to mean "dregs," and in Zhang Jiebin's interpretation, though he does not explicitly refer to these as dregs, he still describes them as being made up of dregs. How could this be possible?

When the ancients sacrificed, they chose the finest to offer up. Imagine using dregs or waste as a sacrificial offering! For this important reason, I distrust both Wang Bing's and Zhang Jiebin's interpretation of this line. The fact that the small intestine receives nourishment that has already been processed and refined by the stomach fits with the notion that *sheng* is actually a fine, sacrificial offering that is being received by the small intestine.

Additionally, if this line is referring to some sort of sacrificial offering, what is being sacrificed to? Of course, it being offered to the five solid viscera, since these store the spirits. The act of taking the purest and most refined elements of the food and offering them up to the five organs is surely a sort of sacrifice. This interpretation fits with the import of the line, and translated in accord with this understanding, it might read: "The small intestine holds the office of receiving sacrifices." From this interpretation, we also know that if the ancients did not know that the small intestine was the main organ for the reception of nourishment, then they would not have used the term *shou sheng*.

I.2.d. The Meaning of Taiyang in Yunqi

We have examined Taiyang with regard to its basic meaning, its meaning in the classics, and the significance of the bowel associated with it. Now we will examine the specific significance of Taiyang in the five movements and six *qi* (*wuyun liuqi*, abbreviated as *yunqi*), the cyclical transformation of universal *qi*. In *yunqi*, Taiyang is cold in the heavens and water on the earth. Together, this is called Taiyang cold water. Taiyang is considered the yang among yang. Why then does it correspond with cold water? Let us consider it from the following perspectives.

I.2.d.1. The Meaning of Water

Everyone should be familiar with the significance of water. We need water every day, and cannot live more than a few days without it. Water is essential to all biological processes, and is the most important substance to life. We may weigh a hundred or two hundred pounds, but most of our weight is water. When we look at a globe or a map of the world, we can see that most of the surface of the earth is covered with water. Laozi said, "Humans take the earth as model," and in contemplating this statement, we should keep in mind that most of the earth is covered with water. From these facts alone, and from our own experience, the importance of water is obvious.

In 1976, there was the Tangshan Earthquake, one of the deadliest earthquakes of the twentieth century. It killed hundreds of thousands of people. Some persons who were buried under earth and rubble were found alive more than a week later. How could they survive so long? They had water. Anyone can live a week or two without food, but no one can live that long without water. Western Medicine has a similar view. When an illness becomes very serious, the focus of treatment often revolves around water. How much has the patient urinated? How much fluid should be administered? Are the electrolyte levels stable? In short, the importance of water to life cannot be overstated. To raise another simple example, the Chinese character meaning "to live" (*huo* 活) has the water radical on the left and the tongue radical on the right. This character seems to say: "as long as you keep your tongue wet, you may yet live."

Water is essential to all life, but it has an even more important facet, and this aspect of water is realized by examining the trigrams and hexagrams of the *Classic of Changes*. The trigram that represents water in the *Classic of Changes* is *Kan* Water (☵). Water is of course the most yin thing there is, so we might expect that it would be represented by all yin broken lines. However, this trigram consists of a yang line between two yin lines. This reveals an essential aspect of water. As long as it possesses this yang element, this water is truly living water, and can be used by living things.

Without this living yang element, the water is the stagnant water of a still pond. Such water cannot sustain life. Li Bai has a famous poem entitled "Invitation to Wine." It includes these lines: "Have you not seen the waters of the Yellow River coming down from heaven, flowing to the sea, never to return?" As a practitioner of Chinese Medicine, when we read Li Bai's "Invitation to Wine," do we have any insights? Do we find ourselves asking questions? Why do the waters of the Yellow River descend from the heavens? Where does water come from in the sky? This is a question of transportation. There is something that transports water up into the sky, and that something is yang, it is Taiyang, the sun. In the *Yellow Emperor's Classic* where it says: "The earth *qi* rises and becomes the clouds," we have an indication of this very process. How does the earth's *qi* rise and become the clouds? Things that are yin always sink downward.

If we read the discussion of the five elements in the *Book of Documents's* "The Great Pattern," we then understand that wood is crooked and straight, fire burns upward, earth is sowed and reaped, metal flays the hide, water moistens and descends. Water always flows downward. People tend to live up on hills, and water always flows downward. You can do a very simple experiment to prove this point. Tip over a bowl of water and see if it flows upward or downward. If water is to ascend upward and become clouds, then it needs the help of yang *qi*, it needs the help of fire. For this reason, if water is to become "living" water, if it is to enter into the endless revolutions of the water cycle, by which water from the oceans is evaporated and descends upon the land as rain to begin its return to the oceans, and whereby it becomes useful to the life we see around us, then it must enjoy the assistance of the yang *qi* of the sun's light and heat.

This necessary assistance of yang is the reason for the solid yang line between the two broken yin lines in the *Kan* Water trigram. This brief examination of the *Kan* trigram deepens our understanding both of water and of Taiyang *yunqi*. It reiterates the absolute necessity of carefully studying the *Classic of Changes* in order to adequately understand the principles of Chinese Medicine.

I.2.d.2. The Meaning of Cold

Logically speaking, after water has been vaporized by the yang *qi*, we would expect that it would steam ever higher. Why then does it condense and precipitate? What influences it to descend? Water rises as it is steamed upward by the yang, but once it reaches a particular height, it encounters a certain influence: cold. The English saying "It's lonely at the top" has a parallel in Chinese poetry: "It's cold in high places," or, more literally: "Attaining a high position does not defeat the cold one finds there."

High places are very cold. If you go to the high plateaus of western China in summer, several thousand meters in elevation, you will find luxuriant green grass rolling right up to the foot of the mountains, but the mountains themselves are decked in pure white. Such a location gives you a clear sense of the strong association between increased altitude and an increase in cold. Water is turned into vapor by yang, but when it reaches the cold of the great heights, it condenses and returns to the earth as liquid. This is the process described in the *Yellow Emperor's Classic* as "the celestial *qi* descending as rain." The waters of the Yellow River most certainly descended from heaven, but Li Bai does not go so far as to tell us exactly where in heaven they come from. We, as Chinese physicians, must clarify this point.

Through the process in which water rises up as vapor and descends again as rain only to be steamed upward again and repeat the cycle, water becomes *living* water; it is "living water that comes from its own source of its own accord." This "living" water is of immense importance. Imagine for a moment if humans had to do all of the irrigation that is required by plants and animals to live. We could not irrigate more than a tiny fraction of what the sky does. Life simply could not exist without the sun and its effect on water. Without the cycling of water, the myriad living things would perish. This cycle consists of three indispensable entities: the sun and its yang warmth that causes water to ascend; the cold which induces water to condense and descend upon the earth; and water itself.

The pairing of Taiyang with cold water is deeply significant. If we look at the Taiyang section of the *Treatise on Cold Damage*, on a subtle level it is discussing the process of the water cycle. In a manner of speaking, whenever this water cycle is in any way interrupted, Taiyang disease ensues. Sometimes the cycle is jammed during the ascension of the water vapor. Sometimes the descent of water in its cycling becomes jammed. For this reason, the Taiyang section of the *Treatise on Cold Damage* refers to syndromes related to the channel and those related to the bowel.

For instance, when we use Mahuang Tang and Guizhi Tang to treat a Taiyang channel syndrome, it is because the ascending aspect of the cycle is hindered. The ascension of the earth *qi* upward to become clouds is inhibited. Therefore, we use methods that induce sweating. Once the sweat is able to freely emerge from the skin, this ascending aspect of the cycle is normalized.

Once the water reaches the heights of the heavens, it changes into clouds and into rain. If during the process of water's descent it becomes inhibited, it often becomes a bowel syndrome, and we should use Wuling San to resolve it. Wuling San is an important formula in the Taiyang chapter of the *Treatise on Cold Damage*. Zhang Zhongjing mainly used it to treat water amassment and dispersion-thirst (*xiaoke*), an illness marked by frequent drinking and urination.

Why is this formula, consisting of herbs that neither engender yin nor specifically increase fluids, indicated for *xiaoke*? How do Baizhu, Fuling, Zexie, Zhuling, and Guizhi treat thirst and frequent urination? Guizhi is acrid and warming and does not increase fluids. How is it able to help cure a dry mouth and thirst? This is a difficult question to answer unless we consider it in light of the larger meaning of Taiyang and in relation to the rest of nature. Once we consider this formula's function as analogous to the process of descent in the water cycle, it is very easy to comprehend.

The earth *qi* ascends to become clouds, and the celestial *qi* descends to become rain. If the celestial *qi* does not descend as rain, then there will be drought throughout the land. What does drought upon the land correspond to in the human body? The land corresponds with earth, the spleen rules earth and its orifice is the mouth. Therefore, this "drought" in the body presents first of all with a sensation of dryness in the mouth, the chief symptom of *xiaoke* disease. Wuling San causes the heavenly *qi* to descend as rain, removing the inhibition in the descending aspect of the water cycle. This is how it treats diseases characterized by thirst.

Laozi said, "Humans take the earth as model; the earth takes the heavens as model; the heavens take the Dao as model; the Dao takes nature as model." This line enlightens us as to why Wuling San is an effective treatment for thirst that is not relieved by increased intake of fluids. Nature as the model or pattern-maker of the Dao represents the highest rung of Laozi's hierarchy; once we have ascended to that lofty plane, everything becomes clear. Those who desire to comprehend Chinese Medicine must also understand what Laozi means by "the Dao takes nature as model." Once this key is comprehended, Chinese Medicine is perfectly clear. But if you do not understand what is meant by this phrase, and instead mistakenly believe that "the Dao takes modernity as model," then Chinese Medicine might as well be a carefully carved mud sculpture of a cow cast into the ocean, sinking out of sight and dissolving in a cloud of formless murk.

The entire Taiyang chapter discusses this central idea of the water cycle in the microcosm of the body. Savor this idea for a moment. Regardless of the formula, whether it is Mahuang Tang, Guizhi Tang, and Wuling San, or Da Qinglong Tang, Xiao Qinglong Tang, and Yue Bi Tang, all of these formulas discuss water. I have gone so far as to have formed a single sentence to summarize the entire Taiyang section of the *Treatise on Cold Damage*: "To treat Taiyang is to regulate water."

I.3. Explaining Disease

I.3.a. *The Chinese Character* Bing

For those in the medical field, disease is commonplace. But how many physicians have genuinely asked themselves what "disease" is? I fear that this particular question has fallen into the blind spot of nearly every physician. An analysis of the composition of the Chinese character *bing* (病), commonly translated as "illness" or "disease," reveals the richness of the Chinese language. The ancients spoke of meditating upon instructions but they also spoke of meditation upon a single word. Within a single word is deep meaning, subtle wisdom, and even the tools whereby we might attain enlightenment. There are times when realizing the inner meaning of a single word unlocks an entire field of study.

If, for instance, you fully understand the Chinese character *bing*, then the study of Chinese Medicine should be no problem at all. Zhang

Zhongjing, in his preface to *Treatise on Cold Damage and Miscellaneous Diseases* wrote: "If one adheres to the information collected here, then one will be able to contemplate more than half [of all diseases]." I boldly confer the meaning of this sentence to my own purpose: if you have fully understood the meaning of the character *bing*, then you will be able to understand more than half of Chinese Medicine.

In the first analysis of the character *bing*, we might immediately presume, as many before us have, that the radical on the left meaning sickness (*ne* 疒) indicates the general category, whereas the radical in the middle (*bing* 丙) indicates the pronunciation of the character. The radical on the left was, in ancient China, a character in its own right, with its own pronunciation: *ne*. The ancient dictionary *Explaining Writing and Analyzing Characters* defines *ne* as: "to recline; the form of a person suffering illness and reclining." When a person is sick, prostration naturally follows. This radical is, therefore, a pictogram showing a person lying down on something, which is exactly how a sick person appears. This is why *Collected Rhymes* (Jiyun) to say that this radical means "disease." We can see that this radical by itself already captures the modern sense of what we now call "disease."

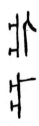 In ancient Chinese writing, this character was a pictographic ideogram: the left side depicted a bed, and the right a reclining figure. Depicting these two together clearly convey the idea of a human figure reclining on a bed. This character evolved into this form (疒), to later become the modern Chinese radical indicating sickness (疒).

Since the *ne* radical already expresses the basic meaning of illness, why was the *bing* radical added to it? Is it merely a phonetic component, indicating how to pronounce the character? This was a topic we discussed in the first chapter of this book. The phonetic marker of a character does not just indicate the pronunciation, but is also closely related to the meaning of the character of which it is a part. One must pay close attention to this fact when researching etymology. There is the pictographic radical *ne* (疒) and a phonetic component *bing* (丙), which together encapsulate the essential aspects of all disease.

The phonetic component *bing* is one of the ten heavenly stems. It is positioned in the South and, of the five elements, it belongs to fire. The ancients paired the ten heavenly stems and placed them in each of the four cardinal directions as well as the center, ascribing to each pair the elemental phase that corresponds to their cosmological position. In this way, the orientation of the *jiayi* stems corresponded with the east and to wood, the *bingding* stems with the south and to fire, the *gengxin* stems with the west and to metal, the *rengui* stems with the northern water, and the *wuji* heavenly stems with the central region and to earth.

As *Explaining Writing and Analyzing Characters* explains: "*Bing* (丙) signifies the south, the direction where all living things mature, and where they stand in abundant light. Here, the yin *qi* begins and the yang *qi* falters. It is composed of one (一), enter (入), and outermost boundary (冂). One is yang." Here, "abundant light" means luxuriant and flourishing; in the *Plain Questions's* "Great Treatise on the Four *Qi* and the Tuning of the Spirit," it says: "The three months of summer are referred to as those of splendorous flourishing." This is referring to the same "abundant light" aspect of *bing*. "The yin *qi* begins and the yang *qi* falters" refers to the emergence of the single yin line in the evolution of the hexagrams. After this line has emerged, yin begins to recover and yang to wane.

What does "one" refer to in this passage? "One" is none other than yang. This is related to the images in the *Classic of Changes*: there is a theory that the origin of Chinese characters is related to the eight trigrams, and this example provides some supporting evidence. The character *jiong* (冂) was explained by the Southern Tang scholar Xu Kai this way: "It is a gate (*men* 門), the gate of the yin and yang of the world." *Bing* is positioned in the south, and it dwells in the months of summer. The summer is when the yang *qi* is in a state of greatest release and must begin to weaken, so as we discussed at some length earlier, after the height of summer, the yang *qi* begins to enter into storage. The phrase "one enters the gate" (一入冂) in the passage translated above describes both the method of creating the character *bing*, as well as describing this process of the yang *qi* going back into storage. The *bing* (丙) radical has profound implications relative to our understanding of *bing* (病), the character for disease.

I.3.b. The Orientation of Illness and Disease

Bing (丙) represents the South, an orientation, a point on the compass. What do the directions do, though? The *Great Commentary of the Classic of Changes* says: "The directions of the compass gather things of their ilk, creatures are thereby gathered together and separated out. The division of the auspicious and the inauspicious emerge from this process." The directions gather things of a certain sort together. The East has eastern things, the South southern things. This combination of the radical *ne* (疒) with the character *bing* (丙) provides us with a very important insight, namely, the correspondences of illness and disease.

Why is this etymological discovery important? It is important because it concerns the central issue of all medicine, regardless of whether it is Chinese Medicine, Western Medicine, Tibetan medicine, or Mongolian medicine. All medical learning focuses on the correspondences of disease. What variable in the human organism brings about disease, and to what is this variable correlated?

The twenty-first century is the century of biological medicine. A great deal of energy in medicine is now devoted to genetics, with the goal of determining the relevance of our genetic code to health and disease. When it comes to most diseases, including AIDS, there is the important issue of susceptibility. One person may be regularly exposed to HIV, but never develops AIDS, while another comes in contact with it but once and immediately begins to develop the disease. Is there a genetic counterpart to the susceptibility of the first person and the resistance of the second? Might it be possible to alter the genetic makeup of the person who is susceptible to HIV infection such that they are no longer prone to contract the disease? If so, HIV could be eradicated. Genetic susceptibility to disease illustrates how the study of medicine, which is the study of the prevention and cure of disease, is the study of correlation between disease and other variables—in this example the correlation between susceptibility to infection and some genetic variable.

Earlier we looked at three patients: one suffered from a malignant tumor, one from sciatica, and one from stomach pain. In the case of all three of these illnesses, the correlating factor was cold dampness. Cold is the *qi* of the north, dampness is the *qi* of the central region. In this way, we can regard the most important variable influencing disease to be a matter of direction.

Biological medicine looks for correlations to disease states in the DNA, and looks for genetic causes predisposing us to particular diseases. Genetics has become the key problem facing those practicing medicine within the biological medical model. Perhaps there will be a real breakthrough in genetics in the second half of the twenty-first century, or the twenty-second century. When that happens, we will find ourselves in a new era of biological medicine, the post-genetic era, with perhaps an entirely new focus.

While biological medicine looks to genetics for correlations to disease states, Chinese Medicine looks at the directions of the compass, the *fang* (方). The *fang* gather together categories of things that are similar, and these categories can be many, even countless. In the categories subordinate to the *fang* can be found the factors that lead to the wide variety of diseases we see. Regardless of how varied and complex a disease may be, it can always be understood in terms of *fang*.

On another note, when we as Chinese Medicine physicians prescribe a formula (also written as *fang* 方), which in Chinese is expressed as *kaifang* (開方, literally "open a direction"), we are opening the same "direction" we discussed above. When you, as a Chinese Medicine practitioner, encounter a disease wrought by pathogenic cold, then the crucial factor causing disease is the northern direction. Of course, you cannot take that cardinal direction by the nose and lead it about, but you can create a formula that addresses that direction, and which is either complementary to it or which harmonizes it.

In the instance of someone afflicted by cold, we can create a "South" formula on the basis of the classical Chinese Medicine maxim of "heat that which is cold," and use our formula to simulate the southern direction to counter the northern one. Once the southern direction holds sway, the effects of the north will naturally fade; summer and winter cannot coexist in the same time frame. Chinese Medicine uses different medicines to create various formulas (*fang* 方) analogous to the many different directions, seasons, and geographical locations. Medicine can be used to simulate the various qualities of time and space. Curing disease is a matter of changing direction, of changing location, causing a person in a state of disease related to one direction to turn to a state of health related to a different direction. In the following chapters, we will discuss this change from disease to health in greater detail.

Direction, or put another way, orientation, is the crucial factor in determining the correlation to disease—in other words, in determining what we can address relative to this disease in order to effect a cure. Why then does the Chinese character for sickness, *bing* (病), use the character *bing* (丙) as part of its composition? The reason lies in this same principle of orientation that underlies all disease from the Chinese Medicine perspective. The directions gather things of like nature together, but how many directions are there? From the most elementary perspective, there are five directions: east, south, west, north, and the center. However, from the perspective of the *Classic of Changes*, the compass is divided into eight basic directions; in terms of the calendar year, there are twelve directions; in terms of the solar terms or calendrical periods, there are twenty-four directions; in terms of the hexagrams, there are 64 directions. When we look at the face of a compass, we see these various levels of directional detail marked out.

A Chinese Medicine physician ought to own a compass. A compass is not merely for the geomancy of the *fengshui* practitioner, it is also important in the practice of Chinese Medicine. At the very least, it can help the practitioner to recognize the different directions, and thereby have some ability to understand the most essential variable connected with the cause of disease.

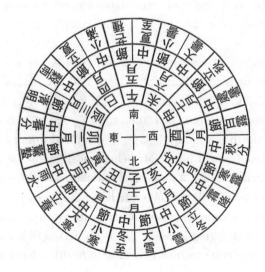

Here, we will first look at the most fundamental division of the compass into the five directions. We will look at each of these directions and examine the class of things each direction gathers.

I.3.b.1. Time

First of all, each of the directions gathers a particular quality of time. The east assembles the periods related to the third, fourth, and fifth earthly branches and the three months of spring. From these, we can deduce the rest. Therefore, time is a very important category related to direction. In the *Plain Questions* chapter "Treatise on the Six Nodes and Visceral Manifestations," we are admonished to "cautiously attend to the timing, for then you will be able to predict the *qi*." It also warns: "If you do not know what each year contributes, the abundance and weakness of the *qi*, and how deficiency and excess arise, then you cannot be a practitioner." These passages emphasize the importance of time in relation to the advent and cure of disease, and the centrality of this concept in Chinese Medicine. A patient afflicted with a malignant tumor who develops this disease in 1994 is different from the one whose disease develops in 1995. Western Medicine pays no heed to what year the cancer arises in. The Western medical physician looks at the results of the CT scan and the biopsy to determine the diagnosis, and does not think twice about the particular year. A Chinese Medicine practitioner who is not concerned whether the disease arose in 1994 or 1995 is wasting his time. Such a Chinese Medicine physician cannot completely understand the disease, because he has not considered an essential factor in its development.

As Chinese Medicine physicians, the year in which a disease arises must always be kept in mind. A disease that arose in 1994 is completely different from one that arose in 1995, because the correlates of the disease are different; "what each year contributes, and the abundance and weakness of the *qi*" make the difference. The Chinese Medicine physician who neglects this aspect of pathology is at a real disadvantage.

Western medical physicians recognize the importance of particular time periods to some extent, for instance in relation to the administration of particular medicines. For example, cardiac glycoside, a class of medications used in the treatment of heart failure and irregular heartbeat: its effects when given in the morning are a hundred times more powerful than when given at any other time during the day. There are certain hormonal medications that must similarly be administered with an eye on the clock. However, Chinese Medicine places a far greater emphasis on timing than Western Medicine does. We will be speaking of the relevance of timing quite a bit more from here on.

I.3.b.2. The Five Phases

The five phases are also assembled by the directions. Thus, the eastern direction gathers wood, the southern direction fire, the western direction metal, the northern direction water, and the central region gathers earth. Disease has a significant relationship with the five elements. This relationship pervades the *Yellow Emperor's Classic*. If you do not talk about the five elements and mistakenly think this facet of Chinese Medicine philosophy is just superstition, then your practice of Chinese Medicine will be shoddy. In the *Yellow Emperor's Classic* as well as in the modern *Fundamentals of Chinese Medicine* textbook, we often find the five phases placed on a par with yin and yang. In fact, the five phases are just different states of yin and yang. The state of yang *qi* emerging is called wood; when it is in a state of growth, it is called fire; when it is in a state of withdrawing and gathering, it is called metal; when it is in a state of storage, it is called water; and the process of transitioning from one phase to the next is referred to as earth. From this analysis, we can see that the five phases are essentially the cyclic transformations of yin and yang. The importance of the five phases to Chinese Medicine is therefore undeniable.

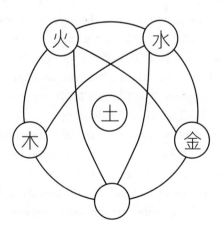

I.3.b.3. The Six Pathogenic Qi

The six *qi* (wind, cold, summer heat, dampness, dryness, and fire) are also assembled according to the directions of the compass. The east produces wind, the south produces fire (and summer heat), the west produces dryness, the north produces cold, and the central region produces damp. In the section about the nineteen disease triggers in *Plain Questions,* it says: "As for the advent of the hundred diseases, they all emerge from wind, cold, summer heat, damp, dryness, and fire." The "hundred" diseases all arise from imbalances of these six *qi,* and all are therefore related to the directions. The "hundred diseases" (not just "one disease") all correlate with the six *qi,* making the six *qi* universally applicable.

I.3.b.4. The Five Qi

The five *qi* are different from the six pathogenic *qi* mentioned in the previous section. The five *qi* refer to the particular orientation of a medicinal substance, whether it is cold, hot, warm, cool, or neutral. The east is warm, the south is hot, the west is cool, the north is cold, and the center is neutral. Previously we mentioned that medicines are able to simulate times, places, and directions; this capacity is related to the five *qi* of the medicinals. A firm grasp of the five *qi* of medicines is an essential part of understanding Chinese Medicine.

I.3.b.5. The Five Flavors

The five flavors, like the five energies, are also arranged in relation to the directions. The east gathers the sour flavor, the south the bitter flavor, the west the acrid flavor, the north the salty flavor, and the central region the sweet flavor. When a Chinese Medicine physician writes a prescription, she relies in no small part upon her understanding of the five flavors and the five *qi* to guide the process. What is the first thing that the *Divine Farmer's Classic of Materia Medica* discusses when introducing an herb? The first thing it discusses are the *qi* and the flavor of the herb. Only after that is the particular effect of the herb discussed. *Qi* and flavor are of first importance, and the herb's particular effect is secondary. The *qi* and flavor are the form; the particular effect is the function. This primary and secondary, form and function relationship between the *qi* and flavor of the herb on the one hand and the particular action of the herb on the other should be clearly understood by those who practice Chinese Medicine.

Presently, many people do not understand this relationship between form and function, and even manage to confuse the primary classification of the herb with the secondary one. They think in terms of particular herbs treating particular illnesses. They treat headaches with Chuanxiong and Baizhi, and tumors with Baihuasheshecao. They completely disregard the *qi* and flavor of the herb. How can this be considered Chinese Medicine?

The *Yellow Emperor's Classic* discusses tonifying and reducing methods for treating excess and deficiency respectively. What does the classic rely upon to tonify and drain? *Qi* and flavor. Therefore, in the classics we read "treat cold with heat, and heat with cold," and:

> When the element of wood is in the dominant position of a given year, it can be reduced with the sour flavor and tonified with the pungent flavor; when fire rules, it can be drained with the sweet flavor and tonified with the salty flavor; when earth is in the dominant position, it can be drained with bitterness and built up with sweetness; when metal prevails, it can be purged with acridity and tonified with sourness; when water dominates, it can be reduced with the salty flavor and tonified with the bitter flavor.

And so, when treating a direction or position with Chinese Medicine, we rely upon *qi* and flavor, because only when we know the *qi* and flavor can we then speak of a medicinal's effect upon direction. How can one possibly use categories such as "invigorates the blood and transforms stasis" or "relaxes tension and stops pain" to treat a direction? Do these categories belong to the northern direction or the southern direction? East or west?

The gathering of things of like nature by directional class is a topic well deserving of further research. In a time when people are eagerly searching for Chinese Medicine topics worthy of research, the directions beg for more attention. Furthermore, this research would be significant to Chinese Medicine. In the last several decades, Chinese Medicine research in China has spent untold amounts of money researching countless topics, but I cannot think of a single one that is of any real significance to Chinese Medicine. All these topics had going for them was that they were easy to get funding for, and therefore easily undertaken. If you propose to study some topic related to directionality, the funding is nowhere to be found.

Researching the five flavors also tells us that disease is closely related to diet. The ancients said: "Disease enters through the mouth, and misfortune emerges from the mouth." This saying certainly resonates with our current understanding of disease. If we look at the deadliest diseases—cardiovascular disease, diabetes, and cancer—they are all influenced by diet. Modern scientific study of nutrition looks at the composition of food: how much fat, sugar, trace elements, vitamins, saturated or unsaturated fat, protein, etc., that it contains. As a Chinese Medicine practitioner, we cannot forget the five flavors.

From the discussion we just had regarding the categories related to the five directions, we can see that the same variables that cause disease are also those that can cure it. This is to say that the same influences that create disease can also cure it. This understanding is in some ways unique to Chinese Medicine. It is one of the major differences between Chinese Medicine and Western Medicine.

Take the example of wind. Wind is an important pathogenic influence: "All sudden rigidity belongs to wind." On the other hand, wind can also cure disease; for instance, it is wind that can overcome dampness. Western Medicine takes a very different stance. Mycobacterium tuberculosis and staphylococcus bacteria are regarded solely as pathogens, never as cures. The Western medical practitioner seeks to exterminate these pathogens with other substances, such as antibiotics. A Chinese Medicine practitioner does not cure with the goal of killing the pathogen. How can one kill wind? We can only strive to harmonize the organism by applying the principles and formulas passed down to us by our ancient predecessors. In a sense, the Chinese practitioner tries to make sure that water surrounding a boat buoys it rather than capsizing it. To use the language of Sun Tzu and *The Art of War*, Chinese Medicine "attacks the heart," rather than "attacking the walled city."

I.3.b.6. The Five Colors

The five colors are blue-green, red, yellow, white and black. The East is blue-green, the South red, the Center yellow, the West white, and the North black. Because color has such a relationship with the directions, we cannot simply dismiss color as something beautiful but essentially meaningless, as merely decoration. Clearly, it is imbued with significance and potential usefulness to the Chinese Medicine practitioner.

If we encounter a person whose earth *qi* is weak and we use medicines aimed at tonifying the earth such as Si Junzi Tang or Li Zhong Tang but they never improve, why is this? Let us say that we notice this individual with weak earth *qi* is always wearing blue or green colored clothing. This is the color of wood, which controls earth in the cycle of restraint among the five elements. We are trying to tonify earth with our formula, but the color of his clothing is undermining earth, so how could he be expected to improve?

The causes of disease are complex and are related to a whole host of influences. If the practitioner only knows about clearing heat and resolving toxicity, or benefiting the *qi* and nourishing yin, or invigorating the blood and transforming stasis, then he only knows the aspects of function and primary indication. When these obvious methods fail, that same practitioner might go so far as to say that Chinese Medicine is ineffective, or that Chinese Medicine theory is not applicable in the clinic. Isn't this issue of limited understanding of Chinese Medicine theory and limited application of its principles worth serious consideration? Shouldn't we make an effort to change this problem?

The five colors are an important factor influencing health and disease. Let me give you an example from my master Zeng Yousheng. He once treated a patient suffering from severe cirrhosis of the liver and subsequent ascites. The patient could not even get out of bed, so he implored Mr. Zeng to come to make a house call. After examining the patient's and writing a prescription, Mr. Zeng did something unexpected. He ordered that the wall at the foot of the patient's bed, which stared back at him day and night, be painted jet black. The patient was directed to continue to take his formula and convalesce in that room. The patient quickly recovered.

The black color is gathered by the north, and to the north belong water and the kidneys, so Mr. Zeng's use of the color must have been to address the kidneys. To treat disease we should not only use the *qi*, flavor, and primary indication of medicinal substances; we can also use the five colors to conform with or adjust the direction. We can draw a lesson from Mr. Zeng on this point.

There are many factors that influence disease. If, for instance, we have a patient in whom the effect of the northern direction is insufficient, and the formula we prescribe is not quite strong enough to do the job, we might consider other factors that influence disease to assist in our treatment. Color, for instance, might be considered. This is an aspect of Chinese Medicine that deserves our attention.

I.3.b.7. The Five Tones

The five tones are *jue, zhi, gong, shang,* and *yu.* The *jue* tone pertains to the East, the *zhi* tone to the South, the *gong* tone to the Center, the *shang* tone to the West, and the *yu* tone to the North. Are the five tones related to disease? Absolutely. The *Yellow Emperor's Classic* speaks of looking, hearing, questioning, and palpating. Those who understand the disease simply by looking are called divine; those who understand the disease by listening are deemed sages.

What do we look at in order to diagnose disease? We look at the complexion and the appearance of the patient. It is very difficult to see the *qi* of the patient; we can only see the physical form. When the *Yellow Emperor's Classic* speaks of understanding a disease by listening, what is being listened to? We are listening to the five tones. We listen to the five tones to determine which tone is strong and which weak, which tone is present and which absent, and how these tones are coordinated. We must be able to distinguish all of these simply by listening. This is a very profound field of study. The ancients said: "in the entire world, there are only a few people who understand the tones." The original meaning of the "tones" was the five tones; it was only later that it came to take on a broader meaning.

When we hear another person's voice, we can understand their situation. This is not too obscure to fathom. There were a number of persons in history who were able to do this. Even when behind a wall, when the patient speaks, the physician is able to understand the nature of his illness. This is what is meant by "to hear and thereby understand the disease is considered sagely." This is because the five tones and disease are related.

If you suffer from a lung disease, then the *shang* tone will exhibit some problem. If you have an illness related to the heart, then the *zhi* tone will have some problem or other. In this way, listening to the tones allows you to understand the patient's health. The only problem is that, practically speaking, we might as well be deaf. We stuff our ears with cheap, lewd songs and have no idea what the five tones even sound like. Some Chinese Medicine physicians are ignorant of the entire concept of the five tones, and some even say that there should be seven notes, not five tones, and discount the system of five tones as unscientific. In my opinion, the five-tone system is a very deep subject, and worthy of arduous research.

Above we discussed using the five tones in diagnosis; using them in the treatment of disease is the same. The five tones, like the five flavors and the five colors, can cure disease. The *shang* tone belongs to the West and to metal. This metal tone can control wood. As a Chinese Medicine practitioner, you should not just know that Lingyangjiao and Gouteng can pacify liver and extinguish wind; the *shang* tone can do the same. At present, in the West, it is quite popular to use music as a form of therapy. This trend is indeed heartening, but the level at which it is practiced is far below that traditionally used in Chinese Medicine. The difference between these nascent experimentations and the high level of expertise wrought by classical Chinese Medicine practitioners is the difference between kindergarten and university. This high level is evident in the most refined music, such as the piece for Chinese zither (Guzheng) called *High Mountain, Flowing Water*. Researching this area of Chinese Medicine will be most fruitful. We are not limited to Xiao Chaihu Tang, or Mahuang Tang, or modern formulas such as Jing Fang Baidu San, and should broaden our horizons a little.

In the twenty-first century, Chinese Medicine has the potential to make great accomplishments. This potential is derived from the vast number of correlations Chinese Medicine has established. These correlations provide fertile ground for profound achievements. Presently, many Chinese Medicine practitioners have gone to the West, but they only do some acupuncture, a little massage, some herbs, etc. The Westerners around them also assume that this is all that Chinese Medicine has to offer. Why not research the five tones and open a convalescent hospital that uses these five tones to cure disease? In the *Book of Music* from the *Records of the Grand Historian*, it says: "music moves and vibrates the blood vessels, causing the essence and spirit to circulate." It is clear that recognition of the relationship between music and the human body and disease is not something that was only found out in modern times! This just goes to show that Chinese Medicine can be practiced by means of countless modalities. We should not be restricted to those few avenues that are popular currently.

I.3.b.8. The Five Odors

There are many topics related to the directions. There are the seasons, the five elements, the six *qi*, the five colors, the five tones, the five flavors, and many others. The odors are different from the flavors; they are perceived by the nose, not the mouth. The five odors are fetid, burnt, fragrant, rancid, and rotten. The odor of the east is fetid, that of the south is burnt, the central region is fragrant, the west is rancid, and the north is rotten.

We may be especially sensitive to smells, and there are some aromas that affect us deeply, for instance fragrant, dry things. Why do people enjoy the smell of things that are fragrant and dry? Even if we do not have much of an appetite, we still like to eat things that are fragrant. Why? Because fragrant odors belong to the central region; fragrance enters the earth and therefore the spleen and stomach, improving transportation and transformation and subsequently improving our appetite.

I remember a story of when old master physician Pu Fuzhou treated an elderly patient whose illness was characterized by emotional agitation, insomnia, anorexia, and constipation in which she had a bowel movement once a week. Her illness then progressed to nausea and vomiting such that whatever she ate, she vomited. If she drank water, she would puke it up. If she took medicine, she would vomit that. The patient's family had already lost all hope of her surviving, and turned to physician Pu with an attitude of last resort.

Physician Pu interviewed the patient at some length and, learning that the only nourishment she could even consider was tea, told the patient to take six grams of dragonwell tea and place it in water that had been boiling for two minutes. This should be brought to a boil twice, and then the patient should sip the resulting decoction a little at a time. The next day, the patient's son and daughter, with joyous surprise on their faces, came to tell physician Pu what had happened: "As soon as the tea was done boiling, our mother smelt it and wanted to drink it. She slowly drank a few sips without vomiting, and she seemed relaxed and free of worry. Then her stomach gurgled loudly and she passed gas a couple times. Next, she passed two dry stools. That night, she was able to sleep soundly, and in the morning she woke up with an appetite for the first time!" Physician Pu advised that the patient should be given thin rice porridge, a little at a time, and after recuperating for a next month or so would be recovered. The fact that a simple prescription of tea leaves was able to resolve this patient's morbid condition, where attempts with other formulas had failed, became a tale told far and wide among physicians of the time.

When I first heard this story, I found it rather unbelievable, and did not understand the logic behind this sudden cure. Today, within the context of a discussion of the five odors, this reasoning is very clear. High-grade dragonwell tea is redolent with fragrance. The special brewing method physician Pu prescribed extracted the maximum amount of this odor from the tea leaves, while minimizing the flavor. This allowed the fragrant *qi* to enter the central earth. This, of course, awoke the spleen and the appetite. The way in which tea alone could restore this patient's digestion lay in its aromatic quality.

There are many examples illustrating the significance of the five odors. In the first chapter in our discussion of the book *A Great Revolution in the Brain World*, we talked about curing bone cancer with regard to the five odors.

I.3.b.9. The Five Animals

There are two different versions of five animals discussed in the *Yellow Emperor's Classic*. In one version, the five animals are common domesticated animals: chicken, goat, ox, horse, and pig. The east is the rooster, the south is the goat, the central region the cow, the west the horse, and the north the pig. Another version is described in the seven chapters of the *Yellow Emperor's Classic*, generally referred to as the seven grand treatises. In this account, the five animals are referred to as the five "worms" or creatures. There are the hairy creatures, the feathered creatures, the naked creatures, the shelled creatures, and the scaled creatures. This system of classification also includes humans, as it applies to living creatures in general.

We here in China find ourselves in a carnivorous era. When I was a child, we might have meat with a meal maybe once a month, and eating meat was a special occasion. Nowadays, every meal consists at least in part of some sort of meat. The ailments we see today are increasingly complex, and strange diseases present in the clinic with greater and greater frequency. Many of the diseases we see are related to the increase in meat consumption in our diets. From a Chinese Medicine perspective, and from the perspective of the five animals, an essay could be written on the subject.

To our discussion of the five animals, we might also append another topic, that of the twelve animals of the Chinese zodiac. Every Chinese person is familiar with these: the rat (representing the earthly branch *zi*), ox (representing the earthly branch *chou*), tiger (representing the earthly branch *yin*), rabbit (representing *mao*), dragon (representing *chen*), snake (representing *si*), horse (representing *wu*), goat (representing *wei*), monkey (representing *shen*), rooster (representing *you*), dog (representing *xu*), and pig (representing the earthly branch *hai*). Several days ago, I read a very interesting article in the *Reference News* (a limited-distribution newspaper in China) that recounted how the Americans dealt with the threat of a poison gas attack during the Persian Gulf War. Besides many high-tech pieces of equipment, the Americans also brought with them live roosters. The roosters, being extremely sensitive to both the smell and effects of poison gas, served as a sort of infallible early warning system for the American soldiers.

One might ask why roosters would be such excellent early warning systems for poisonous gas. From a Chinese Medicine perspective, the rooster is the animal associated with the tenth earthly branch *you*, and the position of *you* is in the west. The lungs are the organs of the west, the orifice of the lungs is the nose, and the sense of smell is of course seated in the nose. From this line of reasoning, we might already assume that roosters possess an extraordinary sense of smell. This particular news article awoke in me the sense that the twelve animals of the zodiac deserve careful contemplation. The zodiac animals are not simply a symbol. There is profound knowledge invested in the animals of the zodiac.

I.3.b.10. The Five Grains

The five grains are wheat, millet, sorghum, rice, and beans. The grain of the east is wheat; the grain of the south is broomcorn millet, also known as common millet; the grain of the central region is sorghum; the grain of the west is rice; and the grains of the north are beans. We discussed the five grains to some extent during the first chapter, with reference to beans. If you remember, beans are associated with the north and have an especially close connection with the kidneys. Therefore, beans are called the grain of the kidneys. If you look at a single soybean, it looks like a miniature kidney. Because of this affinity with the kidneys, legumes and leguminous products have a particularly strong action on the kidneys and the bones and brain that are closely related to the kidneys.

A nutritional supplement derived from legumes that has become popular recently is lecithin. In China, lecithin is used to regulate blood lipids, benefit the cerebrovascular function, improve memory, and abate some types of hair loss. From a Chinese Medicine perspective, all of these effects are related to the northern direction, and to the kidneys. Among the five grains, rice belongs to the western direction. It is the grain of the lungs, and the lungs rule the skin and body hair. From a cosmetic perspective, rice is therefore the most beautifying. One might postulate that part of the reason the hair and skin of people from the south of China is more beautiful than that of those who live in the north is because rice is the staple grain in the south, whereas wheat is the staple in the north of China.

I.3.b.11. The Five Emotions

The five emotions are anger, joy, pensiveness, sadness, and fear. The emotion of the east is anger, of the south joy, of the center pensiveness, of the west grief, and of the north fear. The connection between the emotions and disease is widely understood, so I will not elaborate on it here. The effect on health of too much worry, grief, fear, etc., are all clearly recorded in the *Yellow Emperor's Classic*, showing the close correspondence between emotion and disease. Some diseases are directly caused by emotion, and treating such diseases with herbal medicines will not resolve the illness satisfactorily. The psyche of the person must be addressed. In the ancient medical records, there are many accounts of physicians using the five emotions to cure disease. The five emotions are able to cause disease, and they also possess the power to cure it. Ultimately, this capacity can be traced back to the workings of directionality.

I.3.b.12. The Five Numbers

The five numbers are one, two, three, four and five. These are doubled, however, so we have one through ten. Among these, five pertain to heaven and five to earth; together they are called the "five" numbers. *The Great Commentary of the Classic of Changes* says: "Heaven is one and earth two, heaven is three and earth four, heaven five and earth six, heaven seven and earth eight, heaven nine and earth ten." In other words, the odd numbers one, three, five, seven, and nine pertain to heaven, and the even numbers two, four, six, eight, and ten pertain to earth. The odd numbers are yang and the even numbers yin. As far as the five directions are concerned, the numbers one and six belong to the North and to water; two and seven belong to the South and to fire; three and eight are of the East and of wood; four and nine correspond to the West and metal; and five and ten correlate with the Center and earth.

The way in which the five numbers pertain to the five directions harkens back to the *River Chart* (Hetu). The *River Chart* is one of the most esoteric artifacts of traditional culture, and is said to be understood only by the greatest of sages. Confucius mourned the fact that those great sages had not come again, and once exclaimed ruefully: "The Phoenix does not come and the River produces no Chart, what hope do we have!" In the *Great Commentary of the Classic of Changes,* he made a related statement: "The Yellow River brought forth the Chart, the River Luo produced the Inscription, a true sage will be guided by them." Much of the essence of traditional culture is stored in the *River Chart.*

Here, however, is not the time to expound on the mysterious and obscure aspects of ancient understanding. Let us discuss the five numbers in simpler terms. The most characteristic feature of modern science is its system of mathematical logic. In modern mathematics, numbers are considered to be purely abstract entities, and mathematics is an abstract science. Correspondingly, the most characteristic feature of traditional Chinese culture is its system of yin yang numerical calculations. Within this system, there is a dichotomous understanding of number.

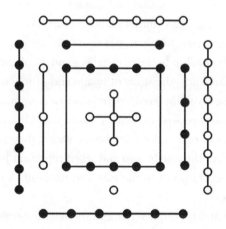

On the one hand, they are abstract. For instance, in our discussion of the categories related to particular directions, we find seemingly completely unrelated things belonging to the same class. How is it that they are gathered into the same category? In the process that the *Classic of Changes* refers to as "directional categories accumulating things of similar ilk," the non-essential aspects of phenomena are disregarded and their most essential attributes abstracted. In this way, seemingly unrelated phenomena, once distilled into their essential attributes, are brought together. The process of categorizing phenomena demands that they be regarded abstractly.

On the other hand, in Chinese yin yang numerical calculations, there are those things that resist abstraction. In modern mathematics, numbers are purely abstract. For instance, the number one is the number one and nothing more. It represents only itself, the number one, and not anything else. It has no concrete, specific implication; it does not represent any phenomena but itself. In modern mathematics, any object of study, any image to which a number refers, must first be distilled into its purely abstract, numerical form.

Not so with traditional Chinese yin yang numerical calculations. Within this system, numbers are also images (*xiang*). Thus, the *Commentary of Zuo* of the *Spring and Autumn Annals* says: "When phenomena emerge, there are images; when images emerge, there are numbers." Within phenomena there are archetypal images, and within each image there is number. Or the other way round, every number has specific images associated with it, and these images are directly related to phenomena.

In line with this idea, traditional Chinese culture actually had a field of study called "image and number study" (*xiangshuxue*), that specifically explored the connection between archetypal image and number and furthermore, the relationship between numbers and all phenomena.

In this field of study, the study of image and number, numbers cannot be abstracted. They contain fixed, correspondent connotations, images that they are immediately related to. This is the profound message of the *River Chart*. The numbers one and six symbolize water; they have the connotation of water, and of the north. Two and seven represent fire and the south. Three and eight correspond to the east and to wood. And so on with the rest of the numbers.

Why do one and six imply water and the north? This correlation is not something that could be arbitrarily decided in the present day and age, but it is most certainly something that had been positively ascertained and was absolutely certain in the minds of the Chinese ancients. For them, it was a point of fact. To overturn this understanding would be tantamount to rebuking the entire culture of Chinese antiquity.

This point brings to light a crucial difference between traditional Chinese culture and modern Chinese culture. Modern-day calculations are based on probability and statistics. Ancient Chinese calculations were based on the relationship between number and image. The study of image and number is not a token field of study. It was a very real and very consequential field of study. It was by means of image and number that the ancients determined the size of formulas, the number of medicines used, and the dosage of each individual herb.

I.3.b.13. The Five Emotional Toxins

In addition to the factors listed above, I would like to add one more, the five emotional toxins: greed, anger, infatuation, sloth, and jealousy. The concept of emotional toxins is a Buddhist one, and I raise the topic here in the hope that it may provoke the reader to consider whether our good and evil, especially the sort of good and evil as it exists in our hearts and minds, has an effect on our health.

The *Commentary of Zuo* of the *Spring and Autumn Annals* says: "A person given to goodness and charity will be happy and fortunate, while a person who lacks such merits will inevitably meet with calamity. The "Treatise on Heavenly Truth in Remote Antiquity" (Shanggu tianzhen lun) from *Plain Questions* says: "Those who are able to maintain a state of tranquility and lightheartedness, without ambitions or preconceptions, will always stay connected to the source of true *qi*, their spirit and essence will be contained and preserved, and no illnesses will develop."

When a person assumes an attitude of peace and does not strive or contend, the five emotional toxins are dispelled. Furthermore, greed, anger, infatuation, sloth, and jealousy create a psychological environment that does not allow for tranquil indifference, or the sort of emptiness that generates equanimity. As soon as the person achieves this tranquil state, the true *qi* blossoms, the spirit and essence can be preserved within the person, and disease cannot come about in such a person. From this point, we can see that morality is not merely a religious or social question; it is also a medical question.

In the above discussion, we made a rough sketch of the meaning of "direction." On the surface, the contents of each category seem to be completely different. However, when one looks at their essential aspects they seem equivalent, even somewhat equivocal. It is precisely because of this equivocal quality that there is so much flexibility and diversity among the diagnosis and treatments of Chinese Medicine practitioners. They seem to be very different and unorthodox, as if each sticks to his own view, and each feels they are right. In fact, this is a sort of great harmony, and each reaches the same goal by different routes. Each has their own way of playing the game, but none violates the principle of direction.

The famous *Dream of the Red Chamber* scholar Zhou Ruchang, in speaking about the particular allure of Chinese culture, cited two superlative qualities. The first is that etymology (literally "to bite off words and chew on single characters" in Chinese) is the highest level of Chinese culture. The second is that Chinese characters are the crystallization of mankind's highest wisdom. From our explanation of the character *bing* (病), and the correlative aspect of this concept, namely its correspondence with *fang* (方) directional categories, we can see the evidence for Mr. Zhou's words.

I.3.c. Why Use the Radical Bing?

In accord with the preceding discussion, the character *bing* (病), usually translated into English as "disease," uses the radical *bing* (丙) as a directional indicator, and thereby reveals the correlative property of disease. If the purpose of this radical, which represents one of the heavenly stems, is only to indicate the directional, correlative aspect of disease, the character *jia* (甲), also a heavenly stem, might just as well be used as *bing*. Why choose *bing*?

The heavenly stems begin with *jia*. All things being equal, if one simply reaches for a heavenly stem, one would naturally grasp *jia* first. If the sages who first created the Chinese language had used *jia* instead of *bing*, then the character for disease would be pronounced "*jia*" instead of "*bing*."

I think that if it is purely a phonetic component, simply a marker of pronunciation, then it would not make much difference. In that case, it would be merely a matter of custom. To draw an analogy from elsewhere in Chinese culture, it is like when a girl, before she is married, calls the mother of her prospective husband "auntie," but as soon as she is married and moves into his household, she calls her new mother-in-law "mother." At first, this feels unnatural. But no matter, after a few months it feels comfortable.

I do not think that the use of the radical *bing* can be explained by mere phonetic convention, therefore.

I.3.c.1. The Heart Holds the Office of the Sovereign and Ruler; Spirit Brightness Originates from It

The use of the radical *bing* (丙) in the character for disease (*bing* 病) most certainly contains very specific information. Among the ten heavenly stems, *bing* belongs to the category of the southern direction, to fire, and to the heart. What is the particular function of the South, fire, and the heart? Those who do not study Chinese Medicine might have difficulty answering this question.

Now let us move our discussion, for the moment, to the "Treatise on the Spiritual Orchid Secret Canon" of the *Plain Questions*. In the *Plain Questions* of the *Yellow Emperor's Classic*, we find various models used as analogics or schema for medical concepts. There are biological models, cosmological models, psychological models, and even societal models. The "Treatise on the Spiritual Orchid Secret Canon" uses societal structure to discuss complex medical concepts.

In such a model, the southern direction and the heart play the most crucial role. The treatise reads: "The heart holds the office of the sovereign and ruler; spirit brightness originates from it." The office of the "sovereign ruler" in this model is analogous to the office of the President in the United States, or the Chairman of the Communist Party in China. These roles embody, in a single agent, the most crucial decision-maker in a country. Thus, after this chapter discusses the particular function of each of the organs, it makes the following summary:

> As for these twelve offices, they must never lose contact with each other.
> If the ruler is bright and clear, there is peace below. To nourish life on
> the basis of this results in longevity. There will be no risk of failure till
> the end of all generations. To rule the world in this way results in great
> abundance.

If the ruler is not bright and clear, the twelve offices are all imperiled. The Dao will be closed off and obstructed, and the physical form will be greatly harmed. To nourish life on the basis of this results in disaster. To rule the world in this way will greatly endanger the ancestral temple. Beware! Beware!

If the ruler is bright, then all below it will know peace. If the sovereign ruler is bright, then the entire body, all twelve officials, will be tranquil. A life lived in such a way results in longevity.

Thus, if you wish to obtain a healthy body and a long life, you should do everything possible to make the ruler bright and clear. This is especially evident when we survey history. When we look back through the millennia, every dynasty and succession that was characterized by a wise monarch was also characterized by tranquility among his subjects, and the people flourished. When fatuous and self-indulgent rulers held the reins of government, there was great disorder and the people suffered hardships.

From the "Treatise on the Spiritual Orchid Secret Canon," we know that the heart, the fire of the south, is the ruler. It is the crux of the entire organism. Health, longevity, and premature death are all related to the heart, to the southern direction. Whether the person is healthy or sick depends upon the heart. Thus, the character for illness (*bing* 病) uses the radical *bing* (丙) because it represents the south. Earlier, we mentioned that Chinese Medicine "attacks" the heart, and not the city. This is an allusion to the Sun Tzu's *The Art of War* where it is stated that "attacking the heart is superior, and attacking walled cities is inferior." If you only know how to attack the stronghold and do not know how to assail the heart and mind, then you are not a true practitioner of Chinese Medicine, or at the very least will never be a physician of the higher order.

What does it mean to "attack the walled city"? What does it mean to "attack the heart"? This is something one must contemplate.

I.3.c.2. The Nineteen Disease Triggers

In addition, there are the nineteen disease triggers to consider. There are five lines for the five solid viscera, and another two lines for the upper and lower body, for a total of seven lines. The wind, cold, and damp disease triggers each receive one line, for a total of ten lines. The remaining nine lines are all concerned with fire and heat pathogenicity. If to these we add the line from the five viscera that is devoted to the heart, we have a total of ten lines discussing fire and heat, which is more than half the total lines.

At the outset of this passage on disease triggers, Huangdi says: "As for the advent of the hundred diseases, they all emerge from wind, cold, summer heat, damp, dryness, and fire." All diseases are related to the pathogenic factors of the five directions. Why then, when Qi Bo arrives at his discussion of the nineteen triggers that cause disease, does he cast all others aside and primarily discuss fire and heat, the pathogens that pertain to the southern direction? This emphasis reflects the role of the heart, and by extension the southern direction, as "sovereign and ruler" in the "Treatise on the Spiritual Orchid Secret Canon."

Disease is related to many factors, but there is one single pathogenic influence that is most decisive and crucial. This is analogous to a country's government: all of the branches and ministries of a government are important. One cannot say that the Ministry of Foreign Affairs is important and that the Ministry of Finance is unimportant. They are all important. However, among these important variables, there is one that is most important.

The sages who created the Chinese characters selected the radical *bing* instead of *jia* or some other radical in accord with this understanding. The selection of this radical has profound meaning. Proceeding from our initial examination of the character *bing* (disease), we explored a number of related topics. At the outset of this discussion, I went so far as to say that once the practitioner of Chinese Medicine truly realizes the meaning of this particular character, one comprehends half of Chinese Medicine. Does this statement seem overblown? I do not think it is.

Any field of medicine researches two things. The first is to which factors the occurrence of disease is related. The second is to which factors the treatment of disease is related. The construction of the character *bing* (disease) references both of these factors, therefore, one should ponder this character carefully and thoroughly.

Let us consider Zhou Ruchang's conclusion that etymology comprises the highest level of Chinese culture and ask ourselves whether or not Mr. Zhou was correct. Etymology can border on the pedantic, looking for problems where there are none. How could it be the highest level of Chinese culture? However, if you carefully ponder this question, then you will realize that without this "biting language and chewing characters," then the highest level simply does not exist. This "biting and chewing" is not a simple affair. It requires deep erudition, attention to a wealth of detail, the application of logic, and the ability to make intuitive perceptions, judgments, and associations. Without all of these, you cannot "bite" into anything, and cannot chew the flavor out of a single morsel.

If you cannot chew and you cannot bite, the limit of Chinese culture cannot even be talked about. Furthermore, we cannot speak of "biting language and chewing characters." The day you are able to bite into and chew at language, and you taste a mouthful of its enduring aftertaste, this high plateau of Chinese culture of which Mr. Zhou spoke will spontaneously emerge before you. This spontaneous emergence is not terribly different from the sort of spontaneous realization that Buddhists speak of. There are those elderly scholars who are utterly steeped in learning, whose every sentence is laden with meaning, and every word they use seems worth a thousand gold pieces in its descriptive power. Such intellects are unsurpassable. Zhou Ruchang's quote about "to bite language and chew words" is a most excellent example of such a use of words.

I.4. Explaining Pulse

I.4.a. The Chinese Character Mai

Let us begin our explanation of the pulse by looking at the composition of the character for pulse: *mai*. In the simplified form (脉), the character consists of the radical 月 plus the character *yong* (永), which means "perpetually, forever, always." In the more traditional and more orthodox form of the character (脈), it consists of 月 plus the radical 辰. The 月 radical in this case originated with the character *rou* (肉), and is identified as such by both *Explaining Writing and Analyzing Characters* and the *Kangxi Dictionary*. The radical 月 can represent either the character *yue* (月) meaning "moon" or the character *rou* (肉) meaning "flesh."

Personally, I think the *Kangxi Dictionary* and *Explaining Writing and Analyzing Characters* are only half right by interpreting the 月 radical to mean "flesh." They are half right because from the perspective of the human form, the pulse is an event which takes place in and of the physical body, the flesh. However, from the perspective of its function, and in the broader sense of the pulse, this emphasis on "flesh" is inappropriate. From this perspective, its radical should be "moon," not "flesh."

The character *yue* (月) refers to moonlight, and *Explaining Writing and Analyzing Characters* explains that the moon is the "essence of Taiyin." In the *Records of the Grand Historian*, it says: "the moon is the gathering of the yin essence." In the *Huainanzi*, it is written: "the essence of water *qi* becomes the moon," which is to say that the moon is the product of the coagulation of the *qi* of water.

Looking briefly at the simplified form of the character *mai* (脉), the original meaning of the character *yong* (永) was "long." When this concept of "long" is placed within the frame of reference of history, it might be taken to mean "eternal." When placed in the context of the natural world, this idea naturally resonates with the image of a river, long and constantly flowing. Therefore, *Explaining Writing and Analyzing Characters* says: "*yong* means long, it resembles the lengthy flowing path of a river." Take for instance the Yangzi River that begins in the Tanggula Mountains and flows all the way to the sea, traversing as it does the entire interior of China from west to east. What is longer than this? The original meaning of *yong* lay in this idea of the main stream of a major river.

The radical 厎, as found in the traditional form of *mai* (脈), is also related to water. It indicates a tributary or branch of a river. Both the character *yong* and the radical 厎 refer to rivers; the first to the main stream of a river and the second to a tributary. In any case then, the character *mai* is closely related to the concept of water.

I.4.b. The Meaning of Pulse

Both the semantic and the phonetic meanings of *mai* (脈) are as we have described, keeping in mind that we are discussing the semantic element of the character with the assumption that it refers to the moon, not to flesh. The moon is yin, and things that are yin are dark rather than luminous. Why then is the moon luminous? The ancients discussed this particular topic and considered the light of the moon to be a result of the sun's light. By this they meant that the moon, being yin, was lightless without the sun.

When, at midnight, we look at the surface of a lake, we might see the moon there. Or, looking in a mirror, we might see a vase of flowers. There is, of course, no moon in the lake nor any flowers in the mirror. These are only reflections. The light of the moon is like this. The moon is like a mirror for the light of sun, a mirror for the yang *qi*.

The phases of the moon, its constant waxing and waning, are the result of the positions of the sun and moon in relation to the earth. From a Chinese Medicine perspective, these phases correspond to ebb and flow of yang *qi*. The changing face of the moon, its endless flow of light and shadow, is purely a reflection of changes in the yang *qi*. As I write this, it is the eleventh day of the lunar month. After another four days, it will be the fifteenth day of the lunar month. For the next four days, the bright face of the moon will become rounder and rounder until it is full on the fifteenth. The moon is yin, so does that mean that when the moon is full, the yin *qi* is at its zenith? No, on the contrary, when the moon is full, the yang *qi* has reached its limit and is at the height of flourishing.

This raises the topic of the cyclical nature of the month. Earlier in this book, we discussed the daily and annual cycles, and indicated that these cycles pertained to the advent of certain diseases. For instance, individuals with certain gastric diseases may only suffer during the spring. During the rest of the year, they may be free of symptoms, but as soon as spring returns so too does their discomfort. In such a case, we should consider that the disease is related to the eastern direction and to the liver and gallbladder as well. When we contemplate the appropriate treatment of this disease, we should keep these factors in mind.

There are also those patients whose disease follows no particular annual pattern but whose symptoms have a definite circadian rhythm. The patient may only feel uncomfortable at nightfall, for instance, and feel fine the rest of the time. From our earlier discussion of daily rhythm, we know that nightfall corresponds to autumn and to the western direction, the lungs, and metal.

Each cycle of the moon, each lunar month, also has its own "spring," "summer," "autumn," and "winter" periods that correspond respectively to the emergence, growth, retrieval, and storage of yang *qi*. The way in which the cycle of the patient's disease corresponds with the lunar cycle provides us with useful information for its diagnosis and treatment.

The *Zhouyi cantong qi* by the Han Dynasty alchemist Wei Boyang made such an impression on subsequent generations of Chinese thinkers that it was lauded as the "Everlasting King of Alchemical Classics." This book uses the hexagrams of the *Classic of Changes* to describe the phases of the moon. For instance, the fifteenth day of the lunar month, when the moon is fullest and the yang *qi* is in its most liberated state, corresponds with the hexagram *qian* (Initiating): "The fifteenth day is embodied by the hexagram *qian*. It symbolizes the fullness of the eastern direction, represented by the first of the ten heavenly stems, *jia*." The correspondence between the hexagram *qian*, consisting only of yang lines, and the full moon indicates that the time of the full moon was considered to be the time when the yang *qi* was purest and most abundant.

Following the full moon, the utmost yang becomes yin, the yang *qi* slowly shifts toward a state of retrieval and then storage. The moon slowly wanes from full to new. As the last quarter of the lunar cycle progresses, the luminous face of the moon withers to a thin sickle, at which point it corresponds with autumn until, at day thirty of the lunar month, the moon becomes completely dark. At this point, we see only a shadowy disc in the sky, what is referred to as the "new moon" in English and the "dark moon" in Chinese.

When the moon is dark like this, where has the moon gone? The moon is still there. If we move the flowers, we can no longer see their petals but the mirror itself remains. That which was reflected is gone, but that which reflects is still there. At this time, the yang *qi* is hidden; it has been stored away. Because the yang *qi* is stored away, the moon becomes dark. This period of lunar darkness corresponds to the season of winter. The whole lunar cycle describes the permutations of yang *qi* in the same way that the cycle of the four seasons or the cycle of a day does.

The phases of the moon represent the phases of the yang *qi*, therefore, the moon can also be called the "mirror of the yang." Whether or not it was specifically called the "mirror of the yang" or not by the ancients, I am not certain. If it was not, then I believe we are entitled to coin the term here. Thus, the phases of the moon render yang's state obvious. Now that we have discussed the significance of the moon, we can return to our discussion of water.

Water belongs to yin. Water is an inanimate substance. It only flows downward. Thus, there is a Chinese saying: "People go upward toward high places and water flows downward to low places." However, there are some exceptions to this general rule. Water rises and falls, for instance with the tides. This exception causes us to contemplate the underlying cause of this rising and falling.

In the past year, there was a popular Chinese television program on the spectacular Qiantang River tidal bore, a wave that is brought in on the tides into the wide, funnel-shaped estuary of Hangzhou Bay. I was especially impressed by the way in which two large tidal waves collided into each other, forming a natural yin yang symbol. This, of course, caused me to recall the famous line: "the Dao takes nature as model." Ancient understanding of how the world worked was not fanciful or imagined. Their understanding had a solid basis, and this basis was nature.

How is water, a passive substance which, left to its own accord will only descend, enticed to surge upward with such vigor? This activity of water is similar to the shining of the moon. The moon is dark and passive, but reflects the light of the sun, making it bright. Water is essentially passive, but the yang influence compels it to move. Therefore, this is entirely a matter of the influence of yang *qi*, and should correspond with the changes and transformations of yang.

The ancients spoke of "viewing the tide when the moon is full," and this referred to the fact that typically the tide is most pronounced during the full moon. When the moon is full, the tides rise, and when it is new, the tides fall. Why is this? Modern scientific understanding of ocean tides recognizes that when the moon is full, the gravitational influence of the moon on the earth's tides is greatest. The rise and fall of the tides correspond to the gravitational influence of the moon. This is the modern scientific explanation of this phenomenon.

However, the ancients did not possess a scientific concept of gravity. What influence did they indicate caused the changes in tidal patterns? Yin and yang are the ultimate agents of change, as was clearly set forth in the *Plain Questions* chapter "Great Treatise on the Correspondences of Yin and Yang." What factor could cause water, this passive, yin, descending entity to rise so vigorously? Nothing other than yang.

Yang rules movement and rising; only by means of the action of yang can water be induced to surge upward. When the moon is full, the yang *qi* is also most abundant. This aligns with the modern scientific explanation. The action of yang causes this passive substance to become active, it causes this descending substance to rise upward. The rise and fall of the ocean tides in fact reflect the changes in yang *qi*. When the yang exerts itself on yin, the tides rise. The level of the tides reflects the presence of yang in the same that the brightness of the moon does; both are the result of yang joining yin.

In the natural world, the oceans are affected by the gravitational pull of the moon's mass, and by the influence of yang *qi*. What about in the human body? On the basis of the mutual correspondence between humans and nature, the human body ought also to be influenced by these phenomena of nature. This influence manifests in the blood and pulse.

Several years ago, there was an article in *China Youth* journal that substantiates the idea that the blood in the human body correlates with the oceans. This article made two main points. The first point was that life arose in the oceans. We will discuss this point in greater detail during the Jueyin chapter. The origin of life is closely related to the *River Chart* and the five elements. The second point was that seawater is similar in many respects to blood. In what way? Human blood is salty, and seawater is salty.

In nature there are rivers, lakes, and seas, and in the body there is the blood and the pulse. Blood is a fluid, like water. Blood is a passive substance, so how is it able to flow through the blood vessels, and how is it able to pulse? The movement of the blood, as science has revealed, is the result of the perpetual beating of the heart. A purely scientific explanation for this movement does not satisfy all our questions. The ancients recognized that it was the beating of the heart that produced the pulse, and understood it as being related to the stomach *qi*.

However, if we wish to place the principle of the pulse within the comprehensive framework of Chinese Medicine, then we must return to a discussion of yin and yang. Trees desire stillness, but the wind never ceases; the yin blood desires quiet, but yang moves it. If we were to take one single sentence to define the pulse, it would be: "Yang joined with yin is called the pulse."

If you understand this essential definition of the pulse, you will easily comprehend why palpation of the pulse is so essential to the practice of Chinese Medicine: because it allows us to understand yin and yang. The *Yellow Emperor's Classic* says: "The pulse allows us to observe yin and yang." The pulse allows us to observe the state of yin and yang, because the shape that the pulse takes and the ways in which it changes possess all of the essentials of yin and yang.

When we feel the pulse, the most basic, the most important thing we are doing is acquainting ourselves with the state of yin and yang. The "Great Treatise on the Correspondences of Yin and Yang" from *Plain Questions* says: "Yin and yang are the Dao of heaven and earth, the warp and weft of the myriad things, the mother and father of change and transformation, the origin of life and death, the palace of spirit brightness. To treat disease, we must seek the root."

In the second chapter, we discussed the question of what the "root" is; it refers to yin and yang. The occurrence, development, and transformation of all phenomena are related to yin and yang; all are brought about by yin and yang. Disease is no exception. As physicians, we wish to understand disease, investigate disease, and understand the underlying cause of disease. Where do we start? Of course, we must start with the essentials. If we wish to begin with the essentials, we cannot neglect yin and yang.

Where can we observe yin and yang? The pulse! Because the pulse so aptly reveals the motion of yin and yang in the body, palpating the pulse is one of the premiere diagnostic methods in Chinese Medicine. Of course, if one possesses the ability to accurately diagnose disease as the legendary physician Bian Que could, then feeling the pulse is not so important. Bian Que could simply look at the patient and know the internal state of yin and yang. Bian Que's method of diagnosis is, of course, very difficult. For most of us, palpating the pulse is the best option for determining the patient's balance of yin and yang.

I.4.c. On the Pulse in the Four Seasons

The study of the pulse in Chinese Medicine is a rich and complex field. Some speak of twenty-eight different pulses, others of thirty-six. These discourses are invaluable, but truly mastering these systems of pulse diagnosis is not an easy task. In the *Yellow Emperor's Classic*, pulse diagnosis is not as complicated as some later physicians made it out to be. That book discusses only the most essential principles of pulse diagnosis.

For example, the *Yellow Emperor's Classic* only discusses one pulse for each of the four seasons, not thirty-six different pulse types. Even so, if the practitioner of Chinese Medicine can aptly discern these four different pulses, then that practitioner has already solved much of the difficulty inherent in pulse diagnosis. In the following passage, I wish to explore the pulses of each of the four seasons.

I.4.c.1. The Wiry Pulse of Spring

The four seasonal pulses are those that correspond to spring, summer, fall, and winter. The spring pulse is "wiry." What does "wiry" mean? The "wiry" pulse is relatively easy to understand. The ancients described the wiry pulse "as if pressing on the string of the Chinese zither." So, if we press down on the patient's pulse and it feels like pressing down on the string of a zither, this is a wiry pulse. The typical wiry pulse feels slightly tense, or "high strung." If it were still tenser, we would call it a "tight" or "tense" (*jin*) pulse.

As a result, many medical charts show the pulse described as "wiry and tight," because many find that the quality of these two sometimes overlaps and is difficult to differentiate. However, there is a way to clearly distinguish between the two. Why is the pulse of spring wiry? Having read the second chapter, we know that in spring, the yang *qi* begins to rise and be released outward. However, at the time of spring, the yin cold has not yet been completely dispelled. This is especially true in the north of China, where the first couple months of spring are still very cold.

During this period, the yang *qi* wants to emerge, but the yin cold obstructs this release, and binds up the yang *qi*. This results in a sort of revolt on the part of the yang *qi*, against the yin cold that thwarts its liberation. This combination of yang struggling against yin presents us with a picture of the typical wiry pulse. Therefore, when we palpate such a pulse, we will invariably receive the impression of being barred or detained. It is cumbersome to try to adequately describe this particular sensation with words and language. One must experience this feeling to grasp it.

Why does this particular dynamic of yang *qi* struggling to emerge against the lingering yin cold manifest as a wiry pulse? It is the very antagonism between yang and yin that produces a wiry pulse. If the yang *qi* were completely unfettered, there would be no wiry pulse. And so the wiry pulse depicts the essential yin yang dynamic of spring. Therefore, if we take someone's pulse during the spring and find it wiry, this is normal and should be expected. However, it should not be too wiry. If it is, the patient is sick.

An overly wiry pulse depicts a scenario in which the struggle between the yang and its yin fetters is abnormally intense. If you wish to understand why the pulse is so wiry, you must discover why the struggle between yang and yin is so fierce. If, on the other hand, the pulse is flaccid during the spring season, without even a taste of tension or tightness, this tells us that the yang *qi* has failed to rise and there is a problem with its emergence. And so, if in spring the pulse is either too wiry or lacks wiriness, we should be concerned. So it is in spring.

If during any other season of the year the pulse is wiry, we must look for the reason. This is especially true of our female patients. If we detect a wiry pulse, we should inquire after their recent emotional state. Have they felt irritated or annoyed? When a person is irritated or annoyed, their pulse will often become wiry. This is because when we are annoyed, we can easily begin to feel down, and this depression in mood inhibits the free flow of *qi* and blood, fettering it. When we encounter a wiry pulse during seasons other than spring, we must discover its underlying cause.

I.4.c.2. The Flooding Pulse of Summer

The pulse of summer is called a "flooding" or "bounding" (*hong*) pulse, or it may be referred to as a "hook" (*gou*) pulse. The pulse of summer is described as "flooding" because the yang *qi* is still rising, continuing the trend begun during the spring. The yang *qi* rises and spreads, ever upward and outward. Unlike the pulse of spring, during summer the yin cold has retreated, and the yang *qi* is entirely uninhibited. Yang spreads its wings and soars through the air with complete freedom. The pulse of summer reflects this flooding upward of the yang *qi*. When we detect such a pulse during summer, it is timely. If we detect this pulse during other seasons of the year, it is untimely.

In the winter of 1982, according to medical records written by my late mentor, he participated in a banquet provided by a friend of his who worked for the railroads. Before the meal, this friend of his asked my teacher to feel her father's pulse. This he did, but said nothing until after the meal was over. Then, as he was leaving, he said to her: "Your father must be careful with his health. If he does not, then next summer he will have a real problem." His friend became worried when she heard this, in no small part because she had personally witnessed many of my teacher's diagnostic prophecies come to pass.

She urgently begged my teacher to help her prevent such an event. My teacher took out a piece of paper and wrote a prescription consisting of two ingredients. The first was Shigao, and the second Sumu. She was instructed to bring these to a boil in water and have her father drink them as tea.

On what basis, you might ask, did my teacher prescribe this simple formula? At the time, it was winter, but the pulse his friend's father exhibited was a flooding pulse. During the winter, the yang *qi* is being stored, but this patient had a pulse that was characteristic for summer, when the yang *qi* is completely liberated. This indicated that the patient certainly had a problem. During the winter, there were natural factors that helped to check this internal disharmony. But, as my teacher warned, once summer came round and there were no inhibitory mechanisms to check this disharmony, the problem could erupt like a volcano.

In Cold Damage theory, this sort of pulse is called a Yangming pulse. Yangming diseases can be treated with Baihu Tang. Therefore, the formula my teacher prescribed was a modified, simplified version of Baihu Tang.

After my teacher left, his friend went to her father and told him that Dr. Li had prescribed a formula to help him maintain his health. Unfortunately, her father was an old veteran cadre, and stubborn as well. He had just undergone a thorough physical examination and was told that he was in fine health. Why should he take any medicine? So he did not take the formula. Summer came and sometime in July, he suddenly experienced a cerebral hemorrhage. He was rushed to the hospital and died within a week.

The story of this patient made a deep impression on me. It made me realize the important usefulness of pulse diagnosis. If one learned this skill well, one can not only recognize disease but also prevent disease. Despite this, many Chinese Medicine practitioners in China only have confidence in computed tomography and magnetic resonance imaging (MRI).

I.4.c.3. The Hair-like Pulse of Autumn

The pulse of autumn is "hair-like" (*mao*) and "floating" (*fu*). By "floating" it is meant that the pulse can be felt with even very light pressure. By "hair-like" it is meant that the pulse feels light and empty. This floating pulse is not to be mistaken with the floating pulse that indicates pathology, which seems overabundant with even very light palpation. The *Plain Questions* chapter "Treatise on Phenomena Reflecting the Status of *Qi* in a Normal Person" describes this pulse as "dainty and delicate, like elm pods falling through the air."

The commentator Wu Kun said: "'Dainty and delicate' indicates that the pulse is fluttering and elegant, floating superficially and fluently." Zhang Jiebin noted: "'Like falling elm seeds' indicates that the pulse is lightly floating, gentle, and mild. This image captures the essential meaning of a fine hair." And according to the Qing dynasty text *Comprehensive Differentiation of Pulse Types*:

> The *qi* of the west belongs to the metal element, it is positioned with the earthly branches *shen* and *you*. It is paired with the autumn season, when the myriad creatures enter into a state of storage. This gathering of *qi* starting from the exterior naturally results from the extreme limit of dispersal, like waves breaking leaving calm behind them, or smoke trailing off after a fire has gone out. In the human body, this *qi* corresponds with the lungs, and this is when we find the hair-like pulse.

I have limited experience with this "hair-like" pulse, but in short, we can describe it as the yang *qi* desiring to be restrained and collected.

I.4.c.4. The Stony Pulse of Winter

In winter, the pulse becomes like a stone (*shi*). Stones sink, and the feeling of this pulse is like that of a stone that has been dropped into water and rests on the bottom. Why do we find this sort of pulse during the winter? For the simple reason that the yang *qi* has been gathered and stored up during the winter months. At this time, the yang *qi* is like the light of the new moon. It cannot be seen. When the yang *qi* has been gathered up, it does not agitate the yin or blood, we do not have a case of yang joining with yin. The pulse naturally reflects this stored state.

In the transformations of the pulse through the seasons, we can clearly see that the form of the pulse reflects the changes in the state of yang *qi*. When the yang *qi* emerges, the pulse floats upward. When the yang *qi* retracts, it sinks back down. With regard to the pulse, we are looking at this very phenomenon.

Once we have clearly delineated the different pulses from a theoretical perspective, we can practice them over time and get to know them better. Pulse diagnosis is not a practice that can be mastered after a couple of tries. One should begin with simple concepts and go from there.

We should first learn to distinguish floating from sinking, and after we can readily discriminate between these two, we will know if the disease is in the three yang or the three yin. If the pulse is floating, the disease lies in the three yang; if it is sunken, it is in the three yin. Once yin and yang have been clearly delineated, we possess the means to find the root of the disease. We also have a general idea of how to treat the disease.

In addition, there are fast and slow, slippery and wiry, big and small pulses. These qualities are relatively easy to distinguish from one another. Besides these, there is also whether the pulse possesses strength or does not possess strength. The aforementioned renowned physician Zheng Qin'an considered this point of particularly high importance. He believed that this was the one and only way to determine whether the *qi* of the pulse possesses spirit (*shen*) or not.

Based on my own experience, I regard this point as profound, and especially when the pulse is large, it is important to determine whether or not it is forceful. If it is forceful, it indicates a Yangming condition, and we should use clearing and draining methods if we wish to be successful. If it is without strength, it indicates deficiency from overtaxation. Clearing and draining methods are absolutely contraindicated in such a case. We should use sweet, warming prescriptions in such an instance. In the clinical setting, should we encounter such a pulse, regardless of the disease before us, we can use the same curative method. For instance, we can use a modified Huangqi Jianzhong Tang or Dang Qi Jianzhong Tang to treat it. Often these formulas achieve remarkable results in such cases.

I.5. Explaining Syndrome

I.5.a. The Chinese Character Zheng

The traditional form of the character *zheng* (證), commonly translated in a Chinese Medicine context as "syndrome," has the component indicating speech (*yan* 言) on the left and the character *deng* (登) on the right. The modern simplified version of *zheng* is similar in that it also has the radical *yan* on the left, though in a simplified form (讠), but on the right it has the character or radical *zheng* (正). These two versions of *zheng* have certain differences, but they also possess subtle commonalities.

I.5.a.1. Language (Yan)

Let us first examine the pictograph *yan* (言) meaning "language," "words," or "speech." *Explaining Writing and Analyzing Characters* explains this character as: "to speak directly is *yan*." To say what one has to say in an open way is *yan* (言). If one says something in an indirect way, obliquely, this is not *yan*. The character *yan* is often used in conjunction with the character *yu* (語)—*yuyan* (語言) or *yanyu* (言語), for instance, both compounds meaning "language" or "speech."

What does *yu* (語) mean? *Explaining Writing and Analyzing Characters* says: "*Yu* is the sort of language one must use in a difficult debate." Thus, when we are discussing a difficult topic, one that requires a degree of careful thought and deliberation, the sort of speech we use is *yu*.

The difference between *yu* and *yan* is that *yu* involves the application of logic. There are times when we speak without any consideration for logic. We simply say whatever thoughts come to mind. In order for those same thoughts to be expressed as *yu*, they would first have to undergo the scrutiny of the logical mind and pass muster. If you wish to raise difficult questions for discussion or debate a particular topic, you cannot proceed without logic. We can see that *yan* and *yu* are different.

In *Explanation of Names* it says: "*Yan* is a sort of proclamation of an individual's opinion." When one declares their particular opinion, this is called *yan*. There is another, more deeply implied meaning of *yan*, namely that espoused by the Han Dynasty philosopher Yang Xiong. In *Laws and Teachings*, he writes that "*Yan* is the sound of the heart."

So what is meant by *yan* and *yu*? What is the "voice of the heart"? The voice of the heart is the sound of the mind, the call of the mind. The sound and call of the mind can be expressed in the form of *yanyu*. The inner workings of the mind of a person cannot be discerned. For instance, what passes through your mind at different hours of the day? I have no way of guessing what sorts of thing your mind is up to. Perhaps, if I possessed a sort of transcendental Buddhist empathy, I might have a chance; but as it is, I can only guess what others are thinking.

However, there is something that allows me to know the workings of your heart and mind, your thought processes. This thing is *yan*. This is what is meant by "*yan* is the sound of the heart." What is in your heart? What sort of thoughts move about in your mind? Of course, if you speak what is in your heart, you must speak with honesty. If you hold one thought in your heart and another in your mouth, this is not *yan*.

Therefore, *Explaining Writing and Analyzing Characters* defines the most basic condition for *yan* as "speaking directly." What does it mean to speak directly? Giving voice to what one thinks in one's mind, this is called *yan*. If one speaks in a way that is counter to what one actually thinks, this is not *yan* but simply falsity.

Yan allows us to know and understand that which we would otherwise not be able to know and understand. It allows us to know things that we could not otherwise know or see. The purpose or use of *yan* should be clearer at this point. I hope that the usefulness of *yan* can be more fully realized by the reader, because it is so important. Things that are kept inside, deeply hidden so that no trace can be found, become clear as day once they undergo the process described by *yan*. Is *yan* not a formidable thing? I believe the key difference between humans and all other animals lies here. This is *yan*.

I.5.a.2. Deng (Zheng)

Now let us consider the component on the right of the character, the phonetic component *deng* (登, as in the traditional form of *zheng* 證) or *zheng* (正, as in the simplified form of *zheng* 证). This is the phonetic marker but, as we have repeatedly emphasized, the phonetic marker is also a key to understanding the meaning of the character. Chinese characters are composites of pictographic and phonetic elements, both of which convey meaning. Sometimes it is the phonetic element that best communicates the particular meaning of a character.

The character *deng* (登) means "to ascend" or "to climb." The original meaning, as explained by *Explaining Writing and Analyzing Characters*, is related to climbing up into a chariot. The chariots of China's distant past were all very high and riders had to climb up onto a step to get into them. The meaning of this character was gradually extended to refer to ascension in general.

In the Chinese calendar, the ninth day of the ninth lunar month is the Double Yang Festival, also referred to as the Climbing (*deng*) High Festival. First of all, it is called "Double Yang" because nine is the most yang of the numbers, and on this day, both the month and the day of the month are assigned this number. In the ancient *Inscription of the River Luo* (Luoshu), the number nine occupies the highest position. What else can a person do on the ninth day of the ninth month but climb a mountain? Climbing a mountain on this day is a way of acting in accord with the prevailing energy.

By climbing to a high place on the ninth day of the ninth month as per Chinese custom, we are according our behavior with the *Luoshu*.

What is the purpose of *deng* ("climbing")? Climbing to a high place allows us to broaden the horizon, to expand our minds, and to see far into the distance. As the Tang Dynasty poet Wang Zhihuang wrote: "If one desires to see a thousand leagues away, one must go up the stairs to the next story." Initially, there are places that we cannot see; we are as short-sighted as a mouse. But when we climb to a high place, we can suddenly see far into the distance.

The simple action of climbing upward expands our field of vision immensely, and allows us to see faraway places and times. This is what is meant by *deng* (登).

The simplified form of the character, now the standard form in the People's Republic of China, is written with the radical *zheng* (正) instead of *deng* (登). The use of *zheng* to simplify the character is also very astute. *Explaining Writing and Analyzing Characters* explains the character's meaning this way: "It means 'right' or 'true'; it is derived from *zhi* (止), meaning 'to halt' or 'restrain,' and *yi* (一), which means 'one.'"

This character, compounded from *zhi* and *yi*, is profoundly significant. If we were to take all of Daoist and all of Confucian thought and distill it into a single character, it would be *zheng*. To "restrain the one" means to "embrace the one." It means to know the one, and by extension, to "obtain the one."

The tenth chapter of the *Classic of the Dao and Its Virtue* (Daodejing) says: "To sustain the eternal sojourn while embracing the one, focus on the breath to bring about softness, like a baby at the breast." In Chapter 39 of this same book, we read:

> That which entities obtain as the most ancient is the one. Heaven obtained the one and became clear. Earth obtained the one and became tranquil. The spirit obtained the one and became intelligent. The grains obtained the one and ripened to fullness. The myriad things are born by obtaining the one. The noblemen and kings obtained the one and thereby all is right under heaven.

And in Chapter 45 of Laozi's book, we read: "With clear and quiet, all is right under heaven."

From these preceding passages, we sense that "restraining the one," "embracing the one," "obtaining the one," and "rightness" (*zheng* 正) concentrate the essence of the Dao.

If we look at Confucianism, we see that it also focuses on the character *zhi* and the character *zheng*. *Great Learning* was one of the "Four Books" of Confucianism and, written posthumously, reflected Confucius's ideals. This book makes its thesis known from the outset:

> The way of great learning lies in illustrious virtue, in one's relationship to one's people, in stopping *zhi* (止) at that which is good. To know when to stop and to then hold fast, to hold fast and to then become quiet, to become quiet and thereby attain tranquility, in tranquility to contemplate, and through contemplation to gain attainment.

"Attainment" of what? Attainment of the Dao of course, the highest aim of the sage. And how is this highest aim achieved? The cultivation of this skill lies in *zhi* (止) and *zheng* (正). In restraint (*zhi*), we cannot depart from the one. If we departed from the one, how could we refer to this as *zhi*? Furthermore, one of the core ideas of Confucian scholarship is to "attain knowledge through the investigation of phenomena" (*gewu zhizhi* 格物致知). We discussed this concept of investigating things to attain knowledge earlier in this book, but what exactly do we depend on to investigate things? The ability to investigate things remains with the attainment of *zhi*. If one cannot stop (*zhi*) oneself, there cannot be investigation. Therefore, *Great Learning* continues by saying:

> Things are investigated and then knowledge is perfected, knowledge is perfected and one's intentions become sincere, sincerity of intention leads to rectification (*zheng*) of the heart and mind, rectification of the heart and mind leads to cultivation of one's self, cultivation of one's self brings about order in the home, order in the home results in proper regulation of the kingdom, and once the kingdom is ordered, the world will know peace.

These are the lofty ideals of Confucianism, but to realize these ideals, the one (*yi* 一) must first be detained (*zhi* 止). If one does not rectify one's own heart and mind, can there be sincerity? You can see that Confucian thought also constantly returns to the concept of rectification (*zheng* 正).

Even if we leave aside an analysis of this character, *Explaining Writing and Analyzing Characters's* explanation of this character as meaning "right" or "true" is extremely incisive. This explanation is related to a discussion of right and wrong, and has the larger meaning of "right and direct"; it has to do with "truth" in the larger sense of the word. The question then, is: How do we attain this "truth"? Other than this concept of *zheng*, there is no other way.

Thus, rectification (*zheng*) can aid us in our perception and understanding of truth. It can help us to clearly understand right from wrong. *Zheng* can even help us to realize the highest ideals. This is how we might regard *zheng* from a philosophical perspective.

From a different perspective, there are three different dynastic time periods that all postulate the "right beginning" of the year (*zheng*), or even seven *zhengs*. There are two different sets of three "correct ways of ascertaining the first month of the year": the first indicates the three *zhengs* of the ancient Xia, Shang, and Zhou, regarded as correlating to the third, second, and first earthly branches: *yin*, *chou*, and *zi*. In this discussion, we will continue to use the *zheng* of the Xia, hence the third earthly branch, *yin*.

The three *zhengs* can also pertain to the sun, moon, and stars. The seven *zhengs* refer to the sun, moon, and the five planets. Therefore, *zheng* can be regarded as an astronomical concept. It is difficult to see most celestial bodies. Modern telescopes and other detectors of astronomical events are vastly more sensitive and far-seeing than the human eye. A modern radio telescope can see events from several billion light-years away.

The ancients did not possess such advanced equipment, so how did they familiarize themselves with distant objects in the sky? They made astrological observations. For instance, they observed the way the length of the sun's shadow changed over the course of the day and then determined the twenty-four calendrical periods of the year. If we observe which direction the handle of the big dipper is pointing, we can know which season we are entering. Or, we can observe the waxing and waning of the moon to determine the relative positions of the earth, sun, and moon. In short, through a process of "rectification," we can comprehend complex astronomical processes.

Additionally, *zheng* possesses another related, implied meaning, namely: "The part of a room that is well lit is called *zheng*" (*Kangxi Dictionary*). Ancient houses and buildings were different from those of today with their large windows and good lighting. With the exception of the greeting room where guests were entertained, which was well illuminated due to a central "sky well," a central aperture in the roof of the structure overlying a courtyard, the windows of the rest of the house were small, meaning the adjoining rooms were relatively dim.

These relatively small windows were insufficient to light the entire room in which they were found, and the portion of the room close to the window, which was relatively bright, was called *zheng*. Due to its brightness, the contents of this part of the room were clearly visible. The other parts of the room that lay in shadow and were not *zheng* could not be observed, and therefore not understood.

I.5.a.3. The General Meaning of Zheng

The preceding analysis of the semantic and phonetic components of the character *zheng*, have provided us with a basic understanding of the word. So, what is *zheng*? At this point, I would guess that even if I do not explain this concept further, the reader has a fair idea of what this character denotes.

First of all, what is *yan* (言)? *Yan* is the means by which the inner workings of your mind, those things that are hidden from the view of others and known only to yourself, are made knowable to others. No matter how deeply it is buried, or how secretly it is concealed, frank speech (*yan*) can lay it bare.

What then is meant by the character *deng* (登), as found in the traditional form of the character *zheng* (證)? By means of ascent (*deng*), our field of vision is broadened. By means of *deng*, we gain a clear, panoramic view of things that otherwise are beyond the range of our vision. By means of *zheng* (正), the alternate phonetic radical in the simplified form (证), those things that would otherwise be secret and hidden from view and mysterious become distinct and definite. Equally important, by means of *zheng*, we can clearly distinguish right from wrong and understand truth.

If we synthesize these three elements, the meaning of the character *zheng* becomes immediately evident. In modern Chinese, the character *zheng* is often used as part of a two-character compound word, such as *zhengming* (to "prove") or *zhengju* ("evidence"). *Zhengming* literally means to prove something and thereby make it clear. After something is proven, it becomes clear and comprehensible; this is what is meant by *zhengming*.

During the Cultural Revolution, the concept of *zhengming* was extremely important in Chinese daily life. During this time, one could not undertake any endeavor without some kind of "proof" or official authorization. One could not even stay in a hotel.

Zhengju ("evidence") refers to providing proof of something such that it then has an established basis to be taken as fact. Thus, the three taken together can clearly be understood to mean the process whereby that which is most innate, deepest and far-reaching, most complex, and most difficult to grasp becomes absolutely clear and comprehensible. In more concrete terms, the phonetic component of the character (*deng* or *zheng*) indicates the practical method by which this process is carried out, and the pictographic or semantic element *yan* indicates the result or outcome of this process.

Now that we have a clear understanding of the implied meaning of the Chinese character for syndrome (*zheng*), we can understand why Chinese Medicine places such an emphasis on the differentiation of syndromes (*bian zheng*), and why Chinese Medicine has its most crucial teachings in the arena of *zheng*.

I.5.b. Specialized Meanings of Zheng

We will primarily discuss the different specialized meanings of *zheng* from a Chinese Medicine perspective, as in Chinese Medicine it is an extremely important concept. It can be said that it is impossible to overemphasize the importance of this concept in Chinese Medicine. Before, we discussed the concept of disease (*bing*). Between the concepts of disease and of syndrome, everything in Chinese Medicine is contained.

In the case of disease (*bing*), the most important thing is discovering relevant correspondences. The syndrome (*zheng*) is that which is drawn from these correspondences. Disease is essentially a discussion of the theoretical process, whereas syndrome refers to the practical method or operation. To borrow terminology from Chinese Buddhist teachings, disease discusses educational principles whereas syndrome refers to proof. The theoretical and the practical, the pedagogy and the proof; together these two characters contain the essence of all Chinese Medicine.

In our discussion of disease, I wrote that once one understands this concept completely, one has "understood half of Chinese Medicine." The remaining half is entailed in the concept of syndrome. If you understand all of the implications of syndrome, and you can clearly determine the particular syndrome pertinent to the patient's condition, then you clearly understand all of the changes inherent in the patient's case. Are you still determined to order a CT? Will you order an MRI? Will you need lab tests? In my opinion, not necessarily!

Once you have determined the correct syndrome, you can be certain. Once you have determined the syndrome, you will know things that lie far afield; you will even be able to foretell when the patient's disease will reach a state of crisis. What more do you want? Once you have discovered the syndrome, you will know. In the history of Chinese Medicine, there are many accounts that illustrate this point.

Huangfu Mi's *A–Z Classic of Acupuncture and Moxibustion* (Zhenjiu jiayijing) records a particular account of Zhang Zhongjing. When Zhang Zhongjing was treating the nobleman Wang Zhongxuan, he examined him and said: "Your highness has a disease. If it is not treated, then your eyebrows will fall out at the age of 40, and then within half a year you will die." At the time, Wang Zhongxuan was young and vigorous and had a high position even though he was only in his twenties. Therefore, Wang Zhongxuan disregarded his advice and did not take the young Zhang Zhongjing's prescription of Wushi San. Ten-odd years passed and, as predicted, Wang Zhongxuan's eyebrows fell out. When this happened, he already knew it was too late, and he passed away within half a year.

One should not dismiss this account as a joke or a fable. It is a true account of actual events. If Zhang Zhongjing did not possess such skill, then he would not have been worshipped by so many subsequent generations of physicians, and I doubt that I would have been so enamored with the *Treatise on Cold Damage*. Why did I choose Zhang Zhongjing as my model? Why not choose Sun Simiao or Tao Hongjing, or the Four Great Physicians of the Jin and Yuan Dynasties, or the Four Greats of the Warm Disease School? These physicians are some of the finest in Chinese Medicine's history. Yet their wisdom cannot compare with that of Zhang Zhongjing.

Therefore, we must have very solid grounds for believing that this particular account is completely true, without even the least bit of hyperbole. How did Zhang Zhongjing know how this particular illness would develop so far into the future? Did he rely on some form of intuitive shamanic insight? Not at all! He knew because he discerned the syndrome (*zheng*). If you have a firm grasp of the syndrome, and you can peer into the essence of the rationale underlying that syndrome, then you can understand not only the disease that lies before you, but also those changes that it will undergo in the future.

The twenty-first century is the century of biology. Developments in genetics will replace current diagnostic methods to greater and lesser degrees in the years to come. When this technology reaches maturity, it will be able to diagnose the disease a newborn or fetus might experience in the next several decades of its life. Diagnosing the diseases that a newborn or even a fetus may experience in the span of its life, is this not prescience?

More to the point, does this modern scientific capacity to predict the course of health and disease conflict with the philosophical tenets of Chinese Medicine we have been discussing? If genetic diagnosis can truly predict with accuracy what will happen ten, twenty, thirty years from now, then we are truly talking about a sort of divination! How does this differ from fortune-telling? In essence, there is no real difference. How should we regard these prescient genetic diagnostics? In the past, we regarded the occurrence of many diseases as happening by chance. A streptococcal infection led to symptoms of wind, damp, or heat; infection with hepatitis B virus or with the AIDS virus, and a case of hepatitis B or AIDS simply emerged. However, actual experience tells us that it is not so simple.

Modern Chinese news media and even China Central Television have latched onto AIDS victims, in stories such as the popularized "Tale of Little Lu." There is a sort of hysteria that currently surrounds AIDS in the popular media. You can see the color in someone's face change with even a mention of the disease. The rate of AIDS infections increases every year, and the route of infection is well known. Fluids containing the virus, such as blood or semen, are transmitted from one person to another, allowing the disease to spread. Despite this, "Little Lu's" wife has never become infected with the disease. Why?

Today, if we look at this issue from the perspective of genetics, we can see that although we previously believed that infection with disease such as AIDS was simply a matter of direct exposure to the pathogen, genetics plays a key role in whether or not this disease takes hold. If you have the gene that predisposes you to AIDS, then even slight contact with the virus will result in infection. If you lack this particular gene, then you will be like "Little Lu's" wife. Regardless of how often and how intimately you come in contact with the virus, you will not become infected.

The preceding analysis tells us that when research occurs on a different level, and knowledge is gained in a different realm, then one's view may also change. At the level of understanding where the ancients worked, it was possible to perform real acts of prescience, but these acts are now dismissed as superstition. However, when it comes to the level upon which we work at in modern times, the realm which we consider to be the most advanced, the same acts of prescience are not dismissed as superstition, but rather appear to us like a new horizon and are embraced as the fruits of scientific development. This, once again, reminds us that we cannot simply disregard traditional scholarship as mere superstition and assume that it can be tossed away without further attention as if it were pseudoscience. The future is full of surprises.

When we gain understanding of different levels and of different realms, why shouldn't our understanding of traditions change as well? Zhang Zhongjing's syndrome differentiation occurred at a different level, in a different realm than ours. If he relied on genetics for his diagnosis, why wouldn't he be able to predict a patient's future? As far as recognizing and grasping the appropriate syndrome, there are at least four levels of ability among Chinese Medicine practitioners: the divine (*shen*), the sagely (*sheng*), the adept (*gong*), and the astute (*qiao*). To know by simply looking, this is divine; to listen and know is sagely; to ask and then to know is adept; to feel the pulse and know is astute. If you practice Chinese Medicine, ask yourself which category you belong to. If you have not yet attained even the level of the astute practitioner, then how can you even begin to infer the level of ability of those practitioners whose skill is divine? You would think that everything they do is impossible, or just superstition. This is as if we were stuck using research methods from the early nineteenth century, in which case it would be impossible to discover genetics, or even understand the idea of genetics.

The syndromes of Chinese Medicine merit our best efforts to understand them. The *Treatise on Cold Damage* talks about differentiating diseases by means of the pulse and syndrome, by which he means that the disease can best be known through the pulse and syndrome. Zhang Zhongjing raises an important principle regarding the treatment of disease: "Observe the pulse and syndrome, know what contrary treatments were performed, follow the syndrome, and treat in accordance with it." Why should we treat in accordance with the syndrome? The answer is obvious I am sure: the syndrome matters a great deal!

The syndrome can tell us everything. Things that are indelible, that are difficult to perceive, are made known by the syndrome. You need not use x-rays or MRI; the syndrome alone can make the patient's situation clear to you. What is the point of modern physical, chemical or biological examination methods? The goal of all of these technological developments is to recognize the correct syndrome, in the Chinese Medicine sense of the word. Syndromes are an extraordinary aspect of Chinese Medicine theory, and not to be underestimated.

Nowadays, many people look down upon the concept of syndromes. If one disregards syndromes, then how can one have regard for the *Treatise on Cold Damage*? Every syndrome described in the *Treatise on Cold Damage*, if thoroughly researched, offers up profound insights.

Not long ago, a patient came to me from the city of Guilin in Guangxi province. She had made a special trip because Western Medicine offered little help for her condition, an aggressive form of malignant melanoma. After surgery on the first tumor, it metastasized to her lungs and her abdominal cavity. For the past three months, she was in intense pain. She took powerful analgesic medications including morphine, but these relieved her pain for a few hours at most. Without morphine or other painkillers, she could not find sleep. Then, nausea began to set in. She had no desire to eat and her mouth was filled with a bitter taste. These symptoms tell us the patient's syndrome. The syndrome is the most crucial aspect of the patient's condition to be understood. The heap of medical records and exam results the patient brought with them were also worth consulting, but mostly because when the patient asks how confident they can be of recovery, you can give a conservative answer and not promise more than you can deliver. Besides this, the records and results that cost the patient so much money have no real significance to the case. This is my opinion at any rate.

This sort of Western diagnostic information may serve as a point of reference for Chinese Medicine. As reference points, they are worthy of contemplation but should be considered neither crucial nor decisive. Still, we cannot disregard such findings. Our ability to differentiate syndromes is not so lofty as that of Zhang Zhongjing, or Bian Que, or Cang Gong. When, after having performed the four diagnostic methods of Chinese Medicine diligently (looking, listening and smelling, asking questions, and palpating), we neither grasp the patient's current danger nor feel confident of a prognosis, Western medical diagnostic tests help us to understand the patient's condition. However, these should merely be viewed as points of reference, and as subsidiary to the decisive variable, the syndrome afflicting the patient. With only the syndrome, as conveyed by the pulse, we can understand the nature of the disease before us, and based on that understanding we can choose the appropriate method of cure. Such is the basis of Chinese Medicine diagnosis! All of the diagnostic testing that Western Medicine has to offer cannot come close to providing such decisive information.

If, on the contrary, you think that the results of such tests can provide you with the basis for deciding upon the appropriate route to curing disease, then you are no practitioner of Chinese Medicine. If you are so startled by the results of an MRI that all you can do is reach for Baihuasheshecao or Banzhilian or some other Chinese herbal medication that is deemed appropriate for combating tumors, how can you possibly be considered a true practitioner of Chinese Medicine? Regrettably, the relative majority of those who claim to practice Chinese Medicine practice in precisely this manner. This is the greatest problem currently facing Chinese Medicine. It is the most glaring shortfall in the way that Chinese Medicine is practiced in the modern age. Modern diagnostic tests are no substitute for the four methods of traditional Chinese Medicine diagnosis: looking, smelling, questioning, and palpating. Nevertheless, the application of these methods is rapidly declining, and the practice of Chinese Medicine languishes. Chinese Medicine cannot dispense with the syndrome differentiation. At the very least, the application of syndrome differentiation cannot afford to repeat the trajectory of decline that has been witnessed in the past period of time.

If we take the preceding case as an example, besides the Western medical diagnostic tests that were performed, we also saw that the pulse on the right side was sinking, fine, and weak, and the pulse on the left side was fine and slightly slippery. What information do we derive from the Western medical tests? What can be clearly known and understood? From a Western medical perspective, this is a case of malignant melanoma. As a practitioner of Chinese Medicine, however, you cannot diagnose this patient's illness as malignant melanoma. That would be entirely incongruous with the principles and practice of Chinese Medicine. Based on the preceding diagnosis, we are however inclined to consider the possibility that this patient's disease is related to Shaoyang, and that this is some sort of Shaoyang disease.

Her tongue coat was white, thick, and greasy, indicating that, of the six pathogenic factors, damp was foremost in her case. I considered her condition to be a case of dampness afflicting the Shaoyang layer. I prescribed Xiao Chaihu Tang and added Pingwei San plus Zhebeimu and Juanbai. The patient took the formula, and three days later the patient's husband called me to say that the medicine had worked wonderfully. The patient's pain was greatly reduced, and she had not needed to use morphine or any other painkiller. Furthermore, she had been able to fall asleep at night and her nausea had vanished.

Setting aside for a moment the ultimate outcome of this patient's serious illness, it must be acknowledged that such a vast reduction in the patient's suffering resulting in a marked improvement in the patient's quality of life is no small thing. The mere fact that Xiao Chaihu Tang together with Pingwei San succeeded where morphine and other powerful analgesics failed tells us something. It tells us how important it is to recognize the syndrome, to differentiate the syndrome accurately, and to treat in accordance with the syndrome.

Another physician might have regarded this patient's case solely from the perspective of her malignant melanoma. To me, she suffered from a Shaoyang disorder. When Shaoyang is encumbered, then the blood and *qi* of Shaoyang become obstructed, and pain is the result. If you adjust Shaoyang with your treatment and resolve the problem afflicting it so that the *qi* and blood of that layer are free of obstruction, the pain will naturally disappear.

How did I know it was a Shaoyang disorder? I knew because I discerned the syndrome. We certainly do not possess the wisdom to completely penetrate the meaning of syndrome, but having analyzed the character, we begin to realize what a wondrous thing it is.

This is especially evident in the *Treatise on Cold Damage*. In the *Treatise on Cold Damage*, the syndrome and the pulse are sometimes discussed together, but more often only the syndrome is talked about. The syndrome alone is discussed far more often than the pulse. Many articles do not discuss the pulse at all, for instance article 96:

> When there is cold damage of five or six days, or wind-strike, with alternating heat and cold, the chest and ribcage feeling bloated and uncomfortable, the patient withdraws and has no desire to eat, is annoyed with a desire to vomit, or there is a feeling of vexation in the chest with no vomiting, or there is thirst, or the center of the abdomen is painful, or below the ribs there is focal distention and hardness, or there are palpitations below the heart and an inability to urinate, or there is a lack of thirst and the body is slightly hot, or there is cough, then Xiao Chaihu Tang governs.

In this article, more than ten syndromes are discussed, but not a single pulse. The *Treatise on Cold Damage* predominantly discusses syndromes, and when pulses are detailed, they are introduced within the larger framework of a particular syndrome. Based on the understanding of syndrome that we introduced here, the pulse is primarily used as a means of recognizing a particular syndrome; it is a method for determining the pertinent syndrome. The pulse is part of the syndrome picture.

Why is it repeatedly emphasized that we become well versed in the *Treatise on Cold Damage* such that we can recite the lines from memory? In order that we become thoroughly familiar with the syndromes, are able to recognize them when we see them, and thoroughly understand them. Regardless of whether a disease is mild or serious, it can be deciphered in terms of syndrome. If you do not understand the relationship between one syndrome and the next, or between the syndrome and the disease or the syndrome and the appropriate formula, how will you determine the correct treatment? It will be very difficult.

This concludes our general overview of syndrome (*zheng*).

I.5.b.1. The Definition of Syndrome

In concrete terms, syndromes can help us to understand the existence of and changes in disease. Sometimes the existence of a disease is readily known. Sometimes the disease lies hidden, without emerging in an evident way, as it did in the case of the nobleman Wang Zhongxuan when Zhang Zhongjing diagnosed him. Changes in the course of pathology make it more difficult for us to recognize the factors contributing to the existence and evolution of a particular disease. However, as we described in our discussion of *zheng* above, syndrome allows us to know hidden diseases and to understand and predict their permutations.

Therefore, every outward sign that corresponds to the existence of a disease, every indication that a disease is changing course, and every clue that points to the factors which cause the disease and instigate its rearrangement, all of these constitute syndrome. If we want to give "syndrome" a precise definition, I think this one will suffice.

If Western Medicine wants to diagnose a syndrome, it has to rely on modern means. It might be said that all of modern science assists the practitioner of Western Medicine to correctly diagnose a syndrome: biology, chemistry, physics, electronics, even nanotechnology. All of these are practically lining up to help the Western physician obtain a diagnosis, or some picture of the presenting syndrome.

As for Chinese Medicine, who or what helps a Chinese Medicine practitioner form a diagnosis? Nothing and nobody. Science certainly will not help you. Science not only will not help you, but I am afraid it may have a word or two to say to you. If so and so is somehow able to diagnose disease simply by looking, they will probably be accused by modern science of practicing superstitious beliefs. So, this is one of the challenges facing Chinese Medicine!

I have already talked about my first master, Li Yangbo. After he passed away, I had an abiding desire to publish his ideas. I believed that his ideas would help not only Chinese Medicine practitioners, but also students of traditional Chinese culture. In 1997, I had the unexpected opportunity to meet an editor at the China Press of Traditional Chinese Medicine. I discussed my idea to write a book about my first mentor, and he was excited about the idea and willing to help me publish it. He insisted that I write a lengthy preface to the book, introducing Li Yangbo to the reader. My former mentor was not famous, and had neither formal training as a physician nor a diploma. I already possessed my PhD at the time, and I suppose that the purpose of my preface was, in part, to establish the legitimacy of Li Yangbo's contribution. In this preface, I attempted to write everything I knew of my mentor, leaving out nothing of import.

After I finished my draft of this foreword, I sent it to various people to get some feedback, and without fail they all said that "It is written very well, but you have really made your master out to be entirely too miraculous. If you do not tone it down a bit, it might have an adverse effect." What can we make of this statement? Although there were times when my master could diagnose simply by looking, or know the nature of a disease by feeling the pulse, these occasional breakthroughs were dwarfed by the abilities exhibited by Bian Que and Zhang Zhongjing. So if you disbelieve these few anecdotes regarding my late teacher's ability, how could you possibly have faith in the accounts of Bian Que and Zhang Zhongjing?

This aptly illustrates the situation we practitioners of Chinese Medicine find ourselves in currently. Not only does science not make any real effort to recognize Chinese Medicine accurately, and offers no assistance in identifying syndromes, it even complains about us and holds us back. Perhaps there are those who would say that Chinese Medicine at present is buzzing with activity. They point to biochemical insights, modernization of methods and theory, and globalization of the practice of Chinese Medicine as testimony to seeming advancement. This busy scene of seeming growth is nothing more than the steroidal glow of a bubble economy buoyed up by sham prospects.

I stand by the above statement; I am confident enough that I have included it in this book for all to see. If you do not believe me, just wait and see what the future will bring. Confucius said, "to be unacknowledged by others and to remain unperturbed is part of noble character." Without this quality, one can do little of merit. Chinese Medicine has no external assistance from other fields; it depends upon the ability of its practitioners to look, listen, ask, and take the pulse in order to arrive at the correct syndrome. There is no other way for us. However, once we are able to perform these with some skill, the results are extraordinary. It is as I illustrated in the last example I gave of the person I treated. Who could believe that a simple Xiao Chaihu Tang could cure with such dramatic effect?

For the past several years, I have felt an increasing affinity with the ancient Chinese saying: "In poverty, cultivate one's own abilities, and in plenitude, seek to benefit the world." My study of Chinese Medicine is always with the goal of realizing the wisdom of this saying. Now that I have the opportunity to say a few things regarding my sentiments, I am inclined to speak my mind.

After this little book is published, there are bound to be a few people who appreciate it; it is bound to have an influence on a few people. And what if you or anyone else has not yet had an opportunity like this? Well then there is no reason not to hole oneself up and ignore what is going on outside. Chinese Medicine theory is a wondrous thing to contemplate, and I, for one, would not rank it second to the theory of relativity. If one has nothing else, he or she can still find joy without poverty in an earnest study of Chinese Medicine.

I.5.b.2. The Basis for Syndrome

As stated earlier, the basis for deriving a syndrome in modern medicine is provided by the theories and technology from the entire field of modern science. What is the theoretical basis for deriving a syndrome in Chinese Medicine? Its basis is that described in the *Yellow Emperor's Classic*: "That which is internal manifests externally." This is the most important basis. Regardless of the internal changes, regardless of their number or their subtlety, these changes will definitely manifest in some outward sign. This is absolutely definite; there is no doubt about this.

The question is, can we see the entire internal landscape from that which can be seen on the exterior? Do we know which external signs correspond with which internal conditions? Are you capable of constructing this system of correspondences in your thinking? This is an area of great difficulty. There are certainly correlations and correspondences, but some are easier than others to perceive. For instance, if your face grows dull and dark, it is easy to guess that you are unhappy. If you are laughing and boisterous, then your heart is light. These are representative illustrations of "that which is internal manifests externally."

How will you detect more subtle, more profound changes? This depends on your ability to "observe something miniscule and thereby know all." This means to see something seemingly inconsequential or minute and thereby discover something profound, something remarkable, or even something from the distant past. As a matter of fact, Chinese Medicine already boasts a complete set of methods for doing just this. Through rational thought and by correlating the internal conditions with the external, we are able to recognize the disease at hand and establish the pertinent syndrome.

These ways of thinking, methods, and techniques aimed at obtaining the appropriate syndrome are together referred to as "differentiation of syndrome." When Bian Que diagnosed disease by observing the appearance of his patients, or when Zhang Zhongjing predicted the occurrence of disease in the nobleman Wang Zhongxuan, these episodes illustrated obtaining an accurate diagnosis through "observing the subtle and thereby knowing the obvious," through the differentiation of syndromes. If we as physicians and students of Chinese Medicine manage to grasp this process, then such feats will be within our grasp.

Not long ago, a long-standing patient and old friend of Dr. Li, my late mentor, came to see me on account of a sore throat. In the southern city of Nanning, most people regard a sore throat as a manifestation of fire afflicting the body. For this reason, this patient treated himself by drinking cooling teas with the result that the more he drank, the more his throat pained him. The patient began to become alarmed and sought me out.

Both his right and left pulses were deep and sunken, and when I looked at his tongue, it was very pale. How could this be the result of fire? Accordingly, I prescribed Mahuang Xixin Fuzi Tang. Two hours after ingesting the decoction, his sore throat was greatly relieved, and after taking the second dose, the patient reported that he was completely recovered.

This old patient recounted to me a story from twenty years before. At that time, he lived a floor up from a 40-year-old woman who had been suffering from abdominal pain for some time. She went to a large hospital where she was examined and told that she had a tumor in her pelvic cavity that needed to be surgically removed. Just as she was preparing to take her things to the hospital in preparation for this surgery, this old patient, who knew my former teacher well, insisted she go to see Dr. Li. The patient took his suggestion and was subsequently diagnosed by my late mentor who told her that the cause of her abdominal pain was not a tumor but worms. If she rid herself of these, she would regain her health.

He prescribed anti-parasitic medication and several days later, she had a bowel movement brimming with long and stringy materials in it. She regained her health and did not undergo surgery. When she returned to the hospital to be re-examined, they could not find any sign of tumor.

This anecdote serves as a reminder that the value of diagnosing the syndrome cannot be overestimated. If you are able to accurately determine the syndrome, you have everything that modern science could possibly offer, and perhaps more.

I.5.b.3. The Difference between Syndrome and Disease

Now let us discuss the relationship between syndrome and disease. Disease refers to the overall malady, described in general terms. The syndrome refers to how it is different from other diseases, and refers both to its individual character and its distinct features. Disease is a rough description, and syndrome a detailed one. For instance, Taiyang disease is a relatively rough and general reference to the pathology at hand. On the other hand, how about Taiyang wind-strike syndrome? This is relatively precise, and indicates a distinct malady.

Moreover, within the individual syndromes one can further differentiate between different levels. Wind-strike is a syndrome, and belonging to this syndrome there are further distinctions such as fever, sweating, aversion to wind, and a floating pulse. These are lesser considerations, being subheadings of the main syndrome. Nevertheless, they help to provide a more detailed and refined differentiation of the syndrome. The syndrome is the reflexive reaction of the individual to the presence of disease and the pathogen within the organism. Every person is different, thus this reflexive reaction is not completely identical from person to person. This is no different from everyday life—people react differently to the same stimulus. For instance, if a group of people were to watch the same movie, each individual's impression of that movie would vary according to personal experience, values, differences in personality, and so on. Some might think the movie was excellent, and others might find it completely boring.

A few days ago, I asked someone what they thought of the movie *Crouching Tiger, Hidden Dragon*. He said, "It stinks!" He said that if he were to give it a score from one to a hundred, it would get a 59. After hearing his criticism, I was a bit surprised. I was afraid that watching the movie I might just be wasting two hours of my life. I gritted my teeth and went to see it anyway. After seeing it, I was flabbergasted that I had almost been taken in by his critique. I love watching martial arts movies anyway, but a movie like *Crouching Tiger, Hidden Dragon* is a real gem.

This example is worth considering when thinking about the relationship between disease and syndrome and how it is different in different individuals. The same disease is different to some degree in each person because each person's reaction to that disease is individual. This is called "the same disease but a different syndrome." The disease may be identical, but the syndrome might be altogether disparate.

For this reason, when we are working out a treatment plan, we must consider not only the disease but also the factors that distinguish the syndrome. In Western medical treatment, emphasis is placed on distinguishing the disease. Emphasizing the disease means emphasizing the general, common factors that characterize the disease. In Western Medicine, if a thousand different people contract tuberculosis, they would all get the same antibiotic treatment. The patients all get the same treatment, but are the patients all the same? Of course not.

Of course, the fact that Western Medicine has arrived at a general understanding of this disease and has identified common elements in all sufferers of tuberculosis is a great and admirable achievement. From a wide range of presentations, Western Medicine has determined the common denominator—admirable indeed! However, having discovered the commonality, it neglects the individuality, and this is its failing. Herein lies the strength and weakness of Western Medicine.

In Chinese Medicine, it is also imperative that, in the course of diagnosis, the disease be determined. The *Treatise on Cold Damage* provides a good example of this, as each section first discusses the disease in question. However, the disease alone is not enough; we must also differentiate the syndrome, and that means that the individual's response to the disease must be determined. If you can figure out both the commonality and the individuality of the disease, then your understanding will be comprehensive.

Contemplating Western Medicine and Chinese Medicine in this way, we have a basis for comparison and evaluation. From a rational perspective, which system is superior? Chinese Medicine is an outstanding medicine. Unfortunately, far from surpassing the standards set out by our predecessors, we have rather distorted Chinese Medicine into something that pains one's heart to see. It is not that Chinese Medicine is deficient. Chinese Medicine is wholly good! We have simply failed to preserve its original integrity.

I.5.b.4. Explaining Syndrome

I.5.b.4.i. "Discerning the Disease, We Have Not Necessarily Determined the Syndrome"

In short, the syndrome is the individual organism's response to a particular disease. Each individual is different, and therefore the way in which that individual responds to a particular disease is also different. Some people respond to a disease in an indistinct or subtle way such that it is difficult to detect the disease clinically. These cases constitute patients "without a syndrome" that can be perceived. We may not be able to make out a syndrome, but they are certainly sick. For example, a person with cancer might not feel the least bit unwell until the cancer has progressed considerably. The patient was already sick, but the syndrome had not yet come into view. Why does the syndrome present so clearly in one person and so faintly in another?

This is the very question we will be addressing in later chapters. The answer to this question reveals that the key to recognizing syndromes lies in the skill of the practitioner. Zhang Zhongjing's incredible skill at recognizing syndromes allowed him to know the course of Wang Zhongxuan's pathology years in advance. At the time Zhang Zhongjing first diagnosed him, Wang Zhongxuan was not completely without disease or syndrome. In his case, his disease had not yet assumed a definite form and his syndrome was very subtly evident. If there were absolutely no trace of disease or syndrome, then this story would be just a myth. Zhang Zhongjing was not relying on clairvoyance, nor was he fortune-telling. He was simply able to know an entire process from very subtle clues.

We can understand this interpretation of subtle clues from the perspective of form and *qi*. To see the subtle (*wei*) is speaking of the *qi*; to know the obvious (*zhu*) is speaking of the form (*xing*). The *qi* of a thing is often very subtle indeed. There is a saying in Chinese: "Chase the wind and clutch at shadows." *Qi* is often not even as tangible as wind or shadows, however. But once the *qi* takes form (*xing*), it becomes remarkably distinct. Once it takes form, it is easy to perceive and the syndrome becomes obvious. The process by which all phenomena come into being follows this course, from *qi* to form. During the *qi* phase, it is not easily evident, and is difficult to detect; but once the form stage is reached, it is not difficult to distinguish.

If you are able to detect the disease and syndrome during the *qi* stage, this is called "seeing the subtle" (*wei*). If the physician is able to recognize this subtle stage of development, then he knows that as this *qi* develops there will at some point be a change in the form, and knowing this change is called "knowing the obvious" (*zhu*). This is what is meant by "seeing the subtle and knowing the obvious." Knowing the process by means of subtle clues is a key topic in Chinese Medicine.

The *Yellow Emperor's Classic* repeatedly emphasizes "the higher physician treats not-yet disease" (*weibing*). What is *weibing*? Is "not-yet disease" the same as "no disease"? If the person has no disease whatsoever and we treat them, we are asking for trouble where there is none. "Not-yet" disease is not synonymous with no disease, nor does treating "not-yet" disease constitute preventative medicine. "Not-yet" disease is disease that has yet to assume a particular form; it is a disease that is still brewing, that exists at the stage of *qi*. If you choose to treat the disease at this time, then it will require only the very slightest effort on the part of the physician.

Once one waits until the disease has taken form, however, once it has formed a tumor or an organic disease, we have a very different story. At this point, treating the disease is like moving a mountain or reeling silk—both long and laborious processes. Thus, the higher-level physician does not treat disease that has already taken form, or she would not be referred to as a "higher" physician. If you treat these sorts of diseases, the higher physician will probably smile and quote the classics: "To begin digging a well when one grows thirsty or to start forging weapons once the battle has begun, a bit late, is it not?"

Some years ago, when relaxing idly, I was leafing through a history book and came across a wonderful passage. At the time I thought I would remember it, so I did not take notes, nor did I place any sort of bookmark. At present, I would love to recount this passage to the reader, but I cannot remember it in any detail, and am not even sure if I read it in the *History of the Early Tang* or some other work. The basic story goes like this.

There were three brothers who practiced medicine. The youngest was the most famous and had many patients. His courtyard was as busy as a fair, and many patients were carried in to see him. His patients came and went like bees. The second brother was not as famous as the youngest. His courtyard was not as busy as his brother's was. The oldest brother's place was almost entirely unfrequented, and no one who was seriously ill went to see him.

One time, a man of noble character took his disciple to survey these three brothers. When they returned, he asked his disciple which of the three brothers he deemed most skillful and which was the most deficient. Without hesitation the disciple replied: "The youngest brother's skill was greatest. Did you see how many patients he had? His curative abilities must be formidable to have acquired so extensive a clientele. The eldest brother's abilities are obviously the least of the three. His place was desolate and all he treats are trifles and minor ailments. What sort of skill is that?"

His master listened and then shook his head emphatically and spoke: "Wrong! Among the three, the youngest was the least skillful. He hasn't even a tenth of the skill possessed by the eldest brother. The youngest brother is a low physician at best, the second brother a mid-level physician. Only the eldest deserves to be called a higher physician. The eldest brother treats disease without leaving a trace. When disease is treated at this early stage of its development, when it has not yet assumed any form, then it will never result in any serious ailment and will never have an opportunity to take form at all. That is why you did not see any serious ailments at his clinic. He had treated just as many patients with serious diseases, only he cured them so that no trace remained, rescuing their health. If disease is not correctly detected and treated during this early stage, and the physician instead waits until the disease becomes complicated and only then an attempt at cure is made, this is nothing but great effort made in vain."

This story might be historical fact, or it might be pure fabrication. Regardless, it warrants deep consideration. If one wishes to treat disease before it has taken form, one must first be able to recognize such disease. If you want to discover disease before it has taken form, you must be very skilled at recognizing the syndrome, and very skilled at knowing the obvious by seeing the subtle. If you can perceive the syndrome where none is clearly evident, then you may truly be counted among the higher physicians. Modern medicine's methods for detecting disease are only able to detect disease once it has taken form. Discovering disease only once it has already progressed to this stage puts modern medicine at a terrific disadvantage. Not until the ability to predict disease based on genetic analysis is available to Western physicians will they be able to treat "not-yet" disease (*weibing*) and be counted among the ranks of the "higher" physicians.

I.5.b.4.ii. If There Is a Syndrome, There Must Be Disease

In order to have a syndrome, there must first be a disease. This is a certainty, and we do not need to spend a lot of time discussing this point. In Western Medicine, however, we often meet with the opposite situation. For instance, where functional disorders of the nervous system are concerned, there are many syndromes that have no corresponding disease. In Chinese Medicine, this situation cannot occur.

I.5.b.4.iii. The Degree of Severity of a Syndrome

A great number of variables contribute to the development of a syndrome, so the severity of a syndrome is not directly related to the seriousness of a disease. There are some patients in which the syndrome is prominent but the disease is actually quite small or slight. A toothache is a good example. There is a Chinese saying that goes like this: "A toothache is not a disease, you say, but the pain is enough to make you pray!" The issue of the complexity of syndromes is worthy of serious contemplation. It is not the sort of thing one can think about once or twice and completely understand.

Whether or not there is a syndrome, and whether it is serious or slight, depends on the degree to which the organism reacts to the presence of the disease. It depends on the organism's sensitivity to the disease. And of course, it depends upon the extent to which the organism resists the disease process. These are all factors that we must consider when researching syndrome.

I.5.b.4.iv. Syndrome Characteristics

A basic outline of the special, characteristic features of syndromes are as follows: First, syndromes generally reflect the location of disease. For instance, pain in the epigastric region indicates that the disease may be located in the stomach. A headache centered on the forehead indicates that the disease is in Yangming. This is to say that there is a correlation between the location of the syndrome and the location of the disease. This is well worth keeping in mind when determining the pattern syndrome.

Second, syndromes reflect the nature of the disease. This is an extremely important characteristic of syndrome. Determining the location of the disease is, of course, also very important. For instance, differentiating the syndrome's location allows one to determine whether the disease is a Yangming disease or a Taiyang disease. However, within the six conformations we must also differentiate the presence of cold or heat, excess or deficiency. If these qualities are not clearly differentiated, and one simply says this is a Taiyang disease or a Yangming disease, it is not nearly enough. For instance, if the patient has a Taiyang exterior disease, it must still be determined whether it is cold damage or wind-strike. How do we differentiate cold damage from wind-strike? By relying on the syndrome to show us the nature of the patient's disease.

If we combine these first two characteristics of syndrome, we have the disease trigger (*bingji*).

Third, the syndrome reflects differences between individual patients; differences in constitution, for instance. Two persons who are afflicted by the same pathogen might respond differently. Take for instance, a case of food poisoning. Jim over here might find himself with a bad case of diarrhea, whereas Tom might vomit incessantly. These differences in syndrome reflect differences in individual constitution. In the above example, perhaps Jim has a relatively weak Taiyin and Tom a relatively weak Shaoyang.

Fourth, syndrome has a dual nature. We must keep an extremely broad horizon when investigating for the syndrome. The syndrome is the external manifestation of disease, so in this sense we hope to find no signs of a syndrome in our patients. From another perspective, the syndrome allows us to detect disease in a timely manner and keeps disease from remaining hidden where it can continue to cause harm. Many diseases, especially those as defined by Western Medicine, are such that by the time they manifest in a noticeable way, they are already at a very dangerous stage of development. Examples of this are cancerous tumors or chronic nephritis. In cases like this, we are wont to complain that the syndrome did not present itself early enough.

So in one sense, syndrome brings us pain and suffering of both body and mind. In another sense, the syndrome can often show us the channel through which the disease might be dispelled. For instance, sweating, vomiting, and diarrhea often constitute a syndrome, but Chinese Medicine also often uses these "syndromes" (sweating, vomiting, purgation) as curative methods by inducing sweating, vomiting, and defecation. Therefore, we should thoroughly investigate these two facets of a syndrome: the syndrome's relationship to disease, as well as its relationship to the disease's cure.

The practitioner of Western Medicine need pay no heed to such particulars. In that system, one can order a series of lab tests to determine all that need be known. However, the practitioner of Chinese Medicine must pay careful attention to these details; she must not let a single syndrome slip past. Every syndrome might be the "primary symptom" (*zhu zheng*) as described by Professor Liu Duzhou. Any and every syndrome might be the one that allows you to cure the disease at hand.

Here is an example from not too long ago. The patient was a 60-year-old female whose chief complaint was insomnia. At its worst, she could not sleep at all during the course of the night, to the point that she would hallucinate, hear things, and mumble to herself. She tried both Chinese and Western Medicine to no avail, for neither helped in the least. Reviewing the efforts of physicians before me, besides the sedatives prescribed by Western doctors, the patient had taken a fair amount of Chinese Medicine to nourish the heart and calm the spirit, build the yin and subdue the yang.

I took her pulses and noted that both were slippery. Presuming that she was afflicted by phlegm turbidity, I began to treat her accordingly and prescribed a modification of Wendan Tang and Gaozhen Wuyou San. To my disappointment, however, this formula produced no results. Afterward, I listened to the patient more carefully and discovered that her insomnia was worst when she was overworked and tired. If she exercised a bit too much, she often had difficulty entering slumber. Most people sleep better when they are tired from exertion, but this patient was exactly the opposite. Once I heard this "syndrome," everything became clear.

Her entire illness became clear in light of my revised symptom picture, with this seemingly contradictory piece of information as its linchpin. The ancients said: exhaustion damages the spleen. From this, I knew that the patient's disease was seated in the spleen, and furthermore in the conformation related to the spleen, Taiyin. I prescribed Guipi Tang for her and after a number of doses, she was able to sleep soundly. It has already been over a month and she has been sleeping well every night without the use of sedatives.

Fifth, let us look at the diseases with the greatest number of syndromes. As we discussed earlier, the relationship between disease and syndrome is very complicated. It is not the case that if there are a lot of syndromes then the diseases are also numerous, or that if the syndrome is serious, so too is the disease. Your understanding of the relationship between syndrome and disease will depend in part on what angle you consider it from. If we study the *Treatise on Cold Damage*, we soon discover that with regard to the relationship between disease and syndrome, as well as formula and syndrome, that some diseases and formulas are associated with very simple syndromes and others are associated with very complex and variable syndromes.

Looking at the entire *Treatise on Cold Damage*, the most complex and variable syndromes are those that pertain either to disease of the "hinge," and diseases in which water *qi* plays a key role. The formulas that correspond to these types of diseases are also those associated with the most complex and variable syndromes. Thus, we have Chaihu preparations that correspond to disease of the "hinge," and formulas that regulate water *qi* such as Xiao Qinglong Tang and Zhenwu Tang. How do we determine which syndromes and formulas are the most complex and variable? It is done by looking for the mentions of "or" in the lists of syndromes in *Treatise on Cold Damage*.

If we look at the 397 lines of the *Treatise on Cold Damage*, of the 112 formulas found within those articles, which lines contain the most "or" syndromes? The highest number appear in line 96 about Xiao Chaihu Tang, line 318 referring to Sini San, line 40 mentioning Xiao Qinglong Tang, and line 316 referring to Zhenwu Tang. Xiao Chaihu Tang treats Shaoyang disorder, with seven associated "or" syndromes. Sini San treats Shaoyin diseases, and has five "or" syndromes. Shaoyang and Shaoyin both govern the hinge mechanism. Earlier, in Chapter Three, we discussed the flexible nature of this hinge, and we can see this flexibility in the number of "or" syndromes associated with the Shaoyin and Shaoyang.

The influence of this hinge mechanism is extensive; the resulting complexity of clinical presentation is a natural result. When, in the clinical setting, we encounter a syndrome that baffles us with its complexity and we have no idea how to proceed, we should consider the possibility that the syndrome at hand is related to this hinge mechanism. The scenario with water *qi* is similar to this, as your own contemplation may make clear.

I.5.b.4.v. The Essential Variables of Syndrome

We have discussed the topic of syndrome at some length now, and so it is helpful, at this juncture, to establish the essential factors of a syndrome. In other words, through the process of establishing a syndrome, what is it that we aim to discover? Besides the elements we have already discussed regarding syndrome, there is another critical and overarching concept that we seek to address: yin and yang. To determine the syndrome, we can use the methods of looking, listening, asking, and palpating. After we have determined, contemplated, analyzed, and evaluated the syndrome, what emerges? What emerges from this process is a picture of yin and yang.

We must put our conclusions into terms of yin and yang, and once we have put it into such a manner of speaking, we can grasp the essence of how to treat the disease. This cannot be forgotten at any point during the process of deriving a syndrome and putting it to use. Yin and yang are the alpha and the omega of the practice of Chinese Medicine. That is as far as we will discuss the topic of syndrome.

I.6. Explaining Treatment

At this point, I do not plan to discuss the character *zhi* (治), translated in this context as "treatment," at great length. The original meaning of the character *zhi* pertained to water. *Explaining Writing and Analyzing Characters* defines *zhi* as: "The water that emerges from Donglai Qucheng, and enters the sea at Yangqiu mountain." The name of the river that follows the course described in *Explaining Writing and Analyzing Characters* is *zhi*. Thus, the pictographic element of this character, the radical comprised of three dots on the left of the character (氵), represents water.

The extended meaning of *zhi* is to "put in order" (*li*). In Chinese, the two characters are often used together *zhili* to mean "to govern" or "to put in order." Why does the character *zhi* have such a close relationship with water? Because water, if regulated, nourishes all living things, but if disordered, it endangers all life. The methods of regulating water include dredging, conducting, drawing, leading, enclosing, storing, and so on, all of which involve taking advantage of water's natural tendencies, and guiding its action according to circumstances. Treating disease involves an analogous series of similar processes, thus the use of the same character, *zhi*, is fitting. Thus, in order to fathom the deeper meaning of the treatment of disease, we must seek to understand it from the perspective of regulating water. This applies not only to the treatment of disease, but also to the regulation (*zhi*) of anything in life.

II. An Outline of Taiyang Disease

II.1. Taiyang Disease Trigger Text

Our discussion of the content of Taiyang disease outlined in the *Treatise on Cold Damage* will focus on the first line of the Taiyang chapter: "When Taiyang is diseased, the pulse is floating, the head and nape of the neck are stiff and painful, and there is aversion to cold." Successive dynasties after Zhang Zhongjing regarded this line as an outline of Taiyang disease. The Qing dynasty cold damage master Ke Yunbo (Ke Qin) therefore came to regard this line as the one that conveyed the Taiyang disease trigger. In his *Collected Writings on Renewal of the Discussion of Cold Damage* (Shanghan laisu ji), he puts it this way: "Regarding the general composition of Zhang Zhongjing's treatise, he established one line for each of the six conformations that reveals its associated disease trigger. This line brings out the essential aspects of this conformation. In order to do so, it was necessary to select the most representative pulse and pattern syndrome and set them as the basic framework [for the text]." "Disease trigger" means the most crucial factor contributing to the emergence of a particular disease. Where do we begin our search for this essential factor? We begin our search with the pulse and syndrome. Therefore, Master Ke frames his discussion of the disease trigger in terms of the representative pulse and syndrome.

Regarding the Chinese word *zheng*, usually translated as syndrome, when I looked up this passage in my 1959 copy of the *Collected Writings on Renewal of the Discussion of Cold Damage*, syndrome (*zheng*) is written 症. The two characters, 證 and 症, pronounced the same way in Mandarin Chinese (*zheng*), are often confused and I feel the need to clarify their distinct meanings. In modern Chinese, the character 症 refers to the symptoms of a disease. This character did not exist in ancient times, nor is it a simplified version of a traditional character, so there is no explanation of it in traditional dictionaries such as *Explaining Writing and Analyzing Characters* or the *Kangxi Dictionary*.

The twentieth-century physician-scholar Qin Bowei expressed the opinion that the two characters 證 and 症 had the same meaning and were interchangeable. However, if we analyze and contrast the construction and connotations of 證 with 症, we find that the two meanings are vastly different. The character 證, as discussed earlier, is broad and extensive in its meaning, while 症 is narrowly defined. The two cannot act as substitutes for each other. Western Medicine in China uses the character 症 but does not use the character 證. It is suitable, therefore, that Chinese Medicine use the character 證 and not use the character 症.

Getting back to the text, since the opening line of each section of the *Treatise on Cold Damage* provides us with the disease trigger, our understanding of this line might be aided by placing its content into a standardized form. The standard syntactical form for discussing disease triggers is provided by the nineteen disease triggers in the *Yellow Emperor's Classic* we discussed earlier. Written in like fashion, this first line might read: "All floating pulses, stiffness and pain of the head and nape of the neck with aversion to cold belongs to Taiyang."

To summarize, this line contains three elements related to the pulse and syndrome characterizing the disease trigger. They are: a floating pulse, a stiff and painful head and nape, and aversion to cold. These three elements distinguish the pulse and syndrome of Taiyang disease. So then, must the patient exhibit all three elements in order for us as physicians to diagnose her with Taiyang disease? If the patient has all three, then they certainly have Taiyang disease, but what if the patient has just one or two of the three? Can this be considered Taiyang disease? This question has been hotly debated for ages. My personal view is that we need only see one or two of these three elements in order to accurately diagnose Taiyang disease.

For instance, line 6 reads: "Taiyang disease in which there is heat effusion and thirst but no aversion to cold is warmth disease." In this case, the line specifically states that the patient does not have an aversion to cold, so one of the three elements is already missing. It would be reasonable to assume this means it is therefore not Taiyang disease, but at the outset of the line it clearly states that this disease is Taiyang disease. This clearly tells us that, of the three elements constituting the disease trigger, the patient need only exhibit one or two in order for us to consider the possibility that the disease is a Taiyang disease. By the same logic, it is implied that every line in the *Treatise on Cold Damage* that is concerned with Taiyang disease can be understood to be associated with the three elements of the opening line. The patient must exhibit at least one of these elements in order to be said to have Taiyang disease, even if the particular line describing the patient's symptom picture does not explicitly mention these elements.

II.2. Explanation of Its Meaning

II.2.a. Floating Pulse

A floating pulse refers to a pulse that can be felt at the surface of the patient's skin. In his book on pulse diagnosis *Lakeside Master's Study of the Pulse* (Binhu maixue), Li Shizhen wrote: "floating on the surface, like wood drifting on the water." Those who practice pulse diagnosis should take care to feel all three positions of the pulse: superficial, middle, and deep. As long as the practitioner avoids going straight to the deep level like an Olympic diver, she should have no difficulty learning to recognize this particular type of pulse. In the following passages, we will explore different aspects of the floating pulse, in order to better understand it.

II.2.a.1. The Location of the Pulse Is the Location of the Disease

We have already discussed the features of a floating pulse, but what causes the pulse to float? It floats on the exterior because the pathogen is afflicting the exterior of the body and the yang *qi* emerges to the exterior in order to combat this pathogen. The pulse follows the yang to the exterior and therefore floats on the exterior of the body. From this, we know that where the pathogen is, there too is the yang and where the yang is, we will find the location of the disease. Therefore, wherever we find the pulse, we find the disease. If the pulse is located in the three yang, then the disease is located in the three yang. If the pulse is stationed in the three yin, then the disease can be found in the three yin.

II.2.a.2. "Humans Take the Earth As Model"

In discussing the connotations of Taiyang disease, we referred to Taiyang ruling cold water, and its position being highest. According to Laozi, we should consider questions we have about human beings in terms of the earth on which we live. On earth, what is the highest place? The Himalayas, of course. The Himalayas are the highest mountain range on earth and, situated on the border between China and Nepal is Mt. Everest, the world's highest peak, with an elevation of more than 29,000 feet. The summit is covered with snow throughout the year. Thus, we know the highest point on earth is not only high, it is cold, and there is always water there. According to Laozi's adage: "Humans take the earth as model," then, if we wish to find a testimony to a Taiyang cold water on earth, there is no stronger proof than Mt. Everest. This is the place on earth with the strongest affinity to Taiyang.

Why is the very element in the description of Taiyang disease a floating pulse? The position of the pulse reflects the position of the disease. In this case, the pulse is floating on the surface; in other words, it is in the highest possible position. Taiyang disease is reflected in the high, cold, water-laden mountaintops. Thus, a floating pulse is the premiere proof of Taiyang disease.

II.2.a.3. Taiyang Emphasizes the Pulse

Each of the six conformations emphasizes determining the quality of the pulse. Each describes the disease, the syndrome, and the pulse as a single, organized whole. However, if we look closely at the opening line (the disease trigger line) of each of the six sections of the book, we discover that the pulse is given special prominence in the case of both Taiyang and Shaoyin disease. The opening lines of the Taiyang and Shaoyin sections both describe the type of pulse associated with the disease. The Taiyang pulse is "floating" and the Shaoyin pulse is "faint and fine." The opening lines of the other four conformations do not mention the pulse.

The emphasis placed on the pulses in the Taiyang and Shaoyin sections underlines the decisive characteristic of the pulse in these two types of disease. In the diagnosis of both Taiyang and Shaoyin disease, the pulse often has the final word. For instance, line 42 says: "Taiyang disease, when the exterior syndrome has yet to resolve, the pulse is floating and weak, it is appropriate to resolve the exterior through inducing sweating, so it is suitable to prescribe Guizhi Tang." Line 52 reads: "The pulse is floating and rapid, sweating can be induced, Mahuang Tang is suitable." And in the Shaoyin section of the book, line 323: "Shaoyin disease in which the pulse is sunken, it is urgent that it be warmed and suitable to use Sini Tang."

Of course, the indication for Guizhi Tang is not solely a "floating and weak" pulse, nor is Mahuang Tang only indicated for a "floating and rapid pulse," nor is the prescription of Sini Tang limited to "a sunken pulse." However, based on the structure of the text, we must recognize the pivotal role of the pulse in arriving at a diagnosis. The pulse is the "trigger" in the text. This is rarely the case with the conformations other than the Taiyang and Shaoyin channels. We rarely see it written that "if the pulse is wiry, it is suitable to use Chaihu Tang" or "if the pulse is large, Baihu Tang is advisable." This shows that the pulse has high specificity in the case of Taiyang and Shaoyin disease.

Why do both Taiyang and Shaoyin disease share this special connection with the pulse? From our previous discussion, we know that the pulse correlates with water and the moon. The pulse is yang joined with yin. Without yin water, the pulse has no substance. Without yang fire, the pulse cannot move. Thus, water and fire, yin and yang, constitute the key elements of the pulse. Taiyang rules water, it is extreme yang within yang, while Shaoyin is the storage of water and fire. The implications of Taiyang and Shaoyin tally perfectly with our understanding of the pulse. Therefore, it is said: "the pulse reflects Taiyang, or the pulse reflects Shaoyin." Hence, changes in the pulse most greatly reflect changes in Taiyang and Shaoyin.

II.2.a.4. Contemplating "The Lungs Face the Hundred Pulses"

Now that we have explained the special relationship between the pulse and both the Taiyang and Shaoyin conformations, it is time to turn our discussion to the relationship between the pulse and the lungs. In "Further Discourse on the Channel Vessels" of the *Plain Questions*, it says: "the *qi* of the channels returns to the lungs, and the lungs face the hundred pulses." In our *Fundamentals of Chinese Medicine* textbook, it explains the phrase "the lungs face the hundred pulses" in terms of the lung assisting the heart to move the blood. This explanation relies upon an awareness of the pulmonary circulation (as distinct from the systemic circulation) in the modern sense.

As the blood courses through the body, it loses oxygen to the surrounding tissues. By the time it returns to the heart, its supply of oxygen has been almost wholly depleted. The blood first enters the right side of the heart, which pumps it through the pulmonary circulation, the system of blood vessels in the lungs that allow for the exchange of carbon dioxide with oxygen. The blood then returns to the left side of the heart via the pulmonary vein, and then re-enters the systemic circulation. The blood must pass through the pulmonary system in order to be re-oxygenated. After passing through the vessels of the lungs, it continues on its way throughout the rest of the body.

From this perspective, "the lungs face the hundred pulses" makes perfect sense. However, this type of understanding introduces a problem: How did the ancients know of the "pulmonary circulation"? How did they know that the "lungs face the hundred pulses?" Did they do experiments? Or did they rely upon logical deduction?

On a separate point, with regard to the original meaning of the "pulse" (*mai*), the pulse is comprised of water combined with the moon. We have already clarified the meaning of water, and discussed the significance of the moon. *Explaining Writing and Analyzing Characters* says: "The moon is the essence of Taiyin." The essay "Patterns of Heaven" of the *Huainanzi* says: "The essence of water *qi* becomes the moon." The essence of Taiyin becomes the moon, and the lungs rule Taiyin. The essence of water *qi* becomes the moon, and the lungs are the upper source of water. Keeping in mind the lung's relationship to both water and the moon, it corresponds perfectly with the pulse. Why does the *Plain Questions* say that "the pulse faces the hundred pulses"? Why does pulse diagnosis, as explained in the *Classic of Difficulties*, rely solely upon the *cunkou* pulse position of the wrist, which is governed by the lungs? The answers to both of these questions lie in the close relationship of the lungs with the pulse, as we have just described.

In the past, when I read the *Fundamentals of Chinese Medicine*, I could not fathom what was meant by "the lungs are the upper source of water." How could the lungs be the "upper source of water"? It was not until the summer of 1996 when I first set foot in the western regions of China and for the first time saw snow-capped mountains, and watched that same snow melting into rivulets to form streams that, descending the mountainsides, became rapids that fed the mighty Jinsha River, that I suddenly realized the meaning of this line from the classics, and all my doubts about it faded away. The importance that the ancients placed on "reading myriad books and wandering myriad roads" became clear to me at that moment. Reading books alone is not sufficient. Reading is how we study, but moving through the world is how we contemplate and think through what we have studied. "To study without contemplation is to be deceived." "Wandering myriad miles" is just as important as reading widely.

Laozi emphasized that "Humans take the earth as model; the earth takes the heavens as model; the heavens take the Dao as model; the Dao takes nature as model." Laozi's description of these four models or patterns reveals a world in which everything is woven into an interdependent, organic whole. Chinese medicine is distinguished by this holistic view of the human body, and a diagnosis based on the patient's overall condition. Many people might talk about this holistic view, but if one has not grasped the "four models" of Laozi, then a truly holistic view cannot be attained. If your study of Chinese Medicine is restricted to the world of the human body, or merely integrated with some scientific studies, there will be many questions that you will not be able to figure out, and you will feel anxious and unsure about Chinese Medicine theory.

Once you place these concepts within the conceptual framework of heaven and earth, into the larger context of nature, many difficulties will be resolved, and your attitude toward Chinese Medicine theory will change. Framed by validating structure of nature, upon which it was patterned, Chinese Medicine theory appears rich, substantial, and completely reliable. The *Plain Questions's* "True Speech of the Golden Cabinet" reads: "the north produces cold, cold produces water." Water initially belongs to the northern direction; how has it suddenly changed its location to the west?

This question raises a couple of important points. First is the mutual engendering concept. Metal produces nascent water. We will discuss this point at greater length later in this book. Another related concept has to do with prenatal and postnatal categories, as understood by Chinese Medicine. For instance, within the *Classic of Changes* system, there are the eight prenatal and eight postnatal trigrams. Among the eight postnatal trigrams, *Kan* is water, and is located squarely in the north. Based on the postnatal configuration, we know that water belongs to the northern direction. That is at least the case from the postnatal perspective.

And where is water located in the prenatal configuration? Among the eight prenatal trigrams, *Kan* Water is not located in the north. Instead, it is located squarely in the west, where we might otherwise expect to find the metal element. The *Kan* Water is located westward. This of course explains the location of the fountainheads of both the Yangzi and Yellow Rivers to the west. It also validates the line: "The lungs are the upper source of water." Therefore, the identification of western metal with water, as well as the lungs with the upper source of water, is related to the prenatal perspective. The prenatal is the form, the postnatal is the function. The prenatal is the source, the postnatal is that which flows from the source. Form and function, source and outflow, spring and brook—it is vital to pay close attention to these distinctions in order to study Chinese Medicine correctly.

In the chapter titled "Treatise on the Microcosm of the Human Body" from the Qing dynasty text *The Source of Medicine*, we read: "In the human body, the lungs are the imperial canopy, located in the highest position." The lungs are associated with metal, the densest material. Why is the densest and heaviest material the one that occupies the position of the "imperial canopy"? Why are the vast majority of the highest mountains located in the west? These are intriguing questions, and contemplating these questions will most certainly help us to better understand Chinese Medicine and traditional Chinese understanding in general.

The lungs are positioned as the imperial canopy, the lungs are the upper source of water, the lungs send forth the hundred pulses; all of these aspects of the lungs strongly correspond with Taiyang. These correlations contribute to the fact that much of the Taiyang chapter of the *Treatise on Cold Damage* is devoted to the diseases of the lungs. Thus, when we consider organs of the body related in some sense to Taiyang, we are not limited to the urinary bladder associated with the Taiyang channel of the leg, or to the small intestine associated with the Taiyang channel of the arm.

The American physicist Subrahmanyan Chandresekhar, who won the Nobel Prize for Physics in 1983, published a book of his lectures titled *Truth and Beauty: Aesthetics and Motivations in Science*. In one of his lectures in that book, "Shakespeare, Newton, and Beethoven or Patterns of Creativity," he writes:

Sometimes we take a particular line of thinking and apply it to seemingly unrelated topics. For instance, we can take our understanding of the movements of particles in a colloidal suspension, what is referred to as Brownian motion, and apply this understanding to the movement of stars within galaxies. It is astounding that these two seemingly unrelated phenomena, the movement of sugars in milk and stars in the Milky Way, can be understood through the same theoretical framework.

Of course, after sharing in Professor Chandresekhar's brilliant insight, don't you feel a similar sense of amazement from our discussion of the fountainheads of the Yangzi or Yellow Rivers, or the Tanggula or Himalayan mountains with regard to the "lungs as the imperial canopy" and "the lungs as upper source of water," weaving these seemingly completely unrelated topics into a single understanding?

II.2.a.5. "The Highest Good Is Like Water"

Before we conclude our discussion of the "floating pulse," we might first pursue the train of thought we touched on before and speak a bit about the concept of water. Chapter 8 of the *Classic of the Dao and Its Virtue* reads: "The highest good is like water. Water benefits the myriad things but does not contend. It dwells in places that the multitude shun. Thus, it is interwoven with the Dao."

Why is it that in Laozi's view, water is a metaphor for what he holds in highest regard? It is because despite water's innate nobility and its benefit to the "myriad things," it is capable of not contending with others and is ready to dwell in places that the masses consider nauseous. What are the places the multitude shun? Put simply: in the lowest places.

People have a predilection for high places. Those who pursue careers wish to be promoted. Those in academia seek to stand out among their fellows. Businessmen who become millionaires strive to become billionaires, and billionaires emulate trillionaires. If we take a look at these rich princes relative to one another, isn't each "a cut above" their peer? Which of them would be willing to live below the other?

Those who are genuinely akin to Zeng Guofan, the suppressor of the Taiping Rebellion, who held himself to the highest Confucian standards, those who intentionally increase the burdens on their descendants for the greater good are far too few. If those in officialdom were truly able to live up to the slogans they shout and act as public servants, it would be remarkable. Greed and avarice make it decidedly difficult to behave in such a way, and equally impossible to be become "interwoven with the Dao."

They do not interweave with the Dao, instead they turn their back on the Dao. How can that which turns its back on the Dao last eternally? The ancients said: "Wealth does not last more than three generations." There is a lot of sense in this saying. You could be Li Ka-shing, one of the wealthiest men of our time, and you still cannot do anything about that particular problem. This is because it is very difficult for a person to become "interwoven with the Dao." It is very difficult to adopt the characteristics of water.

And if you do not possess the character of water, how will you both endure and thrive? If wealth and honor can last out three generations, that is already quite an accomplishment!

Let us examine water in the human body. The masters of water in the body are the kidneys, and the kidneys are the viscera belonging to the element of water. Of the five viscera, the kidneys reside lowest in the human body and yet the efflorescence of the kidneys is the hair of the head, seated at the highest position on the human body. One is the highest and the other the lowest; this paradox is insightful.

The contemporary master physician Dr. Yue Meizhong consulted the classics and preferred to use the herb Fuling by itself as a means of stopping hair loss. I used to find this method puzzling, but today, when I regard it from the perspective of this herb's effect on water and the kidney's relationship to water, I think it is fitting.

II.2.b. "The Head and Nape of the Neck Are Stiff and Painful"

II.2.b.1. Taiyang Position Rules the Head and Nape of the Neck

The Taiyang position is the highest position. Before, when we discussed the floating pulse, we talked about how, among pulse positions, it is the highest. Here we are discussing the head and nape of the neck, which also occupy the highest position. Therefore, in matters of Chinese Medicine it is important that we look not only at the theoretical mechanism involved but also at correlations, that is to say, mutually corresponding areas. Correlations are an important aspect of Chinese Medicine.

Each of the six conformations may present with headache. Why, then, is it that in the lines outlining the six conformations and the pathology of each, there is mention of headache only in the section devoted to the Taiyang configuration? This is evidence of an important corresponding relationship.

II.2.b.2. The Xiang is Taiyang's Special Location

An explanation of xiang (項) in *Explaining Writing and Analyzing Characters* reads: "The back of the head." The *Explanation of Names* says: "Firm. Hard and firm. The place that is received by the pillow." Medical practitioners therefore often refer to the *xiang* as the nape of the neck; that is the back of the neck. The part of the body referred to as the *xiang* is in the posterior;

this point is uncontested. But what portion of the body is it on the back of? The definitions above are slightly vague on this point.

So, what is the most fitting place for us to regard as the location of the *xiang*? If you feel around below your occiput, you will feel a sort of hollow place. This is where rivers join and swell: the water that flows from the high mountain snow enters into wide rivers at this place. I consider this to be the actual location of the *xiang*. It is by means of this point on the body that the *xiang* is able to act as a centralized extension of both the upper and lower aspects of the body.

Taiyang rules water. The Taiyang channel of the leg arises at the point Qingming, travels up along the foremost aspect of the brow, and then descends along the *xiang*, the back of the head and neck. Thus, Wu Renju said, "The *xiang* is the specific position of Taiyang." Taiyang headaches often refer to the back of the head and nape of the neck; this is a notable characteristic of Taiyang headaches. Other types of headaches typically do not extend to the *xiang*.

In this line, besides pain, there is also *jiang*, which is translated as "stiff" in the phrase "the head and nape of the neck are stiff and painful." Gentle and mild are the opposite of *jiang*. Therefore, in one sense, in the event that "the head and nape of the neck are stiff and painful," the nape of the neck loses its gentle pliancy and comfortable aspect. This is most important in relation to cold pathogenic influence, since when living things encounter cold, there is a strong contraction, and when they encounter heat, they become relaxed and pliant.

Another aspect of the stiffness of the nape of the neck is evidenced in the nineteen disease triggers section of the *Yellow Emperor's Classic*, where it is written: "All tetany and stiff nape belongs to dampness." The nape is the joining point of the two rivers, the banks of which require earth to be properly regulated. On account of this aspect of the symptom *xiang jiang* ("stiff nape"), we can see that besides its relationship with the Taiyang conformation, there is also a strong relationship with the earth and damp of Taiyin. Nowadays, we see a lot of cervical spine disorders. All of this cervical pathology can be considered and treated from the perspective of Taiyang and Taiyin.

II.2.c. Aversion to Cold

II.2.c.1. The Most Important Syndrome

When the exterior of the body is affected by a pathogenic influence, there are a number of effects: Taiyang opening mechanism becomes stuck, the yang *qi* is hindered from emerging, and is unable to spread to the external musculature. When these are present, we know that there will be "aversion to cold." This symptom is also referred to as exterior cold, and it is important to note this "cold" is not completely identical to the meaning of a low temperature, as we will discuss in the next section. Aversion to cold is a very important indication of an exterior syndrome, and of the contraction of a pathogen by the Taiyang system. Thus, the ancients said: "If there is aversion to cold, then this is an exterior syndrome." When you see this syndrome, you know that you need to treat the exterior, and treat Taiyang.

II.2.c.2. An Emphasis on Subjective Experience

Earlier when we talked about how to read the classics, I emphasized the importance of all three levels of meaning, especially a cautious, unambiguous reading of the meaning of each character. So it is in the case of "aversion to cold." When cold is prefixed with aversion, there is a very particular meaning that is indicated. What is "aversion"? "Aversion" refers to the likes and dislikes of the human mind, a type of subjective experience.

If you detest so and so or such and such a thing, you find it difficult to stand that person or thing, even for a minute. This aversion that you experience, however, does not necessarily mean this particular person or thing is so detestable in and of itself. Therefore, when we speak of "aversion to cold," we are limited to a subjective experience, without any indication of how cold the actual temperature is, or how far below zero the thermometer reads. This concept must be fully apprehended.

There are some people who contract Taiyang disease on a summer day, when the weather is actually very hot. The sick person will nevertheless get in bed and pull two quilts over them. This is "aversion to cold," and it is completely unrelated to the actual temperature. If at this time you take the person's temperature, it may be 39 or even 40 degrees Celsius (102–104 degrees Fahrenheit). Thus, this "aversion" represents a subjective state or experience and by no means can be understood to convey an objective reality.

In our examination of the meaning of "aversion" above, we encountered an issue regarding subjectivity and objectivity. This is a problem that, as students of Chinese Medicine, we should contemplate carefully. It is a major issue in Chinese Medicine. It also represents, in many respects, a line of demarcation between Chinese and Western Medicine.

Western Medicine is clearly biased toward objectivity rather than subjectivity. For instance, Western medical diagnosis employs methods derived from chemistry and physics to determine particular objective indicators of disease. Furthermore, determination of a disease's advance or retreat also relies on these objective markers. If a person has severe and complicated subjective symptoms, but the objective markers do not reveal anything out of the ordinary, they are often simply diagnosed with a "nervous disorder."

Chinese Medicine is vastly different in this respect and places great emphasis on the subjective experience. For example, the syndrome of thirst. If a person has thirst, a relatively objective feeling, Chinese Medicine is concerned with the underlying, subjective experience: Does the person desire hot drinks or cold drinks? Often, it is these subjective manifestations that afterward serve as the definitive diagnosis of an ailment that was already intimated by the objective signs.

If the person prefers cold drinks, the disease is usually in Yangming; if the person desires hot drinks, then we could very possibly be looking at a disease that resides in Shaoyin. One is Shaoyin, the other Yangming; one is deficiency cold, the other excess heat; the differences between these are simply enormous. These polar opposite diagnoses are made on the basis of what? Quite simply, they are determined according to like and dislike, desires and aversions.

Earlier, we mentioned the late, venerable old doctor Lin Peixiang. Now I would like to refer to a patient treated by Dr. Lin in the 1970s. The patient had suffered from 40 days of incessant fever. He consulted with prestigious doctors of Western Medicine and took every sort of antibiotic, but his fever never decreased. He also took no small quantity of Chinese Medicine, but his condition did not improve.

As the situation progressed, the respected doctors of our college were invited to assemble and discuss the diagnosis. Dr. Lin was one of the invited doctors. All of the doctors gathered together and each, of course, wanted to display his or her skill and offer their own views. Just as everyone was concentrating their attention on the four methods of diagnosis and a differential diagnosis, Dr. Lin was surprised by something the patient was doing.

That particular day was very hot, and so it was hardly unusual that the patient should drink water. However, this patient would pour water from the thermos of boiled water into his cup and then, without waiting more than an eye blink, would drink down the entire cup. Was it possible that his thermos contained only warm water? Dr. Lin quietly touched the drinking cup that the patient had just emptied. The cup was scalding hot. To desire piping hot water on such a hot day would only be possible in the case of severe interior cold.

Thereupon Dr. Liu prevailed over all dissent from his colleagues. They determined that this was a case of Shaoyin illness with an overabundance of internal yin cold repelling yang to the exterior. From this, they derived a treatment plan and prescribed a large dose of modified Sini Tang. The medicine contained the very hot, pungent herbs Fuzi, Ganjiang, and Rougui. After one dose of the decoction, his temperature dropped significantly. After several doses, his body temperature returned to normal.

This case gives us a fine example of the differences between Chinese and Western Wedicine. In Western Medicine, both diagnosis and treatment rely on the exam results using methods derived from the fields of physics and chemistry. While Chinese Medicine also relies on relatively objective findings: the wiriness of the pulse, or its slipperiness, for example; there are also times, however, when Chinese Medicine is more concerned with subjective preferences: likes and dislikes, desire and aversion.

If someone is thirsty, the Western physician may be concerned with how many ounces of water the patient drinks per day, but whether the patient prefers hot or cold water is of entirely no interest to the Western physician. If the patient has a fever, the Western physician is concerned with the exact temperature of the fever, whether it is remittent or continuous. As for whether the patient has an aversion to cold or an aversion to heat, this detail is disregarded.

If a physician of Chinese Medicine disregards these subjective variables, then he or she will miss crucial information. So why is it that Chinese Medicine stresses the importance of subjective experiences? It is because these experiences are under the purview of the heart, and the heart "holds the office of the sovereign and ruler. Spirit brightness originates from it."

Thus, by emphasizing this aspect, we are in fact emphasizing the aspect of the heart, and thereby stressing the importance of that which is beyond form: the metaphysical level of pathology. This is a special territory of Chinese Medicine, and, as physicians, we should learn to know it well. Otherwise, under the name of modernization, or objectification, these subjective variables will be disregarded entirely. As for Chinese Medicine, just like any other matter of importance, we must examine it carefully with our own faculties in order to understand it, judging by our own lights its merits and qualities, not merely parroting the words and ideas of others.

Subjectivity has its limitations. Being swayed by one's emotions and not recognizing that "beauty is in the eye of the beholder" can be blocks to recognizing truth. But there are times when it is important to follow one's feelings. This is true for both the arts and the sciences.

We have discussed the floating pulse, stiffness and pain of the head and nape of the neck, and aversion to cold. There is no question that these three aspects of pathology belong to the Taiyang category of disease. And if the patient's pathology exhibits only one or two of these three signs, one still ought to consider Taiyang disease as a possible explanation for the pathology.

Do not forget that a Taiyang syndrome can be incomplete or that it can exist simultaneously with other patterns. For instance, the patient could have aversion to cold, but the pulse could be sunken instead of floating. This indicates that the disease is not entirely in Taiyang, but also contains elements of the three yin.

When later generations employed Mahuang Xixin Fuzi Tang to treat what they called Tai-Shao (Taiyang and Shaoyin) syndrome, it was because they had surmised there was a simultaneous affliction of both layers. In light of this, we should consider all three syndromes we have discussed thus far, and examine them comprehensively and flexibly.

III. The Timing of Taiyang Disease

At this juncture, we will focus on an explanation of the meaning of line 9 of the *Treatise on Cold Damage*: "Taiyang disease tends to resolve in the time from *si* to *wei*."

III.1. Carefully Attend to the Timing, For Then You Will Be Able to Predict the *Qi*

III.1.a. Timing Lines and Disease Trigger Lines Are Equally Important

Of the *Treatise on Cold Damage's* 397 lines, the longest lines consist of as many as 100 characters, and the shortest of no less than ten. In this, we can see that the transmitters of Zhang Zhongjing's work placed emphasis on the ideas he was conveying and were not sticklers about adhering to a particular verse or format. Despite the relatively free way in which Zhang Zhongjing's work has been passed down, we can nevertheless find twelve lines that share a very similar syntactical pattern. These are the six conformation outlines, all of which include "it is" (*zhi wei* 之為), and the six timing lines, all of which include "a time when it tends to resolve" (*yu jie shi* 欲解時) as key syntactical elements.

In the original text authored by Zhang Zhongjing, each of the six conformations had one line consisting of an outline. These are also referred to as the disease trigger lines. Additionally, each of the six conformations has one line concerned with the timing of the disease. Combining the six lines discussing disease trigger with the six lines explaining their timing makes a total of twelve lines. To find this symmetry in these lines makes them stand out from the rest of the text, and the special format of these twelve lines indicates that they have a special meaning. It is indeed unfortunate that scholars throughout history have placed emphasis on the first six lines of each section, the outlines or disease trigger lines, and greatly neglected the last six, which were concerned with timing. Much of Zhang Zhongjing's arduously constructed legacy was thereby lost.

In Chapter 74 of the *Plain Questions*, "The Great Treatise on the Essentials of Ultimate Truth," when discussing the concept of disease trigger, emphasized that one should "Carefully attend to the appropriate *qi* (*qiyi*), and do not miss the disease trigger"; and "Carefully investigate the disease trigger, and do not miss the appropriate *qi*." This tells us, in no uncertain terms, that we are to think about the disease trigger in light of the appropriate *qi*, and, vice versa, that we should consider the appropriate *qi* while fully grasping the particular trigger of the disease. Both are indispensable to one another.

As for studying the *Treatise on Cold Damage*, we should take this concept to heart and grasp both the trigger of the disease, and the *qi* that is suitable to its resolution with either hand, each hand grasping firmly its contents. Historically, by emphasizing only the six lines concerned with the disease trigger, we have only grasped with one of our hands. What can be said of the other hand?

The contents of the other hand can be found in the text of the six lines regarding resolution times. In Chapter 9 of the *Plain Questions*, "The Six Nodes and the Visceral Manifestations," it states: "When a time period begins, the respective *qi* spreads. . . . Carefully attend to its timing, for then you will be able to predict the *qi*." Although the text of the line that discusses the timing of a disease's tendency to resolve merely mentions "time," once it speaks of time, we should think of *qi* as being contained within this term as well.

Thus, those six passages that contain the phrase "a time when it tends to resolve" (*yu jie shi*), which we can call "timing" lines, are actually passages that are concerned with the "appropriate *qi*." If we simply discuss the lines of the passages that outline the form of the disease and disregard the passages that are concerned with resolution time, how could the picture of the pathology be considered complete? Only when these are included do we have a complete comprehension.

When we look at this unique writing style consisting of six pairs of corresponding lines per passage, in which the first part of each pair speaks of the disease, and the second addresses the "appropriate *qi*," we can see the essence of the meaning of the passage in Chapter 74 of the *Plain Questions*, where it states: "Carefully investigate the disease trigger, and do not miss the appropriate *qi*." Legendary figures in China's history, such as the martial arts masters we read of in Jin Yong's novel *The Free and Easy Life of a Wanderer*, are said to be able to defeat their enemies without leaving a trace of their presence. We can see that, in Zhang Zhongjing's utilization of the classics in his writing, he, like they, has attained such a high degree of skill that he leaves no tracks from which we can easily retrace his steps. Even if based solely on appreciation of this level of skill, the *Treatise on Cold Damage* must merit our delight and our highest praise!

III.1.b. Explaining Time

III.1.b.1. The Chinese Character Shi

The modern, simplified form of the Chinese character *shi* (时) consists of the pictogram meaning sun (*ri* 日) together with the phonogram meaning inch (*cun* 寸). The traditional form of the character *shi* (時) contained the same pictogram on the left side with the phonogram meaning temple (*si* 寺) on the right. The meaning of *ri* is perfectly clear: it signifies the sun. The use of this radical in the construction of the character indicates the close relationship between the passage of time and the movement of the sun. What then of the radical *si* ("temple")? *Explaining Writing and Analyzing Characters* says it means "The royal court, where there are laws." Thus, a character representing the sun and another representing laws were combined to form the character signifying time. This combination is food for thought.

The simplified form of this character uses the radical *cun* (寸) instead of *si*. *Cun* ("inch") was the most basic unit of measurement used by the ancients. By combining the character for sun with that for inch to make the character signifying time, we see the character indicates that the measurement of the sun's movement was an indicator of the meaning of "time." The construction of the simplified character seems simpler to understand than the traditional one. Let us return to reality, to the natural world, and inquire as to whether time is indeed produced by the movement of the sun and whether it can be measured by marking the movements of the sun.

As for the movement of the sun producing the passage of time, it is indeed the case that the relative position of the earth to the sun produces the cyclic changes of the four seasons. The seasonal pattern of time in the natural world, at the very least, is closely related to the position of the sun in the sky, even if it is produced by the revolution of the earth around that fiery orb. The seasons are produced by the relative position of the sun to the earth, but if we wish to know where we are in the cycle of the seasons, we must make precise measurements of the sun's position. Therefore, the left side of the character is the radical *ri* (日) representing the sun, but the right side consists of the character *si* (寺), which is itself a compound character composed of *tu* (土) meaning earth above and *cun* (寸), the most basic unit of measurement, below. Taken as a whole, this character would seem to be an apt signifier of not only the passage of time, but also of the act of determining our position within the passage of time. In this character, we see both a branch of learning and a particular discipline within that branch of learning. Such is the unique beauty of the Chinese written language, that its characters carry rich etymological connotations.

The simplification of Chinese characters has been a boon to the speed and ease of writing our language, but when we look at the simplified version of a character such as *shi*, it loses much without the radical *tu* as a part of its composition, for without the relative position of the sun to the earth, how could we have the passage of seasons? On Mars, what does the passage of time seem like? Our notion of the four seasons is a specifically terrestrial concept.

Regarding the calculation of the four seasons and more specifically the twenty-four calendrical periods, the most classical and authoritative method can be found written down in the *Arithmetic Classic of the Gnomon and the Circular Paths of Heaven*. It says:

> Regarding the eight nodes of the lunar calendar and the twenty-four calendrical periods, the increases and decreases of *qi* [per calendrical period] can be measured as nine *cun*, nine *fen*, and six *fen*. When winter arrives, the measurement is one *zhang*, three *chi*, and five *cun*. When summer arrives, the shadow is one *chi* and six *cun* in length.

The method whereby these measurements are obtained consisted of placing a staff eight *chi* high upright on the ground and, at midday, measuring the length of the shadow it cast upon the ground. The eight lunar nodes and the twenty-four calendrical periods could thereby be ascertained.

On the day the shadow is shortest, namely one *chi* and six *cun* in length, was set as *xiazhi* (summer solstice). At this point, the calculation of nine *cun*, nine *fen*, and six *fen* per calendrical period (there are ten *fen* per *cun*, ten *cun* per *chi*, and ten *chi* per *zhang*; the smallest *fen* is also divided into ten smaller *fen*) could be used to determine the arrival of the next period, namely *xiaoshu* (minor heat). This pattern repeats itself until *dongzhi* (winter solstice), when the maximum length of the shadow, one *zhang*, three *chi*, and five *cun* in length, is reached. Then the shadow begins to shorten again with the same periodicity, punctuated by the regular arrival of distinct calendrical periods until the cycle completes itself, back at the summer solstice.

Let us regard the ancient Chinese process of marking the passage of time and noting the calendrical cycle. First of all, it consists of observing the movement of the sun, namely waiting for the midpoint of the day to take measurements. Secondly, it consists of observing the ground to see the shadow cast upon the ground by the sun. This shadow reflects the relative position of the sun to the earth, and in turn it reflects the relationship between yin and yang, thereby allowing us to establish the degree to which the yang *qi* is being released or gathered back in. And third, the aforementioned process requires that a rod with specific measurements (*cun*) be used. All three of these elements are crucial to determining the passage of time; without any one of these, the process of telling time, and thereby creating a true sense of time, could not be undertaken.

The simplified character, lacking the radical representing earth (*tu*), may save us a bit of work when writing, but it casts aside a crucial etymological aspect: the yin earth aspect. If you cast aside the yin, does the yang become orphaned? An orphaned yang cannot grow and flourish! Whenever I think earnestly of the simplification of characters, I grow worried, anxious, and pained. The written language is the means by which we convey the truth, it is the means by which the Dao is transmitted, the vehicle of civilization and culture, and the courier of consciousness. Written language allows us to both know and transmit culture. By means of the written character, three thousand, even five thousand years of crystallized culture are conveyed up to the present day and into the future.

If we discard one of the wheels of the vehicle of the written Chinese language, can we still expect that car to move forward? At present, in my own generation, there are many of us who have been exposed to complex, traditional characters because we have perused ancient books. As a result, the barriers to inheriting knowledge imbued by our newly amputated system of writing are not as evident as it might otherwise be. What sort of state will we find Chinese culture in after some decades or centuries of persistently using these abbreviated, and therefore obviated, instruments of language? It may be that the pulse of Chinese culture may be completely cut off by the simplification of Chinese characters. The simplification of Chinese characters is not a trivial matter. It is by no means something we might simply leave to the impulses of some individuals in a position of authority, for if we do, then we will find ourselves bound into a bad contract, a mortgage that will ultimately lead to cultural bankruptcy. We must not be so careless!

III.1.b.2. The Significance of Time

Regarding time, and here I mean time as defined by traditional Chinese culture, we must be absolutely clear: time as understood in China by the Chinese is different from that of the West. In the West, time is more of a mathematical concept, whereas in traditional Chinese culture, time is more related to its connotations with physics. Therefore, when the Chinese discuss time, it is connected with the movement of the sun, the relationship between the sun and the earth, the relationship between yin and yang, and weather. When we say "spring" there is an immediate association with "warm," when we say "summer" we immediately think "hot," when we say "autumn" we immediately think "cool," and when we say "winter" we immediately think "cold." Why do we say "when the time period begins, the respective *qi* spreads"? Why should we "carefully attend to the timing, for then you will be able to predict the *qi*"? The reason lies in the close relationship between *qi*, weather/temperature and time.

The establishment of time results in the formation of yin and yang, and once yin and yang are created, *qi* begins. In Western culture, "time" does not carry such connotations. If we examine the topic of time from this particular angle, and redefine Chinese Medicine in terms of this understanding, we see that traditional Chinese Medicine is time-based medicine or, put another way, chronological medicine.

In recent years, with the advent of chronological biology, many people have realized that the Chinese Medicine discipline contains chronological medicine. Following this realization, there has been research into "Chinese Medicine's chronological medicine" or "Chronological Chinese Medicine," exposing the chronological aspects of Chinese Medicine. If we look at this issue logically, we might conclude that there are aspects of Chinese Medicine that are chronological, and other aspects that are not related to time. Is this actually the case? If we consider yin and yang and the five elements as well as the Chinese conception of the organs and the channels as the heart of Chinese Medicine, then Chinese Medicine is utterly and completely a medicine of chronology. It is by no means partially so!

III.2. The Time When It Tends to Resolve

The "time when it tends to resolve" (*yu jie shi*) indicates the time a disease is apt to resolve, or when a person is prone to recover from an illness, or the period in which the disease will tend to be ameliorated. Earlier in this book, when we discussed the implied meanings of the character *bing* ("disease"), we focused on the correspondences of disease, its relationship to periods of time, to directions of the compass, to the six *qi*, and many other factors. We summarized this by saying that it corresponded with yin and yang. Besides the lines outlining each of the six conformations of disease, Zhang Zhongjing's *Treatise on Cold Damage* also contains text outlining the periods in which these diseases tend to resolve (*yu jie shi*). As such, we return to the topic of the correspondences of disease. This return also proves our explanation of the character *bing* ("disease") to be correct.

III.2.a. From Si to Wei

In Zhang Zhongjing's textual discussion of the time periods in which disease tends to resolve, he says that the Taiyang disease resolution time is "from *si* to *wei*." This time period consists of the three consecutive periods related to the three consecutive earthly branches *si*, *wu*, and *wei*. To which aspect of the three time periods does this line refer to? Zhang Zhongjing does not explicitly say, and this tells us that *si*, *wu*, and *wei* have at least three levels of implied meaning. The first level of meaning relates to the three time periods of the day correlating to these three earthly branches, a period spanning from 9 am to 3 pm. The second is the period of time within the course of the month that corresponds to these earthly branches, namely the period before and after the fifteenth day of each lunar month. The third level of meaning are the three periods of the annual cycle that pertain to *si*, *wu*, and *wei*, namely the period spanning the fourth, fifth, and sixth months of the old calendar.

The fact that time periods in which disease is inclined to resolve have multiple levels should make us conscious of the multiple levels involved with Taiyang disease's inclination to resolve. Taiyang disease is a broad category of disease; it includes many externally contracted and internally originating diseases. Within this broad category, there are a great number of subcategories of disease. For this reason, one should not adopt an overly simplistic view of Taiyang disease and thereby mistake it for a simple cold brought on by pernicious wind, or fever resulting from exposure to cold temperatures. Taiyang disease can present as either acute or chronic disease.

In the case of acute disease, the course of disease lasts just several days and so we should consider the period in which the disease will tend to ameliorate or resolve in terms of the course of a single day. If the signs and symptoms of the disease are lessened during the *si*, *wu*, and *wei* period from 9 am to 3 pm, we should consider Taiyang disease as a possibility. If the disease is chronic, lasting more than a month or two, or even a year or two, and furthermore exhibits no clear pattern of change through the course of the day, or is irregular, then we should look for a pattern of amelioration within the course of the month, or even the course of the year. If the disease appears to lessen in intensity during the full moon or the months of summer, then we must carefully consider the possibility of Taiyang disease.

III.2.b. The Essentials of Taiyang Disease

Earlier we discussed the disease trigger of Taiyang disease. Now we have just finished discussing the time correspondence of Taiyang disease, so we should now be able to give a general summary of Taiyang disease, and also take a look at the essentials of Taiyang disease, or at the very least its most common elements.

In my view, the essentials of Taiyang disease are as follows: First, the disease is in the exterior system. The exterior is understood in relation to the interior. Therefore, its scope of meaning is broad in Chinese Medicine, and diseases of the exterior are not limited to the common cold and the flu. Besides these, there are many diseases that can be said to be exterior disorders.

The *Plain Questions* chapter titled "The Great Treatise on the Essentials of Ultimate Truth" tells us: "As for the advent of the hundred diseases, they all emerge from wind, cold, summer heat, damp, dryness, and fire, and from these they change and transform." The myriad diseases are brought on by these six pathogens; they are influenced by these pathogens, and atop the foundation wrought by these pathogens the damaging transformations of internal and external disease occur. The influence exerted by the six pathogens mentioned in this chapter of the *Yellow Emperor's Classic* begins in the exterior system. Hence, the position held by Taiyang in the human body is exceedingly important. This position is reflected in the outline of Taiyang disease by the fact that the pulse of Taiyang disease is a floating pulse.

Secondly, Taiyang disease is characterized by profuse cold. As we mentioned, Taiyang disease is located in the exterior system, and the disease can be induced by any of the six pathogenic influences: wind, cold, summer heat, damp, dryness, or fire. However, the most prominent influence is undoubtedly cold. Why is this? Regarding this point, Zhang Zhongjing, in the section called "Guide to Cold Damage" (Shanghan li), provides an important explanation: "Any of the *qi* of the four seasons can induce disease, but cold damage is toxic, as it is the most lethal and damaging *qi*." Why is cold the most lethal *qi*? If the body is damaged by it in the fall and winter, then the yang *qi* cannot be retrieved and stored. If the damage occurs in the spring and summer, then yang *qi* cannot be properly released. If the retrieval and storage are lost, then the form is damaged, and if the ability to release properly is lost, then the function suffers. In the case of cold, both the form and the function of the body can be injured, therefore it is most lethal. That is why cold stands out from the other pathogens in relation to Taiyang disease.

Third, it is the opening mechanism of the body that becomes diseased. The above discussion provided a general outline regarding Taiyang disease relevant to its location or position, namely the exterior, and this leads us to inquire as to the mechanism that led to this kind of locationality. The entire Taiyang system, or put another way, the entire exterior system of the body, is linked to this "opening mechanism" of the body. The instant this opening mechanism is obstructed in any way, it has an effect on the entire Taiyang system, and the signs and symptoms of Taiyang disease emerge.

III.2.c. The Essentials of Si, Wu, and Wei Time Correspondences

The key correlations with the *si*, *wu*, and *wei* time periods can be discussed from three different angles. First, we can look at the changes associated with each of these time periods by examining their related hexagrams: *qian* (Initiating, ䷀), *gou* (Encountering, ䷫), and *dun* (Retreat, ䷠). Within the *Classic of Changes* system, there are the classical trigrams and the divergent hexagrams. The classical hexagrams are the eight trigrams that are probably most familiar to us. The divergent hexagrams consist of combinations of these eight trigrams, one atop the other, and constitute the majority of the 64 hexagrams.

The two trigrams composing each hexagram have an upper and lower, exterior and interior, inner and outer relationship to each other. After the *zi* period of the day, from 11 pm to 1 am, the hexagrams restart with *fu* (Turning Back, ☷), *lin* (Approaching, ☷), *tai* (Advance, ☷), *dazhuang* (Great Strength, ☳), *guai* (Eliminating, ☱), *qian* (Initiating, ☰), and so on, in such a way that the yang lines are sequentially released from below to above, from inside to outside, from the interior to the exterior. Up until the hexagram associated with the *chen* period, from 7–9 am, the yang *qi* still has not reached the upper position of the hexagram, where it would be spread upward toward the outside and the exterior. It is only after the *si* period, after the *qian* hexagram has appeared, that the yang *qi* reaches the exterior and gains outward and upward expression. Therefore, the three time periods *si*, *wu*, and *wei*, corresponding to the hexagrams *qian*, *gou*, and *dun*, exactly express the process of yang *qi* emerging to the exterior.

Secondly, with regard to the sun, these three earthly branches represent midday and the height of summer, when the yang *qi* is most abundant and when weather is at its hottest.

Third, *si*, *wu*, and *wei* correspond to midday, the summer season, and the period just before and after the full moon and so, in terms of functionality, these three have the strongest affinity with the opening mechanism of Taiyang.

The three essential time correspondences of *si*, *wu*, and *wei* are that they correspond to the time when yang is emerging to the exterior, to the time when fire and heat dominate the air, and the time when the opening mechanism is most abundant. The first essential correspondence explains why, during the period of time represented by these three earthly branches, it is easiest to treat diseases of the exterior; the second explains why it is the best time to treat illnesses wrought by cold; and the third explains why it is the most advantageous time to treat hindrances to the opening mechanism of the body. Besides addressing these three essential aspects regarding the treatment of Taiyang, this explanation also clarifies why it is during the *si*, *wu*, and *wei* periods that Taiyang disease is most apt to resolve.

III.2.d. The Essentials of Treating the Taiyang Orientation

Within this small subsection, we will discuss a very important topic. This particular topic is couched in the content of our earlier discussions, and if the reader keeps that information in mind, this topic will not be too difficult to understand. My former teacher Li Yangbo once transmitted to me a secret of Chinese Medicine. He said that when prescribing a Chinese Medicine formula, we were actually prescribing time. How can we prescribe time? When this secret was first passed onto me, I did not really understand it, much less know how to go about implementing its usefulness. Today, however, I have achieved a basic understanding of this concept. As soon as I understood it, I realized that what my teacher had said was no trivial matter. With one short sentence, he had managed to express a profound mystery of nature. I wanted to do as Huangdi had done at the end of the "Treatise on the Spiritual Orchid Secret Canon," and "choose an auspicious day and store it in the chamber of the Spiritual Orchid so that it could be preserved and transmitted."

Earlier in this book, we discussed how water can both carry a boat or capsize it, and how both success and defeat can be due to a single factor. These principles seem to be especially important in Chinese Medicine. When diagnosing disease, we must begin by seeking its cause in yin and yang. What about when we treat disease? When treating disease, we must also rely upon yin and yang. A true master of Chinese Medicine formulas can be distinguished from a practitioner who has picked up a trick or two here and there by examining how much he or she makes use of yin and yang to guide the selection of the appropriate formula. In this case, the permutations of yin and yang are synonymous with time. For instance, if we diagnose a disease characterized by fire and heat, we might have a difficult time wrestling with the concrete meanings of these seemingly abstract qualities. However, if we think of these qualities within the framework of time, and think, for instance, of a sweltering summer day in the city of Chongqing or Nanjing, we quickly grasp the significance of fire and heat. Once we understand the situation presented by a fire heat disease, how do we deal with it? Again, if we think in terms of time, winter is the perfect antidote to summer.

Nowadays, when confronted with the broiling temperatures of summer, we might retreat into the cool environment of an air-conditioned apartment. Air conditioning is a means of bringing winter into summer. It can safely be said that air conditioning is a convenience developed by science. The heat of summer that fills a room is easily dispelled by an air conditioner, but when this fire and heat present in the body as disease, air conditioning does little to dispel it. For this, we must rely upon the properties of medicine. Just as you can use an air conditioner to transport the coolness of autumn or the cold of winter into your bedroom, Chinese Medicine can instill the qualities of fall or winter in your body in order to cope with a hot, fiery disease. By means of Chinese Medicine, the corresponding qualities of a winter day can be imitated and imbibed. By the same principle, we use medicines that are hot in nature to treat diseases that are cold in nature.

Time, or time's qualities, can be imitated with Chinese herbal formulas as long as the medicine contains the same qualities that characterize the particular time. Regarding this point, when we discussed the implied meanings of the Chinese character *bing* ("disease"), we discussed how medicinal substances have all manner of characteristics, and among these characteristics the most important or guiding characteristics are their *qi* and flavor. If we place this *qi* and flavor within the framework of the four directions and their corresponding seasonal influence, the temporal quality of the formula quickly emerges. Thus, medicines that are cold belong to winter, those that are cool pertain to fall, hot medicinal substances are summer, and warm medicinal substances are vernal. If we add the flavor and other qualities of the medicine to our understanding of their *qi*, we can arrive at a more detailed understanding of the medicine's chronological influence.

When we orchestrate a treatment in Chinese Medicine, why is this process referred to as "opening a direction" (*kaifang*)? Why did my former mentor say that in treating disease we are "prescribing a time"? This is intriguing. In the *Treatise on Cold Damage*, there are three formulas that are especially interesting: Qinglong Tang, Baihu Tang, and Zhenwu Tang. Qinglong, the name for the stellar constellations in the east, is nothing but a reference to the eastern direction; Baihu references the western direction; and Zhenwu (also called Xuanwu) correlates to the northern direction. When the eastern direction is prescribed, we are prescribing the three months of spring designated by the earthly branches *yin, mao,* and *chen*; when the West is prescribed, this is prescribing the three months of autumn, designated by *shen, you,* and *xu*; and when the formula of the North is prescribed, we are of course prescribing the three months of winter, marked by *hai, zi,* and *chou*. So we see, when we prescribe a Chinese formula, we are indeed prescribing a particular seasonal influence, a time.

We mentioned a formula for each of three directions, which might lead certain persons to ask why there is not a fourth formula for the South ("Zhuque Tang" for instance). Zhuque ("scarlet bird") is the group of stellar constellations in the South, but Zhang Zhongjing most definitely did not mention a "Zhuque Tang" in the *Treatise on Cold Damage*. This may have been because of a taboo regarding the use of references to the Emperor, who was identified with the south, or for some other reason. In any case, there are representative formulas for the southern direction, but they are not named after the scarlet bird of the south. Now then, of the 112 formulas listed in the *Treatise on Cold Damage*, which formula might we consider to be the equivalent of a "Zhuque Tang"? This is a question to mull over. In my opinion, the formula we seek must be in the Taiyang section of the book.

Once we link the formulas with particular periods of time, our thinking and our form of expression takes a great leap forward. Nowadays, people talk about the modernization of Chinese Medicine. What is meant by the modernization of Chinese Medicine? Most people believe this modernization should consist of combining molecular biology with Chinese Medicine or applying some other branch of modern scientific understanding to Chinese Medicine, or performing some sort of modern experimental research. Most individuals actively engaged in Chinese Medicine are pursuing this sort of modernization. The modernization of Chinese Medicine depends upon the approval of little white mice and little white rabbits. This can, of course, be called modernization, but when all is said and done, it is only one facet. Can we consider this issue from a different angle, and broaden our conception of modernization to some extent?

For instance, can we take this medicine that was developed within traditional modes of thought and traditional forms of expression, and tug it a little closer to methods of thinking and expression that are more in line with the flavor of modern culture? The aim of such reform would be to make Chinese Medicine concepts easier to understand, more convenient, and thereby gain broader acceptance. This broader acceptance would be not only with patients, but also with the cultural community, with the scientific community, and especially with the elite of both of these communities. It could be a turning point leading to genuine integration and exchange between the traditional and the modern. It should be clear that real meaningful exchange and integration between the traditional and the modern can be created only by the elite experts of each field. This is a matter best handled through close association, mutual respect, and even friendship of highly skilled experts.

Can the present phenomenon of prescribing some heat-clearing herbs along with antibiotics, or performing the four diagnostic methods and then ordering a CT or an MRI, really be called integration between the fields of traditional and modern medicine? I am afraid this sort of arrangement results in nothing but a mess. This sort of integration just wastes resources and will never achieve the desired result. Integration cannot be undertaken by the average practitioners such as ourselves; it must be undertaken by the elite of our fields, the aces. Such an integration between the elites of each field might require a meeting of minds between two close friends, a sort of Watson and Crick moment in the history of medicine. In any case, the concepts and ideas we have presented thus far in the course of this book should, at least, increase the likelihood of such an integration someday taking place. Therefore, if we take the thought process by which Chinese Medicine selects formulas and medicinals and express it in terms of time, or seasons, then the distance between the traditional and the modern shortens considerably.

Is such a shortening of the distance between traditional and modern disciplines a form of modernization? I believe it is a more meaningful and significant form of modernization, a more wonderful sort of modernization. If we look at the Taiyang section of the *Treatise on Cold Damage*, when it says that the time period in which Taiyang disease is apt to resolve is the time from 9 am to 3 pm, this clearly states the significance of time in understanding Chinese Medicine physiology. If we also look at Mahuang Tang in this same section, what do we find the function of this formula to be? Mahuang Tang is hot in nature, and it has a disposition to cause the body to open and emit. After taking this decoction, the body becomes warm and the patient perspires, as if the body has been placed in the fiery heat of the summer sun. Taiyang disease is resolved during the chronological periods of *si, wu,* and *wei,* is it not? Mahuang Tang exerts the same influence as *si, wu,* and *wei.*

If we say that Mahuang Tang's pungent warmth resolves the exterior, opens the lungs and relieves asthma, you might have some difficulty understanding, or you might find this manner of expression unscientific or otherwise unconvincing. But if I say that Mahuang Tang possesses the effect of summer, and that it uses medicinal substances to mimic the energy of the time periods *si, wu,* and *wei,* you might have a very different reaction and you might look at Mahuang Tang with newfound respect. How is it that Mahuang Tang possesses the characteristics of a summer day? How does Mahuang Tang mimic the effects of a summer day? In Chinese Medicine, time can be mimicked; it can be forged from medicinal substances. Is this not a bit strange? Once our train of thought and manner of expression are shifted to chronological terms, what at first glance seemed crude and unsophisticated appears completely transformed. If this transformation is able to inspire a curious and questioning attitude, then intelligent questions and research will naturally emerge. In contrast to the earlier examples of the integration of biomedicine and Chinese Medicine, if we begin our research with these questions as our starting point, then we may be able to achieve true integration between the traditional and the modern.

III.3. The Time When It Tends to Act

Now that we have a clear understanding of disease resolution times, we should do as Confucius has instructed us and, knowing one corner, infer the other three. In this vein, I wish to discuss the time in which the effects of the disease are most noticeable or severe. The time in which a disease is inclined to resolve relates to diagnosis of that disease, and more importantly to its treatment. In diagnosis, the time in which the disease is most likely to resolve certainly has its place. The patient, however, is less interested in the time when the effects of the disease will lessen. The patient is primarily concerned with those periods of time in which the disease grows worse, when the symptoms become more severe, the time at which the disease manifests. The patient tends to be clearer about when the disease worsens than when its intensity abates.

In relation to the time when the disease tends to emerge or intensify, we propose a corresponding concept, that of "the time in which the disease will tend to act" or, put another way, "the time in which the disease tends to become more severe." Taiyang disease has a time in which it will tend to get better, and so logically, it should have a time in which it worsens. It tends to improve in the time period from *si* to *wei*, but when does it tend to worsen? The time in which it tends to worsen must be opposite to the time that improves, namely the time period from the twelfth to the second earthly branches, from 9 pm to 3 am. *Si, wu,* and *wei* directly oppose the earthly branches *hai, zi,* and *chou*. The branch *si* opposes the branch *hai*, the branch *zi* opposes the branch *wu*, and the branch *chou* opposes the branch *wei*. The opposing branches are also those that are contrary to one another; they are contrary in terms of time and also contrary in terms of the pattern of yin and yang that they exhibit.

Therefore, when during the time period of *hai*, *zi*, and *chou*, the yang *qi* is going back inside, being collected and stored. This is wintertime, when the weather is coldest. This is the time when yin is most abundant and yang is sparsest. These three time periods are opposite to those in which the disease tends to resolve, should we not expect the disease to worsen during this time? We must examine the possibility that, just as there are three different levels of times in which Taiyang disease will tend to resolve, that there will also be three different levels of time in which it will tend to worsen from. If a cough or abdominal discomfort go through regular changes during the course of a day; for instance, if they always occur or worsen during the *hai*, *zi*, and *chou* periods, in other words if they occur or worsen in the middle of the night, then we should consider the possibility that they are Taiyang disease. This cough could be a Taiyang cough. The abdominal pain could be Taiyang in origin. Therefore, when it comes to the diagnosis of disease, the time in which the disease will tend to worsen is of greater importance than the time in which it resolves.

III.4. A General View of the Times in Which Disease of the Six Conformations Will Tend to Resolve

Earlier, we discussed the time in which Taiyang disease will tend to resolve. Now let us take a general view of the times in which disease of the six conformations will tend to resolve, and see what the differences between them are from a yin and yang perspective. We can first make two general distinctions between the diseases of the six conformations. First, diseases of the three yang tend to resolve during the period beginning with *yin* and ending with *xu*, nine time periods altogether. The three yin diseases begin with *hai* and go to *mao*. Altogether there are five periods.

Secondly, with regard to resolution of the three yang diseases, Taiyang tends to resolve during the periods *si*, *wu*, and *wei*; Yangming during the periods *shen*, *you*, and *xu*; and Shaoyang tends to resolve during the periods *yin*, *mao*, and *chen*. Each of the three periods adjoins the next, but there is no overlap between the periods in which the diseases tend to resolve. As for the periods in which the three yin diseases tend to resolve, Taiyin tends to resolve during the periods *hai, zi,* and *chou;* Shaoyin during the periods *zi, chou,* and *yin;* and Jueyin tends to resolve during the *chou, yin,* and *mao* periods. Notably, each of these periods overlaps with the next, and they share periods of time. What meaning can we derive from the differences between the three yang and the three yin diseases? I think the significance of these differences can be divided into the following aspects.

First, the path of yang is abundant and the path of yin is wanting. These are technical terms from Chinese astronomy: "abundant" means long or plentiful, whereas "wanting" indicates a shortage or deficit. From Chinese astronomical perspective, the sun is yang and the moon yin. The revolution of the sun is a year in length, whereas the revolution of the moon is one month. The revolution of the yang is far vaster than that of yin. In this respect, the times in which the three yang diseases tend to resolve and the times in which the three yin diseases tend to resolve directly correspond with this notion of the "path of yang is abundant and the path of yin is wanting." We can observe this dimension in other areas as well. In the "Treatise on Heavenly Truth in Remote Antiquity," the rhythm of the life of the male and female is described. The life of the male is series of eight-year periods, and the life of the female is a series of seven-year periods. The male is virile for eight times eight (64) years, whereas the female reaches menopause at seven times seven (49) years. The physiological rhythm of the yang male and the yin female obviously correspond with the notion that yang is long and yin is short.

Equally important is that yang corresponds with day, and yin corresponds with night. The three yang diseases tend to resolve during the light of day, whereas the three yin diseases all resolve during the dark of night. The times in which disease will tend to resolve is based on a profound understanding of the workings of nature. They cannot be briefly summarized and are worthy of close study.

Secondly, each of the yang diseases has three distinct, consecutive two-hour periods in which the disease will tend to resolve, and these do not overlap with those belonging to either of the other yang diseases. If we examine the chapters devoted to each of the three yang diseases, we see that Taiyang disease is primarily characterized by cold on the exterior and Yangming disease is characterized by heat in the interior, while Shaoyang disease is half exterior and half interior. Therefore, Taiyang disease is treated by resolving the exterior, Yangming disease is addressed by cooling the interior, and adjusting the pivot is the treatment for Shaoyang disease. The treatment method for each disease is clearly distinguished from the other and there is no overlap.

The three periods in which each of the yin diseases tend to resolve, despite having different names, overlap and share periods of time. If we take a close look at the three chapters devoted to the yin diseases, we see that although there are small differences between Taiyin, Shaoyin, and Jueyin diseases, they all have internal deficiency cold in common. The Sini family of formulas are not only used in Taiyin disease, but also Shaoyin and Jueyin disease. If we take all of this into account, we can see that, as far as disease of the six conformations is concerned, when the times in which the disease is likely to resolve are distinct, so too are the treatments, and when these times are the same, the method of cure is also similar.

From this, we can see the truth in the line from the *Plain Questions's* "Treatise on Six Nodes and Visceral Manifestations," which says: "If you do not know what each year contributes, the abundance and weakness of the *qi*, and how deficiency and excess arise, then you cannot be a practitioner." These are not empty words. Can we take the rhythms of time lightly? Absolutely not!

That is as far as we shall discuss the outline of Taiyang disease.

CHAPTER SIX

THE ESSENTIALS OF
YANGMING DISEASE

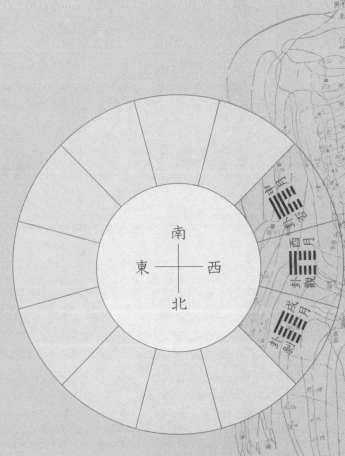

Yangming disease tends to
resolve in the time from *shen* to *xu*.

I. An Explanation of Yangming

If we are to study closely the Yangming chapter, we should go about it just as we did with the Taiyang chapter, and first examine the title of the chapter: "Differentiate Yangming: disease, pulse, syndrome, and treatment." In our explanation of the Taiyang chapter, we discussed the concepts of differentiation, disease, pulse, syndrome, and cure. We will not duplicate that discussion here, but will instead move directly to an examination of the meaning of Yangming.

I.1. The Meaning of Yangming

What is Yangming? In the *Plain Questions* chapter "Great Treatise on the Essentials of Ultimate Truth," it says: "What is meant by Yangming? Qi Bo answered: The two yang unite brightness (*ming*)." What is meant by "unite"? Depending on how this "unite" is interpreted, the concept of Yangming carries various connotations. Does the uniting of the two yang mean that when the two yang are added together, we call this yang brightness (*yangming*)? Is it like a chandelier with more than one light bulb? Turn on one bulb and it is bright; turn on two bulbs and it is even brighter. That is how many understand Yangming today, and many people from previous generations also understood it in this way. The two yang joined together, that is Yangming. Yangming, after all, is bountiful in both *qi* and blood, so this explanation seems to fit.

However, as soon as we examine the subject more carefully and analyze its details, and further place it into the context of the natural world and the cosmos constituted by that natural world, we realize that the above is not an apt explanation of Yangming. In this context, "unite" means "to converge," "to join together," and is the opposite of "to divide," "to open." It does not mean "added." It does not mean to add one to one and get two. It means that yang *qi* begins to gather and draw together, and change from a state of issuing and release to a state of accumulation and storage. This is the meaning of "The two yang unite brightness." This understanding of Yangming gets at the basic meaning of the concept. This concept is equivalent to that of Jueyin, which results from the completion of the exchange of two yin. This is not the adding together of the two yin, but the completion of yin and the emergence of yang. How could Yangming possibly mean two yang added together? Therefore, "unite" and "complete" are equivalent terms. The meaning of "unite" is "to close"; it does not mean "to add." This understanding of Yangming will be borne out by our further discussions.

I.2. The Meaning of the Yangming Channels

Essential aspects of the Yangming channel in Chinese Medicine channel theory refer to the Yangming channel of the arm and the Yangming channel of the leg. The flow of the channel is over the front and center of the body. The *Yellow Emperor's Classic* speaks of the abdomen being yin and the back yang. The front yin descends, and the back yang ascends. The Taiyang leg channel flows along the back of the body, and so Taiyang rules opening and raising, while Yangming rules closing and descending. From the perspective of the course Yangming follows in the body, does the phrase "The two yang unite brightness" mean that the two yang accumulate and then emit their energy with greater intensity? Or does it refer to the converging of the yang, the enclosing of brightness? I will let you ponder this yourself.

I.3. The Meaning of the Yangming Bowels

The stomach and large intestine are the Yangming bowels or hollow organs. The stomach is related to the spleen, and the large intestine is related to the lungs. In the *Treatise on Cold Damage*, the compound word "stomach-intestines" is often used, which is the long form of this term. Sometimes, only the character for stomach is used to convey the meaning of both the stomach and intestines. In the second half of the twentieth century, during the period when Western Medicine doctors in China were ordered to study Chinese Medicine, many found line 215 in the Yangming chapter, "In the stomach there must be five or six pieces of dry stool," to be a strange or even ridiculous statement. However, if they understood that "stomach" is a broad term, inclusive of the whole length of the gastrointestinal tract, they would not think this line so odd or funny.

In the *Plain Questions*, it says: "The six channels are the great rivers, and the intestines and stomach are the seas." This relationship between the six channels and the stomach and intestines, a relationship analogous to waterways and the open sea, is important both in the *Treatise on Cold Damage* and Chinese Medicine as a whole. It is especially crucial to understand

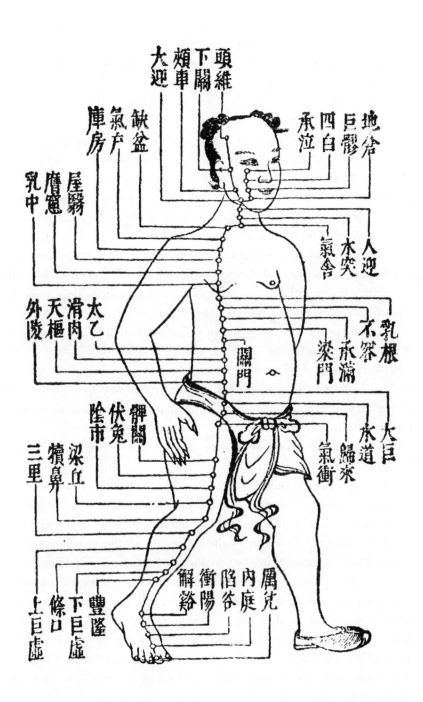

this concept when seeking to treat disease with Chinese Medicine. When treating, this concept makes the difference between success and failure. Why is the downward purgation method of treating disease practically panacean in Chinese Medicine? Why do pathological changes in the six channels, or in any of the organs of the body, collect in the intestines and the stomach, and then gain resolution simply through downward purgation? The theoretical basis for this can be found in this concept of rivers and seas, and crucial to this concept of movement from rivers to seas is the characteristic of descending. It is my belief that once the practitioner fully grasps this crucial point, this secret of success in treating disease, and has thoroughly researched its implications, a great advance in both therapeutic and curative results will be made.

Another important facet of the Yangming bowels is their relationship to the brain. In Chinese Medicine, the brain is the "sea of marrow," and is considered one of the extraordinary hollow organs. In modern medical science, the brain is the primary locus of the central nervous system. Its function and purpose are very clear. If we keep this modern understanding in mind when studying the *Treatise on Cold Damage*, we discover that nearly every syndrome that is characterized by mental or psychological irregularities can be found in the Yangming chapter, and almost every method of curing these syndromes is a Yangming method. Knowing this, we cannot help but think about the relationship between Yangming and the brain. What is the basis of this relationship?

Humans are said to contain "four seas," and the brain is the sea of marrow. If we open a map and look at the four seas surrounding China, indeed all of the oceans of the world, we see that they communicate with one another. Do the four seas of the human body communicate in an analogous way? The September 27, 2000 issue of the *Reference News* contained a research article titled "Humans Have Two Brains" by Professor David Wingate of the University of London. In this article, the author, after years of research, concluded that hundreds of millions of nerve cells are gathered in nerve plexuses in the gut, rivaling the number and complexity of nerves in the brain. Based on this observation, he coined the phrase "gastroneurology" and dubbed the gut a "second brain." I think that Professor Wingate's research is helpful to our understanding of the relationship between Yangming and the brain.

I.4. The Meaning of Yangming in *Yunqi*

There are two facets of the meaning of Yangming in the five movements and six *qi* (*wuyun liuqi*, abbreviated as *yunqi*), the cyclical transformation of universal *qi*. The first we have already addressed, the connection between the lungs and the large intestine. The other aspect regards dry metal. At this juncture, we will discuss the latter aspect. Yangming is dryness in the heavens and metal in the earth. Why does dry metal accompany the uniting of brightness of the two yang? The significance of this is no less than the significance of the association of cold water with Taiyang. We must be clear on this point in order to have a clear understanding of Yangming.

I.4.a. The Meaning of Dryness

The key to understanding the line "The two yang unite brightness" is the way in which we interpret the word "unite." It means to gather together and enclose, and in this case it refers to the gathering together of the yang *qi* so that it cannot be scattered and dispersed.

What then is the meaning of dryness (*zao*)? Looking first to *Explaining Writing and Analyzing Characters*, we read: "*Zao* is dry (*gan* 乾)." *Zao* is *gan*, and so oftentimes in the Chinese language these two characters are used in conjunction, as in *ganzao*, meaning dry or arid. The character *gan* (乾) is also pronounced *qian*, and this pronunciation represents the *Classic of Changes* hexagram or trigram consisting solely of yang lines. Why does this character indicate both dryness and a hexagram or trigram consisting solely of yang lines? This question brings us to a very interesting topic. In the postnatal system of the eight trigrams, *Qian* Heaven represents the northwestern direction. In the northwest of China, we find a vast arid region, the Gobi Desert. For most Chinese, there is a reflexive association of the northwest with dryness. Recently, I flew to the northwest of China to see an American patient. When I boarded the plane, I wore summer clothes, but as soon as I disembarked, I was compelled to put on a wool sweater.

If the weather is cold, it does not affect me much. I just pull on a few extra layers of clothing. The one thing a Chinese southerner such as myself cannot stand, however, is dryness. By the second day, my lips were dry and cracked. By the third day, they were blistered. Why is the northwest so dry? The fact that the same character form is used to represent both the trigram and dryness has deep significance. The opposite of dry or arid is moist, damp, or humid; these two are opposites, just as cold and heat are opposites. Earlier, our discussion of cold was furthered by contrasting it with heat. We can use a similar dialectical method to better understand dryness in relation to dampness. This will allow us to understand it within the larger framework of yin and yang, as well as to gain an understanding of its changes and effects.

Our understanding of the meaning of the character dampness *shi* (濕) begins by looking at the composition of the written character. The radical on the left of the character, the three little dots arranged vertically (氵), represent water, and indicate the obvious relationship between dampness and water. The portion of the character to the right of these three dots, understood to be the phonetic component of the character, is an abbreviated form of the character *xian* (㬎/顯). What does *xian* mean? A character that is often used together with the character *xian* (顯) is the character *ming* (明), consisting of the sun on the left and the moon on the right, and meaning "bright." We have for instance, the combination *xianming* and *mingxian*, both of which mean distinct, obvious, or clear. What allows things to achieve a state of being distinct, obvious, or clear? During the day, we have the sun, and at night we have lights of various sorts. The sun and lights both signify yang, and both make things evident, clear, and bright. And so, yang is in a way synonymous with *xian*, and *xian* synonymous with yang. Once we understand the meaning of the character *xian*, the meaning of dampness (*shi*) is easy to discern. What is damp? How is damp formed? Water added to yang becomes damp. The action of yang upon water, causing it to steam upward into vapor becomes damp. Dampness and water are related. Where, after all, does dampness come from? It comes, quite obviously, from water. Therefore, many places are considered to be watery and damp. However, there is a clear difference between water and dampness, and this difference lies with *xian*, in other words, with yang.

Although dampness is derived from water, it is not the same as water. The water must first be scattered and dispersed by the yang *qi*, vaporized by the force of yang. Only after this takes place can we say that it is "dampness." Yang *qi* is necessary to the formation of dampness. Let us take a simple example. Of the four seasons, spring, summer, fall and winter, which are damp and which are dry? Of course, spring and summer are damp, and fall and winter are not as damp. The southeast of China is yang and is very damp, and the northwest of China is yin and is very dry. What produces such salient differences in moisture? The difference is clearly the result of the effect of yang scattering and dispersing the water, and turning it into vapor and damp. The yang *qi* of summer is relatively greater, therefore its related dampness is also greater, whereas in fall and winter the yang *qi* is united and gathered together, and because it is enclosed, the scattering and dispersing force is minimized. Without this vaporizing force, the basic conditions for the formation of dampness are not met, and the result is a relative reduction in the amount of dampness.

The lack of dampness during fall and winter is directly related to our topic: dryness. Dryness and dampness are opposites, so when dampness is prevalent, dryness is scarce, and when there is little damp, there is naturally a lot of dryness. Why are autumn and winter dry? Why is the northwest dry? In a word, whenever dampness is in scarcity, so too is the vaporizing power of the yang *qi*. When we investigate phenomena, we seek their essence. What is the essence of phenomena? None other than yin and yang. In our discussion of dampness and dryness, a pair of opposing qualities as polar as cold and heat or yin and yang, we are reaching back to the essence of the present topic. This is what is referred to as "investigating the root" in the *Yellow Emperor's Classic.*

Now that dampness and dryness are clearly understood, let us return to the nineteen lines regarding disease triggers we examined earlier. Now, it should not seem so strange that dryness is not mentioned in these lines. As when dampness or heat are mentioned, we gain information regarding dryness. When yang *qi* is released, there is dampness and heat. When it is gathered back in, dryness emerges. Dryness and dampness are different states of yin and yang. The famous physicians Liu Wansu and Yu Jiayan thought they were being quite brilliant by developing a disease trigger specifically for dryness and adding it to the nineteen disease trigger lines, but we can see this was superfluous.

We can also look at dryness and dampness from the perspective of the hexagrams of the *Classic of Changes.* The fifth hexagram in the Zhou sequence of the *Classic of Changes* is called *xu* (Needing, ䷄). This hexagram is composed of the *Kan* Water trigram above and the *Qian* Heaven trigram below. There were originally three systems of ordering the hexagrams of the *Classic of Changes*, and the Zhou sequence is but one of them. Besides the Zhou order, there are also the Lianshan and Guicang sequences. The Zhou sequence begins with the hexagram *qian* (Initiating); the Lianshan begins with *gen* (Keeping Still); and the Guicang sequence begins with *kun* (Responding). In the Guicang system, the hexagram *xu*, with *Kan* Water above and *Qian* Heaven below, is called *ru* (溽). *Ru* is synonymous with dampness. This hexagram deals specifically with dampness.

An examination of the structure of the hexagram as a two-dimensional image reveals the basic dynamic of dampness. Water above and heaven below provide us with an image of water up in the sky. Water filling the heavens is the image of dampness. As we have said before, without the dispersing and enlivening properties of yang *qi*, this water could not possibly be vaporized and thereby fill the air. Without the action of yang upon water, water can only flow downward, and dryness naturally results.

I.4.b. Why Is Dryness Associated with Metal?

In the *Yellow Emperor's Classic*, dryness is associated with metal, and as a result, the term "dry metal" is often used. Why is dryness associated with metal? If we fully understand the preceding discussion regarding dryness, this is not a difficult problem to resolve. Among the five elements, metal is the heaviest. Why is the metal endowed with heaviness? It is this heaviness that causes it to sink and collect deep within the earth. This same tendency to sink and collect downward provides it with the capacity to restrain yang *qi*, and to keep the water from ascending into the air. Dryness naturally results. This is why metal and dryness are associated.

Laozi said, "Being and Non-being produce each other; the difficult and the easy complement each other; the long and the short form one another; the high and the low fill one another; the sound and the voice enclose each other; what comes before and what comes after follow one another." In reality, dryness and dampness share this same sort of relationship with one another. For instance, if we look at the hexagram that corresponds to and follows the hexagram *xu*, we find *song* (Contention, ䷅), the inverse of *xu*, with the heaven trigram above and the water trigram below. Just as the hexagram *xu* represents humidity and dampness, the hexagram *song* must represent dryness. We can see that it represents dryness from two points of view. The first is the one we just mentioned, the inversion of the trigrams: the dryness of heaven is above and water is below, the heavens ascend and water descends, and so there is dryness. Another facet involves the meaning of the character *song* (訟) as "lawsuit" or "to sue," which of the five phases belongs to metal. We have already discussed the relationship between metal and dryness, so we need not reiterate it here. Needless to say, both of these facets of *song*, its composition and the meaning of the character associated with it, show that the hexagram can be understood to represent dryness. When we look at the *song* hexagram paired with the *xu* hexagram, the two the relationship between dampness and dryness is made very clear.

I.4.c. The Qi That Corresponds to Dryness and Dampness

Dryness and dampness correspond with and complement one another. The *qi* that belongs to each of these influences are also complementary. As the yang *qi* slowly gathers, the weather gradually turns cold, water no longer is vaporized into clouds and steam, and dryness emerges as a salient influence. In other words, the essential nature of dryness is coolness. Put another way, the *qi* of dryness is cool. Put in these simple terms, in terms of the process of yang *qi*, we can easily see why autumn is both cool and dry.

During the spring and summer months, the yang *qi* is steaming and vaporizing water into the air. The weather changes from warm to hot, and with it the intensity of this vaporization increases. The yin water rises into the air, becoming dampness. Therefore, although our basic Chinese Medicine textbooks may say that dampness is a yin pathogen, we can see that it more closely corresponds to yang warmth and heat. This point must be clearly understood. As we can see from this example, once we have looked at an issue from the most basic perspective, that of yin and yang, not only do we clarify the issue, but our understanding becomes unwavering. Once our thought is thus anchored, should Huangdi or Qi Bo himself attempt to challenge our understanding, we would not falter. Of course, should Huangdi or Qi Bo actually visit us, they would probably be impressed that we were even attempting to think through such problems, and might deem us worthy of instruction. In any case, the reason spring and summer and the southeastern direction are so damp lies in this simple principle.

Earlier, when we said that the nature of dampness is hot and the nature of dryness is cool, we were speaking from a very fundamental perspective. From this perspective, we can understand how and why the bitter flavor can be used to dry dampness and the pungent flavor can moisten dryness. The nature of bitterness and pungency is clearly defined in the *Yellow Emperor's Classic*: the pungent flavor opens and the bitter flavor descends. By opening is meant the opening and release of yang *qi*, and by descending is meant the descending of yang *qi*.

When I was studying Chinese medicinals as an undergraduate, we learned that Huanglian, Huangqin, and Huangbai share the ability to "dry dampness." We studied Chinese medicinals in our first year of college, so the reason that these three herbs shared this particular ability remained on my mind, puzzling me for some ten years. In *Fundamentals of Chinese Medicine*, it was clearly stated that dampness is a yin pathogen, and so it only made sense that it should be combated with a yang medicinal. After all, it was a fundamental principle that cold be used to combat heat, and heat to combat cold, and yang be used to combat yin, and yin to combat yang. All three of these particular herbs are bitter and cold medicinals. Their natures are utmost yin. To use these three yin herbs to combat dampness would be like frost settling atop the snow. How could it possibly dry dampness? For the life of me, I could not solve this riddle.

It was not until ten years later, when I began to use yin and yang to ponder difficulties in Chinese Medicine, to contemplate the six *qi*, that I realized how simple this problem was, and how easy it is to understand. Bitter and cold herbs are used to cool heat and drain fire. They are used to descend yang. They assume the pattern of fall and winter, and thereby remove the *xian* (羴) which, as we discussed in this chapter, represents the yang aspect of the character for dampness (*shi* 濕). If the fire and heat are purged and the yang *qi* subdued, if the pattern of fall and winter are generated and the *xian*, the yang aspect, of dampness gone, there is no dampness to be spoken of. This summarizes the standard way in which bitter and cold herbs are used to treat dampness. When we consider this simple curative principle, in light of what is said in the *Plain Questions*: "Yin and yang are the way of heaven and earth, they are the guiding principle of the myriad things, the father and mother of change and transformation, the origin of life and death; they provide a container for the living spirit," we realize the profound truth in the *Plain Questions*. When we apply this simple principle to perplexing Chinese Medicine riddles, they undergo a sea change.

Once we understand how bitter and cold herbs are able to dry dampness, understanding the moistening property of pungency presents no difficulty. How do warm, pungent herbs moisten? Warmth and pungency rouse the yang *qi*, cause the yang *qi* to steam upward. Pungency and warmth assume the very structure of spring and summer; they return the *xian*, the yang aspect, to cause dampness to manifest. Once the yang *qi* is stirred up and set in motion, and the pattern of spring and summer are established, once dampness is made manifest, there is no dryness left to speak of.

Wu Jutong developed a formula that was famous for treating dryness called Xing Su San. This is a formula that most Chinese Medicine practitioners have heard of, and probably have had occasion to use in the clinical setting. This formula is composed of eleven ingredients: Zisuye, Banxia, Fuling, Qianhu, Jiegeng, Zhike, Gancao, Shengjiang, Dazao, Jupi, and Xingren. Of the ingredients used in this decoction, besides the moistening aspect of Xingren, all of the other herbs not only have no notable moistening property, but are warm and pungent. Nevertheless, Wu Jutong uses them in this formula to moisten dryness. Previously, I could not understand this formula. From reading our textbook on formulas, it was clear that those who wrote the textbook and taught the course did not necessarily understand how this formula worked either. It was not until I really understood the meaning of *zao* (dryness) that I could understand the principle behind this formula and why it possessed so many warm and pungent herbs. If we compare Xing Su San with Xiao Qinglong Tang, we see that one is a post-classical formula, one is a classical formula; one is mild in action and the other fierce; and both achieve the same wondrous result, albeit by different methods.

I remember how my first master treated a female patient who suffered from a cough. For three years in a row, as soon as autumn arrived, she would cough for a month or two and then stop. She tried to treat her cough with both Chinese and Western medicines, to no avail. In her fourth year of this, the patient came to see my teacher. After diagnosing her, he said: "This is a dry cough. We should use the acrid and moistening method by means of Xiao Qinglong Tang." She took one dose and her cough ceased. Altogether, she took three doses of this decoction, and her cough never returned.

How does Xiao Qinglong Tang moisten dryness? If we only know that it is a warm, pungent formula and that it is able to treat diseases dominated by water *qi*, then it is really quite difficult to understand how this formula is able to moisten dryness. Once we examine the formula in light of the essential significance of dryness, however, we see that there is nothing strange about using it to treat dryness. Why, after all, is it called Xiao Qinglong Tang? The blue-green dragon supposedly rode in the clouds and induced them to descend as rain. Once the rain begins to fall, dryness cannot persist. The Qing dynasty scholar-physician Zheng Qin'an, in his book *The Unbroken Circle of Medical Methods*, writes:

> We must seek evidence of yin and yang. We cannot simply treat symptomatically. We cannot simply see headache and treat the head, see cough and treat the cough. We must always seek the trigger for the increases and decreases in yin and yang. Upon this basis, one will grasp the methods of treating from yin and from yang, and this understanding will free one to apply it to both classical formulas and post-classical formulas. In time, one will become flexible in one's methods and means; one's understanding of the entire circle will be unbroken; one's reasoning will be refined and one's skills practiced; and every action and thought will exemplify the Dao. Even a simple prescription of two or three herbs will be an extraordinary formula arrived at through wonderful means.

Having seen my teacher treat a dry cough with Xiao Qinglong Tang, I realized the meaning of "every action and thought exemplifies the Dao." The study of medicine places an emphasis on clear reasoning, and only when one's reasoning is refined will one's skills become practiced. This particular point is one that we must be perfectly clear about. Do not look down on discussions of basic medical theory, or nod off every time yin and yang are discussed, and only wake up when you hear that such and such a formula treats such and such a disease. If the basic principles are not clear, how can one be skillful? If the basic principles are not well understood, then one's methods cannot be flexible and accommodating, and one's actions and thoughts will not exemplify the Dao.

I.4.d. Dry Heat and Damp Cold

Just now, we discussed the essential nature of dryness and dampness, and this discussion was probably easy to understand once the topic was set against a background of larger natural processes. In the *Plain Questions*, "dry" pathogenic influences were also referred to as "clear" pathogenic influences. To treat "clear" conditions, we are advised by the *Plain Questions* to warm them. In the *Classic of Difficulties's* discussion of the broad definition of *Shanghan*, when dampness is examined, it is discussed in terms of damp heat and not as cold damp. This discrimination harkens back to the basic essence of dampness, and its requisite relationship to warmth and heat. The basic essence is the big picture, the overall view of the topic. However, dryness and dampness also have another side, namely that of dry heat and cold damp.

In the *Classic of Changes's* commentary on the hexagram *qian* (Initiating), it says "Fire is dryness"; and in the *Explanation of Trigrams* (Shuogua) commentary, it says: "Of the myriad things, none is drier than fire." Why is the radical on the left side of the character for dryness (*zao* 燥) the fire radical (*huo* 火)? It would seem to correspond to the close association between fire and aridity. Originally, we stated that coolness is dryness; when the yang *qi* is gathered back in and the weather turns cool, the environment naturally becomes dry. In the fall or winter, if you should travel about a bit in the North of China, you will realize that the phrase "cool is dry" is no empty talk. How then do we suddenly turn around, and assert that "Fire is dryness" and "Of the myriad things, none is drier than fire"? This would seem to be a difficult contradiction to resolve.

However, in reality, these are two entirely different topics. As soon as we differentiate the two, we will be able to clear up this apparent contradiction. The idea that "fire is dry" is something that we frequently encounter in everyday life. If you take something damp and place it near a fire, it will slowly dry. Based on our daily experience, the relationship between fire and dryness is an easy one to understand. When we take something and place it near the fire to dry, where does the moisture that was originally in the object we have dried go? Did the fire obliterate it? I do not believe fire is able to do this. In my hometown, when we had occasion to burn wet firewood, we could see steam and froth emerging from the ends of the wood. It is clear to anyone who has witnessed this event that fire does not destroy the water it heats; all it does is steam it out. If we dry freshly washed clothing by the fire, we might see a bit of steam rising from its exterior, and if we close the windows while drying clothes in this fashion, it will not be long before beads of moisture trickle down the glass. Fire only has the ability to move moisture about, to transport it a little ways off from its flames. Near the fire becomes dry, but elsewhere, dampness is generated. Therefore, dry heat is only part of the story. It is a description of a localized event, not the overall picture. It is a superficial description that disregards the larger scenario.

The relationship between fire and dryness leads us to think of an issue affecting our entire planet at the moment: global warming. Every year, glaciers around the world recede and the polar ice caps dwindle at a rate never seen before. The world's climate grows steadily warmer. What has brought about this situation? It is clearly related to the emission of greenhouse gases. Can our air conditioners and refrigerators ultimately cool the atmosphere? Of course not. All they do is cool a small area while increasing heat elsewhere. We are stealing from Peter to give to Paul, or as the Chinese put it: "tearing down the eastern wall to build one in the west." Therefore, the more we use air conditioning, the warmer the atmosphere becomes; and the warmer our climate becomes, the more we will be induced to turn on our air conditioners. We have entered into a vicious circle. From this perspective on the relationship between fire and dryness, we can clearly see that wherever fire goes, dryness follows.

In warm disease theory, diseases are differentiated into *wei* (defensive *qi*), *qi*, *ying* (nutritive), and *xue* (blood) levels. Once the heat pathogen has entered into the nutritive and blood levels, the blood becomes hot and this heat in the blood leads to dryness in the blood. Once dryness in the blood emerges, wind is generated. This wind will only be generated if the heat pathogen enters into the blood level. Therefore, we cannot use the term "blood dryness" casually. A deficiency of blood, in the Chinese Medicine sense, is not synonymous with blood dryness. We must be clear on this point.

Earlier in our discussion of dryness, we examined Xing Su San. A converse formula is Sang Xing Tang. This formula consists of Sangye, Xingren, Shashen, Zhebeimu, Dandouchi, Zhizi, and Lipi. The *qi* and flavor of this formula is the opposite of that of Xing Su San: it is used to treat dryness of the blood, the dryness induced by fire (dry heat). It is relatively simple to treat dryness: First we remove the fire and once the fire is removed, the dryness will naturally depart; this calls for "clearing heat." At the same time, also it is necessary to restore the moisture that has been driven off by the fire; this calls for "nourishing yin." Now we have arrived at the goal of "moistening dryness," a goal which both formulas share. One formula treats dryness with warmth and pungency, the other with sweet, cold herbs.

Although both are used to moisten dryness, they use converse methods. This topic is deserving careful contemplation. Once we have contemplated it and gained clarity on this topic, we will have made great strides in our comprehension of yin and yang.

It follows, then, that our analysis of cold damp should follow similar lines. We have already made it clear that the basic nature of dampness is heat. Therefore, if we wish to treat dampness, we must clear heat. In warmth disease theory, it is said that when dampness departs, heat is orphaned. As a matter of fact, we can see that the opposite is also true: when heat departs, dampness is left alone. During the humidity of spring and summer, the air becomes muggy, and the very ground is moistened. In the south of China, when the humidity is at its worst, there is no way to dry the floors or walls. As soon as a cold front from the north pushes through, however, and the north wind blows, the air becomes pleasantly cool and the ground is immediately dry. Why does everything dry out as soon as the wind from the north blows, and the more the weather from the south persists, the damper everything becomes? It is because the north wind brings with it cold and descent, whereas the south wind carries with it heat and ascent. From this perspective, it is easy to understand dampness, and it is also easy to understand how one dries dampness with bitter and cold medicinals.

However, if we now turn to the treatment of cold dampness, not only can we not use bitter and cold medicines, but on the contrary, we should use bitter and warm or bitter and hot herbs. At first glance, this method does not seem to make sense. We must look at this problem in the same way we looked at dry heat. Dryness and dampness are opposites, and we can understand their converse natures in light of their essential nature, as well as their outward nature. The outward nature of dryness and dampness are also opposite to one another; the outward nature of dryness is heat, and that of dampness is cold. Thus, dry heat and damp cold are also opposites. Once we have established the converse relationship of dry heat and cold damp, we can see that the process by which damp things become dry when placed in close proximity to fire is none other than the process of drying cold damp.

Fire is dryness, the flavor associated with fire is bitter, and its nature is hot. Therefore, when we speak of using bitter and warm or bitter and hot herbs to transform dampness or dry dampness, we are actually speaking of the same way in which "fire is dryness." "Fire is dryness" actually addresses two issues: one is the process by which dry heat assumes form, and the other is the process by which we treat cold damp.

This is a good way to contemplate dry heat and cold damp.

I.4.e. The Dryness of Yangming Disease

An important aspect of Yangming disease is dryness. Whether this dryness refers to its essential nature, cold, or its outward nature, heat, warrants clarification. The essential dryness of Yangming is cool dryness, as we have already discussed. Therefore, the *Yellow Emperor's Classic* calls this "clear *qi*." Of course, if it becomes excessive, it becomes a pathogen ("clear" pathogen). This conforms to Yangming governing uniting, gathering, and descending. What, then, is Yangming disease? Yangming disease is disease characterized by disruption of Yangming's normal uniting, gathering, and descending. That which is most damaging to Yangming's usual function, that which most easily disrupts the essential nature of Yangming, is fire and heat.

The nature of fire is to blaze upward, and this is precisely contrary to the physiological role of Yangming. Thus, the action of fire directly opposes the restraining and subduing function of Yangming. Thus, the dryness of Yangming disease is in complete opposition to the cool, physiological dryness that is so closely tied to Yangming's normal functioning. The dryness of Yangming disease is the outward nature of dryness; it is a hot dryness, or put another way, it is dry heat. To treat this sort of dryness, we should use Baihu Tang, or one of the three Chengqi decoctions. What do Baihu Tang and the Chengqi decoctions do? They are clearing formulas, descending formulas, and fire-draining formulas. Once the fire and heat are drained away, the essential nature of Yangming dryness naturally returns. Thus, the central theme of Yangming disease is alienation from and return to the normal function of Yangming.

Furthermore, we must consider that matter is not destroyed. If here we have fire, and all the moisture has evaporated away, then elsewhere we will have dampness. And vice versa. Nature's climates are also like this. After a great flood, there will be a great drought, and after a great drought, there will be a great flood. Why does one follow the other? This is nature's balance, it is the harmonization of natural forces, and ultimately, it is based on the principle that material properties cannot be destroyed. It cannot rain forever. How could there be so much rain to fall? Aridity, by necessity, follows heavy precipitation. A long period of dryness, in which water is being constantly evaporated, does not mean that the water has departed for the Milky Way or some far off star. Therefore, it steams to a certain degree, the water rises to a certain height, and then it encounters influences that induce it to descend, and it precipitates. If it rises for a long time, then it must descend for a long time. If the amount that rises is great, then the amount that descends must also be vast. That is why a great flood follows a great drought, and vice versa.

Laozi speaks of being and non-being, the difficult and the easy, the long and the short, the high and the low, the sound and the voice, before and after, all emerging from one another, completing one another, forming one another, benefiting one another, enclosing one another, and following one another. Likewise, cold and heat, dryness and dampness, droughts and floods, day and night, and east and west are like this. Yangming disease is characterized by an overabundance of heat in the qi level; it is an overabundance of heat in the stomach and intestine. When there is an overabundance of Yangming heat, it evaporates the fluids of the stomach, drying the stomach and intestines, and resulting in a disease of stomach family fullness. If we follow our previous train of thought, where does the fluid that is dissipated by the heat of Yangming disease go? Some of it is lost through the interstices of the body. Thus, Yangming disease is characterized by heavy perspiration, and streaming sweat from the hands and feet. And the rest of the fluid? The rest rises upward and becomes dampness. When the production of this dampness becomes excessive, it obscures the clear orifices, and the result is changes in the psychological state of the patient, delusions, unconsciousness, and/or delirious speech.

In days of old, it was said that when heat is excessive, unconsciousness ensues, and when heat disturbs the light of spirit, the spirit itself becomes obscured. How does heat induce unconsciousness? How does it obscure the spirit? These are difficult questions to answer, but contemplating it from the perspective we discussed earlier should help us to understand them. The Tang dynasty poet Meng Haoran's "Spring Morning" is fitting to our topic:

> In spring I slept unconscious of the dawn,
> From everywhere there was the song of birds.

The sound of wind and rain came with the night;

Who knows how many petals had been dropped?

Why are we unconscious of the dawn when sleeping in the spring? Why are we drowsy throughout the morning? When I am teaching in the spring semester, a large number of my students drop off by the third or fourth period in the morning. I do not think that this is from a lack of diligence on the part of my students, but rather a direct result of a grogginess that is difficult to overcome. Why is this? It is because of the increase in the activity of yang *qi* during the spring and summer, causing humidity to increase both within and without the body. This increase in dampness rises until it influences the clarity of the orifices. Of course, the impact of this dampness is still within tolerable physiological limits, and most people tolerate it with little cause for complaint. We become a little fuzzy and drowsy, and that is all. In any case, it has some effect: it causes us to be "unconscious of the dawn." However, once this influence exceeds our normal physiological limits, then we get into the range discussed in Yangming disease.

The above discussion also leads us to the question of root and branch, or essential and outward nature. In the *yunqi*, why are Yangming and Taiyin thought to have a root and branch relationship? We should ponder this for a time. In the six *qi* method of treating disease, Shaoyang and Taiyin are treated at their root; Shaoyin and Taiyang are treated from root and from the exterior, and Yangming and Jueyin are treated at the level of the intermediary *qi* between the root and branch. Why is Yangming treated at this intermediate level? We can relate this to our understanding of the relationship between dryness and dampness. Yangming disease, as we have just recounted, is the result of excessive fire *qi*. When the fire *qi* is excessive, Yangming's essential function is disturbed. When this occurs, we should treat with Baihu and Chengqi.

Have you ever wondered why formulas that contain Dahuang, Mangxiao, Zhishi, and Houpo are called Chengqi ("support the *qi*") decoctions? What *qi* is being supported? It is Yangming *qi*, the descending *qi*. Once heat ensues, and Yangming can no longer descend, the goal is to support the *qi* by inducing it to resume its descent. My late teacher used to call Chengqi Tang by the name Shunqi ("follow the course of *qi*") Tang, and the reason is clear from the perspective of this purpose. It causes Yangming *qi* to resume its normal course of flowing downward. If the opposite were the case, and the function of Yangming were too intense, then this is another reason for pathological dryness to occur. This type of dryness, however, would be the dryness of Yangming's essential nature, simply overshooting its goal. The *Plain Questions* calls this sort of dryness "wanton dryness." When this wanton dryness exists in the interior of the body, it is regulated primarily by means of bitter and warm herbs, with the assistance of sweet and pungent herbs. When we encounter this sort of dryness in the clinical setting, it would be a grave error to administer Chengqi decoction. To do so would be to further dry an already pathologically dry patient, adding insult to injury. Instead, we should prescribe warm and pungent or warm and bitter herbs to moisten dryness. Yangming section of the *Treatise on Cold Damage* references Wuzhuyu Tang, for instance. Wuzhuyu Tang is specifically designed to counter wanton dryness. One should not get stuck on the fact that the herb Wuzhuyu is acrid and drying, as the formula as a whole is able to cure dryness, to moisten dryness. Ultimately, theory provides the crucial element in this understanding. Once the principle underlying these medical concepts is clearly understood, the rest is simple. Why is it that Wuzhuyu Tang cannot be used to treat dryness that is cool? Why is it useless for a dry cough? It can be used to treat both of these conditions. This is called using what is near at hand, and recognizing that the Dao is everywhere.

Another point relates to the fact that this year (2000) is a *gengchen* year, and there has been an especially large amount of rain in the south. Why? Is this related to the contribution of this particular year? I believe it must be related. I invite the reader to his or her own contemplation regarding this point, but we have already discussed the principle at work here. Undoubtedly, it is a case of one rising when the other falls, one emerging and one entering, one hot and the other cold, fire followed by water, and so on. If we were to summarize this process, it is simply a matter of yin and yang.

II. An Outline of Yangming Disease

Let us first examine the first line of the Yangming section of the *Treatise on Cold Damage*, line 179. It reads:

> With regard to disease, there is Taiyang Yangming disease, Zhengyang Yangming disease, and Shaoyang Yangming disease. What is the meaning

of this? Taiyang Yangming disease is the same as the disease spleen constraint; Zhengyang Yangming disease is fullness of the stomach family; Shaoyang Yangming disease, after inducing perspiration and disinhibiting urine, is characterized by dryness, vexation, and fullness in the stomach, and difficult bowel movements.

We can discuss this line from four different perspectives.

II.1. General Meaning

II.1.a. The Different Routes of Yangming

At this point in our discussion, we will examine the three Yangming: Taiyang Yangming, Zhengyang Yangming, and Shaoyang Yangming. In other words, there are at least three routes by which Yangming disease can come about, and the three routes discussed are limited to the three yang. In this discussion of the three yang, Taiyang is the exterior, Yangming the interior, and Shaoyang is half interior and half exterior. As diseases of the three yang progress toward Yangming disease, in terms of the patient's condition, the location of the disease, and the patient's condition, this progression toward Yangming is a progression toward greater severity. Thus, it was Zhang Zhongjing's intention that his work allows the physician to interrupt the routes by which this disease can develop as early as possible. Once these three routes are blocked, there is no spleen constraint, no fullness of the stomach family, and no difficult bowel movements.

Besides these three routes, are there other routes whereby Yangming disease may come about? For instance, besides Taiyang Yangming, Zhengyang Yangming, and Shaoyang Yangming, is there a Taiyin Yangming, a Shaoyin Yangming, and a Jueyin Yangming? This is a question we must contemplate together. From the clues Zhang Zhongjing provides, it would seem that these three Yangmings must exist as well. For instance, line 278 of the Taiyin chapter reads: "on the seventh or eighth day, although there is severe irritation when urinating, after the tenth day it will cease of its own accord. This is a result of excess of the spleen family, and requires the elimination of rotten materials." The ancients said: "If the patient's illness is excessive, then it is a Yangming disease, and if it the illness is deficient, then it is a Taiyin disease." Thus, this line illustrates a case of Taiyin disease progressing to Yangming disease, and is an example of Taiyin Yangming disease.

In addition, can it be said that the "three urgently purgative syndromes

of Shaoyin," made known in lines 320, 321, and 322, depict Shaoyin Yangming conditions? In the Jueyin chapter line 374, can it be said that the use
of Xiao Chengqi Tang is in relation to Jueyin Yangming disease? As mentioned above, the three yang leading to Yangming disease appear to result
in an increase in the severity of the patient's condition. What about when
the three yin progress toward Yangming disease? These two would seem to
be completely different issues.

II.1.b. Contemplating Downward Purgation from a Modern Perspective

Earlier, we discussed the importance of the Yangming channel. Why is it so
important? It is where the precious treasures are stored, the food we ingest.
It is also where the dregs and waste products from digestion are kept,
where the feces are held before leaving the body. Yangming is where both
the *crème de la crème* and the dross and dregs are found. It contains both
healthy and unhealthy influences, dwelling in the same domicile. From a
modern perspective, the place in which both gems and filth reside, where
the healthy and unhealthy dwell together, can be considered in a number
of different ways. For instance, the human body contains a great number of
bacteria. The weight of these bacteria is greater than two pounds, and the
volume is about the same of the liver.

What is the primary residence of these bacteria? They dwell in the
organs related to Yangming, the organs of the digestive tract. Some of these
organisms are pathogenic and when conditions are ripe, they incite disease.
Some of these bacteria, on the other hand, are beneficial to the human
organism and produce essential nutrients, such as vitamins, that are used
by the human body. Furthermore, these beneficial bacteria help to defend
the body from pathogenic ones. At present, many persons are unaware of
the biological function of bacteria, and mistakenly assume that all bacteria are harmful. For this reason, bacteria are largely considered to be the
chief enemy of human health, whereas antibiotics are considered to be sort
of a salubrious talisman. Among the general populace, whenever anyone
becomes ill, they consider antibiotics to be the most necessary and efficacious medicine to return them to health. Furthermore, physicians feel that,
regardless of the disease, if they do not prescribe some antibiotics they have
been somewhat negligent. This is the present situation in the medical world
in China, and constitutes one of the greatest fallacies of modern medicine.

Americans have reflected deeply upon the various influential medical misconceptions of the twentieth century. Among these misconceptions, perhaps the greatest misunderstanding is related to the abuse of antibiotic therapy. To safeguard against the abuse of antibiotics, American health officials have instituted a number of protocols. Today, in America, it is more difficult to procure antibiotics than it is to buy a firearm. This would seem to indicate that American health officials recognize that the potential of antibiotics to cause harm to human health exceeds even that of firearms. Water can keep a boat afloat, but it can also capsize it. Americans seem to be aware of this fact. In China, people seem to be confused on this point.

How then can we optimize the "treasures" of Yangming and the functions that are analogous with these treasures? How do we minimize the harmful effect of the "dregs" found in the digestive tract of Yangming? It is crucial that we look to the functioning of the Yangming system. The functioning of Yangming is primarily manifested through its unobstructed descent. The most obvious sign of this unobstructed descent can be found in the downward and outward elimination of the contents of the intestines, the elimination of the feces. For this reason, ensuring that the elimination of feces is unhindered is crucial to maintaining overall health.

The unobstructed descent particular to Yangming allows us to make a comparison with tidying up a table after a meal. It is easy if we are able to simply throw away the waste. This "tidying up" is analogous to the downward purgation method, and it is the operative principle of the three Chengqi formulas. As soon as the illness progresses to the Yangming stage, it can be done away with by means of downward purging. For this reason, a prerequisite of using the downward purgation method is that the pathogen inhabits the Yangming system, and it must present as Yangming disease with the characteristic Yangming pattern. If the pattern of the disease is not a Yangming pattern, if it does not assume the characteristic form of Yangming disease but the downward purgative method is used anyhow, this is referred to as "erroneous downward purgation." Erroneous downward purgation can cause problems. I think the recent news about Hu Wanlin, who practiced medicine without a license in China for years and prescribed unsafe doses of Mangxiao resulting in numerous deaths, is a prime example. Mangxiao is an effective purgative, but inappropriately prescribed, it can kill. However, we must consider both sides when looking at the case of

Hu Wanlin; we cannot act as if the case is entirely cut and dry or be overly brusque in our judgment of him. His bold use of the downward purgative method enacted a great number of impressive cures. His successes should lead us to consider the principle underlying his success. His failing was in apprehending the degree of moderation necessary to safely enact a cure, and he did not fully understand the prerequisite Yangming pattern for prescribing the downward purgative method.

This prerequisite is exceedingly important. If the disease is not in Yangming, is there a way that we can induce it to enter Yangming so that it can be purged? Is there a method to assist in the formation of a Yangming pattern and then purge it? In my opinion, in theory, this is totally possible. Furthermore, a number of ancient medical practitioners, such as Zhang Congzheng, have performed a number of explorations and tests in this regard. Borrowing from these explorations and experiences, we can develop such a technique and perhaps perfect it. Now, when we raise this particular question, when we begin our contemplation of the matter, we suddenly realize that we are considering a very traditional and classical issue but that we are over two thousand years from the time this question first arose. If we use modern thinking to consider this ancient problem, and contemplate it from a new perspective, are we engaged in the modernization of Chinese Medicine? I believe this question is very worthy of our contemplation. It especially should not be disregarded by the administrative departments in our field.

When one mentions modernization, most people immediately think of modern scientific methods and equipment. Some believe that without experiments, laboratories, genetic research and a thorough application of the laws of physics to every aspect of its theory, Chinese Medicine cannot be modernized. This is not modernization. We do not need a nod from little white rabbits and mice in order to modernize Chinese Medicine. At present, however, if you propose doing research without modern methods and equipment, you will have a hard time getting any funding. Of course, such research should and must be undertaken, but it is only one facet of modernization. If all of our talents, resources, and attention went into such research, it will be hard not to make mistakes.

At present, we are discussing modernization, and like the purgative method, it has important prerequisites. It is like negotiating with Taiwan.

As long as a unified China is the premise, everything else is on the table. Without this premise, there is nothing to talk about. The modernization of Chinese Medicine is also like this: it is only possible when the premise is maintaining the integrity of the field. The director of Guangxi University of Chinese Medicine where I teach, Professor Wang Naiping, has repeatedly emphasized this point: "Should we depart from the premise of Chinese Medicine in order to pursue modernization, the result would be that the more modernization occurs, the quicker Chinese Medicine dies." Director Wang's judgment shows great depth of both philosophy and strategy. It reminds me of the parable of King Yingdi in *Zhuangzi*:

> The Emperor of the South Sea was Emperor Shu, and the Emperor of the North Sea was Emperor Hu. The Emperor of the Central Region was Emperor Hundun. Sometimes, Emperor Shu and Emperor Hu would meet up where Emperor Hundun dwelt, and Emperor Hundun enjoyed extending his hospitality to them. Shu and Hu discussed their host's merits and remarked that all other persons had seven orifices with which to see, hear, eat, and smell—only Hundun lacked these apertures. "Let us chisel these openings for him!" they agreed. Each day, they chiseled a new orifice in Hundun. On the seventh day, Hundun died.

It is true that Chinese Medicine must modernize, that it cannot remain a musty, stodgy old set of superstitious practices. The aim of modernizing Chinese Medicine is to increase the usefulness and service of Chinese Medicine to modernity. However, if we do a sloppy job of modernizing Chinese Medicine, it may be that Chinese Medicine will die at our hands, just as Hundun did. This is a real possibility. To preserve and further the true character of Chinese Medicine is a beautiful and meritorious undertaking. If done incorrectly, however, it is nothing but pie in the sky. Modernization of Chinese Medicine and preservation of its traditional character often seem to be mutually exclusive goals. Grasping at one, we lose our grip on the other, and vice versa. How many persons are there who can gain ground in the laboratory while at the same time unearthing treasures from the *Yellow Emperor's Classic*? How many have an equally good grasp of the laws of physics and the *Yellow Emperor's Classic*? It is similar to the "material and spiritual civilizations of socialism" proposed by Deng Xiaoping, we should grasp both and grip them hard. However, very few people can achieve this. The vast majority grasp molecular biology but have no real concept of the

Yellow Emperor's Classic. This is a point I brought up in the first chapter of this book. Why is it that there are so few Chinese Medicine doctors who even glance at the *Yellow Emperor's Classic* or the *Treatise on Cold Damage?* They are caught in a dilemma. I am the same way. My mind is buried in the *Yellow Emperor's Classic* and the *Treatise on Cold Damage.* I cannot simply grow another head and stick it in the laboratory. Nonetheless, I follow modern developments with great interest, and I often use contemporary concepts to contemplate issues that pertain to traditional Chinese Medicine.

After a great deal of time spent paying close attention and contemplating, I have arrived at two fundamental opinions on the issue: First, modernization of Chinese Medicine is, in the first place, a modernization of Chinese Medicine ideas, thought, and expression. To modernize these, we must enter into the introspective laboratory of the mind, and not the laboratory in which little white rats are experimented on. Secondly, the merging of the modern and the traditional must be done by the most talented individuals of each field. Only if these masters of the traditional and masters of the modern join together will we achieve meaningful results. In years past, we have attempted to conjoin the traditional and the modern by instilling both in a single person and then letting the essences of each intermingle and integrate in his or her mind. This method would seem to be the most expedient, but has yet to prove its efficacy. The integration of Chinese Medicine with modern science must be undertaken as two separate endeavors. Developing talent in modern scientific thought is not difficult, because modern society is constantly training these individuals *en masse.* Developing talent in Chinese Medicine is a far more difficult endeavor. Therefore, if we wish to achieve a fusion of traditional Chinese Medicine and modern medical science, we in this field must focus our efforts on traditional thought. I believe that is the most important prerequisite.

Can Chinese Medicine make use of modern medical methods? Can it benefit from a CT or an MRI? Of course it can, no problem! I believe Chinese Medicine practitioners can utilize just about every modern medical method, but we should not fool ourselves into thinking that this constitutes modernization! If you mistake these for the modernization of Chinese Medicine, then this integration will never be comprehensible from a logical or rational point of view. The current situation cannot be called modernization of Chinese Medicine. At best, it is simply Chinese Medicine implementing modern technology. Chinese Medicine may trade its traditional apparel for a Western suit and leather shoes, but a change of clothing does not change Chinese Medicine. It is the same Chinese Medicine wearing different clothes. These are two different things, and I hope that everyone can see the difference.

In the first chapter, I provided the example of how my late teacher treated a hemothorax with a decoction of Chenpi, Baizhu, Yuzhu, and Dazao. After taking the decoction, the patient experienced a large downward purgation, and after this bowel movement, the blood that was filling the pleural space was quickly reabsorbed. The patient experienced diarrhea, and then his hemothorax resolved. Did a channel suddenly open between the patient's pleural space and large intestine, allowing the fluid to drain away? Or was it immediately reabsorbed by the blood? Why is it that the diarrhea that results from gastroenteritis does not have a similar effect? Why did my former teacher not use Xiao or Da Chengqi Tang to purge the patient, and instead used these everyday herbs that one would not normally even think of as purgatives to treat the patient? The problem of the lungs was able to pass to its associated hollow organ, the large intestine, and was then able to exit the body. Can other afflictions be passed from one part of the body to the next via the channels and the relationships between organs, find their way to the large intestine of Yangming and then exit the body? If this method works, then many difficult maladies could be resolved.

If we can think in the above manner when studying this line, we can provide fodder for countless research into both traditional and modern medicine. Is this sort of contemplation not a form of modernization? We must not be too mechanical or rigid in our contemplation of modernization. We need only open our eyes and look a little further afield. There are many issues that have already "received the nod" of two thousand years of history, and we need not wait for the approval of little white laboratory rats!

II.2. Spleen Constraint

Spleen constraint is Taiyang Yangming. Why is it referred to as "spleen constraint"? In the sixth edition of the standard *Treatise on Cold Damage* textbook in China, it explains the meaning of this term as follows: "Spleen constraint: the stomach is hot, the intestines dry, and the fluids damaged such that there is constipation." Others explain it by saying there is stomach

heat and damage to fluids, which thereby constrains the spleen and prevents it from carrying out its function of moving the fluids of the stomach,
and thereby causing dryness of the intestines and constipation. I have never
had much confidence in this explanation of spleen constraint or in the
many others that are similar to it. If the constipation were brought about in
such a way, the ancients could have given it a different name, such as "fluid
damage" or "dry intestines" or "stomach heat." Why should it be given
an irrelevant title such as "spleen constraint"? What is the relationship
between spleen constraint and Taiyang Yangming? If we apply the above
explanation, then a logical connection between the described condition
and Taiyang Yangming eludes us. The signs of spleen constraint are dryness of the intestines and a hardening of the feces. This much is certain.
The question is, why is this dryness of the intestines and constipation called
"spleen constraint"? Furthermore, why is the Taiyang Yangming condition
called spleen constraint?

The fact is that this question is both complex and simple. When we say
that it is complex, we are referring to the fact that in over a thousand years,
no one has managed to come up with an adequately clear and succinct
description or explanation of the condition. When we say that it is simple,
this is because it can easily be comprehended once it is placed within the
context of dryness and dampness. We have just discussed the relationship
between dampness and dryness. As far as the spleen and stomach are concerned, the spleen is ascribed to dampness and the stomach to dryness.
What does "constraint" (*yue* 約) refer to? *Yue* means "to tie up and bind."
Spleen constraint means that the dampness related to the spleen is bound
up. Once the spleen dampness is bound, the stomach's dryness naturally
comes to the fore, and constipation naturally arises. This term might
appear to be just a roundabout way of saying intestinal dryness, but there is
more to it than that.

As soon as the spleen is constrained, dryness emerges as a matter
of course. This is what is meant by "spleen constraint." However, why is
the Taiyang Yangming called "spleen constraint"? Let us look at line 247
of the *Treatise on Cold Damage*: "If the yang pulse of the instep is floating
and rough, we should consider the floating as a sign that the stomach *qi* is
strong, and the fact that it is rough as a sign that there is frequent urination. Together, a strong and rough pulse indicates that the feces are hard,

and the spleen is constrained; Maziren Wan governs the condition." This line highlights the importance of frequent urination in the advent of constipation. An increase in urination leads to a dryness in the intestines and the feces then become hard. Thus, increased urination causes a progression to Yangming disease. The urinary bladder is a Taiyang organ, thus it is called Taiyang Yangming.

But why does an increase in urination lead to spleen constraint? This can be understood by looking at the relationship between water and earth. Normally, earth constrains water, and checks its flow. When the function of the earth, as exercised by the spleen, is itself constrained, then the flow of water is unchecked, and there is frequency of urination. Thus, Taiyang Yangming is closely associated with spleen constraint. In addition, besides constipation as a result of frequent urination, in the clinic we also encounter instances where excessive sweating leads to constipation. Perspiration is controlled by the *couli*, referred to as the striae of the flesh, or the interstices of the flesh. The *couli* are governed by Taiyang. Can the condition characterized by excessive perspiration leading to dryness in the stomach and subsequent constipation also be called Taiyang Yangming? Can it be treated in accord with the same principles as spleen constraint? This is a question that I hope we can contemplate together.

II.3. Zhengyang Yangming

II.3.a. Explanations of the Physicians of Previous Dynasties

The explanations of Zhengyang Yangming offered by the physicians of various dynasties differ. For instance, the sixth edition of the standard *Treatise on Cold Damage* textbook says: "The external pathogen enters the interior, and directly violates Yangming and then assumes form; this is called Zhengyang Yangming." The Qing dynasty physician You Zaijing describes Zhengyang Yangming as: "The heat pathogen enters the stomach, binding up the waste matter there, causing Yangming to spontaneously become diseased." Others have explained that Yangming is fundamentally dry, thus, the dry constipation associated with Yangming disease is a manifestation of disorder related to its own basic *qi*. Thus, it is called Zhengyang Yangming disease. Here, *zheng* (正) means "basic," "direct," "fundamental" or "orthodox." Zhang Xiju, of the early Qing dynasty, understood it to be like this. Others have explained that Yangming disease that is neither Taiyang nor Shaoyang is Zhengyang Yangming. Wang Hu, also of the Qing dynasty, shares this idea. The reader can refer to these different explanations.

II.3.b. The Meaning of Zhengyang

The word Zhengyang is not used independently in the *Treatise on Cold Damage*. It is only used in conjunction with Yangming as part of the term Zhengyang Yangming. Does Zhengyang refer to any Yangming syndrome not falling into the categories of Taiyang Yangming or Shaoyang Yangming? Or does the word Zhengyang have its own connotation? This is a question that our previous explanations have not directly addressed.

We can recognize that Zhengyang does not necessarily just indicate Yangming or, in other words, that orthodox Yangming is called Zhengyang. Zhengyang must have its own particular implications. We can understand its connotations from a philological perspective by examining the character *zheng* (正). In the *Kangxi Dictionary*, we find "Four months are also called *zheng* months," as well as the following classical references—*Classic of Poetry*: "In the *zheng* months, there is much frost"; Zheng Xuan's *Commentary*: "The fourth month, that of summer; the months that establish *si*"; Kong Yingda's *Explanations*: "Those that are referred to as the *zheng* months are during the time that *qian* (Initiating) exerts its influence, the months of the *zheng* pure yang"; Du Yu's commentary on the *Commentary of Zuo*: "The months of *zheng* yang establish *si*." Therefore, the Zhengyang is the *qian* yang, the yang that establishes the months of the sixth earthly branch, *si*. The month that is related to this earthly branch is the fourth month of the year, when the *qi* of summer begins to exert its influence. What is the *qi* of summer? It is the *qi* of fire and of heat. The *qi* of heat and fire puts the greatest imposition on Yangming and most readily causes Yangming disease. Because the nature of fire and of heat is to blaze upward, the very opposite of the descending nature of Yangming, it is most likely to cause Yangming disorders. If fire and heat are the *qi* of the Zhengyang, and fire has the capacity to induce Yangming disease, then Zhengyang Yangming disease is the name of Yangming disease induced by fire. Thus, Zhengyang Yangming disease is more specific than simply any Yangming disease that does not fall into the classification of Taiyang or Shaoyang Yangming disease.

Besides understanding the meaning of the term Zhengyang from examining the characters, as we just did above, we can also look at the lines from the *Treatise on Cold Damage* that deal directly with Zhengyang Yangming disease. Let us look at line 168 of the *Treatise on Cold Damage*, where Baihu Jia Renshen Tang is discussed. Following the formula, it is noted that "This formula should only be prescribed after *Lixia* (Beginning of Summer) and before *Liqiu* (Beginning of Autumn)." Baihu Jia Renshen Tang is a major Yangming formula. Why should it only be prescribed during the summer? The three months of summer is the period of time in which fire and heat are the most prevalent, and the Zhengyang exerts its strongest influence. It is the period of time in which Yangming disease is most easily brought about by fire and heat. The fact that Baihu Jia Renshen Tang can only be given during the summer months validates our interpretation of the meaning of Zhengyang Yangming disease.

II.3.c. Fullness of the Stomach Family

Zhengyang Yangming is also referred to as fullness or excess of the stomach and its family (*wei jia shi* 胃家實). Below, we will examine the meaning of *wei jia shi*.

II.3.c.1. The Stomach

What does the stomach represent? In the first place, it represents the hollow organ we are all familiar with. Beyond this, in the *Plain Questions's* "Great Treatise on the Correspondence of Yin and Yang," there is an important summary of the stomach: "the six channels are the great rivers, and the intestines and stomach are the sea." The relationship between the six channels and the stomach is analogous to the relationship between the river and the sea. What is the relationship between the river and the sea? The saying goes: "The sea receives a hundred rivers, a hundred rivers return to the sea." To say that the "hundred rivers return to the sea" indicates that all rivers have either a direct or an indirect connection to the sea. If there were no connection, how would the water contained by the rivers collect in the sea?

This river and sea analogy indicates the communication between the channels and the stomach and intestines. The pathogenic processes afflicting the six channels can be brought to the stomach and intestines and then flushed out of the body. Why is it that the downward purging method is able to dispel the "hundred diseases"? The reason lies in this relationship between the channels and the gastrointestinal tract. Earlier, we discussed the topic of a "contemplating downward purging from a modern perspective." From this understanding of the relationship between the rivers and the sea, between the channels and the stomach and intestines, we can see that our observations of the curative capacity of the downward purging method are entirely plausible. The six channels circulate through the entire body. There is nowhere they do not travel. They are able to take pathogens and disease from any part of the body, even in the case of very serious disease, and guide them to the gastrointestinal tract, to the sea, where they can then be cleared from the body. Our earlier contemplation is based in large part on this important relationship between the channels and the stomach and intestines.

In 1992, the Hualing Press published a book called *Secrets of Treating Cancer* by Sun Bingyan. This book describes his thirty-four years of experience treating cancer patients. His so-named "secrets of treating cancer" primarily constitute a number of different purgative methods. The wisdom of Dr. Sun's experiences is truly praiseworthy. As soon as they are placed into the framework of the Yangming chapter, and as soon as we contemplate them in the context of "The six channels are like rivers, the stomach and the intestines are like the sea," their theoretical underpinnings can be easily resolved. The difficulty lies in how we go about bringing these pathogens to the Yangming phase. For, once the pathogens have entered into Yangming, they can easily be purged out of the body. If the pathogens are not in Yangming, however, application of the purgative method can do more harm than good, or can even be detrimental to health. Thus, the pathogen must reside in Yangming in order to use the purgative method. That is, as we stated earlier, the prerequisite to using the downward purging method. This is to say that we must see certain signs in order to employ the purgative method effectively.

If the pathogen is in Shaoyin, how can it be led into Yangming? If it is in Jueyin, how do we induce it to enter Yangming? What degree of symptomology is required in order to be certain that it has entered the Yangming phase? For this, we must have concrete signs, and these involve specific diagnostic techniques. To arrive at a clear understanding of these difficulties, we can review what has been said in the classics as well as what is offered by the experiences of our contemporaries. In addition, we can forge new paths and perhaps thereby develop new methods. I believe this sort of contemplation is very meaningful. Any way you look at it, it conforms with the idea of modernizing Chinese Medicine.

From another perspective, the stomach (*wei* 胃) is not just a concept in the field of visceral manifestations in Chinese Medicine; it is also a concept in astronomy. *Wei* (Granary) is one of the twenty-eight constellations in Chinese astronomy. To be more exact, it is one of the constellations found in the seven western constellations, those constituting the White Tiger Constellation (*baihu su*). The west governs descending, as does the white tiger, as does the stomach and Yangming. Why is the representative formula used to treat Yangming disease called Baihu Tang (White Tiger decoction)? Why is the Granary constellation found in the White Tiger group of constellations and not in, say, the Green Dragon (*qinglong*) of the east, or the Scarlet Bird (*zhuque*) of the South, or the Black Warrior (*xuanwu*, or *zhenwu*) of the north? Why is Yangming disease referred to as "fullness of the stomach family"? Once we answer this series of questions, you may suddenly feel that Chinese Medicine is a complete and comprehensive system of thought. It is interwoven with astronomy above, geography below, and the human being between the two. If Chinese Medicine were focused only on the human body, could it ever become such a vast and intricately integrated system? Of course not.

Wei (Granary) is one of the seven constellations of the west. The *Book of Celestial Offices* in the *Records of the Grand Historian* by Sima Qian says: "*Wei* is the celestial storehouse." In the commentary on this passage, it is written: "*Wei* governs the granaries and storehouses, it is the palace of the five grains. When the ruler is bright and clear, there is peace under the heavens and the five grains are plentiful." In the *Plain Questions* chapter titled "Treatise on the Spiritual Orchid Secret Canon," we find: "The spleen and stomach hold the office of the granaries. The five flavors originate from them." We can see that the use of the title "Granary" for one of the seven constellations of the west is not a hollow gesture; it carries real significance, and this significance corresponds with the function of the spleen and stomach governing the granaries and storehouses. Heaven and human correspond with one another. More specifically, the constellations and the organs of the human body correspond to one another. The Granary is the celestial storehouse. The Granary constellation reveals whether there is peace under the heavens and whether the five grains are in plenitude. The stomach and spleen are the officials of the granaries and storehouses in the body; if the spleen and stomach are strong, then the body will be healthy and carefree, and the five flavors will emerge from the spleen and stomach. The Granary constellation of Chinese astronomy and the stomach of human physiology share analogous functions within the larger system of relationships in which they play a part. This observation is worthy of our earnest contemplation and investigation.

Several days ago, one of my elders, also high in the administration at the college where I teach, who was compelled both by his concern for me and a desire to encourage me, told me: "Here at this college, there are very few who have delved so deeply into the classics as you have. However, there is something you must pay careful attention to: in the classics we find both pearls and dregs; you must get the pearls but do away with the dregs." This elder's intended meaning was very clear. On one hand, he expressed his respect for my study of the classics. On the other hand, he expressed his concern that I might mistake dregs of ignorance for pearls of wisdom. He expressed his opinion very well, and it is a point that is widely applicable. It is not only the classics that must be studied with a degree of intellectual discrimination, all fields of study deserve such discernment. In every course of study, we should keep the pearls and do away with the offal. In modern scientific study, are there only pearls and no dregs? Not in the least. Modern science also has its errors. But in the current climate of Chinese Medicine, the problem of mistaking dregs for pearls is not nearly so great as the problem presented by the fact that so many persons, especially those of high rank in our field, consider the classics to consist mostly of dregs with a few pearls tossed in. If there are no pearls to be had, why should they deign to study them? This is why our doctoral graduates draw only upon modern scientific data, the findings of experiments in particle physics and laboratories full of white mice. It is why they scarcely glance at the classics. They fear they will find only dregs therein. Who wants to labor in vain?

The urgent threat at this point is not that we are unable to tell the difference between the weeds and the wheat, or that we might mistake dregs for pearls, but that we have lost all confidence in the classics, and have lost all reverence for them. For instance, should we cast away the correlation between the Granary constellation and the stomach of the human body as worthless bit of dregs, a superstition? Or should we research this correlation from many different angles? Among the constellation of the twenty-eight lunar mansions, there is also a constellation named the Heart. The Heart constellation is located in the seven constellations of the east. Is the position of the Heart different from its prenatal orientation among the eight trigrams? This is a question that deserves further study. Why is it that among all of the constellations of the twenty-eight constellations, only the heart was chosen from the five viscera and only the stomach from the six bowels? The heart is the ruler of the five viscera and the stomach the ruler of the six bowels. Why are the rulers of the viscera and bowels selected to name constellations in the twenty-eight constellations? This question is equally worthy of deep deliberation.

II.3.c.2. The Stomach Family

In the discussion of Zhengyang Yangming, it does not say that there is fullness of the stomach, but rather fullness of the "stomach family." What is the meaning of the term "stomach family" (*wei jia* 胃家)? There are rich connotations of the character *jia* in Chinese language, and several ways to translate it in English. Almost any Chinese person can outline these connotations. In China, if you are single, even if your dwelling is over a thousand square feet in area with three side rooms and two large living rooms, when you go back to your place, you cannot be said to be "returning home" (*hui jia*). You are just going back to your living quarters. In order to be a *jia*, there must be at least two persons living there. A *jia* can consist of two, three, and the old days maybe ten or more persons. Here, where Zhang Zhongjing uses the term "stomach *jia*," he is clearly indicating that there are other players besides the stomach that must be accounted for. Otherwise, it could not be called a *jia*. Thus, the stomach family of Yangming disease includes the intestines as well as the stomach. Otherwise, lines like "in the stomach there must be five or six pieces of dry stool" would be unintelligible and cause for ridicule.

II.3.c.3. Excess or Fullness

When we say that there is fullness or excess of the stomach family, what exactly do we mean by excess (*shi* 實)? Here the character *shi* has two meanings. In the *Plain Questions* chapter "Treatise Thoroughly Deliberating upon Depletion and Repletion," it says: "When the pathogenic *qi* is overabundant it is excess (*shi*), when the *jing* and *qi* are stolen away, this is called deficiency (*xu*)." So then, does the "excess" of the stomach family carry this same meaning? The majority of our predecessors have held this view. Once the disease progresses to the Yangming stage, the pathogenic *qi* is abundant, but the upright *qi* is not yet deficient. Therefore, their reasoning follows that "excess" of the stomach family indicates this idea of the pathogenic *qi* being excessive. This explanation should be considered, but it is not comprehensive. *Extensive Rhymes* defines *shi* as "genuine; full." *Additional Rhymes* defines it as "abundant; the opposite of empty (*xu*)." Thus, *shi* also carries with it the meaning of full, abundant, as well as the opposite of *xu*. If we combine these meanings, we see that it means substantial, replenished, full and complete.

So then, among the two meanings of *shi*, which is the most appropriate, the clearest and most concise? If we look at the first of the two meanings, that of an abundance of pathogenic *qi*, it is based on the etiology of the disease, the cause of the disease. But the etiological perspective is certainly not the correct one in this instance. This is because all of the outlines of the six conformations discuss only signs and symptoms; that is, all of them deal with the outcome of the disease, not the cause. For instance, in the Taiyang outline, there is a floating pulse and painful stiffness of the head and nape; in the Shaoyang passage, there is a bitter taste in the mouth, a dry throat, and blurry vision; in the Taiyin passage, the abdomen is bloated, there is vomiting, and the patient cannot eat; in Shaoyin outline, we read of a thin and delicate pulse and somnolence; in Jueyin, there is illness marked by frequent drinking and urination, the *qi* ascends and collides into the heart; and so on. All of these passages discuss the consequences of the disease, and from these consequences, the cause is sought. Why should the Yangming outline be an exception?

Thus, the first definition of *shi*, that of an "excess" of pathogenic *qi*, is illogical. It must be discussing the syndrome, the outcome of the disease. The second possible meaning, that of "fullness," seems far more appropriate and logical. In the *Plain Questions* chapter titled "Further Discourse on the Five Viscera," we read: "The six bowels transmit materials without storing them, thus they can be full (*shi*), but not solid (*man*). The five viscera store the *jing* but do not purge or drain, thus they can be solid, but not full." Furthermore, it says: "The six bowels alternate between emptiness (*xu*) and fullness (*shi*); when the stomach is full, the intestines are empty, and when the intestines are full, the stomach is empty." The five viscera store the *jing* and *qi* and do not allow them to be drained away, so in health, they can only be solid, never full. The six bowels transport and transform materials without storing them; they principally have the function of transmitting. They can only be filled, but cannot be solid.

If, in health, the six bowels can be full but cannot be solid, and the stomach is the chief of the six bowels, here when we speak of the stomach family fullness, it corresponds with the fullness of the six bowels as described in the *Plain Questions* chapter "Further Discourse on the Five Viscera." This fullness should correspond to the normal state of health. Why is it that in line 179 of the *Treatise on Cold Damage* and in subsequent lines regarding Yangming disease, this "fullness" indicates pathology? The secret to understanding this passage lies in understanding Zhang Zhongjing's use of the word "family." We have already discussed the meaning of this character: there must be at least two members to make up a family. Thus, here in this instance, the stomach family indicates that it is not only the stomach but also the intestines that are full. It is the stomach together with the intestines that forms the stomach "family." If the stomach and the intestines are full at the same time, this breaks the ordinary state of affairs described in "Further Discourse on the Five Viscera" where it states that there is an alternation between fullness and emptiness of the stomach and the intestines: "When the stomach is full, the intestines are empty; when the intestines are full, the stomach is empty." Once the physiological pattern is broken, then we of course have entered into a state of disease. In the first and the fifth chapters of this book, we wrote at some length concerning the meaning of particular characters in the classics. We must be meticulous, even pedantic in our interpretation of characters used in the classics. There is little room for our own personal bias. As our forefathers said: "To understand each character correctly solidifies things like a boulder." Each character in the classics is like a huge boulder, and so the interpretation of each and every character is no small matter indeed. So it is as well with the character *jia* that we just finished examining. A correct understanding of this character is just as important as a huge boulder, is it not? Without the character *jia*, the meaning of this line changes completely. The use of the character *jia* indicates that both the stomach and the intestines are full. If the character *jia* were not used, it would simply be a description of the normal physiological state, not of sickness: the stomach full and the intestines empty. Just as "To understand each character correctly solidifies things like a boulder," we also have the saying "discerning a single meaning is as wondrous as seeing the stars in the sky."

II.3.c.4. To Format As a Disease Trigger Line

In the above line, excess of the stomach family was the focal point. In line 180 that follows, fullness of the stomach family is also the focus. Clearly, "fullness of the stomach family" is a central concept of the Yangming disease trigger. Just as from a five viscera perspective, the central tenet of heart pathology is "pain and itching," from the six conformation pathology perspective, the Yangming disease trigger is centered around "fullness of the stomach family." Fullness of the stomach family is the result; the cause of Zhengyang disease is fire and heat; and Yangming is the trigger. The cause, trigger, and result are all related to one another, but each has a different central focus. We need to integrate the three, but we must also be careful not to confuse them. If we take this generally recognized outline of Yangming disease and rewrite it to match the format of the nineteen disease triggers from the *Yellow Emperor's Classic*, we could write it out as: "All fullness of the stomach family belongs to Yangming."

That is as far as we will discuss the Zhengyang Yangming and the outline of Yangming disease.

II.4. Shaoyang Yangming

II.4.a. Three Yang Therapies

"Shaoyang Yangming disease, after inducing perspiration and disinhibiting urine, is characterized by dryness, vexation, and fullness in the stomach, and difficult bowel movements." This first line lists the prerequisites to Shaoyang Yangming disease as the promotion of sweating and urination. Put another way, sweating and urination are related to the development of Shaoyang Yangming disease. Why does the promotion of sweating and urination lead to dryness, vexation, and fullness of the stomach? Why do they lead to the difficult bowel movements of Shaoyang Yangming disease? It is very clear that the use of diaphoretics or diuretics are contraindicated in the treatment of Shaoyang disease. This urges us to examine the differences between the therapies pertinent to each the three yang diseases.

II.4.a.1. Taiyang Disease Therapies

The two primary treatment methods for Taiyang disease are promoting sweating and urination and, in addition, promoting vomiting. Promoting sweating is primarily directed at syndromes of the Taiyang channel syndrome, exterior syndromes, and the method described in the *Plain Questions's* "Great Treatise on the Correspondences of Yin and Yang": "If the person is afflicted by an external pathogen, induce sweating by immersion in hot liquid; if the pathogen is located in the skin layer, release it with diaphoretic measures." The representative formulas are Mahuang Tang and Guizhi Tang. Promoting urination is primarily a method for treating a Taiyang bowel syndrome, and is an excellent method for opening up the yang. It is as Ye Tianshi has said: "To open up the yang, we do not warm the patient; instead, we disinhibit urination." Therefore, promoting urination is not only a method of "drawing downward and eliminating," but is also included as a method of "sweating and effusion."

Furthermore, promoting vomiting is also a method for treating Taiyang disease. With regard to the location of Taiyang disease, it is not only on the exterior of the body, it is also located high up in the body. As it says in the aforementioned treatise: "when the disease is high up, vomiting can be used." The representative formula for this method is Gualou San, described in the Taiyang chapter. In the first chapter, I introduced Dr. Zeng Rongxiu. Dr. Zeng once shared with me one of his personal experiences. More than ten years ago, he contracted a case of trigeminal neuralgia. The pain was so immense he could hardly stand it. The thought of striking his head against a concrete wall appealed to him. None of the medicine he tried did any good. Dr. Zeng used to smoke a lot of cigarettes, and it created a fair amount of phlegm. Every morning he would have a bout of coughing up this phlegm. However, as soon as his trigeminal neuralgia began, the phlegm suddenly lessened. In the morning, he did not need to expectorate. This change sparked Dr. Zeng to begin thinking. He was still smoking as he had before. He had not made any changes in his dietary habits. So where was the phlegm going? It must be going to his trigeminal nerve! The phlegm obstruction was blocking the channels and network vessels of the area that the trigeminal nerve was ascribed to, blocking the flow of *qi* and causing the pain. Right! That must be it. How should he cause the phlegm to come back out? Dr. Zeng selected the late Qing dynasty physician Zhang

Xichun's method of inducing vomiting by stimulating the point above the suprasternal notch known as Tiantu (CV 22).

The result was that Dr. Zeng vomited up a half a spittoon of sticky phlegm. As soon as he was done coughing it up, the pain in his face was lessened. He induced himself to vomit a few more times, and the pain remitted. As you may know, trigeminal neuralgia is a very stubborn disease. Regardless of what medicine is ingested, the results are not ideal. Some are faced with no alternative but to get surgery and have the nerve severed. To sever the trigeminal nerve in order to alleviate the pain is hardly an elegant method. Dr. Zeng managed to cure this obstinate condition in just a few minutes through promoting vomiting, without spending a single cent. Chinese therapeutic methods like this should not be taken lightly! Vomiting as a form of therapy may appear to be a bit crude, but it can actually cure certain complex diseases.

In summary, Taiyang therapeutic methods (promoting sweating, urination, and vomiting) are all methods that open upward and outward. This shared characteristic corresponds with the fact that Taiyang governs opening in the body.

II.4.a.2. Yangming Disease Therapies

The therapies used to treat Yangming disease can generally be summarized as clearing and downward purging. The clearing method is exemplified by Baihu Tang, though if we analyze the issue a bit more closely, it also includes the methods exemplified by Zhizi Chi Tang and Zhuling Tang. Our forefathers considered the three Chengqi decoctions to be the representatives of the downward purging method, but in Zhang Zhongjing's own words, strict delineations can be drawn between these three. Of the three Chengqi decoctions, only Da Chengqi Tang can be said to be truly downward purging formula, as such it is considered the representative formula of the downward purging method. Zhang Zhongjing describes Xiao Chengqi Tang as a harmonizing rather than a downward purging formula. In line 208, he says:

> Yangming disease in which the pulse is slow, even though there is sweating and no aversion to cold, there will be heaviness of the body, shortness of breath, fullness of the abdomen, gasping for air, and tidal heat; this indicates that the exterior is about to resolve, and the interior can be

attacked. When sweat suddenly emerges from the hands and feet, this means that the stool has hardened and Da Chengqi Tang governs the syndrome. If there is copious sweating with mild heat effusion and an aversion to cold, then the exterior has not resolved. The heat of this pattern is not tidal, and Chengqi decoctions cannot be prescribed. If the abdomen is bloated and blocked up, Xiao Chengqi Tang can be given to subtly harmonize the stomach *qi*. But do not induce great downward purging!

Or again, as line 209 says: "Afterward there is heat effusion, and the stool becomes hard and scanty; use Xiao Chengqi Tang to harmonize it." Or as it says in line 250: "Taiyang disease, after promoting vomiting, downward purging, or sweating, when there is mild vexation, frequent urination, and subsequently a hardening of the stool, give Xiao Chengqi Tang to harmonize and the patient will recover." As the preceding lines from the *Treatise on Cold Damage* reveal, Zhang Zhongjing used Xiao Chengqi Tang to harmonize, and not to induce downward purging. Xiao Chengqi Tang is an example of a harmonizing, not a downward purging, formula.

In addition, Tiaowei Chengqi Tang was not used by Zhang Zhongjing to induce downward purging. After introducing when to use the formula, he notes: "Take warm as a single dose to regulate the stomach *qi*." Thus, Tiaowei Chengqi Tang does just what its name suggests; its main goal is to regulate (*tiao*) the stomach (*wei*). This is a prescription to regulate the stomach, not to induce downward purging.

If we look at all three Chengqi ("support the *qi*") formulas, we must ask what *qi* these formulas are supporting. They are supporting the *qi* of the stomach family, of course. The natural flow of the stomach family *qi* is a downward flow, so all three of these formulas have the ability to restore a downward flow. It is just that the degree of downward flow that these formulas induce is not the same, and so the name of the sort of therapeutic method ascribed to each formula is different: Tiaowei Chengqi Tang is able to regulate the stomach *qi*. Xiao Chengqi Tang is able to harmonize the stomach *qi*. Finally, the degree of downward flow induced by Da Chengqi Tang is sufficient to cause downward purging. Thus, the degree to which each formula supports the *qi* and induces downward flow is not the same. Likewise, their actions and the type of therapeutic result they induce are entirely different.

Therefore, once we thoroughly grasp this difference in degree, we have apprehended a crucial technical problem. If we look at what is noted after each individual formula, we see that after Tiaowei Chengqi Tang, it says that we should "Warm and quaff a dose of it to regulate the stomach *qi*." Of Da Chengqi Tang, it says that it "should be divided into two parts and served warm; once the downward purging has occurred, do not give it again." With regard to Xiao Chengqi Tang, the instructions are: "After first taking the decoction there should be a bowel movement; if there is not, give the rest of the dose. If at any point during the administration of this formula the patient defecates, give no more of it." Among the three Chengqi decoctions, Tiaowei Chengqi Tang says nothing of downward purging, nor does it mention anything about bowel movements. It only speaks of "regulating the stomach *qi*." Da Chengqi Tang speaks frankly of "downward purging." Xiao Chengqi Tang says: "there should be a bowel movement." It is interesting that the term that is used in the original Chinese lines about Xiao Chengqi Tang does not directly say defecation nor bowel movements. Instead, it speaks only of "changing the clothes," an expression that referred obliquely to this normal physiological process.

If the patient suffers from delayed bowel movements, Xiao Chengqi Tang should be used. After taking this medicine, the patient should "change their clothes" and return to regular bowel habits. Thus, "to change one's clothes" and "to obtain downward purging" are very different affairs. From this examination of Zhang Zhongjing's notes on the formulas, we can see that the language he uses is in no way ambiguous. Every word carries a very specific meaning. The differences between these passages reflect their theoretical, logical, and clinical significance very precisely. Zhang Zhongjing's precise use of language reminds us that "to understand each character correctly solidifies things like a boulder."

II.4.a.3. The Role of the Six Bowels Is of Passage

Above, we discussed the Taiyang methods of promoting sweating, urination, and vomiting. We also discussed the downward purging, harmonizing, regulating, and clearing methods of Yangming. Among these therapeutic methods, the sweating method allows passage through the interstices and sweat pores; the urination method opens up the process of *qi* transformation through the urinary bladder; the vomiting method promotes unimpeded flow in the upper burner; and the downward purging, harmonizing, and regulating method all assist with the downward flow of the stomach family.

Although these curative methods are all different, none of them depart from the concept of *tong* ("passage"). It might be said that all of them are centered upon the concept embodied in the Chinese character *tong*, and develop from there. This "passage" method is the most direct way of treating the six bowels. Because the function of the six bowels is passage, only if this aspect of the six bowels returns to normal can their basic capacity of transporting and transforming material without storing be realized. For this reason, the Taiyang and Yangming curative methods are in fact "passage" methods: methods aimed at benefiting the six bowels.

II.4.a.4. Shaoyang Disorders Are Not Governed by Passage

At the beginning of the passage on Shaoyang Yangming disease, we mentioned that the methods of promoting sweating and urination are in no way indicated for Shaoyang disease. Now, as we enter the Shaoyang chapter, and begin to examine its contents, we realize that we not only cannot use sweating or urination, but vomiting and downward purging are also contraindicated in Shaoyang disorders. Sweating, urination, downward purging, and vomiting are all methods that rely upon "passage." Why is it that once we arrive at the Shaoyang bowel, we are forbidden to use passage methods? Is it the case that the role Shaoyang plays is not of passage?

Shaoyang governs the hinge mechanism. Among the six bowels, it is ascribed to the gallbladder. Besides belonging to the category of the six bowels, the gallbladder also belongs to another category, explained in the *Plain Questions* chapter "Further Discourse on the Five Viscera":

> The brain, marrow, bones, blood vessels, gallbladder, and womb; all six of these are produced by the earth *qi*. All of them store within yin and their image is of the earth. Thus, they store but do not drain and are called the extraordinary bowels.

The bowels drain but do not store. Because they drain but do not store, their role is of passage. If the six bowels did not allow passage, how could they possibly drain without storing? Thus, the passage method is the orthodox method of treating disorders of the six bowels. Now, in the above passage from the *Plain Questions*, we learn that besides its characteristics as one of the six bowels, another of the characteristics of the gallbladder is that it stores but does not drain. The bowels should drain but not store. The viscera store but do not drain. Now we are told that this particular bowel, the gallbladder, stores but does not drain; it is a bowel that behaves like the viscera. Strange. Thus, the gallbladder is referred to as an "extraordinary" bowel. The Shaoyang bowel stores but does not drain, so of course we should not use the "passage" method. Therefore, the methods that are suitable to the other bowels (sweating, urination, downward purging, vomiting) cannot be used to treat disease of Shaoyang. If these methods are applied incorrectly in an attempt to treat a Shaoyang disorder, problems may arise. The characteristic Shaoyang Yangming signs and symptoms: "Dryness, vexation, and fullness of the stomach, and difficult bowel movements," should not be treated with these methods either. Therefore, in order to treat Shaoyang disease or gallbladder disorders, we must have an adequate understanding of the extraordinary bowels that "store but do not drain."

In the clinic, we frequently encounter maladies directly related to the extraordinary bowel nature of the gallbladder. For instance, let us compare gallstones with kidney stones. Kidney stones are usually relatively simple to resolve, because the method of promoting urination can be applied. Gallstones, on the other hand, are difficult to resolve. Why is this? Because we cannot use a simple therapeutic "passage" technique, such as urination, to treat the difficulty. If urination is not an appropriate way to treat gall stones, then what method can we use?

This is as far as we will discuss Shaoyang Yangming.

III. The Timing of Yangming Disease

This section primarily focuses an explanation of line 193 of the *Treatise on Cold Damage*: "Yangming disease tends to resolve in the time from *shen* to *xu*."

III.1. From *Shen* to *Xu*

The time from *shen* to *xu* is comprised of the three time periods: *shen*, *you*, and *xu*. There are at least three distinct levels to *shen*, *you*, and *xu*. The first level of meaning relates to the time of the day, namely from 3 pm to 9 pm; the second level of meaning is related to the time of the lunar month, namely before and after the last quarter of the moon; and the third level is that of the year, namely the seventh, eighth, and ninth months of the lunar calendar. These three levels of meaning, related to the time that Yangming has a tendency to resolve, can be understood in much the same way that we discussed the three levels of significance related to the time period in which Taiyang disease tends to resolve. These three levels are only a general outline, and we could make still more precise and more detailed divisions in this period of time. We need only get a firm grasp of the principle of "using the identical image" (*tongxiang*), as discussed in the chapter on the three yin and three yang, and we can then make finer and more sophisticated differentiations. In a word, there are months within days, days within months, seasons within a day, and, of course, seasons in the course of a year. Regardless of whether we make a rough or a precise determination, of whether the period of time is long or short, all of the transformation of yin and yang are equivalent to the cycle of emerging, growth, collection, and storage. Therefore, the principles related to different levels of significance can be interchanged. For instance, according to the *Plain Questions*: "When the moon is new, do not drain; when the moon is full, do not tonify!" This of course is referring to the principles of tonification and draining related to the lunar cycle, but these principles of tonification and draining can just as easily be applied to the levels of the daily cycle or the annual cycle. The meaning of the line from the *Plain Questions*, which says do not drain when the moon is new, and do not tonify when the moon is full, can be extended to mean: "When the moon is new, tonify; when it is full, drain." The new moon is analogous to the winter season in the annual cycle. Most people in China seem to know that one should tonify during this part of the year. Tonifying during the winter has become common sense in China, but this common sense originates in the *Yellow Emperor's Classic*. If one wishes to make more sophisticated divisions and delineations in the cycles of the year, this same principle can be applied, after the time period's position in the cycle of yang's release and storage has been determined. I invite the reader to contemplate this topic on his or her own.

Within the framework of the year, the time periods *shen, you,* and *xu* correspond to the three months of fall. If we were to sum up the function of these three months in a single word, it would be "collection." During the three months of autumn, the yang *qi* is being collected, and the "myriad things" gathered back in. The collection of yang *qi* manifests as coolness and dryness. How do the "myriad things," the myriad living creatures, "collect"? Among plants, this "collection" takes the form of a seed. In the fall, we harvest crops. What part of the crops do we harvest? We harvest their fruits, their seeds. From a practical perspective, seeds are a concentration of life, a sort of memory of the life process. This is true whether we are talking about the "seeds" of animals, or the seeds of plants. The sowing of these seeds in the spring is nothing but the renewed amplification of this concentrated life force, the process of the release of these stored memories. Of course, this sort of concentration and memorization are related to "storage." Thus, we often connect the two characters together in the Chinese language. Storage is, in fact, an extension of the process of collection.

If we relate this to the human body, we might view human memory as a process of this sort. Human memory is closely related to the Yangming conformation, and Yangming disease processes often have a notable impact on human memory: hindering it and inducing forgetfulness. Why is this forgetfulness only discussed in the Yangming chapter of the *Treatise on Cold Damage*? Why does the *Divine Farmer's Classic of Materia Medica* say the herb Huanglian, taken over a long period of time, can prevent loss of memory? This is a very interesting question, and one worthy of further research. Memory loss is a common characteristic of many senile diseases. The twenty-first century is the century of skyrocketing prosperity and power for China, but it is also a century that will be characterized by an aging population. We cannot avoid the fact that there are more and more elderly persons in China, and with that aging population comes an increase in geriatric disease. Might it be possible to thoroughly investigate the Yangming chapter of the *Treatise on Cold Damage* to discover new cures and therapies for geriatric conditions, such as memory loss? I believe that this is entirely possible. In this way, we would raise the quality of research on Yangming to a world-class level.

III.2. The Essentials of Yangming Disease

Yangming is the ruler of the six bowels. When Yangming is diseased, the stomach family is in a state of fullness. This fullness of the stomach family is manifested in three main ways:

First of all, the open passageway of the six bowels is obstructed.

Secondly, the descending aspect of Yangming is lost. The descending of Yangming and the passage (*tong*) of the six bowels are rooted in one another. If there is no passage, then there can be no descent; and if there is no descent, then there will be no passage. We can either speak of these two aspects separately or combined as one.

Thirdly, the cool nature of Yangming is lost. The nature of Yangming is cool, as we discussed earlier in this book. This coolness is produced by the descending of the yang *qi*. Thus, the coolness of Yangming and its descending nature are inseparable; they are two sides of the same coin. Just as the coolness and descent of Yangming are interlinked, so too are the descent and openness of Yangming. The three are separate manifestations of the same central theme, the collection of the yang *qi* exemplified by autumn. This is the crux of "fullness in the stomach family" and is also the crucial aspect of Yangming disease.

III.3. The Essential Correspondences of the Tendency to Resolve

The time in which Yangming disease has a tendency to resolve is the period of *shen, you,* and *xu.* This time period is represented in the course of the year by autumn, and in the course of the day by the time when the sun descends in the west. We know that this is characterized by descent, coolness, and passage. If at this time the cooling, descending, and passage function of Yangming is naturally assisted, there will of course be a recovery from disease of Yangming. This is one aspect, but we can also consider this same time period from a spatial rather than a temporal perspective. The *Illumination of Time* section of the *Principles of the Innate Disposition and the Lifespan* (Xing ming guizhi) says:

> The prenatal *qi* of human beings follows the course of the day:
>
> during the *zi* time (11 pm–1 am), the *fu* (Turning Back) *qi* arrives at Caudal Defile (GV 1);
>
> during the *chou* time (1–3 am), the *lin* (Approaching) *qi* arrives at Kidney Hall;
>
> during the *yin* time (3–5 am), the *tai* (Advance) *qi* arrives at the Mystic Pivot;
>
> during the *mao* time (5–7 am), the *dazhuang* (Great Strength) *qi* arrives at Spinal Handle;
>
> during the *chen* time (7–9 am), the *guai* (Eliminating) *qi* arrives at the Kiln Path (GV 13);
>
> during the *si* time (9–11 am), the *qian* (Initiating) *qi* arrives at Jade Pillow (BL 9);

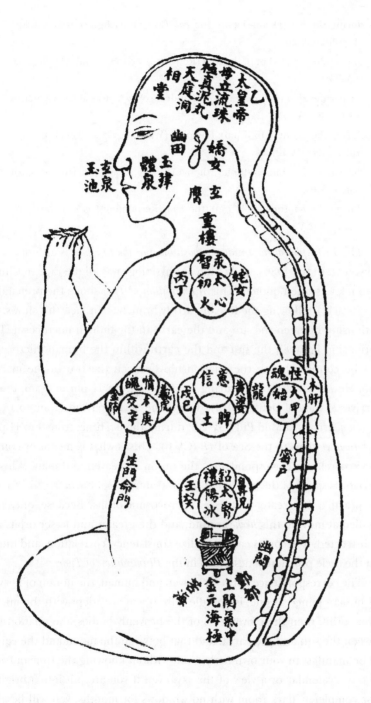

during the *wu* (11 am–1 pm), the *gou* (Encountering) *qi* arrives at the Mud Pill (GV 20);

during the *wei* (1–3 pm), the *dun* (Retreat) *qi* arrives at Hall of Brilliance (GV 23);

during the *shen* (3–5 pm), the *pi* (Hindrance) *qi* arrives at the Center of the Chest (CV 17);

during the *you* time (5–7 pm), the *guan* (Watching) *qi* arrives at the Central Venter (CV 12);

during the *xu* time (7–9 pm), the *bo* (Falling Away) *qi* arrives at Spirit Gate (CV 8);

during the *hai* time (9–11 pm), the *kun* (Responding) *qi* returns to the Sea of *Qi* (CV 6).

The *Principles of the Innate Disposition and the Lifespan* is an important Daoist text. In the 1980s, when human physiology was all the rage in China, this book was often quoted. This *Illumination of Time* shows the prenatal *qi* (*yuanqi* 元氣) following the line of earthly branches. In fact, this shows the relationship between the sun and the earth in the human microcosm. The relationship between the sun and the earth within the human microcosm must be consistent with the relationship between the two in the macrocosm. How is it consistent? During the *zi* time from 11 pm to 1 am, the *fu qi* arrives at Caudal Defile (GV 1); during the *wu* time from 11 am to 1 pm, the *gou qi* arrives at Mud Pill (GV 20); during the *hai* time, from 9 to 11 pm, the *kun qi* returns to the Sea of *Qi* (CV 6). This is what is meant by consistency: correlative correspondence, the union of heaven and man. Why do the Daoists speak of the revolution of the Water Wheel (*heche* 河車)? Why do they practice the greater and lesser microcosmic orbits? Because, once one is skilled at moving this *heche* around, and the greater and lesser orbits are unobstructed, it becomes easy to realize consistency, correlation, and union with the cycle prenatal *qi* described in the *Illumination of Time*.

The correspondence between heaven and human, the notion of heaven and human joined as one, is not idle talk. If you are adept with the microcosmic orbit, then the movements of the heavenly bodies, the relationship between the sun and the earth, and that between the moon and the earth, will be manifest in your own body. Even without knowing the time outside, without a calendar or a view of the sky, even if you are put into a brightly lit or completely dark room with no windows for months, you will be able to know the phase of the moon and the time of the lunar cycle's end. Why? Because the relationship between the moon and the earth are in precise step with your own microcosmic orbit, and that information can be found within you. If you are adept, you can perceive this microcosmic orbit, and you can express what you perceive. This sort of skill was possessed by the ancients, and there are those today who possess it also.

Thus, when we say that "heaven and human are joined as one," this is not merely an intellectual inference or a theory, nor is it an empty phrase; it is a very real thing. Most Chinese know that the central mean (*zhongyong* 中庸) of Confucianism is a lofty achievement. What is this *zhongyong*? Confucious's disciples elaborated upon this idea. Chengzi explains: "That which does not lean is called the mean (*zhong*), that which does not change is called the commonplace (*yong*). The mean is the orthodox way of the world. The commonplace is the universal principle of the world." Zhuzi also explains: "The mean is the name for that which is completely impartial, without overstepping or falling behind. The ordinary is that which is commonplace."

This central mean would seem to be very easy to implement. It is simply impartiality, ordinary and commonplace. But in reality, it is very difficult to attain. Therefore, in Chapter 8 of the *Doctrine of the Mean*, Confucius says: "You might be able to level the rank of all the kingdoms on the earth, you might forgo all rank and walk barefoot on naked blades, but you will not achieve the central mean." When we look back to the past, we get the feeling that we "will not achieve the central mean." If we look on the events of our current era in China, hardly anything seems impartial, from the backyard furnaces of the Great Leap Forward, daring to say that desolate mountains can be fertile farmland, daring to tell the sun and moon to find a new sky, from the People's Republic of China's "theory of the unique importance of class origin," from the public-office-only-with-degree period and the advent of ageism, to the *qigong* scandals of the past decade, and the exploits of the great debunker of *qigong* fakes, Sima Nan, to the formulated regulations governing the practice of Chinese Medicine in China—there are too many examples to count, and all of them make us feel that the central main is truly unattainable. But, having experienced all this, we only cry out more urgently than ever for the "central mean."

We know that those who in the past years have blindly followed tradition, those who have been fanatic about *qigong*, even the phenomenon of Sima Nan in recent years, that none of these exemplify the central mean, none of them are the orthodox way of the world, none of them represent unchanging principles. Regarding tradition, or the unity of heaven and human, or the circulation of the cosmic orbits, we cannot be biased toward their existence. If we are biased, it will only make trouble. Let us put you in a dark room for a week, a month, for as long as a year, and see if you can tell us whether the moon is full or whether it is new. If you cannot say, then we know for certain.

However, we also cannot be biased toward the non-existence of such things. If we are biased that they do not exist, then all the traditions, all of Chinese Medicine, suddenly becomes devoid of merit. Regarding tradition-al knowledge and understanding, regarding the study of Chinese Medicine, can we learn the method espoused by the legendary Emperor Shun and "Examine opposing views, using what lies between the two for the good of the people"? I believe that Chinese Medicine needs such a method.

The prenatal *qi* moves through the Caudal Defile during the *zi* time, through Kidney Hall during the *chou* time, through Mystic Pivot during the *yin* time, through Spinal Handle during the *mao* period, through Kiln Path during the *chen* time, through Jade Pillow during the *si* time, and through Mud Pill during the *wu* time. When the *yuanqi* is moving from the *zi* time through to the *wu* time, it travels through Caudal Defile, Spinal Handle, and Jade Pillow.

These three points are called the three "closed gates." When practic-ing the movement of the Water Wheel, it must move through these three points. Of these three gates, it could be said that each is more difficult than the other, but each gate has its own realm. Once the Jade Pillow gate has been smashed open, the prenatal *qi* enters Mud Pill. At this point the person feels invigorated, as if spring has just arrived. Mud Pill, also called Mud Pill Palace, is an important part of the body for Daoist practices and is the highest point on the human body. After Mud Pill, the prenatal *qi* rushes downward: during the *wei* period, it is at Hall of Brilliance; during the *shen* period, at the Center of the Chest; during the *you* period, at Central Venter; during the *xu* period, at Spirit Gate; and during the *hai* period, it returns to the Sea of *Qi*. As the Water Wheel moves from Caudal Defile to Mud Pill, the process resembles plowing and weeding, extremely arduous and bitter, without any pleasure to speak of. But from Mud Pill to the Sea of *Qi*, it is a process of harvesting, and the feeling is indescribably pleasurable. Whether we are practicing *qigong* or whether we are examining the issue from a purely academic perspective, the nature of the process is the same. Without the bitter cold of winter biting us to the bone, the plum that blossoms in spring is not fragrant; the exhilaration of harvesting results from the toil of sowing.

From the Center of the Chest to Spirit Gate, the points traversed during the periods *shen*, *you*, and *xu* are in Yangming territory. This territory includes the thorax and abdomen; the lungs and the "stomach family" are all found here. The regulation of this particular region of the body is decided by the function of Yangming. If Yangming function is good, then the prenatal *qi* can traverse this area of the body without hindrance. If Yangming function has some problem, then the *qi* will have a difficult time moving smoothly through this area. If the prenatal *qi* is blocked or detained in this area, then it will affect its ability to reach other areas of the body. If the circulation of the prenatal *qi* is detained in its course through the microcosmic orbit, it will not be able to correspond with the macrocosm, the patient will not enjoy health, and disease will arise.

In accord with this line of thought, as the prenatal *qi* circulates through the microcosmic orbit, it receives the functions and influences of the six channel systems separately. For instance, during the *shen*, *you*, and *xu* periods, when it is passing through the particular area of the body associated with these times, the prenatal *qi* primarily receives the Yangming function. To be more specific, the prenatal *qi* receives the influence of the Yangming functions of passage and descending. In this way, the influences of each function are spatially and temporally integrated into the entire body. We read earlier, during our discussion of application and principle, the example of the pneumonia patient who was treated by the external application of a decoction. Why was a decoction applied to the outside of the body at Shenque (CV 8) able to treat a serious case of pneumonia? How could the application of medicine to Shenque cause the patient to make a rapid and complete recovery? In the light of the integration of the Yangming function we just looked at, we have new insights into the way in which such a treatment exerted its effect.

The external application of medicine to treat internal disorders is a technique that merits heavy emphasis. The Qing dynasty physician Wu Shiji's book *Topical Remedies in Rhyme* (Liyue pianwen) focuses on such external applications of medication, and by means of such applications, any disease can be cured. Wu Shiji's book is well worth reading. There is a folk remedy used to treat cancer: an animal product is placed onto the Shanzhong (CV 17) area of the body, in the center of the sternum. The animal product is placed there once or twice, or even repeatedly. The affected area then begins to improve, and eventually the cancer completely remits. Why does this method work? Beneath Shanzhong lies the thymus, which, especially before puberty, is an active organ of the immune system that produces viable T-lymphocytes. There is a direct relationship between the activity of T-cells and the emergence of cancer. Why do the majority of cancers begin after the age of 40? Because after the age of 40 (in women a little earlier), the thymus withers, and the production of T-lymphocytes gradually declines; there is a loss of T-cell related immunity, and the population of these cells is ravaged. The location of Shanzhong is in Yangming territory. According to the *Plain Questions's* "Treatise on the Heavenly Truth in Remote Antiquity": "At the age of five times seven (thirty-five years of age) the vessels of Yangming decline, the face darkens, and the hair begins to drop out." Does topical application to Shanzhong in the Yangming part of the body strengthen Yangming, and turn on the function of the thymus? It is a question worthy of further study.

There are so many potentially significant research topics in Chinese Medicine, one hardly knows where to start. Why is scientific research only directed at one or two areas of study? If you open up a Chinese Medicine research journal, all you find is articles examining the effect of such and such a medicine on such and such a disease, or this formula on that condition, and so on. They are limited to one or two types of study. Everyone is crowding into the same route, hoping for the same sort of success establishing the efficacy of a particular herb or formula. No one dares to leave the beaten path, for who wants to expend effort without the hope of some success? The fear of pursuing a dead end is too great for these researchers to dare to take a new path. I cannot understand why we are so fixated on the same sort of studies over and over, while neglecting such potentially significant and influential research. Why is our concept of what is possible so limited? Why not look a little further on?

III.4. The Essentials of Treating the Yangming Orientation

The inherent qualities of Yangming are passage, descent, and coolness, and Yangming disease is characterized by the loss of these three qualities. Thus, when treating Yangming disease, i.e. when designing Yangming formulas, the goal is to restore Yangming's innate passage, descent, and coolness. If we look at the representative Yangming formulas, Baihu Tang and the Chengqi decoctions, we see that each of these restores these Yangming functions. The three Chengqi decoctions are all cool in nature, and they all open and descend. If used appropriately, their application can restore the Yangming function. This is simple to understand.

But what about Baihu Tang? When those who have not studied Chinese Medicine hear the name of this formula, they find it strange. Once the name is explained to them, they usually find it fascinating. The *baihu* (White Tiger) is the west, the earthly branches *shen, you,* and *xu,* and the three months of autumn. Why does Yangming disease require the use of the white tiger of the west, *shen, you,* and *xu,* and the three months of autumn? As we know, the main pathogenic influences that cause Yangming disease are fire and heat. It is heat and fire that cause the loss of the passage of the hollow Yangming organs and the failure of Yangming to descend. When Baihu Tang is administered, the *qi* cools and is no longer warm, and the normal function of Yangming recovers. Therefore, Baihu Tang not only represents the west, it also represents the three months of autumn, which overlap with the three time periods in which Yangming disease tends to resolve.

When, in Chinese Medicine, we say that we prescribe a formula, why don't we also say that we are prescribing a particular time? For in truth, that is precisely what we are doing, prescribing a particular quality of a specific juncture in the rhythmic cycling of time. We can look at Baihu Tang from several different angles. First, there are the herbs that make up the formula. The formula is constituted of four herbs. Why four? The *River Chart* says: "The four of earth produces metal, the nine of heaven completes it." The number four is the number of metal; it is the number associated with the west. This correlates with the name of the formula, as well as *shen, you,* and *xu.* Secondly, the sovereign herb in this formula, Shigao, is white in color and pungent in flavor. White is the color of the west, and pungency is its flavor, and these correspond with both the western direction and the earthly branches with which it is associated. Third, we have the amounts of each herb used in the formula: one pound of Shigao and six *liang* (a traditional unit of weight in Chinese Medicine, of approximately 50 grams or 1.8 ounces) of the minister herb, Zhimu. What do the numbers one and six represent? The *River Chart* says: "The one of heaven produces water, the six of earth completes it." Knowing that one and six are the numbers associated with water, in other words, the numbers of the north, we can surmise that the cooling and fire-extinguishing properties of Baihu Tang are conveyed by the cold water of the north, by the cooling and clearing properties of the north. The west using the numbers of the north is not only a case of the "son saving the mother," it also exemplifies the mutual engendering of metal and water. By making use of the function of these numbers, the potency of Baihu Tang achieves a manifold increase. The assistant herb in this formula, Jingmi, which is round-grained non-glutinous rice, is also prescribed in the amount of six *he*. The function of Jingmi is to produce fluids and secretions, therefore the number associated with water is used.

The last ingredient in the formula is licorice, in the amount of two *liang*. What does "two" represent? Two is the number of the fire of the south. Why is this fire number used in a formula that is aimed at purging fire? The formula employs the cold herbs Shigao and Zhimu, both of which are able to clear heat and fire, but these are also capable of damaging the physiological fire of the central yang. The use of the two *liang* of Gancao is to moderate the cooling action of the Shigao and Zhimu and protect the central yang. The Gancao in this measurement allows the formula to exert a strong west and north influence without harming the central earth element.

To summarize the functions of these key Yangming formulas, both Baihu Tang and the three Chengqi decoctions exert the effect of the periods defined by the earthly branches *shen, you,* and *xu.* Why does Yangming disease tend to resolve during these periods? The reason is clear, but if we wish to substantiate this rationale, if we wish to gain real benefit from this understanding of prescribing formulas as if prescribing qualities of time, it requires real dedication and hard work. You must first look things over, taking a broad view and integrating this understanding into every aspect of Chinese Medicine theory. Then you will have received real benefits.

If we take a moment to reflect on Yangming, and the emphasis on warmth and heat as the crucial pathogenic factors inducing Yangming disease, it comes to mind that there are many who feel the understanding of Warm Disease developed out of Yangming disease. I think this is a reasonable conclusion, to an extent. From a horizontal east–west perspective, when we go forward from Yangming it looks like the defensive aspect of Warm Disease, and backward it looks like disease wrought by a pathogen at the nutritive and blood level; from a vertical south–north perspective, above it looks like an ailment of the upper burner, and below like one of the lower burner. The Four Stages (defensive, *qi*, nutritive, and blood stages) and the Triple Burner pivot are all found in the Yangming chapter. Did Zhang Zhongjing only discuss cold, and did Ye Tianshi, Xue Shengbai, Wang Mengying, and Wu Jutong, the renowned progenitors of warm disease theory, only discuss warmth? Obviously not, though each specialty certainly has its own particular expertise. This only prods us to think of our earlier discussion regarding the "central mean" of Confucianism. The central mean is the way of kings, not of subjects. In other words, the central mean is a concept intended for leaders, not for ordinary people. Can scholars and specialists make use of the central mean? If you are a scholar or a specialist in some field and you strive to attain the central mean, then you will be destined for mediocrity, and will not amount to anything worthwhile.

This morning, I watched a television broadcast of an important lecture by the Nobel Prize–winning physicist Professor Yang Zhenning called "Beauty and Physics." The subject was two important figures in twentieth-century physics, Paul Adrien Maurice Dirac and Werner Heisenberg. If we compare these two figures of the last century, we find their styles and personalities to be irreconcilable. In their days, their research was considered tantamount to heresy. When Dirac published his equation, it was met with derision and ridicule from the great physicists of the time. Their "heresies" turned out to be breakthroughs that revolutionized physics in the twentieth century. Whether you are a specialist or a scholar, you must have a particular orientation, and after you have picked your direction, you must pursue it wholeheartedly. This orientation becomes your angle of attack, despite the fact that it also makes you biased. If you do not have such an angle of attack but hem and haw looking for an unbiased perspective, you will not amount to anything. You will give up halfway! As a scholar or a specialist, or really anything else, you must be completely absorbed in your point of view, you must rigidly adhere to your chosen perspective.

For instance, in the study of Chinese Medicine, there are undoubtedly two different paths that one can take. You can either pursue the route of modernity, and study molecular biology, and look at everything from a modern perspective, and understand Chinese Medicine from an entirely modern perspective, and transform Chinese Medicine into something new, something that conforms to this modern perspective, and thereby develop Chinese Medicine. Or, you become absorbed in the classics, and you see everything in terms of the classics, you delve deeply into the classics, and perhaps you will find them to not be at odds with modern science, and if you modify them slightly perhaps they will fit with modern science just fine, and perhaps the ancient will even be able to instruct the modern. Of course, becoming absorbed in the classics does not hamper you from paying close attention to the present. In fact, you must take interest in that which is new and modern, but you must also pay attention to the traditional while doing so.

To take interest in something and to become absorbed in something are two different things. The modern and the traditional are polar opposites. You can only grasp one of these polarities. You cannot be both an outstanding expert on the classics and a great physicist. Take for instance Professor Yang Zhenning. His focus is modern physics, specifically theoretical physics. However, Professor Yang Zhenning also takes great interest in traditional Chinese culture, as well as traditional Chinese Medicine. But could Professor Yang, this highly gifted intellect, be both a Nobel Prize–winning physicist and an expert in Chinese Medicine? Absolutely not! As Mencius suggests, one cannot have both fish and bear paws at the same time.

However, leaders and politicians face a very different scenario. They must have fish and bear paws on the same plate; they must take into account different and opposing points of view. To see both poles and make use of what lies in the middle is the highest achievement of the central mean, and the utmost that a king or ruler can achieve. If you were a leader, someone who sets policy, and you took the stance of the specialist, only allowing Chinese Medicine doctors to study modern advances or only allowing them to study the classics, then I think Chinese Medicine would quickly deteriorate. I invite the reader to answer on their own, whether or not this was previously the situation with Chinese Medicine.

Let us take a very simple example. In the recent past in the People's Republic of China, when rising up in rank as a Chinese Medicine doctor, you could either take a test in a foreign language or one in classical medical Chinese. These were your two choices. This had its strong point. If you studied the classics deeply, then you had no time to learn a foreign language, and you could take the classical Chinese test. On the other hand, if your focus was in the modernization of Chinese Medicine, and your foreign language ability was strong, then you could take the foreign language test. This sort of setup smacks of the central mean to some extent. If you like the classics, then you study the old scriptures and there you go, all is well; you can become absorbed in the traditional world of Chinese Medicine. You have the green light to study the classics; you need not worry that by studying the classics, you might end up in disfavor and lose your professional standing. At the same time, if you want to pursue the modern, well then good! Go ahead and focus on modernization. In this way, Chinese Medicine practitioners could dive head first into their chosen path of study. I think that the politicians and the makers of policy should turn in their own points of view. If, prior to becoming a policy maker, one has a particular point of view or a specialty that one is passionate about, then it must be set aside. In its stead, the maker of policy should create an environment in which both traditional and modern take on Chinese Medicine, and research into either branch of the field have bright prospects. Funding must be divided equally between the two camps, so that research into both traditional Chinese Medicine and the modernization of Chinese Medicine have an opportunity to flourish. If only such an environment with such an ambience of equality were created, it would create the best possible circumstances for allowing Chinese Medicine to emerge from its current predicament.

Unfortunately, the situation at the moment is different. Classical Chinese language ability counts for nothing. In order to get a promotion, one has to perform well on a foreign language test. If not, even if one's skill in Chinese Medicine is outstanding, there will be no promotion to director or appointment to the position of professor. It is not my intent to suggest that Chinese Medicine practitioners do not need to study foreign languages; it is just that the way the policy has changed has send out a signal that there are fewer and fewer "green lights" for the study of the classics.

The modernization of Chinese Medicine, on the other hand, is the general trend, and is the popular sentiment, and the irresistible tide of history. When I started to write this book, I was still harboring inordinate ambitions, but Confucius has made me too wise for that now. Within the Chinese Medicine profession, the vast majority are devoted to the modernization of Chinese Medicine, whereas only a tiny handful of practitioners are devoted to the classicization of Chinese Medicine. Take, for example, my classmates from my doctoral program. Some have gone to China's burgeoning metropolises of Guangzhou or Shenzhen, others to Beijing or Shanghai; some have even ventured off to foreign countries. All of them have been chasing after the modernization of Chinese Medicine. Only I, this villager from the mountains, have returned to the backwaters of Guangxi province. From comparing my situation with that of my classmates, I think you can discern the current condition of Chinese Medicine. Those who pursue the modernization of Chinese Medicine are not satisfied going simply to Beijing and Shanghai; they are compelled to venture as far afield as New York and London. Whenever they have a long sabbatical, however, where do they rush to? They go to Yellow Mountain, or Mount Tai, or Jiuzhaigou National Park in Sichuan. They all go to little villages in remote and mountainous areas. The current state of Chinese Medicine is reflected in this dynamic.

So here I wish to express encouragement for my colleagues that study the traditional aspects of Chinese Medicine. While you should not expect everybody in our field to focus on the traditional, you also need not worry that there is nobody who is interested in this aspect. If we take New York and the mountain hamlets of Western Sichuan as polarities analogous to modernized and traditional Chinese Medicine, then we have hope. Extremes produce their opposite, after all. Professor Gu Zhengkun of Peking University's English department gave a lecture called "The Internet with Regard to Chinese and Western Culture." At the end of this lecture, Professor Gu came to an interesting conclusion: when the internet age has truly arrived, "there may be a population shift from cities to small villages. The ruins of cities will remain only to act as reminders of the polluted environment in which our backward ancestors subsisted." I think that the end of Professor Gu's lecture may very well predict the future of Chinese Medicine. Perhaps in the not-so-distant future, there will be a return to tradition, to classical Chinese Medicine. Of course, this return will not be a return in the materialistic sense. Instead, it will be a sort of spiritual and intellectual return.

III.5. The Time When Yangming Disease Tends to Act

We will examine two levels of meaning of the time at which Yangming disease tends to flare up. First, we will look at the conventionally indicated times, and second we will look at a very unique aspect of Yangming's time correspondence.

III.5.a. From Yin to Chen

The times at which Yangming disease is likely to worsen are opposite to the times that it tends to resolve, just as we saw with Taiyang disease. Yangming disease tends to resolve during the time period from *shen* to *xu* (3 pm to 9 pm), so the time in which it is likely to act up is of course the opposite end of the cycle, *yin* to *chen* (3 am to 9 am). The time period comprised by the three earthly branches *shen*, *you*, and *xu*, corresponds to the three months of autumn, and to the west. The nature of these three governs coolness and descending, the physiological nature of Yangming. *Yin*, *mao*, and *chen* are the eastern direction; they are warm in nature, and they govern ascent. In short, the nature of these three is exactly contrary to the physiological function of Yangming. For this reason, these three can easily contribute to Yangming disease, and during this period of time, Yangming disease will tend to be aggravated. Knowing this characteristic time correspondence becomes very helpful when diagnosing Yangming disease.

III.5.b. Tidal Fever at Sundown

A feature of Yangming disease is its association with the *ribusuo* (日晡所), the time period of late afternoon. Specifically, it has a tendency to exhibit tidal fevers during that time in the late afternoon or early evening. Two characteristic features define tidal fever. First, it is periodic. This period is the *ribusuo*, the period defined by the earthly branches *shen*, *you*, and *xu*. Secondly, tidal fever is a high fever. This is an important point. It is not the case that any fever that periodically occurs during the time in question is a tidal fever. If you mistakenly hold to this understanding of Yangming or Yangming bowel syndrome, then you will have problems. It is called "tidal fever," but it is not an ordinary fever; this fever has a truly tidal quality. The ripples made by stone thrown into a pool of water are not equivalent to flooding ebb and flow of a tide. A tide is a mighty thing; it has force and momentum. An ordinary fever, or a low fever, cannot be called a tidal fever.

Tidal fever that emerges around the time of sunset is of great importance to our ability to diagnose Yangming disease, especially Yangming bowel disease. If we open to the Yangming chapter, we find references to "tidal fever" throughout. Our forefathers discriminated between two types of Yangming disease: Yangming channel and Yangming bowel. Tidal fever was instrumental to the definitive diagnosis of Yangming bowel excess disease. Furthermore, in the Yangming chapter, determining the appropriate use of the two Da and Xiao Chengqi Tang, especially Da Chengqi Tang, depended first and foremost upon the presence of tidal fever as a symptom. As it says in line 208: "If the fever is not tidal, then Chengqi Tang is not indicated." The tidal fever of Yangming bowel disease is characteristically one that presents at in the late afternoon. It is fitting, then, that we discuss the term *ribusuo*. The *Jade Discourse* (Yupian) of the Song Dynasty defines *ribu* as "The time of *shen*," which means 3–5 pm. In the *Huainanzi* essay "Patterns of Heaven," we read: "When the sun reaches the sentimental valley, that is the time of *bu*." If we look at the etymology of the term *bu* (晡), we find that the phonetic element on the right half of the character (甫) connotes eating, thus it is combined with a mouth radical and a flesh radical to form the characters meaning "to nurture" (哺) and "dried meat" (脯). So, what does it mean when it is combined with a sun radical (日)? The meaning is clearly that the sun is being devoured, the time when the sun disappears behind the ragged, mountainous horizon. Moreover, we read in *Explaining Writing and Analyzing Characters*: "*Fu* (甫) is a laudatory title (*meicheng*, literally 'beautiful title') for a man." The sun is yang and therefore male, thus 日 together with 甫 describes the beauty of the sun. When the sun begins to disappear, it is the most beautiful time of the day, thus the time of sundown is also referred to as *ribu* (日晡).

Here, the term *ribu* is used in conjunction with the character *suo* (所). *Suo* is a character with a fairly broad range of meanings. It can represent time or place. When we understand it to represent time, it of course represents the time discussed above, and the *Jade Discourse* definitively set it as the time of *shen* (3–5 pm). Other sources seem to have a more flexible denotation of the term, which might be due to the fact that the sun disappears behind the mountain ridges occurs differently and at different times depending upon such factors as latitude and longitude, topography, and season, to name a few.

What then of *suo* as denoting place instead of time? In nature, where does the sun set? It sets in the western hemisphere. From the eastern hemisphere it appears to be descending, and in the western hemisphere it appears to be ascending. Where do these processes take place within the human body? Where does the "sun" of the human body set? It sets, of course, in Yangming. We can observe this directly in the character of the time period *you* (酉), which is composed of the character for "west" (西) plus the character denoting the number "one" (一). What does the number "one" represent? Here, it represents the unbroken yang line of the *Classic of Changes* hexagrams. The character *you* (酉) represents the time when the "one," the yang, the sun, enters the west, for when we see the sun in the west, we know that it is in the process of descending. Furthermore, *shen*, *you*, and *xu* are the three earthly branches ruled by Yangming. For this reason, the yang descends in Yangming, where else? In addition, *Explaining Writing and Analyzing Characters* says: "*Suo* is the sound of trees being cut down." And from the *Classic of Poetry*: "Cutting down trees, *suo . . . suo. . . .*" It is metal that is able to cut down trees. Thus, the customary meaning of *suo* as "place" might be replaced with "metal." Using *ribu* in conjunction with *suo* is a further indication that *ribu* occurs at the time of metal. Because it indicates metal, it of course includes the three periods of *shen*, *you*, and *xu*. This harkens back to what was said by Fang Zhongxing, the Ming Dynasty Cold Damage scholar: "If there is heat only during the *shen*, *you*, and *xu* periods, and if in all the other periods of time there is no heat, then it is tidal fever."

When we discuss tidal fever, it is important for everyone to keep two important characteristics in mind. First, it is characterized by its timing. This time, of course, is sundown (*ribusuo*), namely *shen*, *you*, and *xu*. Second, it is characterized by degree. This second characteristic is especially important, as it is easy to ignore. The first characteristic of timing by itself is not enough to completely define tidal fever. If timing alone is used to understand Yangming and Yangming bowel syndrome, there will be problems. With a name like tidal fever, we know that it does not refer to a regular fever; we have to emphasize the "tidal" aspect. If you throw a stone into a pool and make some ripples, this is not called "tide." Even great waves or flooding cannot be called "tidal." This is because of the second characteristic: that of degree, or of momentum. Regular fever, and especially low fever, cannot be called tidal fever. If we take another look at the quote in the preceding paragraph from Fang Zhongxing, we can see that he only described half of the picture.

Earlier, we discussed tides at some length. The tides swell when the moon is full. Thus, there is the Chinese saying: "When the moon is full, 'watch' the tide." But during what part of the year are the tides the greatest? During the eighth lunar month. The hexagram associated with the eighth month is called *guan* (Watching). Why is the hexagram associated with the eighth month of the year called *guan*? An interesting question! Why do the tides ebb and flow? Earlier, we discussed this in terms of being the result of the function of yang *qi*. When the yang is joined with the yin, this is called a tide. If the tides are the result of a process related to yang *qi*, why is the largest tide not during the summer? Why is it not when the yang *qi* is fullest? Why instead is it during the eighth month of the year, when the yang *qi* is beginning to subside? This is a result of the two forces that contribute to the formation of a tide. There is the force that pushes forward, the yang force. There is also a force that resists this yang movement, and acts as an obstruction to its forward momentum. This force is a function of yin.

If there were only the forward momentum, could it possibly form a tide? It could not form a tide. The most this unopposed force could produce would be the swift and uneventful flow of water, like a waterfall, not like a tide. To produce a tide, the forward thrust must be met by resistance. When the force of the forward thrust and the resistance to that thrust are perfectly equal, when the function of yin and yang are nearly perfectly matched, the strongest tide is produced. This is why the tide is strongest during the eighth lunar month. When the concept of a tide is clearly understood, then tidal fever is easy to explain. Both the timeliness and the degree of tidal fever must be taken note of.

When our predecessors discussed Yangming, they primarily talked about it with regard to its channel and its associated bowel. With regard to disease of the Yangming channel, they spoke of fever. To Yangming bowel syndrome, they also ascribed fever. What is the difference between these fevers? The difference lies in whether the fever is tidal or not. No mention is made of tidal fever with regard to Yangming channel disease; Yangming bowel disease exhibits tidal fever. Thus, the tidal fever of Yangming bowel disease is the primary distinction between the two. We talked about how the fever of the Yangming channel was related to a loss of the physiological coolness and descent of Yangming. We also discussed a third characteristic of Yangming, that of "passage." The level of the loss of this "passage" on Yangming channel disease is not high, but not so with Yangming bowel disease. When we discuss the bowels, the necessity of passage to their healthy function is paramount, and a loss of passage is a great hindrance to their normal physiological functioning. For instance, in the Yangming chapter, we find the line: "In the stomach there must be five or six pieces of dry stool." When dry excrement blocks the way of Yangming, and Yangming heat is also abundant, we have both the forward thrusting and obstructing forces that cause the tidal fever of Yangming bowel syndrome. Thus, whether the fever is tidal or not, along with the intensity of the heat itself, depends upon the extent to which there is an obstruction in the pathway of the bowel.

Why is it said that "If the fever is not tidal, you cannot administer Chengqi Tang"? This is because if there is no tidal heat, then an obstruction in the Yangming bowel is not an important factor. And if there is no significant obstruction of the Yangming bowel, why in the world would one use any of the Chengqi decoctions? Chinese Medicine concepts may seem loose and carefree, but in actuality they are strict and rigorous. Take, for example, the syndrome associated with tidal heat. It is strictly and rigorously defined in relation to Chinese Medicine theory.

III.6. Contemplating Hypertension

The time of sundown (*ribusuo*) is originally the period in which Yangming tends to resolve, but the tendency for tidal fevers at this time is not only the time Yangming disease tends to become more severe, but it is also a key to correctly diagnosing Yangming bowel excess syndrome, as well as a key to knowing when to administer the Da or Xiao Chengqi Tang. Clearly this aspect of Yangming is quite unique, and this uniqueness can lead us to ponder some other related issues.

Some years ago, I came across a Japanese report that stated a strong connection between hypertensive arteriosclerosis and the "large pulse" of Yangming disease. This connection was substantiated by the progress patients made when taking a Baihu formula consisting primarily of Shigao.

At the time, I did not think much of the conclusions made in this report. I felt that drawing a connection between Shigao, hypertensive arteriosclerosis, and Yangming was far too rigid. Up until I began writing this chapter on Yangming, that is. Then, the significance of the connection between Shigao and arteriosclerosis suddenly became as clear as day. What is the purpose of the blood pressure? Why are so many people hypertensive in our present age? Let us first contemplate these questions in terms of the laws of physics.

The purpose of the blood pressure is to ensure a steady flow of blood to the tissues. Every minute, every second, the organs of the body require a certain amount of blood flow for the delivery of oxygen and other nutrients, and the removal of waste products, like carbon dioxide. A certain degree of blood flow is required to maintain normal human metabolism. Normally, blood pressure is maintained at a particular level and is fairly constant, but blood pressure can change in response to particular stimuli throughout the course of the day. Thus, blood pressure has a normal range of fluctuation in the healthy individual. For instance, diastolic pressure between 60 and 90 mmHg (millimeters of mercury) and systolic pressure between 90 and 120 mmHg are considered normal blood pressure readings by most physicians in China.

Why does blood pressure become elevated beyond these normal ranges? In short, blood pressure is elevated in response to decreased perfusion of the tissues of the body with blood. When the bodily tissues do not receive adequate blood flow, certain hormones are released that result in an increase in blood pressure. Elevated blood pressure is the result of the body attempting to maintain the adequate perfusion of blood to the tissues of the body. So why has the flow of blood to the tissues decreased, resulting in an increase of blood pressure? Why is the perfusion of blood not the same as before? Obviously, this is the result of impedance to the flow of blood through the circulatory system of the body. The flow of blood is impeded by a thickening of the blood vessels, by a narrowing of the arterial lumen, or by other obstructive processes. If the blood pressure were to remain constant despite this impedance to flow, the result would be inadequate perfusion of blood to the tissues.

How do we resolve this contradiction? The obstructions to the flow of blood found in the circulatory system cannot simply be removed, but the flow of blood to the tissues must also be maintained at the appropriate rate. The human organism has no choice but to raise blood pressure, but this results in a vicious cycle of an increase in the thickening and narrowing of the blood vessels in an effort to resist the increased blood pressure and an increase in the blood pressure to counter this increased resistance of the blood vessels.

This depiction of hypertension is a rough sketch of the disease, nevertheless it points out the etiology of hypertension: occlusion of the blood vessels and an impedance of the normal flow of blood. For this reason, the basic principle to cure high blood pressure is not to decrease the blood pressure directly. If we prescribe anti-hypertensive medications, the body may simply respond by further increasing the blood pressure in order to ensure adequate perfusion of the tissues with blood. So how do we cure high blood pressure at its root? We must remove this obstruction to the flow of blood. If the obstructions to blood flow are reduced or removed, the blood pressure will decrease on its own, without the use of calcium channel blockers or diuretics. Why is the incidence of hypertension higher every year? Why does the population of hypertensives grow younger every year? It is because of an increasing incidence of obstruction (a lack of "passage," an essential characteristic of Yangming) in our circulatory systems. We must not forget to include behavioral and even social contributors to the advent of high blood pressure.

How do we remove the hindrances to the flow of blood? How do we defeat hypertension at its very root? This is a question that must be answered by Chinese and Western Medicine, hand in hand.

That is as far as we will discuss Yangming disease.

CHAPTER SEVEN

THE ESSENTIALS OF SHAOYANG DISEASE

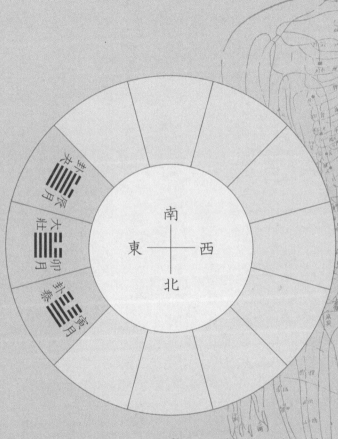

Shaoyang disease tends to resolve in the time from *yin* to *chen*.

I. An Explanation of Shaoyang

We have already discussed certain basic aspects of Shaoyang in earlier chapters of this book. In this chapter, we will discuss four different aspects of the connotations of Shaoyang.

I.1. The Meaning of Shaoyang

What is meant by Shaoyang? *Shao* (少) carries the same meaning as the character *xiao* (小), "small," i.e. not yet big. Thus, if we look at the meaning of the characters alone, we know that Shaoyang is the yang that has just been born, the yang that is not big yet. It is along these lines that the *Yellow Emperor's Classic* has an additional name for Shaoyang, namely "first yang." This is the initial level of Shaoyang's meaning.

The second layer of meaning pertains to Daoist descriptions of the monarchs of the four directions. The monarch of the eastern direction was called Shaoyang. Ascribing the name Shaoyang to this god of the east, we see that the east was clearly associated with Shaoyang. If Shaoyang is associated with the east, then it is also associated with the three months of spring, and with the time periods of *yin, mao,* and *chen.* This orientation certainly tallies with the basic nature of Shaoyang. Thus it is said: "Physicians and Daoists are governed by the same precept." This is certainly a truthful statement!

The third level of meaning relates to the element associated with Shaoyang. If Shaoyang is related to the east, and to emerging yang, and to the yang that is not yet big, then it is certainly also related to the wood element. But in terms of the five movements and six *qi (wuyun liuqi)*, Shaoyang is related to the ministerial fire. This makes it clear that in the classics, Shaoyang has a dual nature and is related to both wood and fire.

This dual nature actually reflects the difference between the form and function of fire. If we look at the pre- and postnatal trigram sequences of the *Classic of Changes,* we see that the trigram *Li* is ascribed to fire, and in the postnatal arrangement it belongs to the southern direction. The south is related to fire, and this orientation reflects the functional aspect of fire. In the prenatal sequence, the *Li* trigram is oriented in the east, in the wood direction. This is related to the form of fire, its origin. Fire comes from wood. In ancient times, fire-starting was much different than it is today, as there were no matches, no lighters, no electronic igniters, etc. The ancients relied on the wood-drill method to start their fires.

In still earlier times, before the advent of the hand drill, how did we humans acquire fire? We got it from lightning. After the third solar term, the third of the twenty-four calendrical periods, called *Jingzhe* (Awakening of Insects), thunder sounds and lightning strikes, setting fire to dry grass and dry wood. This is the most natural, most primeval kindling of fire. Thunder belongs to spring, spring belongs to wood, and this reinforces the connection between wood and fire. Thunder belongs to spring, the dragon also belongs to the category of spring; thunder belongs to the east, and the people of China call themselves the "dragon" and consider themselves to be descendants of the dragon. So then, what is the "dragon," after all? Does the dragon simply refer to a dinosaur? Absolutely not! Is the dragon real or unreal? Only when thunder peals and lightning flashes can we catch glimpses of the dragon's form. Is there a real connection between dragons and lightning? The descendants of the dragon must determine the answer. But when the ancients spoke of Shaoyang fire and called it the "fire of the thunder dragon," this was related to the source of fire in the natural, pre-technological world.

The dragon thunder fire, the wood fire, the fire within wood, fire emerging from within wood—these ideas explain the dual nature of Shaoyang.

I.2. The Meaning of the Shaoyang Channels

In terms of the channels and collaterals, there is the Shaoyang channel of the arm and the Shaoyang channel of the leg. In this case, the significance of the Shaoyang leg channel stands out. The Shaoyang leg channel covers the two sides of the body, the Taiyang leg channel spreads across the back of the body, and the Yangming leg channel courses across the front of the body. Once again, the "Treatise on the Separation and Union of Yin and Yang" in the *Plain Questions* says: "Taiyang opens, Yangming closes, and Shaoyang pivots." This relationship between opening, closing, and pivoting is reflected in the areas of the body related to each of the three yang channels.

Shaoyang is on either side, just as the hinges of a traditional Chinese gate were on either side. The hinges of the gate governed their capacity to open and close, just as Shaoyang governs the ability of Taiyang and

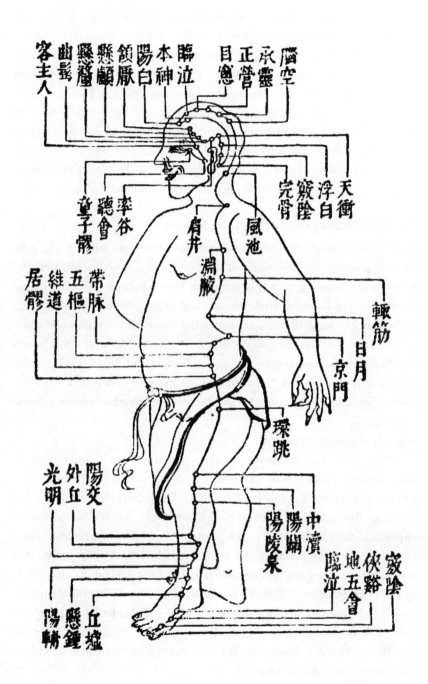

Yangming to open and close. If we define it in more detail: the left is yang, the right is yin. The yang governs opening, and the yin governs closing. Thus, the left Shaoyang is primarily responsible for the opening of Taiyang, and the right Shaoyang is primarily responsible for Yangming's opening. For this reason, if the left Shaoyang becomes diseased, it primarily impacts Taiyang, and it should be treated by addressing Taiyang. In the *Treatise on Cold Damage*, we find the Chaihu Guizhi Tang is designed for this purpose. If the right Shaoyang becomes diseased, it will primarily impact Yangming. The corresponding formula in the *Treatise on Cold Damage* is Da Chaihu Tang, though Xiao Chaihu Jia Mangxiao Tang is intended for this as well.

I.3. The Meaning of the Shaoyang Bowels

The Shaoyang bowels are the gallbladder and the triple warmer. The gallbladder is one of the six bowels of the body, and is an especially peculiar bowel. Why do we say that it is peculiar? The gallbladder, stomach, large intestine, small intestine, triple burner, and urinary bladder constitute the six bowels, but none of them are categorized as both bowels and "extraordinary" bowels except the gallbladder. If we look at the viscera and bowels from a functional perspective, the viscera are yin and the bowels are yang. Viscera and bowels are different in that the five viscera primarily store the *jing* and *qi*, but do not drain, whereas the six bowels primarily transport and transform the contents, but do not store. One stores and does not drain, the other drains but does not store.

The gallbladder is different from all the other viscera and bowels, in that it exhibits properties of both bowels and viscera. It is able to both drain without storing and store without draining. The gallbladder is a bowel that possesses the capacity of both a bowel and a viscus. It is not biased toward either, and thus truly dwells in the position of righteous centeredness and balance. It is unique among the viscera and bowels in this regard. It is precisely because of the unique ambivalence of the gallbladder that it says in the *Plain Questions's* "Treatise on the Six Nodes and Visceral Manifestations": "All eleven of the organs depend on the gallbladder." Thus, it says in the "Treatise on the Spiritual Orchid Secret Canon" in the *Plain Questions* that the gallbladder "holds the office of centered righteousness. Decisions and judgments originate from it."

Referring to the gallbladder as the official of "centered righteousness" is no casual statement. If one wishes to be truly impartial, then you must reside in the center, in a state of equanimity. If the gallbladder drained without storing, or stored without draining, it would be biased, and that would hardly do for the "office of centered righteousness" who issues the decisions. Only if it possesses this prerequisite impartiality can it be capable of making right decisions, otherwise the result will be bribery, fraud, corruption, and abuse of the law! For this reason, in the *Plain Questions's* "Treatise on the Spiritual Orchid Secret Canon," the gallbladder is ascribed with this particular attribute of impartiality. This designation is significant not only to human physiology, but also to social harmony.

Furthermore, if we look at the composition of the simplified character for gallbladder (*dan* 胆), we see that the phonetic component (*dan* 旦) consists of the sun emerging from the earth, the sun rising in the east, illuminating every corner of the land with brilliant light. Thus, this component of the character means brightness. It is precisely this brilliance that enables it to handle decisions. If you are not bright but instead are dim-witted and fatuous, if you are lost in lust for riches, or power-hungry, how can you possibly possess equanimity? How can you make important decisions in an impartial way? One must be bright to make correct decisions. This meaning is contained within the composition of the character.

The gallbladder is the official of centered righteousness, it rules brightness and brilliance, and it is also the "clean" official. We can use four words to sum up the gallbladder: upright, just, incorruptible, and intelligent. But in reality, only if it is "upright, just, incorruptible, and intelligent" can the judgments it passes truly be fair and impartial. For this reason, our discussion of the gallbladder is not simply a discussion of human physiology, life sciences, or biology, but also a commentary on very important social issues. As our study delves into physiology, it brings to light social issues, just as the recognition of social iniquities furthers our understanding of physiological topics. This is the social medicine model revealed in the "Treatise on the Spiritual Orchid Secret Canon."

Let us proceed to an examination of the triple burner. The official position of the triple burner, as defined in the "Treatise on the Spiritual Orchid Secret Canon," is: "The triple burner holds the office of clearing the canals. The paths of water originate from it." What is meant by "clearing the canals" (*jue du*)? *Jue* means to dredge, to flow, to open up what is blocked.

Thus, the *Spiritual Pivot* chapter "Nine Needles and Twelve Sources" states: "Even if blocked up for a long time, it can still be dredged."

What exactly is meant by *du*? *Explaining Writing and Analyzing Characters* says that *du* is an "irrigation canal; ditch." A ditch is a small canal (*du*). Thus, we read that the "Yangzi, Hu, Huai, and Yellow River are the four canals (*du*)." Thus, to clear the canals means that this official is in charge of keeping the irrigation canals and ditches open and unimpeded. Hence, "The triple burner holds the office of clearing the canals. The paths of water originate from it." Only if the waterways are open can it be ensured that water will benefit the myriad things and not do them harm. For this reason, this official of clearing the canals is extremely important to both the health of the body and the prosperity of a nation and its people.

Why does the triple burner (*sanjiao* 三焦) assume the office of clearing the canals? This is a complicated question and the subject of much debate. It would seem that I also lack the ability to clarify it. In light of this, I would like to relay some related views on the matter. First, let us look at the character *jiao*. The meaning of this character is relatively clear. The four dots at the bottom (灬) of the character represent fire, so it is clearly related to fire. When we roast something over a fire, it has a burnt (*jiao*) odor to it. Thus, the "burnt" odor is the smell associated with fire. The "burnt" or "scorched" quality is a manifestation of the function of fire. If we look at the five movements and six *qi*, and realize that Shaoyang is related to the ministerial fire, the connection between the triple burner and fire becomes more definite.

The office of clearing the canals is assumed by the triple burner. The opening and clearing of the waterways is accomplished by the triple burner. What does this tell us? This tells us that the full function of water depends upon the action of fire, and reiterates the principle we discussed in the Taiyang chapter.

If we clearly understand the meaning of *jiao*, and correctly assume that it is related to fire, why is it called the "triple" burner? The number three (*san* 三) in *sanjiao* refers to the three characteristics of fire. There are three origins of fire. Broadly stated, there is celestial fire, terrestrial fire, and the fire of human beings. To put it in narrower terms, there is the fire of the upper burner, the fire of the middle burner, and the fire of the lower burner. The fire of the upper burner is primarily the yang of the heart and lungs, the fire of the middle burner is primarily the spleen yang, and the fire of the lower burner the yang of the kidney.

Let us remember for a moment what was said about edema in the standard *Chinese Internal Medicine* textbook: water metabolism is primarily related to the interplay of the lungs, the spleen, and the kidneys. The natures of fire, the origins of fire, are three in number. For the same reason, if we look at the water that is acted on by these three fires, we see three distinct subjects: the upper burner acts upon the heaven water, the middle burner acts upon the earth water, and the lower burner acts upon the water of water.

If we place this discussion into the larger context of the natural world, we see that the celestial water is rainwater; the lungs act as the heavens among the five viscera, the lungs are the upper source of water. Thus, the water ruled by the lungs is related to the celestial water. The terrestrial water is the water that flows below ground, the unseen pathways of water through the earth. The spleen rules transportation and transformation, the spleen belongs to earth, earth controls water; thus, the water governed by the spleen corresponds to the terrestrial water. The water of water refers to large bodies of water, rivers, lakes, and seas. The kidney is the water viscera, and the water ruled by the kidneys corresponds to this water of water.

These three categories of water—the upper burner water, the middle burner water, and the lower burner water—can be seen as three distinct entities, or they can be seen as a single entity, since water is constantly flowing from each of these three categories into the other. Among the three waters, we must pay particular attention to the water of the middle burner, which is the unseen subterranean water, which flows to become what was traditionally called the "dragon vein." The "dragon vein" is not only an important issue in the practice of Chinese *fengshui*. It is also an important aspect of modern ecological interests. Why is the vegetation in some places so lush and verdant while in other places, nothing grows but the desert sands? The difference between these two depends upon the presence of "dragon veins."

If there are dragon veins, if there is water flowing below the ground, then the myriad creatures, the "myriad things," will flourish, and the mountains will be thickly decked with greenery. If there are no dragon veins, no water flowing beneath the surface of the ground, then the many creatures will not thrive, and the mountains will be barren and desolate. In Chinese, there is a phrase that describes a lush landscape: "cyan mountains and crystalline green water." The crystalline water is the prerequisite for the cyan mountains, covered with foliage. If there is no clear green water flowing, then the mountains will not be covered with foliage; instead they will be barren.

This green water is sometimes water we can see flowing in streams and brooks, and other times it is the water that flows beneath the ground, in the dragon veins. Human efforts to cultivate forests should pay attention to this fact. If a forest is planted in an area with dragon veins, it will easily grow and mature. If there is no subterranean flow of water, however, it is wasted effort to plant trees there. Reforestation requires more than mere enthusiasm. We must pay heed to science. We must take note of the winds and waters, the *fengshui*. *Fengshui* techniques include a method to determine the presence of dragon veins. If you understand these dragon veins to be the subterranean pathways of water, the hidden system waterways below the surface of the earth, then seeking the dragon veins turns into a scientific endeavor. In point of fact, many of the ancient disciplines were scientific, but their names lead us to consider them superstitions at first glance. For this reason alone, it is worth considering changing some of the old names for certain concepts to make them more modern and scientific.

The terrestrial water of the middle burner is important to the health of the entire ecosystem. At present, China is placing great emphasis on the restoration of the ecology of her westernmost provinces, currently under the threat of rapid desertification following decades of intense deforestation and a burgeoning population that overtaxes the water table. Our efforts will come to naught if we do not take notice of the water beneath the earth and its impact upon the ecosystems on its surface.

In addition, if the subterranean water continues its serious decline, what impact will this have on the middle burner of humankind? We should ponder this issue deeply. At present, the effects of social and psychological variables on human health are widely understood and studied. Sooner or later, the health effects of the natural environment, of the surrounding ecology, will also be acknowledged.

I.4. The Meaning of Shaoyang in *Yunqi*

In our earlier discussion of the Shaoyang channel, we noted that the position of this channel on the body was very closely associated with its theoretical function as a pivot. This reminded us once again of the comprehensive nature of concepts presented in the classics. They do not only present a model for understanding the functional dimensions of the body, but simultaneously involve its structural reality. We should therefore be serious and conscientious toward every detail related by the classics, since the truths conveyed in them tend to be multidimensional. No word or line should ever be taken for granted. The concepts conveyed by the classics are as broad as they are deep. No amount of interpretation exhausts their possibilities, and certainly none of the modern standardized TCM textbooks have come close to illuminating all the complex layers of meaning packed into the sentences of the medical classics. We have seen multiple editions of the government's TCM textbook series published, and more are being ushered in every few years with great fanfare—when there is really nothing new in them at all. It remains, therefore, a viable question to ask: Is Chinese Medicine education a field that can benefit from standardized textbooks? Do we really need to busy ourselves with updating them to ever new editions?

Every concept within the classics must be vigorously investigated and explored. This book is titled "Contemplating Chinese Medicine" in Chinese. In essence, it is a compilation of contemplations on certain key concepts in Chinese Medicine. It is especially focused on expounding and elucidating major concepts in the *Treatise on Cold Damage*. By clarifying certain fundamental concepts in Chinese Medicine, every vein and artery of Chinese Medicine may appear clearer before your eyes. At this point, whether you work in the field of Chinese Medicine or not, and regardless of the prevalent societal attitude toward Chinese Medicine, your understanding of Chinese Medicine cannot be shaken. In Buddhism, this sort of confidence is called faith. Faith cannot be easily acquired, but once one has attained it, it cannot be easily shaken. If you wish to study Chinese Medicine in the modern age, you absolutely must have faith in it.

Regarding its role in the five movements and six *qi* (*wuyun liuqi*, abbreviated as *yunqi*), the cyclical transformation of universal *qi*, Shaoyang governs the ministerial fire. The creation of the concept of ministerial fire is of great importance, but I fear that this piece of writing you are reading now cannot completely clarify this concept. The best that I can do here is to proceed from the elementary toward the profound in an effort to explicate it.

Ministerial fire is defined in opposition to imperial fire. An adequate explanation of ministerial fire must proceed from an understanding of how these two differ, and the relationship between ministerial and imperial fire. With regard to the *yunqi*, the ministerial fire belongs to the triple burner and the pericardium, whereas the imperial fire pertains to the heart and small intestine. Let us set aside the triple burner and the small intestine for the time being, and take a close look at the heart and the pericardium.

Outside the heart is an organ independent of it, the pericardium, which has its own channel, the hand Jueyin channel. It holds a unique place in Chinese Medicine physiology. Besides the heart, do any of the other organs have an independent organ that surrounds them? Is there the equivalent of a pericardium for the liver, spleen, lung or kidney? No. Only the heart has such an organ surrounding it. The intimate relationship between the heart and the pericardium reveals the close association between the ministerial and imperial fire. We have touched upon a fascinating subject here.

In the past, certain Chinese Medicine physicians, especially those of the Jin and Yuan dynasties, have simplified this concept. They argued that fire was categorized as imperial and ministerial, that the one was divided into two subcategories. However, considering the two as two distinct fires disrupted the one-to-one ratio of each element to the next. There is one wood, one water, one earth, one metal; how can there be two fires? How can one water control two fires? Consequently, the view that "Yin is constantly deficient, yang is constantly in excess" emerged, and the Nourish Yin and Drain Fire schools of treatment came into being.

But ministerial fire and imperial fire cannot be explained so simplistically as saying that fire possesses imperial and ministerial aspects just as the heart possesses central and surrounding aspects. One is discussed in terms of the five elements and the six *qi*, and the other in terms of the solid and hollow viscera. There are differences between the five elements. Fire and water are different in that one is cold and the other hot. The heavens and the earth are different in that the heavens are high and the earth is low. We can speak of differences between water and fire or heaven and earth, their particular qualities of temperature and altitude, but we cannot say that one is more plentiful than the other. That is ridiculous.

It is incorrect to think of the heart and the other four viscera and fire and the other four elements as being at the same level. They are unequal, and they are different. If you do not recognize this inequality, if you fail to acknowledge these differences, then you have a distorted view of nature. Therefore, I maintain my own view on the equality of the sexes. Men and women cannot possibly be equals. They can only be equal if you can induce men to menstruate and bear children. It is women who menstruate and bear children. If you wish to make men and women equals, do you think it will turn out well?

If we look at long-term benefits and advantages of "equality of the sexes," women are certainly at a disadvantage. Women have gained more rights in recent years, but the burden they bear seems to grow heavier every day. They are between a rock and a hard place. They have gained greater equality in some senses, but overall, they are more unequal than ever. These differences, these inequalities, are still more salient when we compare the physical with the metaphysical. "Beyond the form is called the Dao, the form is called a vessel." We discussed the ramifications of "beyond form" and "form," the Dao and the vessel, in the first chapter of this book. We spoke of how the heart holds the office of the sovereign and ruler, and resides in the realm that lies beyond form. The other organs are vassals to the heart, and reside in the physical realm.

If we look at this relationship between ruler and vassal from the perspective of the five elements, it can be readily comprehended. Among the five elements, fire belongs to the heart. The other elements—metal, wood, water, and earth—belong to the lungs, liver, kidney, and spleen respectively. What is a major difference among the five elements? It is the difference between fire and the other elements. If you let fire go, it moves upward, because fire burns in an upward direction. If you let any of the other elements (metal, wood, water, or earth) go, they simply fall down. The distinction between the physical and the metaphysical is obvious when we regard the five elements. There is no need to expend any amount of mental effort to differentiate them: fire goes up and the rest go down all on their own.

The metaphysical are the Dao, and the physical are the vessels. What is the difference between the Dao and vessels? Besides the distinction between form and formless, and between rising and falling that we have just discussed, there is another intrinsic, essential difference. Vessels, things, change with time, rise and fall, come into being and expire. So it is said in the "Great Treatise on the Six Subtleties" of the *Plain Questions*: "Therefore, rising and falling, coming out and going in only pertain to vessels. Thus, the realm of change and transformation is the realm of vessels. As the vessel disperses, generation and transformation cease." If there are vessels, physical objects, then there are the changes associated with life, and these changes lead to a state of changelessness following the dissolution that results from change. If a thing exists, then it will rise and fall, emerge and lapse. If there is rise and fall, coming out and going in, then the rise and fall will eventually come to an end. The coming out and going in will eventually fall apart. This is an extremely dialectical axiom. Since things come into being, they will also lapse into non-being—"as the vessel disperses, generation and transformation cease." If there is transformation, then there is changelessness. Put into Buddhist terms: if there is life, there is also death; life and death circle one another.

Where is the source of transformation and changelessness? Where do life and death originate? Obviously, these are related to the realm of vessels, to the sphere of the physical. Thus, things that pertain to the world of objects, the things of the physical realm, are subject to change, to the arc of life and death. If there is change and transformation, if there are life and death, then there is fluctuation. Regardless of whether we are discussing the *Classic of Changes* or medicine, both emphasize that "success and failure are born from one another." Therefore, vicissitudes arise. Success and failure, rise and decline, come into being and so too does their constantly revolving flow of alternations. If you wish to attain to that which is perpetual, you absolutely cannot find it in the physical world, for this world is one of change, of life and death. If one wishes to attain that which is eternal, how should one go about it? The only way is to contrive some way of escaping emergence and transformation. Without life and death, without emergence and transformation, it will naturally be without fluctuations and alterations. If it is completely unmoving, how will there be success or failure? How will there be a rise and fall? Such a state is perpetual and eternal.

The possibility of such a state of perpetuity is clearly addressed by the Yellow Emperor in this same chapter of the *Yellow Emperor's Classic*:

> The Yellow Emperor said: "Good! Is there a state without emergence and without change?"
>
> Qi Bo said: "A superb question! In union with the Dao, only then as an immortal."
>
> The Yellow Emperor replied: "Good!"

Thus, a state of changelessness is entirely possible; it is conditioned upon being "in union with the Dao," upon oneness with the metaphysical realm. Because it is at the level beyond the world of form, at the level of the Dao, at the level of the heart, there are no objects, and there is no coming into being and no transformation, and so it is "neither born nor does it perish, does not increase nor does it decrease, is neither soiled nor pure." The goal of the Buddhist and the Daoist, that which they pursue, that to which their ideals aspire, is the realm of the metaphysical, the realm that transcends physicality.

Laozi put it this way: "The path of learning is to gain something more every day; the path of the Dao is to lose something every day. Losing and losing, until there is nothing left and the state of non-doing (*wuwei*) is achieved." What is being "lost" here? What is being lost or decreased are the things of the physical world, of the world of vessels and of objects. If the rigors of the physical world, of the world of things, press upon you less and less due to your persistent efforts, then you will naturally attain to "beyond form," to the world above the world of form.

The Buddhists say: "See through it; set it down; comply with circumstances; be at ease." See through what? Set down what? See through the physical world, set down the world of things. In the world of things, in the world of objects and phenomena, we are fettered at every turn, and endlessly hindered. How can one possibly be at ease? If you really want to be at peace, then you must "see through it, set it down." Buddhist ascetics speak of "clearing the mind to see the essential nature of things," and those who practice Daoism of "cultivating one's mind to nurture one's essential nature." We can see that these are primarily practices deriving from the metaphysical world.

From this, we can see that the physical and the metaphysical are not only divisions between the Dao and vessels, and between the sage and the ordinary man, they aptly categorize the differences between Chinese and Western culture respectively. If you wish to produce a comparative study of Chinese and Western cultures while ignoring the topic we just discussed, what will your comparison consist of?

When we speak of the difference between imperial and ministerial fire, we must also pay attention to the distinction between the physical and metaphysical, between the metaphysical and the physical. Since the imperial fire conforms to the metaphysical level, occupies the position of the ruler and sovereign, and does not possess physical form, how can its activities be integrated with those of the other solid and hollow organs? How can this fire ripen and rot food? How can it steam the fluids of the body? How can it dry the skin, fill the form, and add luster to the hair? It has no choice but to delegate these activities to the ministerial fire, and charge the "ordinary" fire with these duties. Thus, the advent of the concept of ministerial fire arises from this logic and from this actual necessity. Thus, from the metaphysical and physical perspectives, the imperial fire belongs to the metaphysical realm, and the ministerial fire to the physical realm. Because it is metaphysical, the imperial fire is bright; because it is physical, the ministerial fire has an actual position.

The *Great Commentary of the Classic of Changes* says: "The spirit has no set direction." The spirit is without pattern or direction, but the ministerial fire has a particular direction and pattern, since it holds a specific position. It can be said that the spirit is without a particular orientation of position, but merely appears whenever appropriate. But in the physical world, everything must have a place or position, and so the ministerial fire is the fire that has a place or position. Earlier in this book, we talked about how the key difference between human beings and animals is that we spontaneously use fire. Behind this ability to use fire lays a more fundamental difference between animals and humans: our ability to think and reason. The heart fire governs the spirit brightness, and so fire is closely related to the intellect. Fire is related to the mind, and the mind is ruled by fire.

Now that we are dividing fire into imperial and ministerial distinctions, dividing it into physical and metaphysical quotients, we are left to question: Can the intellect also be divided into imperial and ministerial fractions? Within the territory of the intellect, within the territory of consciousness, which parts correspond to the metaphysical and which to the physical? Do the subconscious, the unconscious, and the intuitive faculties pertain to the metaphysical realm? Do the logical processes pertain to the physical sphere?

The intellect and consciousness are subjects of increasing interest and attention in modern scholarship. This is especially true of the thought processes behind those intellectual advances that change the course of history. The harmony and earth-shattering nature revealed in these thought processes were startling and deeply moving. Past scientists have all discussed these processes, and attempted to understand the truth hidden within. How do those things which are buried so deeply in the recesses of the mind come forth into the world? Where do those things that wake in the mind come from? With respect to this question, Plato, in *Phaedrus*, writes: "These things that awaken within do not enter us from without; rather, they come straight from the deep recesses of our unconscious mind." Johannes Kepler, who revealed the revolution of the planets about the sun, was deeply moved by the harmony revealed by this discovery. In his *Harmony of the Worlds* (*Harmonices Mundi*), he wrote:

> People can investigate those things that they do not yet know, but if they do not yet understand the harmonious relationships between bodies within their own mind, how can they possibly deduce such relationships between elements of the outside world? It is my view that those who comprehend truths, who discern harmonious relationships between seemingly disparate phenomena, already possess this understanding within their own minds. They do not arrive at such understandings through a process of internalization, rather they are produced from a sort of innate intuition.

The famous physicist Wolfgang Ernst Pauli put it even more precisely:

> When one analyzes the preconscious step to concepts, one always finds ideas which consist of "symbolic images." The first step to thinking is a painted vision of these inner pictures whose origin cannot be reduced only and firstly to the sensual perception but which are produced by an "instinct to imagining" and which are reproduced by different individuals independently, i.e. collectively. [. . .] But the archaic image is also the necessary predisposition and the source of a scientific attitude. To a total recognition belong also those images out of which have grown the rational concepts.

An act of creativity, a brilliant idea, a theory that stirs the soul—these originate as a sort of latent, awakening imagery in our minds. This primeval imagery is not imported from the outside world. It is not even a product of the machinations of the conscious mind. It stems from the unconsciousness, or "preconsciousness." These prototypical pictures are not brought forth by contemplation; they are sensed, the way one senses imagery. In his *Great Commentary of the Classic of Changes*, Confucius has a passage that reads: "The Changes are free of any thought, and require no effort. They are quiet and unmoving, but once they are perceived, it is as if the hidden workings of the world were laid bare." The creations of this proto-imagery can be different, and the thought created can be different as well; but, astonishingly, the understanding and description of such imagery would seem to be the same across millennia and continents.

Such a revelation instills in us the feeling that the sages of yesterday and today, of east and west, are guided by the same principles. We cannot help but ask what sort of study the *Classic of Changes* really are. Why do the Confucians place the *Classic of Changes* as first and foremost among the classics? Is the *Classic of Changes* an investigation into the imagery referred to by Wolfgang Pauli? As the Chinese song goes: "The stars are still the stars, the moonlight is still the moonlight, the mountains remain mountains, the mountain ridge is still the same mountain ridge." Up until now, the great anthropological theories that seek to explain some asymmetry in nature or between one part of nature and another, in the end all reveal nature's hidden harmonies. Science has yet to create anything that does not already exist in nature, nor has it subtracted anything from nature. The stars are still the stars, moonbeams are still moonbeams. Science has simply made ample use of the balance and harmony inherent in the natural world.

At this point, we suddenly realize Chinese Medicine is not quite the same as modern science in one important respect. Science discerns the harmonies between one part of nature and the next, but Chinese Medicine propounds the harmony between man and nature, and does so with consummate skill.

II. An Outline of Shaoyang Disease

An outline of Shaoyang disease is best discussed with reference to line 263 of the *Treatise on Cold Damage*: "When Shaoyang is diseased, there is a bitter taste in the mouth, the throat is dry, and the eyesight is blurry." Our discussion of this line is separated into two parts.

II.1. Overview of Shaoyang Disease

II.1.a. Shaoyang Disease Trigger

This line describes the disease trigger of Shaoyang disease, as we discussed in our examination of the Taiyang and Yangming chapters of the *Treatise on*

Cold Damage. Because the text is focused on the disease trigger, its implications assist our understanding of the entire Shaoyang chapter. This line merits our most diligent effort to fully understand it. In order to emphasize the importance of the disease trigger, we will rewrite this line to match the format of the nineteen disease triggers of the *Yellow Emperor's Classic*: "All bitterness of the mouth, dryness of the throat, and blurriness of vision belongs to Shaoyang."

II.1.b. The Three Orifices That Characterize Shaoyang

In the outline of Shaoyang disease, we find three extremely simple signs: "bitterness of the mouth, dryness of the throat, and blurry vision." These three signs are not characterized by obvious signs of disease, such as pain or itching, so how is it they form the outline of Shaoyang disease? A bitter taste in the mouth, a dry throat, some blurry vision—these are hardly worrisome symptoms. We must keep in mind that these seemingly insignificant symptoms may carry far greater importance, and, as we have seen before: "to understand each character correctly solidifies things like a boulder"; and "Discerning a single meaning is as wondrous as seeing the stars in the sky." We must be aware that the seeming simplicity of these three signs belies their complexity.

These three signs are related to three orifices: the mouth, the throat, and the eyes. For now, let us set aside the bitterness, dryness, and blurriness these three exhibit, and focus instead on the three orifices where they present. Orifices are holes that things can go into or come out of. Whether we are talking about a cave in the landscape or a nostril, we must keep this basic characteristic in mind. Exiting and entering are ultimately related to opening and closing. If we look at the orifices of the human body, which are the keenest and most sensitive? Which open and close most frequently? The mouth, the throat, and the eyes. Furthermore, the opening and closing of these three orifices is the most directly evident, and the easiest to perceive. When we speak, our mouth is constantly opening and closing. When we eat or speak, breathe or swallow, the throat is constantly opening and closing; it is just that this action is slightly more subtle than that of the mouth. The opening and closing of the eyes is even easier to perceive.

Therefore, the chief characteristic of the mouth, throat, and the eyes, and one that is easiest for us to perceive, is their ability to open and close.

What do opening and closing depend upon? They depend upon the presence of a hinge. The more frequently something opens, the more agile its ability to open and close, the more nimble the hinge must be. The more salient this opening and closing, the more obvious the state of the hinge becomes. For this reason, what sort of problem do the mouth, throat, and eyes make most obvious? They make problems of the hinge more obvious; they make problems with Shaoyang more obvious.

If your mouth, throat, or eyes experience difficulties opening or closing, where can we surmise this change in "opening and closing" or in "positioning" comes from? It stems from the hinge, of course. Thus, if we speak of the mouth, the throat, and the eyes, then we are speaking of the hinge that is governed by Shaoyang and the ministerial fire from which positions originate, exhibiting signs of disease. Is there any other aspect of human physiology more appropriate for the outline of Shaoyang disease? Is there any that better exhibits the action of a hinge? I hope that you feel as I do, that there are really none more suitable than the mouth, throat, and eyes to demonstrate the hinge mechanism. It is not that the mouth, throat, and eyes govern Shaoyang in some way; it is simply that they best represent the central tenet of Shaoyang, its hinging. There is a saying in Chinese that refers to the ancient custom of drinking in pavilions and surveying the surrounding scenery, such as plum blossoms in the moonlight: "when drunk, one's attention is not on the liquor." The exemplification of Shaoyang by the mouth, throat, and eyes, is equally elegant in its circuitousness.

II.1.c. Bitterness, Dryness, and Blurriness

Now let us examine bitterness, dryness, and blurriness. What is bitterness? Bitterness is the basic flavor of fire; fire's flavor is bitter. What about dryness? Whatever is close to fire becomes dry, thus dryness is a characteristic of fire. Blurriness is as it is described in the *Explanation of Names*: "Indistinct, when the eye's vision is disturbed, as if watching a dangling object that is moving all the time." What possesses the characteristic of being "indistinct and moving"? Wind (which pertains to wood) and fire both possess this characteristic. Thus, the presence of bitterness, dryness, and blurriness in this line should not be taken to mean that these three are only present in Shaoyang disease. Rather, these three reveal the wood and fire nature of Shaoyang: its ministerial fire nature.

We can expand upon our discussion of Shaoyang by examining the broader Shaoyang category. For instance, bitterness belongs to the fire element, and so it says in the *Plain Questions*: "The south generates heat, heat generates fire, fire generates bitterness, bitterness generates the heart." Bitterness is not only the flavor of fire; it is related to the heart. If we delve a little deeper, we discover that pain, which is closely intertwined with bitterness in Chinese thought and language, is also related to the heart. Thus, we read in nineteen disease trigger section of "The Great Treatise on the Essentials of Ultimate Truth" of the *Plain Questions*: "All pain with itch and sores belongs to the heart." Pain and bitterness are related to the heart, but when we look at the five emotions, we see that happiness and joy are also related to the heart. Pain and bitterness belong to the heart, and emerge from the heart just as happiness and joy do. This relationship between bitterness and pain and happiness and joy serves to illustrate a universal enigma of human life.

Bitter taste and pain are, at their root, physiological events rather than psychological, but as there is deep mutual influence between physiology and psychology, it is very difficult to separate the two. For this reason, we should not distinguish between the physiological and psychological when looking at pain and pleasure. Humans are afflicted with suffering in countless ways. Can we attribute the many faces of suffering to a single source? Or, put another way, is suffering, at its root, a single problem? In the simplest terms, at its essence, this is completely possible. This single point of origin, this problem, is bitterness and joy. Whatever angle we look at it from, the bulk of human effort is directed at resolving this central problem.

Throughout human history, in ancient times and the modern age, all of science, art, and religion have been directed toward somehow reducing suffering and increasing joy and pleasure. All human behavior, all diligence and effort, are directed toward this common aim. When we look at human intention, at what is desired subjectively, there are certainly no exceptions to this axiom. It should be possible then, to simplify the complex and multifarious causes of suffering by focusing our attention upon and contemplating the conundrum of bitterness and joy. After we have simplified and validated humanity's problems by resolving this fundamental question, we can evaluate it in a straightforward way.

There is no doubt that if this fundamental problem could be resolved, it would lessen suffering and increase joy, or perhaps even allow us to leave suffering altogether and attain a state of pure pleasure, to obtain the ultimate goal of the human species, the goal that has persisted from ancient times until the present day, and will presumably persist far into the future. There are, however, two disparate camps working diligently in an effort to resolve this problem. The one camp is concerned with the metaphysical realm, and the other with the physical world. To put it another way, there are those who approach this problem from a materialistic perspective, and those who approach it from a spiritual, heart-based perspective.

Once these two distinct approaches are acknowledged, and their differences accurately established, many things become clear. Modern science firmly adheres to a materialistic, physical view of the issue. Science attempts to change material circumstances in order to benefit humanity; it uses its materialistic methods to assist humankind to escape from suffering and obtain joy. Can techniques that allow us to alter material circumstances truly allow us to leave bitterness and arrive at happiness? Of course. If one is hungry and is given food, or if one is cold and is given warm clothing, if one is able to depart from a state of starvation and coldness with such simple, materialistic methods, their suffering is instantly banished. Once the person is warm and fed, however, these materialistic methods are limited in their ability to alleviate suffering and bring joy. I assume that most persons reading this have had similar experiences. A millionaire or a billionaire is still vexed by the same host of headaches that plague most persons. Their money does not make them immune to worries, anxieties, and suffering. If the removal of material difficulties were enough, then they should be completely free of troubles, but clearly wealth is not enough to leave suffering behind and attain a state of constant happiness.

Why are material means limited in the extent to which they can relieve human suffering? It is because, as we have said in earlier passages of the chapter, the source of human joy and human suffering, the source of bitterness and joy is the heart, the organ that pertains not to the physical realm but to the metaphysical realm. Thus, this problem cannot be easily solved by material, physical means. This is an indirect solution that will take one in circles. If it is a matter of warming someone who is freezing, or feeding someone who is overcome by hunger, material methods works beautifully. But once the basic necessities of life and human comfort are attained, the usefulness of this method is limited. It is like trying to scratch an itch from outside one's boot. If we wish to solve this problem, it must be addressed directly at its foundation; it must be pulled up at its roots if we wish to eradicate it. The roots are undoubtedly in the metaphysical realm.

At this point, we suddenly realize why the traditional Chinese schools of thought—Confucianism, Buddhism, and Daoism—have all emphasized the importance of "cultivating the heart," and why they emphasized the metaphysical level: the heart level. Only in this way can the most fundamental problem confronting human existence be solved. Take, for instance, Laozi's *Classic of the Dao and Its Virtue.* In that work, Laozi does not entreat us to seek material wealth, or to ceaselessly pursue techniques aimed at gaining mastery over the physical world. Instead, he entreats you to be content with what you have. And why is this? Because Laozi knew that happiness is not derived from material wealth. If one is not happy with what one has, then even if one has billions of dollars and immense social status, one cannot escape bitterness and suffering.

If one follows the path of mastery over the physical world to its very end, even if one can fly out into outer space and beyond, one cannot solve the basic problems confronting humankind. When one finally awakens to this, when one must turn their head and look back to where they went wrong, the only option that remains is to follow the road of the metaphysical, the route of the root. Laozi saw this important point, and saw through the emptiness of material gains. For that reason, he did not encourage people to pursue material gains; he simply said that to be content with what one has is enough: "If one is content with one's lot he will not be disgraced, if he knows when to stop he will not encounter danger." Why should one expend his or her energy pursuing a thankless task?

From this perspective, we can see why China did not take the lead toward modernization, and why it did not attempt to maximize its mastery over the outside world. At a critical juncture in its history, it was content with what it already possessed. To understand Chinese Medicine and its true worth, we cannot limit our investigation to a single disease; we must examine it more broadly. The ancients said: "The highest physicians treat the nation, the mid-level physicians treat the people, and the lowest level physicians treat disease." From our examination of the lines that outline Shaoyang, from the implications of our expanded contemplation of bitterness, we can see that Chinese Medicine contains all three of the levels we just mentioned. It is really just a matter of whether you are able to grasp them, if you are able to benefit from them.

II.2. The Specialized Meanings of Shaoyang Disease

II.2.a. The Characteristics of the Five Orifices

The outline of Shaoyang disease mentions the orifices of the mouth, the throat, and the eyes. These lead us to think about the five orifices as a topic in their own right. Of the five orifices of Chinese Medicine physiology, it is said that the heart opens into the tongue, the spleen into the mouth, the lungs into the nose, the kidneys into the ears, and the liver into the eyes. What is an orifice (*qiao*)? *Explaining Writing and Analyzing Characters* says: "A cavity, an empty space." In *Conveyance of Rites* from *Record of Rites*, it says: "The basic nature of the earth is seen in caves (*qiao*) in the landscape." *Explanations* calls them: "Where the earth grasps the yin *qi*, there are holes in the landscape to exhale and inhale its *qi*."

If we were to summarize what has been said in *Explaining Writing and Analyzing Characters* and the *Record of Rites*, then the *qiao* are holes or cavities, what we might call caves. What is the purpose of these caves? They allow earth *qi* to enter and exit. Although the earth is yin, although it stores without draining, it still engages in exchange both with the heavens and with yang. The earth breathes. This exchange, this breathing, takes place through the caves of mountains and rivers. Every aspect of the natural world is engaged in some useful process. Nothing is idle, though one might mistakenly think so.

Now that we understand the meaning and significance of orifice (*qiao*), we can understand the importance of the orifices associated with the five viscera. First of all, in Chinese Medicine, only the five viscera are associated with an orifice, none of the bowels have an orifice associated with them. The reason for this is that the six bowels are yang, and the five viscera are yin; the six bowels correspond to heaven, and thus they drain but do not store; the five viscera correspond to earth, and so they store but do not drain. The basic nature of the heavens is that they are empty; holes or cavities cannot be found in an immense, empty space such as the sky.

The earth is solid, dense, and deep. It needs holes in order to communicate its interior with the outside world. It is worth reiterating the foundation of Chinese Medicine: ultimately the fabric of Chinese Medicine theory is one with the cloth of nature, and its threads run back to the fabric of the cosmos about us. When discussing Chinese Medicine, the backdrop of the natural world cannot be forgotten. If you have a thorough understanding of the natural world, your foundation in Chinese Medicine will be sound and your understanding can progress. Furthermore, an understanding of the natural world will strengthen your faith in Chinese Medicine, for the two resonate with one another. This is not a blind faith; it is a confidence that is guided by direct observation of the world we live in.

If we look at the orifices that correspond with liver, spleen, lungs, and kidney, we see that all of these correspond with the description laid out in *Explaining Writing and Analyzing Characters* and the *Record of Rites*. All of them are stationed on the "landscape" of the head and body, and all are cavitary in nature. The liver corresponds with the eyes, the kidneys with the ears, the lungs with the nose. All three of these correspond with orifices that are paired left and right. The spleen appears to be an exception, but for the fact that the mouth consists of an upper lip and a lower lip. Only the orifice associated with the heart truly stands apart. Its orifice (the tongue) is solitary, without right or left, upper or lower. Furthermore, it is not an opening that leads to the outside world, nor is it even an empty cavitation.

Among the five viscera, the liver, spleen, lungs, and kidneys are all solid but their orifices are empty. The heart is essentially empty, but its orifice is solid. Among the five viscera, the heart is the sovereign ruler. The ruler is alone and companionless, for it is not part of a left-right or top-bottom pair. All of the other officials are to some extent expendable; there is another above or below, to the left or to the right. This characteristic of the five viscera allows us to see both an important aspect of physiology and of social structure. Ultimately, these two aspects would appear to be inseparable.

II.2.b. Organization of the Nine Orifices

Now that we have examined the five orifices, it is time to take a look at the nine orifices. The nine orifices are the two ears, two eyes, two nostrils, the mouth, the anterior yin (the genitals), and the posterior yin (the anus). The organization of the nine orifices is interesting. There are three orifices consisting of pairs, and three that are solitary. The paired orifices (the ears, eyes, and nostrils) are above, and the solitary orifices (the mouth, genitals, and anus) are below. The paired orifices resemble the yin lines (- -) of the trigrams and hexagrams. The solitary orifices resemble the unbroken, yang lines (—) of the trigrams and hexagrams. Furthermore, even numbers are yin, and odd numbers belong to yang. The three yin lines above form the trigram *Kun* Earth, and the three solid yang lines above form the trigram *Qian* Heaven. What hexagram is formed by this combination of *Kun* Earth above and *Qian* Heaven below? The hexagram *tai* (Advance, ☰). The nine orifices naturally form the hexagram *tai*. What is it that links the upper and lower trigrams together? It is the space between the mouth and the nose, where we find the acupuncture point Renzhong (GV 26).

The significance of the name Renzhong ("human center") may have seemed obscure to the student of Chinese Medicine in the past. It is, after all, situated in the philtrum between the nose and the upper lip. Why is it called "human center"? In fact, this name points to an esoteric fact of Chinese Medicine physiology. It resembles a sort of key that, once understood, opens the door to a wealth of understanding. Why is it called "human center"? Because heaven is above, and earth below, and between the two, according to Chinese cosmology, we find human beings.

Heaven nurtures humans by means of the five *qi*. Earth nurtures humans with the five flavors. The five *qi* enter the nose and are stored in the heart and lungs. The five flavors enter the mouth and are stored in the stomach. The nose and mouth act as important links between heaven, earth, and man. The celestial *qi* joins with man via the nose and the terrestrial *qi* via the mouth. The classics say: "Humans are born of the *qi* of heaven and earth." How is man created from the *qi* of heaven and earth? How does the *qi* of heaven and earth create man? Clearly, the mouth and nose play an important part in the process.

The nose is the orifice of the lungs, and the mouth the orifice of the spleen. The lungs are ruled by heaven and the spleen by earth. Thus, the nose and mouth are referred to as heaven and earth. Since the nose and mouth are heaven and earth, then the trough between the two must be called Renzhong ("human center"). No other name would do. The "Great Treatise on the Six Subtleties" in the *Plain Questions* says: "When we speak of heaven, we refer to the source or root. When we speak of earth, we refer to location. When we refer to human beings, we speak of the exchange of *qi*." Investigating the intercourse of *qi* in the human form is a matter of great importance.

What is meant by the "intercourse of *qi*"? The intercourse of *qi* refers to the intercourse between the *qi* of heaven and earth, the interchange between *qi* of yin and yang. The celestial *qi* descends, the terrestrial *qi* rises. The yang *qi* comes down, the yin *qi* up. The intercourse of *qi* is this downward movement of the heavens and the upward movement of the earth. It is through the intercourse of *qi* that the myriad creatures are created, and through this same process, humans are brought into being. Thus, it is said: humans are born of the intercourse of *qi*. This interchange is the commingling of the descending *Qian* Heaven *qi* and the rising *Kun* Earth *qi*. What does this pattern remind us of? It is the very pattern of the hexagram *tai*.

Thus, the organization of the nine orifices, with the three paired orifices above and the three solitary orifices below, represents the commingling of celestial and terrestrial *qi*, and embodies the pattern we find in the hexagram *tai*. This would seem to be a coincidence, and at the same time, it would seem to be no coincidence at all. In any case, it makes us stop and wonder. Heaven and earth must commingle, yin and yang must intercourse. This interchange of *qi* requires a thoroughfare, and the point Renzhong lies in the middle of the trough-like philtrum between nose and lip, like a canal or gully. The philtrum is aptly designed as a thoroughfare, is it not? That which is within requires that which is without. Although the Renzhong thoroughfare is on the outside of the body, it corresponds to the inherent interchange between heaven and earth, and the commingling of yin and yang. For this reason, the structure of the philtrum and its appearance is very important. Those who are able to read a person's health from their appearance can predict a person's longevity from the appearance of their philtrum.

This is because the structure of Renzhong corresponds with the pattern of *qi* interchange in the body. What does the condition of a person's body, their health and longevity depend on? It depends upon the interchange of *qi*. Those whose interchange of *qi* is good have a firm foundation for health and longevity. If the interchange of *qi* is not good, if the *qi* of heaven and earth do not engender you, if the four seasons do not fill you with their unique energies, how can you possibly find good health? Where can you get longevity? If you do not have a foundation, if the very basis for longevity is lacking, you cannot obtain health and longevity.

When we look at the philtrum, we are looking at the interchange of *qi*, and when we examine the process of this interchange, we are able to perceive the very foundation of the life process. If you can see the foundation of the person's life force, then you can of course predict their health and longevity. Judging a person's longevity by their appearance is not mere superstition. When Sun Simiao said that a great physician is able to understand physiognomy, this was not without reason. If health and longevity can be ascertained by examining one's genetic code, then I am certainly entitled to perform my own research into the appearance of Renzhong.

Is it really the case that genetic analyses are science but deriving information by examining the philtrum is superstition? I do not think so. Why is it that only the most prevalent theories are permitted? The important thing is whether the method is effective. If it is ineffective, then you have every right to declare it a superstition. But if it is just as accurate as genetic assessment, then it should be taken seriously. Such a simple yet effective method does not require validation from some outside source; it does, however, warrant our respect and admiration.

It is simple, so there is no wonder that it has been deemed unscientific and uncouth. It is unadorned, so there is hardly any wonder that those who prefer sophisticated techniques dismiss it as banal. The irony of such disregard brings to mind the Latin phrase *simplex sigillum veri*—"simplicity is the sign of truth." What is it that science pursues? It seeks truth, does it not? Simplicity is an indicator of truth. The more true it is, the simpler, and the simpler the truer. If something is complicated, sometimes the only explanation is complicated as well, but complicated explanations often lose track of the truth. Laozi said: "A violent wind does not blow all morning, a sudden torrent does not fall all day." Whether or not this is simple, the truth is simple enough. It is precisely because it is so simple that it cuts to the truth of the matter. The truth of human life and of society is contained within this concept of simplicity. But it is precisely because of this simplicity that it is so difficult to recognize.

Is it human nature to prefer complexity? We come into the world stark naked, and without a care in the world, but people find this simplicity unappealing. They deem sophistication better. You take their pulse and determine the nature and cause of their disease, but the patient is unsure and would like to have some sophisticated scientific tests performed. Furthermore, if you were to open a hospital and your diagnostic methods consisted solely of the traditional looking, listening, asking, and palpating, and in addition to that you prescribed some Chinese herbs, even if your patients got better, your little hospital would go out of business. Why? Because you would not make enough money! Lack of funds would force you to shutter up. Such a hospital could never prosper in China, though it might fly in a foreign country, I suppose. To be profitable, at least in China at the moment, you need an array of modern diagnostic equipment and the state-of-the-art lab tests. You also need to prescribe Western pharmaceuticals. This is just the reality in China at present, if a Chinese Medicine practitioner wants food to eat and a roof over her head, she had better toe the line.

People are the product of the interchange between the celestial and terrestrial *qi*. This exchange takes the form of the *tai* hexagram, and the nine orifices of the body follow the model of this hexagram. What then is the course, the pathway, where this interchange takes place? It is the philtrum between the nose and the mouth, Renzhong. If the philtrum is deep, long, and broad, then the interplay of celestial and terrestrial forces, the very source of life, will correspond. Many people in China know that if a person faints or falls unconscious, they can be rescued from that state by pinching this philtrum. Countless people have been roused from a state of shock by means of this single pinch, brought from a state of close to death to one safely in the lap of life. Why is this? The thoroughfare by which *qi* interchanges has been opened up, the exchange of *qi* resumes, and so the life force naturally resurges, returning to its original state.

Is Renzhong an important trigger? Does the name "human center" reveal a secret of Chinese Medicine? I invite you to contemplate these questions for yourself.

II.2.c. Exhaustion of Pi Is Followed by Tai

The distribution of the nine orifices mirrors the organization of the hexagram *tai* (Advance). The hexagram *tai* represents the basic conditions whereby life can exist, and the external physical form of human beings represents this pattern beautifully. If we wish to penetrate into the mysteries of life's inner workings, we must pay close attention to this innate process. The structure of the *tai* hexagram is exactly opposite that of the *pi* hexagram (Hindrance). These two hexagrams represent completely opposite processes. They are as opposite as benevolence and malevolence, good and bad, luck and misfortune, the small, mean-hearted person and the magnanimous sovereign. The *tai* hexagram represents that which is good and desirable, and the *pi* hexagram that which is undesirable.

What underlies this difference between the two hexagrams? A look at the *Classic of Changes* commentary on these two hexagrams informs us. The hexagram *pi* has the *Qian* Heaven trigram consisting solely of yang lines above and the *Kun* Earth trigram of three broken yin lines below. The commentary on this hexagram reads: "*Pi* represents a rascal, someone who will not benefit the noble person. Greatness departs and pettiness arrives." Shang Binghe's commentary says: "Yang ascends, yin descends. When yang is above and yin is below, then the two will grow further and further apart from one another. When heaven and earth stop exchanging with one another, becoming *pi*. *Pi* means obstruction."

In the *Commentary on the Judgments* (Tuan) of the *Classic of Changes*, it says:

> The rascal represented by *pi* does not bestow benefit in return for the ruler's loyalty, thus the great are at a loss and the small profit. As a result, heaven and earth do not communicate with one another, and the myriad living things, the myriad things are hindered, the world is filled with disorder. The inside is yin, the outside yang, the inside soft, the outside hard, the person is small and mean inside but noble and magnanimous outwardly. The small person finds an open road and the great person cannot proceed.

Shang Binghe's commentary reads: "The root of celestial *qi* leaps upward and is exterior. The source of terrestrial *qi* falls downward and is internal. They grow further and further apart as they move, thus the *qi* can no longer exchange. The *qi* does not exchange and so the myriad things are hindered, dying." From this, we know that the key reason that *pi* represents all sorts of maladies and misfortunes lies in the loss of interplay between heaven and earth.

Let us contrast this with the commentary and discussion of *tai* (Advance). The hexagram *tai* is composed of the trigrams *Kun* Earth above and *Qian* Heaven below. The phrase associated with this hexagram is "*Tai*: the small departs and the great comes; auspiciousness; success." Shang Bing-he comments: "Yang naturally rises, yin naturally descends. Because yin is above and yang is below, their *qi* transmits and exchanges, becoming *tai*. *Tai* means unobstructed passage." In the *Commentary on the Judgments*, we read:

> *Tai*: the small leaves, the great comes; auspicious, successful. Therefore, heaven and earth exchange and the myriad things are connected. Above and below exchange and their wills are united. The inside is yang and the outside yin. The inside is strong and the outside is smooth, a sovereign within and a petty person without. The ruler's path is long, and the small person's path dwindles.

From this, we know that what makes *tai* so auspicious, harmonious, and peaceful is the intermingling of heaven and earth.

From the descriptions of the images of *tai* and *pi* we just read, we can see that the intrinsic meaning of *pi* and *tai* is both extremely deep and broad. Aspects of it relate to natural science, and others to the social sciences, and still others to the humanities. Such rich and fertile significance and meaning entices us to research this topic more deeply and endeavor to put what we find into practice.

Regarding the natural world, the *Great Commentary of the Classic of Changes* says: "Heaven and earth's misty union; all living things are transformed by it and develop. Male and female commingle their essence, and all living things thereby procreate." How is it that the myriad things achieve fertile harmony, and male and female commingle their essences? They do so by means of the state of affairs described by the hexagram *tai*. On the contrary, if the heaven and earth find themselves in the pattern illustrated by the hexagram *pi*, then there are no harmonious vapors, and no mingling of essences, no fomentation of the vital force, and no emergence of living things. Without these, life cannot flourish and perpetuate itself.

If we were to describe life in terms of normal and abnormal circumstances, the best description might be the contrast between the hexagrams *tai* and *pi*. *Pi* represents the state in which health and vitality are lost; it is also the state of disease. *Tai*, on the other hand, obviously represents a state of health and prosperity. From a Chinese Medicine perspective, one of the chief goals of medicine is to convert the state represented by *pi* to the state represented by *tai*. The hexagram *pi* has heaven above and earth below, in a state in which the two are not inclined to mingle or exchange. When yin and yang do not combine with one another, the prenatal energies of the five viscera cannot flow unimpeded, and a whole host of pathological processes are gradually engendered.

How can we convert *pi* to *tai*? One method is to induce the yang of the *Qian* Heaven trigram to descend. Another is to cause the yin of the *Kun* Earth trigram to rise. Ultimately, the best method at resolving the *pi* pattern lies in dealing with the factors that have contributed to its existence in the first place. When heaven and earth are in harmony, after male and female have mingled their essence, living things ought to be in this *tai* state of peace, a state of health. Why then have they entered into a state in which *pi* predominates? In the final analysis, it is a problem of yin and yang, a problem of rising and falling. It could be a case of excessive yang, rising out of control. Or it could be a case of too much yin so that it sinks and cannot rise. A still more important factor could be some defect in the hinge mechanism. Such a defect can easily lead to a *pi* scenario. Of course, there are times when there are compound factors that bring about a *pi* state, times when there are a complex of contributors to the problem at hand.

The specific way in which *pi* changes to *tai* is clearly illustrated in the Taiyang chapter of the *Treatise on Cold Damage* in its discussion of the treatment of *pi* (痞), usually translated as "lump" or "glomus." This *pi* syndrome is an apt illustration of the *pi* (否) state manifesting in the body. *Pi* ("glomus") can manifest in the body in countless ways, but in the *Treatise on Cold Damage*, these countless manifestations are collected into a single type: the "below the heart" type (*xinxia pi* 心下痞). Why should such an important category of syndrome be summarized by a single, "below the heart" variety? This "below the heart" does not mean below the heart as in the heart of the five viscera. It refers to the large region below the xiphoid process and above the lower abdomen. This area is referred to as "below the heart" (*xinxia*), and is the area of the body in which the spleen and stomach reside.

What is the significance of this area as the place where the spleen and stomach are found? It is crucial to note that rising and falling pivot around this place. If the spleen and stomach are afflicted, then rising and falling the body will certainly experience some difficulty. When rising and falling are hindered, then the *qi* of heaven and earth cannot meet or exchange, and we have the very picture of *pi* (Hindrance). Therefore, *pi* ("glomus") of the epigastric region illustrates the crucial problem presented by the *pi* hexagram. To treat glomus syndrome, the *Treatise on Cold Damage* uses Xiexin Tang, of which there are five different variations: Dahuang Huang-lian Xiexin Tang, as well as the other four other Xiexin decoctions named after their lead herbs: Fuzi, Banxia, Gancao, and Shengjiang respectively. Why is Xiexin Tang used to treat glomus syndrome? Here, draining (*xie*) does not refer to "drain" in the context of tonifying or reducing, but rather to opening the passageway (*tong* 通) inhabited by the spleen and stomach, the place in which the pivot of rising and falling resides. When this place is stopped up, how can rising and falling proceed? When this area of the body is congested, glomus will automatically result. *Xiexin* (to "drain the heart") resolves this blockage, clears out the obstacle, and allows the physiological rising and falling that make for the very picture of *tai* (Advance) to resume. When that which has ascended can descend, and that which is in a low position can rise, then harmony in the body begins anew. We can see that Xiexin Tang is a formula that converts *pi* (Hindrance) to *tai* (Advance).

Of the five Xiexin Tang, the Dahuang Huanglian Xiexin Tang formula descends the yang. All Yangming syndromes in which the stomach will not descend are, as a rule, syndromes characterized by a lack of descent of the *Qian* Heaven yang. When the *Qian* Heaven yang will not descend, *pi* arises. To treat this, use Dahuang Huanglian Xiexin Tang. This formula induces the *qian* Heaven yang to descend, producing the salubrious *tai* pattern. The Banxia, Shengjiang, and Gancao Xiexin decoctions are all formulas that both induce the yang to descend and induce the yin to rise. All syndromes characterized both by a loss of physiological descent in the Yangming stomach such that the *Qian* Heaven yang cannot descend, and a loss of the normal rising function of the spleen such that the *Kun* Earth yin cannot ascend, resulting in a state of *pi*, can be treated with these three formulas. If the formula employs Huangqin or Huanglian, then it descends the yang. If it uses Renshen, Shengjiang, Gancao, and Dazao, then it raises the yin. Banxia is used to open up blockage and allow for communication between the upper and lower regions. Giving this decoction naturally causes the yang to descend and the yin to ascend, changing *pi* to *tai*. Fuzi Xiexin Tang also descends the yang and ascends the yin, turning *pi* to *tai*.

Pi (Hindrance) means obstruction. There is obstruction and so heaven and earth cannot interact. Xiexin Tang clears away this obstacle, allowing heaven and earth to communicate. By using it, one allows "Heaven and earth to commingle and the myriad things to move freely, above and below to interact and their wills to become unified." By using it, we enable the "Sovereign's path to be long, and the small person's way to dwindle." Although there are only five Xiexin decoctions, if we can expand upon the principles they convey, and include herbs from other categories of action, then we can eliminate any illness characterized by congestion between heaven and earth and resulting in this *pi* pattern.

I remember a patient I saw last year, a Tibetan-Chinese. He had some type of liver disease and after developing severe diarrhea, he felt a heat in his chest like fire, but below the waist he felt as cold as ice. After treatment in his local county's Western Medicine hospital, his diarrhea was stopped, but his other symptoms did not change. During the day he was vexed, and at night he could not sleep. His chest full of burning heat and feet as cold as ice led me to believe that the yang was not descending nor the yin rising. It was clearly a picture like that of *pi* (Hindrance). I prescribed Banxia Xiexin Tang with additional Rougui. I added the warm, sweet Rougui so that it, together with the bitter, cold Huanglian, could set the stage for the interaction of the *tai* pattern. This use of Rougui harkens back to ancient times when it was combined with Huanglian, together with other herbs, to make what was called Jiaotai ("intercourse of *tai*") Wan. The patient took this medicine for a little over two weeks and the heat in his chest normalized, his feet grew warmer, and the rest of his symptoms disappeared as well. The *pi* left and *tai* returned.

III. The Timing of Shaoyang Disease

We have discussed the way in which Shaoyang governs the orifices of the body, and we broadened this discussion of the orifices to include a discussion of *pi* (Hindrance) and *tai* (Advance). It should be said that the hexagrams *pi* and *tai* make an apt starting point for discussing Chinese Medicine in general. Regardless of the health problem, regardless of the disease, you can analyze and approach it in terms of *pi* and *tai*. The idea that "exhaustion of *pi* is followed by *tai*" is applicable not only to the affairs of a person's life and to society. It is equally, if not more, applicable to the field of medicine, where this concept takes on an immanence and applicability not found in other fields.

In Chapter Three of this book, we discussed the timing of the opening and closing of yin and yang as a starting point for analyzing disease processes. We can also use *pi* and *tai* as models to describe physiology and pathology. Whether we use opening and closing, or *pi* and *tai*, we are in possession of a comprehensive model. This exemplifies an interesting facet of Chinese Medicine, and one worth discussing.

"All roads lead to Beijing." From Nanning, we take the T6 Express Train to Beijing. If we are in Chengdu, you cannot take the T6; you have to take the T8. No matter where you find yourself, you can find the way (Dao). There is only one Dao, whether it be the Dao of Chinese Medicine, or of Confucianism, Buddhism, or Daoism, it is all one Dao. However, there are many means by which we glimpse this Dao, and by which we make it evident to ourselves and others. In Buddhism, there are 84,000 different doors to enlightenment, 84,000 methods, or put another way, 84,000 starting points. Any one of these starting points will take you on the path to understanding the fundamental truths of the universe and of human existence. In light of this, the many different schools of thought throughout the course of Chinese Medicine history do not seem too strange. Zhang Zhongjing sets forth from the three yin and the three yang. Li Dongyuan begins with the spleen and stomach. Ye Tianshi analyzes disease in terms of the four levels: defensive, *qi*, nutritive, and blood. Wu Jutong explains physiology and pathology in terms of the three burners. Following any of these methods to their final destination, we arrive at an accurate understanding: we "arrive at Beijing." All of these methods reveal the truth, the Dao.

Furthermore, all of these methods, all of these starting points are worth having. One model is no better than the next; each brings us to the truth. If no model is better than another, why is it that I keep emphasizing the Chinese Medicine classics? A discerning person can see what the classics really are. The classics are like the goal to which these other methods lead; they are the destination, the "Beijing" toward which all roads lead. The accomplished physicians of later generations produced many different schools of thought and branches of study. Some physicians were prolific and so broad in their views that they seemed to be all-inclusive, but all of them emphasized the classics and claimed that their views were the direct product of the classics. I am afraid this is not simply a matter of fishing for fame and praise, and feeling it necessary to claim a sage as their progenitor, but rather it is that after pursuing a particular model or theory to its end, the practitioner eventually has a flash of insight and realizes that it leads back to its source—back to the classics!

We already discussed this relationship between the classics and the various, later schools in Chapter Two. It is, in fact, a matter of form and function, of theory and practice. The classics are the form, the theory, and later models are the function, the practice. Without a form, there is nothing to make use of, no function. Without function, without being put into practice, the form remains unknowable. Form and function are so closely interwoven as to be inseparable.

The relationship between these two must be clearly understood. If you are not clear on this point, then you will be uncertain how to proceed. You will find yourself following this theorist for a while, and then following that one for a while, but all the while you will be in the dark and at a loss. You could swim forever like that and never find shore. You cannot amount to much like that, and will certainly never found your own school of thought. Form and function, the relationship between the classics and the later schools, is a topic that must be attended to by the student of Chinese Medicine. Once you are clear on this point, then you will see that the many different theories are not as disparate as they seem, and methods that seem alien to one another on their face are actually close cousins. Then, you can heed your own proclivities in selecting the best method. Or, better still, you can proceed directly from your personal understanding of the classics. You can practice from the original theory and allow function to follow the classical form. Or, you can take the more circuitous route and discern the form through the veil of its function, practicing in accord with the teachings of later physicians.

I believe that both of these methods are acceptable. There is no disagreement between them. My first teacher worked directly from the classics. More often than not, physicians practice using the second method: working from the teachings of later physicians. The most important thing is that one gains mastery in whatever method one employs, that one achieves the stated goal. My only fear is that the student might not follow a particular route all the way to its end, stopping halfway. Such persons end up saying one thing and practicing the other, and say that theirs is the only true style. If one practices assiduously and gains mastery, then one is a descendant of Qi Bo and Huangdi, how there be only one true style? If you take a close look at Ye Tianshi's *Case Records as a Guide to Clinical Practice* or at Wu Jutong's *Systematic Differentiation of Warm Pathogen Diseases*, you will know for yourself of what I speak.

III.1. From *Yin* to *Chen*

In this section, we will discuss the times that correspond with Shaoyang configuration. Our discussion must, of course, also include a look at the time in which Shaoyang disease has a tendency to resolve. In line 272, it says: "Shaoyang disease tends to resolve in the time from *yin* to *chen*." In the Taiyang and Yangming chapters of this book, we discussed a number of topics pertinent to this discussion of the time period in which Shaoyang disease has a tendency to resolve, and regarding the particular time period, the period from *yin* (3–5 am) to *chen* (7–9 am), there are a number of particular characteristics we should look at.

If we look at the cycle of a single day, this time period includes the three two-hour periods of *yin*, *mao*, and *chen*. These three periods stretch from the pre-dawn hour of 3 am to 9 am in the morning. If a particular disease lessens or shows signs of resolving during this time period, we should consider the possibility that this disease is a Shaoyang disease. It will behoove us to discuss this particular part of the daily cycle in relation to the picture of Shaoyang that we have already illustrated in this chapter.

Yin, mao, and *chen* are not merely a matter of time; they are correlated with a number of other phenomena, and in accordance with these correlations, we can make certain inferences. The process of making inferences based on what is stated in the classics is a necessary part of studying and researching Chinese Medicine. For instance, *yin, mao,* and *chen* also include the eastern direction. If a disease, whether it be vertigo, a disorder of the stomach or intestines, or anything else, discomforts the patient terribly when at her home in Nanning, in the Southwest of China, but whenever the patient travels east to Shanghai or Zhejiang, of a sudden she becomes comfortable and at ease, free of vertigo, or indigestion, or whatever it is that ails her, you should consider the possibility that this patient is suffering from

Shaoyang disease, because it has a tendency to resolve in the geographical region related to *yin, mao,* and *chen.*

If we look at the lunar cycle, *yin, mao,* and *chen* relate to the period around the first quarter of the waxing moon, directly opposite the time period in which Yangming disease has a tendency to resolve. This discussion of the lunar cycle brings us to a topic related to women's health. An obvious but important difference between men and women is the menstrual cycle. One of the most notable aspects of the menstrual cycle is described in the *Plain Questions's* "Treatise on Heavenly Truth in High Antiquity": "The moon's affairs are timely." This time includes two different levels of meaning. At the first level, a woman's menstruation is periodical. Secondly, the interval between one period and the next is typically one month.

Why does the name of this physiological function of the female refer to the moon? It has to do with the second level of meaning related to this phrase from the *Yellow Emperor's Classic*: its relation to duration of the lunar cycle. A woman menstruates once a month, just as the moon is full once a month. Earlier in the book, when we spoke of tides, we discussed how the tides are strongest when the moon is full. The Chinese word for tide (*chao* 潮) can also be used to refer to menstruation. The phases of the moon, the female menstrual cycle, and the tides of the oceans—if you can understand the connection between these three, you can understand much in Chinese Medicine. This is especially true of our female colleagues. They have the opportunity not only to understand this topic from an intellectual perspective, but to know of it firsthand from a physical or even emotional perspective. Those who can can realize a great deal about what is meant by "heaven and human are one." In this respect, I believe that female students of Chinese Medicine have a particular advantage because this aspect of Chinese Medicine theory plays itself out in your very body. Monthly menstruation is a profound and obvious response to a basic cosmological cycle. It is a concrete physiological event in response to one of the basic rhythms of our cosmos. Besides noting that the cycle lasts one month in total, it is worthwhile to observe the details of this cycle, the specific time of menstruation. Does menstruation coincide with the full moon, the new moon, the first quarter, or the last?

I once read a study that focused on the timing of menstruation and its association with fertility. The study concluded that those who menstruate at or near the time of the full moon had very low rates of infertility. Those who menstruated at other times, for instance, those who menstruated during the new moon, had high rates of infertility. Furthermore, other gynecological disorders were considerably higher in those who menstruated at the time of the new moon. Why should there be such a discrepancy?

It is a matter of correspondence versus a lack of correspondence. In Chinese, there is a saying: "One who achieves the Dao receives much support, one who loses the Dao finds little support." This is nothing more than correspondence to the intrinsic order of things versus a loss of correspondence to the intrinsic order of things. That which corresponds in such a way receives support. If you consider the power of the cosmos, the power of nature as a whole, and you resonate with that power such that the cosmos can assist you, is there any problem you cannot solve? Naturally, you will be very healthy. And so it is that in the "Great Treatise on The Four *Qi* and the Tuning of the Spirit," it says: "So it is that yin, yang, and the four seasons are the beginning and end of the myriad things, the root of life and death. If you go against them, you will bring about disaster. If you accord with them, no severe illness will ever arise. This is called achieving the Dao." This is even more amply evident in the case of the female body.

Menstruation is the result of a shedding of the inner lining of the uterus. The shedding of this inner lining, in turn, reflects changes in the female hormones. This causes us to see that the secretion of female hormones is cyclical, and this cycle coincides with the lunar cycle. The sun is yang, the moon is yin; men are yang, women are yin. The fact that female hormones have a lunar periodicity is a matter of yin corresponding to yin.

Do male hormones exhibit a similar periodicity? And, if so, does it correspond to the solar cycle? This is a matter worth investigating. It is an example of traditional science posing a question to be answered by modern science. Deeper research into this question has the potential to solve some of the issues encountered by modern science.

"The moon's affairs are timely" also refers to the fact that the time of menstruation varies from individual to individual, and also varies as the person ages. When we discuss disease of the six conformations in relation to their time correspondences, we can divide the lunar cycle into six parts, each corresponding to one of the six conformations. After establishing these six subdivisions of the lunar cycle, the timing of the aforementioned "timeliness of the moon's affairs" can easily be correlated with these six subdivisions. Once these correlations are clearly defined, it would be possible to bridge the six conformation disease theory of the *Treatise on Cold Damage* with gynecological treatments. Such a bridge would provide important insights and would no doubt assist us in treating gynecological disorders.

Chinese Medicine not only differentiates between syndromes, it also differentiates between particular types of disease. The disease is general, and the syndrome is specific. It is only once we have a general idea that we can proceed to a more specific one. From this perspective, the trend of emphasizing "syndrome differentiation" and deemphasizing "disease differentiation" leaves us with an incomplete picture of Chinese Medicine.

Of course, diseases are differentiated differently in Chinese and Western Medicine. For instance, the process of dividing the lunar cycle into six parts and thereby making connections between gynecological disorders and the six conformation is essentially a process of differentiating diseases, from a Chinese Medicine perspective. When we differentiate disease, we are essentially determining the direction of the disease. If we do not know the direction, how can we possibly choose a route? Determining the disease is a relatively clear and objective process. We look at the time, the place, the five elements, the six *qi*—all of these factors are clear and obvious. Once we have organized this information, it is relatively easy to determine the disease. If it has been raining for a period of time, continuously overcast and rainy, what do we have? We have dampness, an indicator of Taiyin disease. There is no need to do any lab tests or perform a CT to apprehend such indicators. However, it is these very easily obtainable pieces of information that Chinese Medicine practitioners too often turn their noses up at. They would rather mouse around for dislodged sesame seeds on the tabletop than pick up a big watermelon set before them. As a result, despite the fact that they have studied Chinese Medicine for years, they remain blunderers.

Western medical practitioners have no interest in these sorts of indicators of disease. A lobar pneumonia contracted during the coldest days of winter, and one that sets in during a long, wet spring are treated with the same antibiotics and anti-inflammatories. If you practice Chinese Medicine and neglect such signs, however, you will be seriously challenged. Why is it that the formula that so successfully combated an outbreak of encephalitis

B in Shijiazhuang, the capital of Hebei, was useless a year later in Beijing? Is it that the efficacy of Chinese Medicine treatment cannot be reduplicated? Of course not! It is because the disease indicators, and therefore the very nature of the disease, have changed. If the disease has changed, then the treatment must also change if it is to be effective.

In terms of the lunar cycle, the earthly branches *yin*, *mao*, and *chen*, are as we have just described. Where do we find these three in the course of the solar cycle? They are the first, second, and third months of the year in the lunar calendar. If we look at the passage of years, the sequence of revolutions around the sun, we have the *yin*, *mao*, and *chen* years of the twelve-year cycle. We must consider the ramifications of these correlations.

III.2. The Essentials of Shaoyang Disease

Earlier, when we discussed the two defining characteristics of Shaoyang function, we said that one of these characteristics was its hinging aspect. When we speak of hinging, we are also speaking of opening and closing, for this is the very purpose of a hinge. As we investigate and study the *Treatise on Cold Damage*, we must keep the relationship between the hinge and opening and closing constantly in mind, for it is an excellent method for understanding this text. Another crucial aspect of Shaoyang function, which we discussed in the beginning of this chapter, is its relationship to the ministerial fire.

Shaoyang rules the hinge. In order for the hinge to function properly, it is important that it is able to move freely and smoothly. The hinge, by moving, regulates opening and closing. If the hinge becomes frozen, opening and closing are lost. For this reason, the hinge benefits from being unimpeded and shuns being bound up. If it is not free, if it is instead bound up, then it cannot open and close and disease arises. In its other aspect, that of the ministerial fire, Shaoyang also requires freedom. Fire tends to blaze upward. Its predilection is to spread, unfettered. It is not predisposed to being constrained, and if forced into an enclosed space, it can cause a violent explosion.

In summary then, a key factor inducing Shaoyang to become irregular and to give rise to pathology is this constraint and binding up, this inhibition of its preferred freedom of movement.

III.3. The Essentials of Shaoyang Timing

Now that we have delineated the essential factors behind Shaoyang disease, we can take a look at the time in which Shaoyang disease has a tendency to resolve. Why does Shaoyang disease have a tendency to resolve during the *yin, mao,* and *chen* periods? In my opinion, one important reason lies in the way in which this time of year alleviates the constraint and inhibition that is so inimical to the health of Shaoyang. The *yin, mao,* and *chen* months of the year are the three months of spring. The spring belongs to wood, and the movement of wood is free and unrestrained. During this period in which freedom and fluency reign, the hinge can move without impediment and the ministerial fire is not subjected to the constraints it despises.

Furthermore, we must keep the time correspondences of the six conformations, the time periods correlated with the three yin and the three yang, in mind at all times and endeavor to integrate these with the time periods related to the five elements. Although yin and yang and the six conformations are two separate things, when we place the two side by side, we see that they are the same thing. Why do we say this? The answer should be clear from the discussions we held in earlier chapters of this book. After all, what is wood? Wood is the state of yang *qi* in a state of release. Of course, while in this particular state, not all of the yang has been liberated; it is fettered by a strand or two of yin. It is not until we reach the time of fire, of summer, that all of the yang is completely liberated. If the yang were not completely liberated at this particular time, could fire be generated? No, it most certainly could not.

When we reach autumn and the metal element, the release of yang has already shifted to its storage. Another way of putting this is that the yang *qi* gradually goes inward and becomes yin. As we progress further and enter the time of water, the time of winter, yang is in a complete state of storage. Ice and snow aptly demonstrate this complete storage of yang *qi*. At present, the global climate is gradually growing warmer. The polar ice caps and the glaciers of our mountain ranges are slowly disappearing. From a Chinese Medicine perspective, from a classical Chinese cosmological perspective, what does this say? It indicates that, on a global level, the storage of yang *qi* is gradually weakening and the release of yang *qi* is gradually increasing. The current era is an era of perpetual opening and release. All day long, every day of the week, we emphasize the release and liberation of yang *qi*, and not its storage. How can we expect to keep the glaciers from melting? In my opinion, it is inevitable. If we look at the problem from the perspective of Chinese Medicine theory, from a five-element perspective, it is completely obvious.

When we speak of metal, wood, water, and fire, what are we actually referring to? We are referring to different states of yin and yang. If you discuss the five-element theory divorced from the context of yin and yang, you will have difficulty making sense or use of this theory.

However, what is the "earth" of the five elements? What state of yin or yang does it represent? It represents an extraordinary state. Dong Zhongshu, a scholar and statesmen who was instrumental in establishing Confucianism as the state religion of China, wrote in his *Luxuriant Dew of the Spring and Autumn Annals* that the earth element was the master of the five elements. The metal, wood, water, and fire of the five elements would not be able to achieve their proper function without the earth element. Yin and yang depend on the earth in order to transition from the storage state of water to the release state of wood. By the same token, the earth element is needed to go from wood to fire, from fire to metal, and from metal to water. Yin and yang depend upon the earth element to change, fluctuate, and cycle. In Chinese Medicine, the earth element is extremely important, extremely special.

Why are the spleen and stomach, the two earth organs, considered to be the root of postnatal *qi*? In its discussion of the pulse, why does the *Plain Questions* say: "If there is stomach, the patient will live; if there is no stomach, the patient will die"? These questions are closely related to the significance of the earth element, and merit further research and study.

The five elements are expressions of different states of yin and yang. Each element flourishes, assists, rests, sequestrates, and severs in its turn. Flourishing refers to the stage of exuberance and prospering. Every element, every particular configuration of yin and yang, when at its zenith, is said to be in a state of flourishing. Assisting facilitates the flourishing; it is the element that must be undergone in order to achieve the phase of flourishing. Resting refers to the fall and decline of the state of flourishing. Sequestration is also a state of decline, but deeper and longer than resting. In the stage of severance, the element is completely finished.

If we take the fire element as an example, it flourishes during the summer, assists during the spring, rests during the eighteen-day periods before the beginning of spring, summer, fall, and winter, is sequestered during the autumn, and is severed in winter. Spring consists of the periods *yin, mao,* and *chen.* Fire reciprocates during the spring, thus fire assists during *yin, mao,* and *chen.* The character we are translating in this context as "assist" is *xiang* (相), which is the same character translated as "ministerial" in "ministerial fire" (*xianghuo* 相火), so if we take look at this another way, spring is the period of assisting (or "ministerial") fire.

We can see that *yin, mao,* and *chen* amply embody the nature of both Shaoyang and ministerial fire. When Shaoyang becomes diseased, when its normal physiology is lost, it may return when the patient enters the spatial or temporal domain of *yin, mao,* or *chen.* This is the reason why Shaoyang disease often resolves during the *yin, mao,* and *chen* periods.

III.4. Shaoyang Formulas

The main Shaoyang formula is one that is familiar to virtually any practitioner of Chinese Medicine, Xiao Chaihu Tang. Let us take a look and see if the curative properties of this formula are in accord with our previous discussion of Shaoyang physiology and disease.

III.4.a. Numerology of the Formula

Xiao Chaihu Tang uses seven ingredients, so let us begin our discussion with the number seven. What sort of number is seven in the classical Chinese understanding? Seven is the fire number. Thus, it says in the *River Chart*: "The two of earth produces fire, the seven of heaven completes it." The *River Chart* and the *Inscription of the River Luo* (Luoshu) should be carefully studied and even memorized by students of Chinese Medicine. These diagrams are of crucial importance, and the essentials of traditional numerology are contained in these pictures. Without mathematics, modern science would fail to be scientific. Without mathematical calculations and expressions, how could it possibly become sophisticated?

In truth, Chinese Medicine is the same; it is also, of necessity, mathematical, or put another way, numerological, and so these two diagrams are indispensable. Both the *Yellow Emperor's Classic* and the *Treatise on Cold Damage* use these two diagrams. Sun Simiao once said, "If one does not know the *Changes*, one cannot become a great physician." Now we do not expect everyone to "know the *Changes*," but understanding a little bit is not too much to ask.

Xiao Chaihu Tang uses seven ingredients. This indicates that it employs the fire model in its construction, fitting with its ministerial fire aspect. Now, let us examine each herb in this formula. The first ingredient is Chaihu. When we look at formulas in the *Treatise on Cold Damage*, we must first pay attention to the sequence of each formula's ingredients, which comes first and which last. This sequence is very intentional. The first ingredient is usually the emperor herb, the second the minister, and the following herbs are most often the assistant and envoy herbs. Nowadays, when writing a formula, the order of the herbs is often random, without regard to the role the herb plays in the formula. When prescribing Xiao Chaihu Tang, the physician may first write Renshen or Shengjiang instead of Chaihu. This is muddling. "As soon as the expert makes a move, we know whether they are truly an expert or not." If you write a formula like this, it goes without saying that people will know what sort of physician you are.

Chaihu belongs in the first position, for it is the emperor herb in this formula. Huangqin is second, the minister herb. What quantity of these herbs is used in the formula? Eight *liang* of Chaihu and three *liang* of Huangqin are used in this formula. Three and eight just so happen to be the numbers of the east, the numbers associated with *yin*, *mao*, and *chen*. These amounts of the emperor and minister herbs outline the function of Shaoyang, and highlight the time and place in which Shaoyang disease has a tendency to resolve. We can see that Zhang Zhongjing was remiss in nothing. Nothing is arbitrary or casual. If you prescribe Xiao Chaihu Tang and do not prescribe Chaihu in eight *liang* and Huangqin in three, is it still Xiao Chaihu Tang? It is not at all. If you use such a formula to treat a Shaoyang disorder, you may run into problems.

The same is true for Guizhi Tang. If you increase the amount of Guizhi in that formula from three *liang* to say five *liang*, we no longer have Guizhi Tang; instead you have Guizhi Jia Gui Tang, used to treat "running piglet" *qi*. By changing the amount of this one ingredient, the great sage is reduced to a witless commoner. The importance of the amount of a particular herb is evidenced by this use of numerology.

In the suburbs south of Tianjin, there is a blind physician who specializes in treating difficult disorders. People from far and wide come in admiration to request his help. Because he is blind, he cannot rely on visual observations for his diagnosis. Instead, he asks questions and takes the pulse. And after he has diagnosed the disease, what "medicine" does he prescribe? The "medicine" he prescribes is nothing other than the food-stuffs Chinese people eat every day, like mung beans, red beans, raisins, daylily buds, and so on. Regardless of your disease, he prescribes these everyday comestibles. The only difference lies in the number of each that one is instructed to eat. This lady over here is told to eat twenty mung beans and twenty raisins. That fellow over there is told to eat twenty-one mung beans and twenty-one raisins.

From the modern person's understanding, there is no difference between eating twenty mung beans and eating twenty-one mung beans. When all is said and done, it is just mung bean soup, is it not? If we were to use modern methods to analyze the constituents ingested in each case, the two doses are virtually identical. And unless the size of the beans is carefully controlled, it is quite possible that twenty beans could be equal in weight to twenty-one beans. So why is it so different in Chinese Medicine? This blind physician uses number to treat disease, and if we trace the roots of his practice all the way back, they lead us back to Zhang Zhongjing, the progenitor of the use of number to treat disease in Chinese Medicine.

The use of Dazao in formulas is an interesting example of this. In Guizhi Tang, twelve pieces of Dazao are prescribed, and the same number is prescribed in Xiao Chaihu Tang. In Shizao Tang, ten Dazao are prescribed; in Zhigancao Tang, thirty Dazao are indicated; and in Danggui Sini Tang, twenty-five Dazao are used. It is easy to understand why ten or twelve Dazao might be used in a decoction. But when we get to the examples of Dang-gui Sini Tang and Zhigancao Tang, why use twenty-five and thirty pieces respectively?

What do twenty-five or thirty Dazao represent? I ask this question, hoping that even if you do not search for the answer yourself, you sense that something unusual is at work in the prescription of such quantities. Zhigan-cao Tang is used as a formula in the final stages of disease to finish it off. It is used to treat cases characterized by "a bound and intermittent pulse and severe heart palpitations." In the early 1980s, the *Shanghai Journal of Traditional Chinese Medicine* published a series of installments by Professor

Ke Xuefan called *Gathering Flowers in the Forest of Medicine* (Yilin duoying). Later, the separate installments were collected and published as a book of its own. This book used a serial fiction style of writing to introduce principles of medicine and medical cases interwoven with a story line. The book had an entire chapter devoted to the use of Zhigancao Tang.

Zhigancao Tang is used to treat stubborn cardiac arrhythmias like atrial fibrillation and, when used appropriately, is often able to correct such irregularities. This appropriate use includes two aspects. First, we must correctly diagnose the syndrome. It must first be determined whether Zhigancao Tang is appropriate for the case at hand. Regardless of the sort of arrhythmia afflicting the patient, we must first distinguish between yin and yang in the patient and determine whether the syndrome is yin or yang in nature. To be more specific, we must determine if it is a case of yin deficiency or yang deficiency.

When we analyze the ingredients constituting this formula, we see that almost every yin-tonifying herb in the *Treatise on Cold Damage* can be found in this formula. There is little doubt that this formula is suitable for a case of yin deficiency. This formula, a great assembly of yin-tonifying herbs from the *Treatise on Cold Damage* also includes yang ingredients such as Guizhi, Shengjiang, and Qingjiu. It is reminiscent of the traditional yin yang picture, in which there is a bit of yang within the yin and a bit of yin within the yang. This image is clear in Zhigancao Tang.

Zhigancao Tang is suitable for a diagnosis of cardiac arrhythmia of the yin deficiency type. That is the first requirement in the appropriate use of this formula. The second requirement is using the correct amounts of each ingredient. This point is one that Professor Ke specifically mentions. Let us say that you use this formula to treat a patient whose symptom picture fits the indications for Zhigancao Tang perfectly. They have yin deficiency–induced atrial fibrillation, and all the other signs. But when you give the formula, the results are poor. Why is this? The reason lies with the amounts of the ingredients you use.

There is a saying among Daoists who concoct "pills of immortality": "Pass on the medicines used but do not pass on the fire." In other words, they might tell you which herbs are used in a particular formula, but they will not tell you what temperature or duration of time the herbs are cooked at, for this part of the process is far too important. Likewise, the ingredients of each formula may be taught, but the amounts of each ingredient are not passed on lightly. The amounts are like the cooking time and temperature that the Daoist alchemists guard so closely. This is the information that holds the key to either success or failure, so of course it cannot be passed on lightly.

Zhang Zhongjing is an exception. He is a sage of Chinese Medicine and as such keeps no secrets. Zhang Zhongjing reveals not only the formula but also the ingredients, and even the exact amounts of each ingredient.

When discussing the amounts used in the *Treatise on Cold Damage*, we need to look at two different measurements. One is the weight of each ingredient, and the other is the number of pieces. These two are related, but are essentially different. If the weights used are different, then this can result in qualitative changes. If the numbers used are different, this can induce qualitative changes. With regard to a change in weight, we can easily understand how this can cause a change in the action of the formula. A change in the mass, of the physical amount of an herb means more of that material substance. When we consider the second type of qualitative change, however, that which is induced by a change in the number of pieces of a particular herb that is not necessarily accompanied by a change in the overall amount of that herb, this sort of change is not easy to understand, nor can we easily have confidence in it.

When modern textbooks explain the weight measurements used in the *Treatise on Cold Damage*, they equate three grams with a single *liang*, and the standards set in the official modern materia medica are more or less the same. However, based on a large number of official, state-sanctioned bronze and iron weights that were used during the Eastern Han dynasty, Professor Ke Xuefan and associates have determined that the actual weight of a *liang* during that period was not three grams, but 15.625 grams! That is a five-fold increase from the current, conventional estimate of the amount. For instance, if we look at the archaic *jin* of Shengdihuang in Zhigancao Tang, and convert it into grams, the official modern conversion would make it roughly equivalent to 48 grams in weight. Using the archeologically corrected rate of conversion, it would be closer to 250 grams!

The *Treatise on Cold Damage* is commonly accepted to have been written during the last years of the Eastern Han Dynasty. Because it was written during this time period, the weight measurements must be converted in accord with the system of weights and measures prevalent at that time. When we correct our conversion, we are confronted with more problematic questions. A quarter of a kilogram of Shengdihuang, or 93.75 grams of Mahuang (if we convert the six *liang* used in Da Qinglong Tang), exceed the safety limits set out in the official *Materia Medica of the People's Republic of China*. If you use the actual dosages set out in the *Treatise on Cold Damage* and cure a thousand people of what ails them, then good for you! But if even one of them develops a problem from prescribing such high dosages, you will not be able to just walk away from the legal consequences. You will be regarded no differently from Hu Wanlin, who was jailed after patients died from the large dosages of Mangxiao he prescribed. You will find no support for your actions in the official pharmacopeia, nor is there any law or statute for you to fall back on.

Old Professor Ke knew quite well that the amounts prescribed in the *Treatise on Cold Damage* were those that were conventional during the time of the Eastern Han dynasty. This knowledge has more than just an archeological basis; it also has a clinical basis. For, if we use Zhigancao Tang converting one *liang* to three grams, it cannot cure a case of atrial fibrillation. As soon as we use the measurements from the Eastern Han dynasty, however, and use 250 grams of Shengdihuang, the very same formula but with the correct amount, the atrial fibrillation is quickly resolved. Nevertheless, Professor Ke has stressed the following: "Herbal medications must be given in dosages that accord with the Official Chinese materia medica and by Chinese Medicine pharmacology textbooks." If he failed to stress this point, and someone encountered a problem that might be related to the higher dosages of herbs, no amount of help would keep Mr. Ke from lawsuits and penalties.

The question of dosage is an important one. If the dosages remain ambiguous, then half the wealth bequeathed by Zhang Zhongjing might be lost to the wind. Even if your diagnosis is absolutely accurate, and the formula you choose is perfectly suited to the case before you, if the dosages in that formula are incorrect, the curative effect of your treatment will be unsatisfactory. In the end, the blame will fall on Chinese Medicine, and it will be considered poor and ineffective.

I myself have experienced the importance of the correct dosage first-hand. In 1990, when my wife Zhao Lin was 40 days into her pregnancy, she developed an extrauterine hemorrhage. At that time, for a number of reasons, we chose to treat her condition conservatively with Chinese Medicine. We immediately called my teacher in Nanning, Li Yangbo, to tell him what was happening. My teacher gave me a formula over the phone and also told me to immediately go and buy ten grams of Zanghonghua and take it as a decoction. My teacher said that Zanghonghua is the best medicine in the world for internal bleeding.

The next day, my teacher personally came to see us in Guilin. After taking my wife's pulse, he prescribed the following formula: 180 grams of Baishao, 30 grams of Yinyanghuo, and 15 grams of Zhishi to be decocted in water and taken once a day. After administering these two formulas, an ultrasound was performed the following day. Not only had the bleeding stopped, but much of the blood that had spilled into her abdominal cavity had been reabsorbed, and, to our surprise, there was still a fetus in her uterus, alive and intact. I could not help but stroke my wife's forehead as we quietly celebrated this triumph. If we had chosen surgery instead of Chinese Medicine, would we have our daughter today? Whenever I think of this event, I cannot help but feel a surge of renewed gratitude for my former teacher.

The ingredients in the second formula were nothing special, so why did they produce such outstanding results? It would seem that what was remarkable was the dosage of the ingredients. We typically use Baishao in dosages of 10 to 20 grams, and not more than 30 to 50 grams. Using 180 grams is practically unheard of. However, if such a high dosage were not given in this case, it most certainly would have failed to cure my wife. It is clear then, that the amount used in a formula is of crucial importance, and I entreat the reader to research this topic thoroughly, and hope that governmental agencies devise a strategy that allows practitioners to use Chinese Medicine in its full potency. If every practitioner were to voice their concern regarding this issue, I cannot help but think the Chinese government would take heed. If the dosages used in the *Treatise on Cold Damage* during the Eastern Han Dynasty truly were as Professor Ke Xuefan has discovered, then perhaps we will have to reconsider both the practice and efficacy of Chinese Medicine.

Now, let us consider how the number of a particular item, not just the amount, might induce a qualitative change in the formula. The two formulas my teacher prescribed to help my wife with her condition adequately illustrate the way in which a change in the quantity of a particular ingredient can affect the potency of a formula. Let's look at Zhigancao Tang. As we said earlier, this formula nourishes yin. Zhang Zhongjing indicates that thirty Dazao should be used as part of this formula. What does the number thirty signify? Thirty is the number of "a gathered crowd of yin." Of the ten basic numbers, the five even numbers (two, four, six, eight, and ten) are deemed yin. When we add up these five numbers, the result is thirty, and so it is called the "gathered crowd of yin." The use of such a number in Zhigancao Tang obviously accords with its ability to nourish yin.

Another formula the student of Chinese Medicine should be familiar with is Danggui Sini Tang. This formula is described in the Jueyin chapter of the *Treatise on Cold Damage*. The syndrome pertinent to this formula is described as "reversal cold of the hands and feet, and a pulse that is fine and verging on expiry." Considering the composition of Danggui Sini Tang itself as well as its indicated use, we can be certain that it is a formula that warms and nourishes the yang *qi*. In this formula, twenty-five pieces of Dazao are prescribed. Twenty-five is referred to as "a gathered crowd of yang" and, parallel to the "gathered crowd of yin" number, is the sum of all the odd or yang numbers from the basic number set: one, three, five, seven, and nine. Thus, twenty-five is a number in perfect accord with the action of this particular formula. The first number is a gathering of yin, the second a gathering of yang. Why didn't Zhang Zhongjing do it the other way around and put twenty-five jujubes in Zhigancao Tang and thirty in Danggui Sini Tang? Clearly, he did not use number in a vague or careless way. When the number changes, so too does the formula's image (*xiang*). If its image changes, then its effect on yin and yang will also change, and when this changes, the formula's entire nature changes.

Thus, number is not a small issue: it is every bit as important as the previously discussed issue of weight. Numbers in traditional Chinese Medicine are not purely abstract entities without actual impact. There is image (*xiang*) within number and number within image; image and number are one. When number changes, the image changes, and when the organized totality of the formula changes, so does its effect on yin and yang. This is because yin and yang express their function through image. Thus, there is a chapter we have already referred to in the *Plain Questions* called "Great

Treatise on the Correspondences of Yin and Yang." In this chapter, which uses the term *yingxiang* (應象, literally "corresponding image") in the title, we see that through image (*xiang*) we can perceive the principles underlying yin and yang, and from form we learn the function of yin and yang.

Of course, it is difficult to convince people of numerology's validity. We tend to question the real difference between twenty-five and thirty Dazao. We tend to doubt there is any real difference. Despite our doubts, why not give it a try? Experimentation is the standard method of any scientific investigation, so why not experiment a bit and see if number makes a difference. As a practitioner, one might take a number of similar cases, such as patients in the early stage of chronic heart disease. If the practitioner has a number of such patients, she might divide these patients into two cohorts: those with heart yang deficiency, and those with heart yin deficiency. Those with heart yang deficiency might decoct twenty-five Dazao a day, and those with heart yin deficiency might decoct thirty jujubes a day, and then be monitored to see if there is any change. When there is a noticeable effect, and the changes have stabilized, then the practitioner might further the experiment by giving the yin deficiency patients twenty-five jujubes a day and the yang deficiency patients thirty pieces of Dazao a day, and see if the effect of the treatment changes. If there is a change, then we know that numerology is not simply an empty superstition with no bearing on reality, and that numbers contain something that has an effect on the world around them.

So what is this thing that numbers contain? Is it information? Is it some sort of charm? We can research this further once we have established the effect of number as an actuality. If we negate its existence outright, then understanding it is futile. This as far as we will take the discussion that began with an explanation of the use of three and eight in Xiao Chaihu Tang.

III.4.b. The Physical Level

From the use of measure in Xiao Chaihu Tang, we see a particular method. This formula uses three and eight, the numbers that correspond with the earthly branches *yin*, *mao*, and *chen*, the time in which Shaoyang disease tends to resolve. When we diagnose a syndrome and prescribe a formula, it is in order to induce an illness to resolve, is it not? Thus, correspondences with the pattern that induces resolution are a crucial point in the study of Chinese Medicine. The question of number is ultimately a question of image (*xiang*). Although *xiang* has a definite meaning, and there is no reason to have doubts about it, one always has a feeling that this meaning is not terribly clear.

With this in mind, we have a few concrete topics we can discuss, things that relate to the physical level, the level of "things." If we investigate both modern science and traditional Chinese Medicine from the perspective of image (*xiang*), number, and phenomena, then we can see that the area common to both Chinese Medicine and modern science is the level of phenomena, of things. At this level, we must affirm that modern science has gone further and done a better job than Chinese Medicine. In terms of knowledge at the level of things, modern science can detect things that are smaller and subtler; it is more concrete, and it possesses a greater number of techniques.

Has modern science expanded its comprehension of the world to include understanding at the level of image (*xiang*) and number? In other words, has the materialistic research of science expanded to the point that it includes investigation into the realm of image and number? In terms of traditional Chinese Medicine images and numbers, it would appear that science has yet to expand to this point. Yet on these two levels, on the level of image and at the numerological level, traditional Chinese Medicine has already gone a long way. We can see that both traditional Chinese and modern Western Medicine have their own strengths and weaknesses.

In terms of images, we can see that Chinese Medicine is strong, but when we consider its understanding of the physical realm of things, it falls somewhat short. This is because at the time Chinese Medicine was forming, our mastery of "things" was lacking. Two thousand years ago, what sorts of things were there? Furthermore, if you wish to investigate into things, you need special things or devices with which to do it. If you reflect for a moment on the way in which modern science currently investigates phenomena, this should be clear. If you wish to understand a particular material substance, if you wish to uncover the basic composition or structure of a substance, what do you need? You need very precise equipment. You need a particle accelerator, a superconducting supercollider. If you do not have these, you will not be able to break apart the tiniest particles and discover what they consist of.

Once the path of investigating things with things is taken, the traveler finds himself on a long and winding road. The more you investigate things, the more dependent upon things you become; the higher your level of understanding of phenomena, the greater your dependency is upon physical equipment. Once we are following this long and tortuous path into greater and greater dependency on more and more sophisticated and cumbersome equipment, the role that the heart and mind play begins to pale. Modern man uses things to know things, whereas the ancient person used her own mind to know the world around her.

They used their own minds, their hearts, to know the world around them. They investigated things, and studied the phenomena of nature. It was as described by Confucius in the *Great Learning*: "Knowing when to stop, they became determined; becoming determined, they became quiet and reposeful; after quietude came peace, and in this peaceful state, they were able to deliberate at length, and this deliberation allowed them to obtain that which they pursued." Obtaining their aim was last, and revealed that "things and the mind originate from one source."

This illustrates the difference between traditional Chinese and modern scientific methods and techniques for obtaining knowledge. If we are to investigate both modern science and traditional Chinese Medicine, if we are to place them both at the same pinnacle of civilization, then we must recognize these differences. Traditional Chinese Medicine is weaker in terms of its mastery of the physical world, of the world of "things." In this respect, Chinese Medicine will benefit from assimilating methods and techniques from modern science. This is, in fact, the main project Chinese Medicine is currently undertaking as it modernizes. We might ask ourselves: What aspect of traditional Chinese Medicine is in most need of modernization? Only the world of things, physical phenomena, benefits from modernization. How can "numbers" or "images" be modernized? On the contrary, in this respect these categories, rather than being modernized by Western science, can "traditionalize" modern science. It is not simply the case that the traditional can only be modernized; the modern can also be traditionalized!

What is the advantage of such "traditionalization"? Perhaps it could provide breakthroughs in developing certain scientific models, or provide the key to escaping from certain dead ends in modern scientific theories. Certain fields of modern scientific research have already entered into strange territories. For instance, research into the elementary particles of matter have brought us to the land of quarks. What do quarks signify? It will not be easy to find still smaller particles. If it is this hard to glimpse quarks, then how difficult will it be to look still deeper into the fabric of the physical world? Thus, in the material world, in the physical world of "being," you can dissect things into smaller and smaller pieces, but once you get to a certain point, you cannot go any further. At a certain point, if the investigation is continued, "being" becomes "non-being." If we wish to proceed beyond this juncture, then there must be a fundamental change in our way of thinking. I personally believe that traditional Chinese thinking could be exceptionally helpful at this juncture. It is only at this point, at the point at which "being" shifts toward "non-being," that the metaphysical understandings of Chinese Medicine, those of "number" and "image," might find acceptance in modern science.

I often find myself thinking that those who have made Chinese Medicine their profession should practice a little *qigong* and cultivate temperance. They should not seek to modernize everything—there is really no hurry! Chinese Medicine is not a matter of modernization; it is a matter of proper study. If you study Chinese Medicine well, not only can you go wherever you like, but you can also act as a mentor to modernity. In the *Analects*, Confucius says: "Do not be anxious if you have no position; only concern yourself that you are fit to hold one." These words by Confucius are worthy of the student of Chinese Medicine's attention. We need not feel anxious about the position of Chinese Medicine in the future. In other words, we should not fret over Chinese Medicine's market share, or the ability of this profession to line our pockets. We need only worry about our own earnest study of Chinese Medicine, our own efforts to thoroughly understand the wealth of knowledge it affords.

Understanding and fully grasping "image" and "number" is relatively difficult, so we should begin at the level of physical phenomena. From this level, we can see that the emperor herb in Xiao Chaihu Tang is Chaihu. The flavor of Chaihu is bitter, and its *qi* is neutral. Its main actions are clearly described in the *Divine Farmer's Classic of Materia Medica*. In addition, the famous Qing dynasty physician Zhou Yan wrote a book called *Records of Thoughtful Differentiation of Materia Medica*, in which he describes and discusses this herb in vivid and authentic detail. He describes the action of

Chaihu as "From yin emerging yang." How are we to understand this? If we think of the quality of time characteristic of *yin, mao,* and *chen,* this description makes perfect sense. We can think of yin and yang as north and south, or winter and summer, or water and fire. Winter is yin and summer is yang, and spring, the time of *yin, mao,* and *chen,* is when yang emerges from yin. Chaihu corresponds with *yin, mao,* and *chen* perfectly. Since it corresponds with *yin, mao,* and *chen,* it also corresponds with Shaoyang, the time in which Shaoyang disease tends to resolve, and the direction used to treat Shaoyang disease.

The next ingredient in the formula is Huangqin. Huangqin clears heat and eliminates fire. Why must heat be cleared and fire eliminated with this formula? In the discussion of Shaoyang disease in this chapter, we talked about how fire does not wish to be constrained or pent up. If it is constrained, what happens? Those who have lived as farmers in China certainly know the answer to this. Back when I was a farmer, when I lived on a commune as part of the Chinese Commune System that was established during the Great Leap Forward, we rarely used chemical fertilizers. A portion of our fertilizer was "night soil" from the cities, and another large portion was cow and pig dung. At regular intervals, every month or two as the case might be, once the stables were full of dung, we would arrange a work party to come and "bring out the cow dung." We would then pile up the dung in a designated spot in the village. When spring came and it was time to fertilize the fields, we would take the dung from this pile to the fields.

Whenever we would start digging into this pile, it would seethe with hot steam. We had to work the manure into the bin with a long-handled rake to avoid being scalded. It was hot enough to cook an egg. This pile of manure would spontaneously produce heat and fire. It was not the sort of fire that one makes with kindling; it was heat that came from constraint. Once things are enclosed in a small space, they very easily produce heat and fire. Chaihu is able to undo this sort of confinement and constraint, and unblock the path whereby heat rises and is expressed. But from another angle, the heat has already been produced, and this heat must be cooled and eliminated. This is the purpose of the Huangqin in the formula.

The next ingredient in the formula is Renshen. Renshen is able to moisten and nourish the five viscera and tonifies *qi* and yin. In the long term, Renshen promotes longevity, and in the short term it increases energy and overall vitality. The Chaihu helps to raise upward and unblock the congestion and confinement of this upward movement. In essence, Chaihu restores the natural functioning of Shaoyang. It causes yang to emerge from yin, but it needs some assistance in this effort, and Renshen provides that assistance. The action of the remaining four herbs in the formula—Banxia, Zhigancao, Shengjiang, and Dazao—can be surmised by the reader.

III.4.c. Selecting the Appropriate Time to Administer Medication

In our earlier discussions of Taiyang and Yangming disease, when we discussed the times in which these types of disease will tend to resolve, we did not discuss the best time to administer the medicine. Administering medication at the appropriate time is highly important. Let us say that the physician diagnoses a particular disease and then writes an appropriate prescription, for example Xiao Chaihu Tang, then adds that the herbs are to be decocted in water and taken three times per day. This method is fine, but with regard to Shaoyang disease, there is an optimal time at which to take the medication. Furthermore, the physician can achieve twice the curative result with half the effort if this optimal time is taken advantage of. Modern medicine also observes the correct timing in which to prescribe particular medications. For instance, the effect of digitalis on the heart varies with the time of the day, and modern medical physicians pay attention to this timing when treating heart patients. Around 4 am, the effect of digitalis is far higher than at other times of the day. Anti-diabetic medications show similar characteristics. The very same medication given at different times of the day demonstrates a notable change in efficacy. Studying the best time to administer a particular medicine is a matter of learning when to get the maximum effect with the minimum dosage. In Chinese Medicine, there are many research papers or theses that could be written on this subject. There are two aspects that could be written about: the first is searching through the classics for writings on this topic; the other is to search for areas of convergence with modern research on the subject.

From the traditional point of view, we read in the "Great Treatise on the Four *Qi* and the Tuning of the Spirit" of the *Plain Questions*: "Thus, the sages nourished yang in spring and summer, and nourished *yin* in autumn and winter, each according to its root." Their timing was based on the changes of yin and yang. Attention to the flow of yin and yang must be integrated into every aspect of our practice. To put it in simple terms, when should we give medicines that nourish the yang? When should we give herbs that nourish the yin? This should already be clear from the *Plain Questions* passage above. We might compare the principle of these efficacious times to be similar to watering a plant. If we apply the water directly to the roots of the plant, we get more bang for our buck. However, I should warn the reader that Chinese Medicine is not a rigid system. If we actually waited until autumn and winter to administer the yin tonics or spring and summer to nourish yang in the patient, the results would be poor. Are there not four seasons in a day, so to speak? We need not wait until spring or summer to administer medicine that nourishes the yang; we need only wait until the time of the earthly branches *yin, mao,* and *chen,* or the earthly branches *si, wu,* and *wei.* When taking yin tonics, we simply wait until the time period associated with the earthly branches *shen, you,* and *xu,* for these are autumn in the daily cycle, are they not? *Hai, zi,* and *chou* represent winter in the course of a day, just as they do in the course of a year, do they not?

Now that we have explored the topic of when to administer medication to some extent, let us return to the topic of when Shaoyang disease tends to resolve. Why does Shaoyang disease resolve during *yin, mao,* and *chen?* Why does Taiyang disease resolve during *si, wu,* and *wei?* And why does Yangming disease improve during the hours of *shen, you,* and *xu?* It is simply a case of "nourishing yang during spring and summer, and *yin* during autumn and winter." But here it is the firmament, the cycling energies of nature, that are assisting the human form. Once this is recognized, the physician realizes that for all of the six conformations, the time in which the disease has a tendency to resolve is also the correct time to administer the appropriate medication. For instance, take Mahuang Tang used to treat Taiyang cold damage. Taiyang disease should be treated during the period in which Taiyang disease has a tendency to resolve, the period consisting of the earthly branches *si, wu,* and *wei.* When we give this medicine during this time, the medicine and the prevalent cosmological energy work synergistically, "each in accord with the root," and twice the result is achieved with half the effort. Administering this medication during other parts of the day can still be done, as necessity or convenience dictates.

Regarding modern research, we can also incorporate some basic insights derived from research into chronology, so that the ancient and the modern might benefit and inform one another. For instance, we gave the earlier examples of both cardiotonic and anti-diabetic medications that are most effective around 4 am, during the time period of the *yin* earthly branch (3–5 am). Because of this time connection, we could see that diabetes and heart disease have an internal connection to the categories of Jueyin, Shaoyin, and Shaoyang disease. Not only do these three diseases share *yin* as a period that they tend to resolve, it is the only trigram associated with the time periods of the six conformations that contains two yin lines and one yang line. For this reason, the time period of the earthly branch *yin* deserves earnest research and contemplation, both from traditional Chinese Medicine and modern scientific perspectives. For instance, if you contemplate the internal connection of diabetes with Jueyin disease, then I guarantee that you will have new insights and perhaps even breakthroughs with regard to treating this illness. Chinese Medicine and Western Medicine can be complementary. We need only pay close attention to how they might best complement one another. Taken to the highest level, adversaries can become friends, all the more so with Chinese and Western Medicine.

III.5. Two Unique Herbs in *Divine Farmer's Classic of Materia Medica*

In the *Divine Farmer's Classic of Materia Medica*, there are two herbs that raise an interesting question. The first herb is Chaihu as used in Xiao Chaihu Tang, and the second herb is Dahuang used in Da Chaihu Tang. Chaihu is considered a "higher" herb in this herbal classic, and Dahuang is considered a "lower" herb. The *qi*, flavor, and action of Chaihu and Dahuang were described as follows in the *Divine Farmer's Classic of Materia Medica*:

> Chaihu is bitter and neutral. It primarily treats bound *qi* in the heart, abdomen, intestines, and stomach; accumulations of food and drink; and pathogenic *qi* of cold or heat. It aids in ridding the old and bringing in the new. It lightens a body that has grown weary, brightens the eyes, and benefits the *jing*.

> Dahuang is bitter and cold. It descends blood stasis blockages in the blood, cold and heat, lumps in the abdomen that cause distention and pain, and accumulations of stagnant food and drink; it wipes clean the intestines and the stomach; it pushes out the old and restores the new; opens the passageways through which digested food travels; regulates the center and transforms food; and quiets the five viscera.

Chaihu and Dahuang are different in terms of their *qi*, their flavor and their action, but when we take a close look at what the *Divine Farmer's Classic of Materia Medica* says about these two herbs, we see that they actually share a number of traits. They both break up stagnated accumulations and open up the passageways of the intestines and stomach. The two are different in the intensity with which they break up these accumulations, and each has its own particular sphere of influence in which it is able to break these up. We will discuss this particular point at greater length later. A shared aspect of these two herbs is the ability to "push out the old and restore the new." According to my investigation, there are only three herbs that are given this particular description, the third one being Xiaoshi. Xiaoshi is rarely used, and we need not discuss it here. Now, let us take a closer look at the shared traits of Chaihu and Dahuang.

III.5.a. Phase Transition

Let us first discuss "pushing out the old and restoring the new." Old and new are opposing concepts. "Old" means a thing or a state that is already established. "New" represents the opposite state. To overturn an old or established state and set up a new one, this is what is meant by "pushing out the old and restoring the new." In addition, to encourage one thing to transform into something entirely different and new is also within the scope of "pushing out the old and arriving at the new."

At the forefront of modern physics is an extremely important field of study about the "phase transition point." We are not going to discuss this field of study from an expert's perspective here, but will rather look at it as more of a general observable phenomenon, giving us an opportunity to more directly engage with the questions it presents.

A simple explanation of phase transition is a change in the state of something. In Chinese Medicine, such a change of state can be described in terms of yin and yang: it is said that "yin and yang are the father and mother of transformation." The changes and transformations of yin and yang are discussed in terms of their archetypal image (*xiang*). Thus, the *Yellow Emperor's Classic* refers to the type of transformation we just described as "change of image" (*xiang bian*). When a thing shifts from one phase or state of matter to another, it must undergo a process of transformation, and during this process there is a critical point, or critical state, where the question of whether or not the transformation will take place and what particular direction it will take are determined. The change that occurs in this state is called the critical point phase transition. Thus, the critical point as well as the transition of phase determines the outcomes of the transformation situation.

The change that occurs in the critical point affects a thermodynamic system's entire arc of change. Whether a thing can traverse from "old" to "new" is determined by this phase transition. From this perspective, it would seem that the function of both Chaihu and Dahuang, which get rid of the old and bring in the new, influence this phase transition state. This is worth contemplating. Suppose Chaihu and Dahuang actually have an effect on phase transition and influence the likelihood of a phase transition state. This would have profound and far-reaching implications. Disease is a state, just as health is a state. At times we go from health to disease, and at others we return to health from disease. How does this change come about? There are different phase transitions, and the direction of the transition also varies. As a result, we have these different states of health and disease. When disease shifts to health, it is as we wish, as we desire. When a state of health changes to sickness, it is not as we had hoped. Might it be possible to find a method of using the common action of Chaihu and Dahuang, along with the appropriate accompaniment of other herbs, to influence the direction of "phase transition" and take a patient from a state of sickness to health? This question is worth looking into, and is one that is especially pertinent when it comes to diseases that come about suddenly, such as the metastasis of malignant cancers.

III.5.b. The Correct Way

Making a connection between the "changing old to new" action of Chaihu and Dahuang and the modern scientific study of phase transition may not be exact, but it allows for an interesting segue between the traditional and the modern. Besides sharing this action, another shared aspect of these herbs is their function of breaking up bound *qi*, accumulations, blood stasis, and obstructions to the flow of blood. Put another way, Chaihu and Dahuang are able to clear away obstacles. After all, bound *qi*, accumulations of morbid matter, blood clots, and blocked circulation are the obstructions that plague the five solid and the six hollow organs, the "four limbs and the hundred bones," the channels and course ways of the channels and collaterals. The ancients said: "Only if the original authenticity of the five viscera remains unobstructed and clear will none of the hundred diseases arise." The myriad disease states arise from blockages in the five viscera. Therefore, if you can remove these obstructions and blockages in the body, you can resolve a crucial contributor to disease. Chaihu and Dahuang share the ability to remove such blockages, but there is a very important difference in the sort of "thing" that is removed.

The connotations of the Chinese word for "thing" (*dongxi* 東西) are not aptly represented by the term's English counterpart. *Dongxi* literally means east-west. *Dongxi* can mean virtually anything, regardless of size or type. The English word "thing" has a much narrower range of meaning. So what defines *dongxi*? Earlier, when we discussed the part of the body referred to as Renzhong ("human center"), we talked about how it contained a sort of Chinese Medicine secret. The Chinese word *dongxi* also contains such a secret, but its implications are far wider than those of Renzhong.

The Chinese understood phenomena to be inseparable from yin and yang. According to the *Plain Questions's* "Great Treatise on the Correspondences of Yin and Yang": "Yin and yang are the way of heaven and earth, the warp and weft of the myriad things, the father and mother of change and transformation, the origin and source of life and death, the palace of the spiritual light." Yin and yang can be understood as we have summarized them earlier in this book: "yang brings forth and yin grows, yang kills and yin stores." What is yang emerging? The east is where yang emerges. What is the withering effect of yang? The west, where the sun sets, of course. Only if something is born can it grow, and only if it is killed can it be stored. Hence, *dongxi* aptly conveys "birth, growth, death, and storage." Thus, the meaning of *dongxi* is very deep; it cannot be adequately translated with the English word "thing." This is akin to the common translation of *Honglou-meng*, usually translated as *Dream of the Red Chamber*. This translation conveys one possible meaning of these three characters, but it fails to convey all of the other possibilities inherent in the Chinese. The result is a flat, one-dimensional translation of a title that is as rich and varied as the imagination. Within the Chinese word *dongxi*, there is birth and death, change and transformation, impermanence, and much of the basic traditional worldview. Why did Confucius emphasize that "The nobleman eats without seeking satiation, rests without seeking quiet"? Why was Laozi so prudent in his speech, when he constantly reiterated: "Being contented with one's lot is no disgrace, knowing contentment one is constantly happy"? Because everything must come to an end, and nothing is permanent. If you look for something permanent in this world of impermanence, or something constant in this world of perpetual change, you will be disappointed until the day you die. Once you recognize this, you would do your best to change course. Do not center your life on material gain; instead, focus your efforts on the Dao. There is much that we can learn simply from *dongxi*!

From the perspective of "vessels" that we spoke of earlier in this book, the *Plain Questions* says: "Rising and falling, coming out and going in only pertain to vessels." That which rises emerges, like the east. That which descends enters, like the west. Being a "thing" (*dongxi*) means rising and falling are an inherent part of it. Rising and falling, exiting and entering— these categories of movement and the larger patterns of activity that they entail are absolutely essential to life and health. In the *Plain Questions* chapter "The Great Treatise on the Six Subtleties," we read: "When exiting and entering are ruined, the transformation of the spirit trigger perishes; when rising and falling cease, the *qi* is orphaned and endangered. Without exiting and entering, there can be no cycle of birth, growth, adulthood, and old age. Without rising and falling, there can be no birth, growth, transformation, retrieval, and storage." Why should exiting and entering cease? One important reason these might cease is that the thoroughfares whereby entering and exiting take place can become obstructed, and thereby hindered. If the passageways are not open, how can exiting and entering take place? How can rising and falling occur? There is nothing to do but quit in such a situation.

These thoroughfares or passageways are two in number: one on the east that allows for rising and emerging, and another on the west that allows for entering and descending. Both of these passages must be entirely open, and the rising and falling, entering and exiting functions thereby ensured, thereby preserving the proper workings of the spirit-mechanism of nature and the appropriate positioning of *qi*. Health naturally results. When there are blockages and obstructions, the spirit-trigger is extinguished, and the proper positioning of *qi* becomes abandoned, how could the person possibly be healthy and strong? The only way to restore health is to devise a way to dredge these obstructed channels.

Earlier, when we spoke of how Chaihu and Dahuang clear away obstructions, we mentioned that these two herbs were similar in some ways, but different in certain important respects. What are these differences? They are different in the paths they open. Chaihu opens up the eastern path and clears the way for rising and emerging, whereas Dahuang clears the western path and removes obstructions to entering and descending. Sometimes disease is caused by an obstruction of the eastern path, sometimes by an obstruction in the west, and sometimes it is caused by obstructions in both paths. We can determine where the obstruction lies through the pulse and the overall syndrome picture. If the eastern path is obstructed, then we must use Chaihu; if the obstruction lies in the west, then Dahuang is indicated. Of course, if both paths are hindered, then we should use both Chaihu and Dahuang, as we see in the Da Chaihu Tang. The function of both Xiao Chaihu Tang and Da Chaihu Tang should be clear to us. Xiao Chaihu Tang clears the eastern path, and Da Chaihu Tang clears both the eastern and the western paths.

From this particular perspective, that of east and west, we can derive a paradigm, a "Correct Way," that might be applied to almost any problem or contemplation in Chinese Medicine. This is called the east-west paradigm, or the rising and falling method paradigm, or even the emerging and entering paradigm. All disease states can be understood in terms of this paradigm. The disease may be the result of a problem with the east path, or the west path, or both. Regardless, the importance of Chaihu and Dahuang in treating disease according to this paradigm is clear. When my late teacher was still alive, he placed special importance on these two herbs. Once he said, "Chaihu and Dahuang, when used correctly, are without equal in this world." To the perspectives on these two herbs we have already explored, those of "pushing out the old and arriving at the new" and "critical point phase transition," we can add this east-west paradigm.

In the Yangming chapter of this book, we spent some time discussing high blood pressure. In that discussion, we saw how high blood pressure is essentially a disorder caused by obstruction of the vessels through which the blood moves. When we touch on the topic of obstruction, we are quickly reminded of the notion of east and west we just discussed. When we discussed this obstruction in the Yangming chapter, we did so in a general way. Now that we have examined Shaoyang, and the paradigm of east and west, the topic of obstruction becomes clearer. When we speak of obstruction, we are speaking of obstruction of either the eastern or the western route. In the Yangming chapter, it was primarily obstruction of the western, descending path, and with regard to Shaoyang, it is primarily obstruction of the eastern, ascending way. Whether it be obstruction of the eastern or western path, any obstruction can result in elevated blood pressure. It is only required that we differentiate the two before we choose our method of treatment. Currently in China, many Chinese Medicine practitioners seem unable to think outside the Western model of high blood pressure. As soon as they encounter a hypertensive patient, they immediately conclude that it should be treated by calming the liver and subduing wind. How is this treating the disease in accord with the differentiation of the syndrome? It is not. This is called mistaking the slave for the master. If there are no guiding principles in Chinese Medicine, upon what can you rely to decide your method of cure?

When a Western medical physician treats high blood pressure, anti-hypertensives are used, and that use is absolutely in accord with the principles of Western Medicine. But if a Chinese Medicine physician behaves this way, it is farcical. What sort of "thing" (*dongxi*) is hypertension? What is it that you are "dropping" when treating a hypertensive patient? In the clinical setting, there are patients for whom Western anti-hypertensive medication is unsuitable, but who got no results from the piles of liver-calming, liver-subduing, wind-extinguishing herbs they took. If we take the pulse, we might immediately see yang deficiency and water-rheum. If you warm the yang of these patients and transform the rheum, their blood pressure will gradually come down. Why is this? Because once the yang *qi* is warmed and the water-rheum transformed, the eastern path is no longer obstructed. In Chinese Medicine, we clearly distinguish between the root and the branch, the primary and the secondary. We cannot let ourselves be led about by Western Medicine's penchant for giving a particular symptom a disease name. If we allow ourselves to be shepherded by this convention, we will lose the essential nature of Chinese Medicine.

III.6. The Shaoyang Pulse

Let us take briefly discuss the two Shaoyang pulse types we most often encounter, in simple terms. The two most common Shaoyang pulses are evident in the *Treatise on Cold Damage*. Line 265 reads: "In cold damage when the pulse is wiry and fine, the head painful with heat effusion, this belongs to Shaoyang." And according to line 266: "When Taiyang disease does not resolve, but instead proceeds to become Shaoyang disease, the area below the ribs becomes hard and full, the patient retches and cannot eat, heat and cold alternate, and neither downward purgation nor vomiting have been induced, the pulse is sunken and tight, treat it with Xiao Chaihu Tang." One pulse is wiry and fine, and the other sunken and tight. Either pulse indicates that there is Shaoyang disease. Why is this? If we remember our earlier discussion, we will recall that in Shaoyang disease, there is constraint or inhibition that results in stifling. When constrained and stifled in this way, the *qi* of the pulse cannot rise up and smooth out. Whether it is wiry, or fine, or sunken, or tight, it comes about the same way. It is as the Qing dynasty physician Zhou Yan said: "Should it be the case that after the completion of yin, yang emerges, the patient will still be beset by yin, and will easily become constrained by cold, which will prevent the yang from extending outward, and causing it instead to contend with yin." Thus, the pulse becomes wiry and fine, sunken and tight.

That is as far as we will discuss Shaoyang.

CHAPTER EIGHT

THE ESSENTIALS OF TAIYIN DISEASE

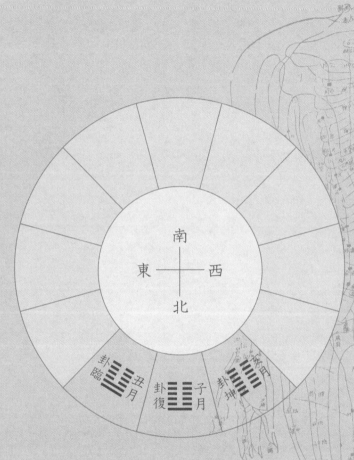

Taiyin disease tends to
resolve in the time from *hai* to *chou*.

Beginning with this chapter, we will be looking at diseases of the three yin conformations. Let us begin by looking at the chapter on Taiyin in the *Treatise on Cold Damage*. The Taiyin chapter is the chapter with the fewest lines in the *Treatise on Cold Damage*, consisting of only eight lines. In these eight lines, it primarily discusses the issue of Taiyin spleen earth, and does not touch upon Taiyin lung metal.

There are eight lines in the Taiyin chapter, and here we are discussing Taiyin disease in Chapter Eight of this book. This was an unwitting coincidence. I have simply been writing and it turned out like this. The inadvertent can, at times, seem intentional. Shao Kangjie of the Song dynasty was a great master of the *Classic of Changes*. He wrote a famous book called the *Plum Flower Calculations for the Changes*. In this book, he discussed the relationship between the eight trigrams and numbers. Thus, *Qian* Heaven is related to the number one, *Dui* Lake to the number two, *Li* Flame to the number three, *Zhen* Thunder to four, *Xun* Wind to five, *Kan* Water to six, *Gen* Mountain to seven, and *Kun* Earth to eight. *Kun* is Earth and its number is eight. And so, the number of lines in the Taiyin chapter of the *Treatise on Cold Damage* agrees with this piece of numerology. Numbers are truly marvelous.

Below, we will discuss the first question with regard to the Taiyin chapter.

I. An Explanation of Taiyin

I.1. The Meaning of Taiyin

Taiyin belongs to the spleen and to earth, that much is clear. However, to flesh out the basic meaning of Taiyin, we will need to expand on this point a bit. Does the name Taiyin refer to anything else besides "earth"? Indeed it does! It also refers to water, since Taiyin is directly related to the concept of "damp." Therefore, we must look not only at earth but also at water; indeed, it would behoove us to consider the two together, as a joined entity. This union of water and earth is essential to life on earth. It is almost impossible to imagine our world or human life, if water and earth were not almost constantly wedded to one another. It would be a world of dust and deluge and nothing in between. In order to discuss the essential meaning of Taiyin, it is of great importance that we make the relationship between water and earth perfectly clear.

I.1.a. Taiyin Refers to Spleen Earth

Taiyin rules the spleen earth, and this is pointed out in a number of classical sources. Thus, there is plenty of support for this supposition in the classics. For instance, we find it in the following *Plain Questions* chapters: "Treatise on Taiyin and Yangming," "Treatise on The Essentials of Diagnosis and On Exhaustion in the Channels," "Great Treatise on the Five Regular Policies," as well as the "Great Treatise on the Policies and Arrangements of the Six Principal *Qi*."

Furthermore, the "Treatise on the True Words in the Golden Cabinet" also discusses the issue of spleen earth. However, in this chapter, spleen earth is not discussed in terms of Taiyin; it is referred to as the "extreme yin within yin" (陰中之至陰). Why is spleen earth referred to as "extreme yin" (*zhiyin*)? Or, put another way, how is the "extreme yin" earth? There are two interpretations of this.

First of all, what is *zhi* (至)? *Zhi* means "utmost," "ultimate," or "maximum." This Chinese character is roughly equivalent to the English suffix "-est"; it indicates the superlative. Thus, the *zhiyin* is the utmost yin, the yin beyond which there is no more yin. That is an apt definition of *zhiyin*, but can we define it in more concrete terms? To do this, we must rely upon the *Classic of Changes*. If we look at the trigrams of the *Classic of Changes*, which trigram represents the *zhiyin*? It is the trigram that contains no yang lines whatsoever, the trigram that consists solely of yin lines. It is, of course, the trigram *Kun*. The *Kun* trigram is earth. Thus, the utmost yin is earth and this is clear when we look at the trigram.

Secondly, what other meanings are attributed to *zhi*? In Chinese, we say "... from Nanning '*zhi*' Kunming." What does *zhi* mean in this context? In this context, *zhi* means "to arrive at." Based on this understanding of the word, *zhiyin* means to arrive at yin, to get to the yin. What is yin? If we look at the four seasons of the year (spring, summer, fall, and winter), spring and summer are yang, and fall and winter are yin. Autumn is the beginning of this yin period, so the *zhiyin*, the arrival at yin, is also the arrival or beginning of autumn. What time of year do we arrive at autumn? We arrive at autumn in late summer, and late summer is the time of year associated with earth. This is another understanding of the association of *zhiyin* with earth.

Yet another meaning is that spoken by the ancients: Taiyin is the moon. What is the moon? The *Gongyangzhuan* commentary on the *Spring and Autumn Annals* says: "The moon is the essence of the soil and earth." From this perspective, too, Taiyin is ascribed to earth.

I.1.b. Taiyin Refers to Kidney Water

Just now, in our discussion of Taiyin as related to earth, we briefly touched on three ways in which we could understand the connection between the two. Now, we will look at Taiyin as related to water, and we will also look at this relationship from three corresponding perspectives.

First from the Taiyin perspective, as we see it in "Nine Needles and Twelve Sources" of the *Spiritual Pivot*, which says: "The kidneys are *taiyin* within yin." This definition of Taiyin as the kidneys is very straightforward and we need not belabor the point.

Secondly, Taiyin is the same as *zhiyin* ("extreme yin"), but there is yet another interpretation of *zhiyin*. This is the interpretation that can be derived from the *Plain Questions* chapter titled "Treatise on Acupoints to treat Water and Heat." Here we learn that "The kidneys are the *zhiyin*, *zhiyin* refers to the plentiful abundance of water." And in the chapter titled "Treatise on Explaining the Profound," it says: "The accumulation of water is the *zhiyin*, that which is *zhiyin* is the essence of the kidneys." Both pieces of writing are very clear about the position of the *zhiyin*. For this reason, there is little doubt that the *zhiyin* belongs to the kidney water. Secondly, there is an acupuncture point named Zhiyin (BL 67). The acupuncture point Zhiyin is the well point of the bladder channel. Thus, according to the *Spiritual Pivot* chapter "Conveyance of the Root" (Benshu): "The bladder emerges at Zhiyin. Zhiyin is the point at the tip of the smallest toe, it is the well metal point." The urinary bladder holds the office of regional rectifier, and the body liquids are stored in it. The fact that the well point of the bladder channel is the one that is called *zhiyin* reaffirms the connection between *zhiyin* and water.

Furthermore, the term Taiyin is directly associated with the moon. *Explaining Writing and Analyzing Characters* says: "The moon is the essence of Taiyin," and the *Huainanzi* tells us "The essence of the water *qi* is the moon." Taiyin is the moon, and the essence of water *qi* is also the moon. Once again, Taiyin is connected to water.

I.1.c. The Union of Earth and Water

The union of earth and water is evident from the preceding discussion. In medicine, Taiyin is related to spleen earth, just as the *zhiyin* is related to spleen earth. This is clear. There is an equal amount of evidence that Taiyin is related to kidney water, and that the *zhiyin* is related to kidney water. Outside the realm of medical texts, we also read that "Taiyin is the essence of soil and earth," and then we read that "Taiyin is the essence of water *qi*." This is enough to confuse people. It is apparent contradiction like this that causes people to think that Chinese Medicine concepts are a chaotic mess of inconsistencies. Grandpa says it belongs to earth, Grandma says water— how confusing! At first glance, it is confusing. Once you overcome this confusion and see through to its essential quality, however, it no longer seems confusing. Then you will sense that there is profound significance in this "confusion" of water and earth, namely the union of water and earth that we mentioned earlier.

The union of earth and water is of paramount importance. Without this union, there would be no humanity, and what sort of place would the earth be? This planet we live on has people; it has life and up until now, no life has been discovered anywhere else in our solar system. Is there life on some planet somewhere else in space? Perhaps, but so far human eyes or modern scientific methods have been unable to detect it. Why is there life only on earth? Why are there people only on our planet? It is because of the union between water and earth. Are water and earth joined together on any other planet? No, of course not. Absolutely not.

If you remember, several chapters ago, I recommended two texts by the famous Qing dynasty physician Zheng Qin'an of Sichuan: *The Unbroken Circle of Medical Methods* and *True Transmission of Medical Principles*. On page 5 of *True Transmission of Medical Principles*, there is a sentence that reads: "The union of water and earth is the world's greatest achievement." What a truly wonderful line! From a Chinese Medicine perspective, this is a line that penetrates into the very Dao. The concept of Taiyin, the meaning of which is conveyed by its own name, simultaneously implies both water and earth. There is no confusion between the name and what is signified. The concept, the name, of Taiyin refers to the very center of life and existence. All other aspects of our existence depend upon this relationship between water and earth. If water and earth were not harmonized, if water and earth were not joined, then how can we even start to talk about other things?

The relationship between water and earth is central. It is as central to the discourse of Chinese Medicine as the Dao is to Laozi's teachings. Can water be discussed separately from earth? Would it do to have water and earth as separate entities? Of course not. Water and earth must be conjoined; this is the world's great achievement.

From the union of water and earth, the world we know is made and humanity is made. Conversely, it is the responsibility of humanity, born of this union, to safeguard it. Why have we expended such effort to preserve traditional culture for thousands of years? To a large extent, it has been to safeguard this very union. In the current era, as traditional culture and thought is pushed aside, and everything is modernized and made scientific, no one gives two hoots about such unions. However, if humanity disregards this most basic prerequisite for its own existence, and does not endeavor to safeguard and take care of it, tending only to science and the products of science, then humanity is burning a very crucial bridge. Ultimately, it will be humanity that suffers the loss. There is a saying in Chinese: "If the person is about to lose their scalp, they are foolish to worry about their hair." Science should exercise more foresight! We think only of the present, and disregard the future consequences. We idle away our time seeking pleasures, while squandering the inheritance of our children and grandchildren, leaving them nothing but inestimable debt. If this is the type of behavior that science inspires, then perhaps we should reconsider some of the ideas that science has furnished us with.

The union of earth and water is obviously very important, but why do earth and water join? The answer is provided to us by the *Classic of Changes*. The trigrams of the *Classic of Changes* can be divided into pre- and postnatal sequences. How are the prenatal trigrams organized? *Qian* Heaven is the south, *Kun* Earth is the north, the east is *Li* Flame, and the west is *Kan* Water. The south, north, east, and west are called the four seats of honor, and these seats are occupied by *Qian*, *Kun*, *Li*, and *Kan*; heaven, earth, water, and fire respectively. *Qian* Heaven is yang, *Kun* Earth is yin, *Li* Flame is yang, and *Kan* Water is yin. *Qian*, *Kun*, *Li*, and *Kan* occupy the four cardinal points, and so heaven, earth, water, and fire occupy these positions as well, and because these occupy such positions, so too do yin and yang. In the prenatal pattern, the trigram *Kun* Earth occupies the northern cardinal point. When the prenatal pattern concludes, the heavens rotate to the left, and the earth to the right, and the postnatal pattern emerges. What is the format of the cardinal points in the postnatal pattern? *Li* Flame is in the south, *Kan* Water is in the north, *Zhen* Thunder is in the east, and *Dui* Lake is in the west. During the postnatal period, heaven and earth give up their thrones, and fire and water assume these positions.

Why do heaven and earth abdicate? After their rotation, after the intercourse of *qi*, the myriad things come into being and having achieved their goal, they step down. This process is referred to as "hidden virtue" because it "is brought into being but does not take possession, acts without presumption, grows but does not oppress." The perpetuation of heaven and earth depend upon this "stepping down after success," this "hidden virtue." After heaven and earth have given up their positions of power, and the *Kan* Water has moved to the position of *Kun* Earth, water and earth cohabit, providing the foundation for the union of earth and water. We can think about the union of water and earth from this perspective. If heaven and earth do not intertwine, then water and earth will not be able to come together. If heaven and earth do not give up their thrones, the union of water and earth will also be difficult. When heaven and earth give up their thrones, the *Kan* Water makes its home with *Kun* Earth, and we say that water and earth live together. Is there evidence to support this sort of saying? In the *Classic of Changes*, there is a hexagram called *tongren* (Seeking Harmony, ䷌) composed of the trigram *Qian* Heaven above and the trigram *Li* Flame below. Why is a hexagram consisting of heaven above and fire below called Seeking Harmony?

The *Master Shang's Study of the Zhou Yi* (Zhouyi shangshi xue) discussion of the hexagram *tongren* reads: "Xun Shuang says: *Qian* Heaven resides with *Li* Flame, abiding harmoniously. The *Jiujia* commentary says: *Qian* Heaven resides with *Li* Flame, both acting like the sun, the sky and the sun sharing the same brightness, thus they are called *tongren*. It is the case that *Qian* Heaven resides in the south, as the Han Dynasty scholars have already explained. Xun Shuang also commented on the meaning of yin and yang being coupled with that of the sun and moon by saying: *Qian* Heaven resides with *Li* Flame, and the two abide with the sun. *Kun* Earth resides with *Kan* Water, and the two abide with the moon." To say that *Qian* Heaven resides with *Li* Flame means that in the postnatal pattern, *Li* is in the south, but in the prenatal pattern, *Qian* is in the south. *Qian* and *Li* both live in the south, thus it is said that "they abide with one another." This is why, when these two trigrams form a hexagram, the hexagram is called *tongren* (Seeking Harmony).

In the same way, *Kun* Earth resides with *Kan* Water. *Kan* resides in the same position as *Kun*, so how could it not be the case that the two "abide in harmony with one another"? Thus, saying "water and earth reside together," and "the union of water and earth" have a firm basis in the logic of the classics. When the trigrams *Qian* Heaven and *Li* Flame are joined, it forms the hexagram *tongren*. When the trigrams *Kun* Earth and *Kan* Water are joined, the hexagram *shi* (Multitude, also translated as "teacher") is formed. *Kun* is above and *Kan* is below in this hexagram, which is commonly called *Dishuishi* (Earth-Water Multitude, ䷆). The hexagram *shi* is placed seventh in the hexagram sequence of the *Classic of Changes*. Seven is the fire number; it resides in the south, in the position of the sovereign. Thus it is said: "The one who recognizes and employs the multitudes is a king; the one who employs friends is a tyrant; and the one who employs followers will be lost." Thus, the way of teaching the multitudes is the way of the king. Since it is the path the king must take, it makes perfect sense that it occupies the position of the sovereign.

In the past, in the south side of the reception hall of every house, five characters could be read. Whether it was a small house in town or a shrine, these five characters read the same: "Heaven; Earth; Sovereign; Relatives; Multitudes (*shi*, also translated as 'teacher')." From this, we can see the dignity of the teaching profession, a dignity that cannot easily be destroyed.

There is a firm basis for the union of water and earth in the *Classic of Changes*. We need only keep our eyes open to find a basis for it in nearly every corner. Take, for example, the radical *yue* (月) often used in the construction of Chinese characters. This radical also exhibits a union of water and earth. This radical can be written with four brushstrokes in the form 月 (*yue*, "moon"), or it can be written with six brushstrokes as 肉 (*rou*, "flesh"). What is the moon? Earlier in this book, we discussed the relationship between the moon and water, and how the moon and water are conjoined.

What about flesh? The spleen governs the flesh, the spleen belongs to earth, and so flesh is the same as earth. We can see that the *yue* radical also connotes the union of water and earth.

I.1.d. Soil Erosion

The union of earth and water is undoubtedly an issue of great importance. Soil devoid of water is nothing but wasteland; how can it support life? This is easy for the reader to understand. Water without soil is equally unthinkable, but perhaps a bit more difficult to comprehend. Nevertheless, we will discuss this issue in the following passages.

Soil erosion and water runoff, literally "water-soil flow loss," is a topic that fills the newspapers and airwaves in present-day China. The country is faced with a massive soil erosion problem, such that immense tracts of land become desolate every year, and the pace of this erosion increases with each passing year. Soil erodes when vegetation is lost. During the 1950s, the Chinese Communist government instituted a policy of increasing grain production, and made the cultivation of grain the highest agricultural priority. Vast forests were cut down, and grasslands and lonely mountains were put to the task of producing cereal crops. The result of this policy was an overall reduction in vegetation in these areas, and massive decimation of the country's forests. According to the five-element theory, wood controls earth. So it is little surprise that a significant reduction in the vegetation and "wood" resulted in soil erosion. The five-element theory has a wide scope of application. When we speak of wood failing to control earth, you should be able to think of more than disease of the spleen and stomach, Xiaoyao San, or Chaihu Shugan Tang. These are merely prominences in the role that this aspect of the five-element theory plays in Chinese Medicine's treatment of disease. You should think too of soil erosion and of desertification. If you think of such things, you are aligning yourself with the old saying: "The superior physician treats the country."

It is only once vast tracts of land have turned to desert wasteland that we think to ban clearcutting and attempt to reforest fields that have been plowed under. Of course, it is better to come to this conclusion late than never, and it is never too late to do something. Once we destroy the native vegetation, we can shift from agriculture to forestry.

The relationship between soil and wood is highly important. Those who have traveled outside China, especially to places such as North America, Japan, and Europe, know that the vegetative ground cover in these parts of the world is very good, and anywhere there is a plot of ground, there is something growing on it. I was amazed to find that I could polish my shoes but once a month to keep them looking clean. In China, if I polish my shoes in the morning, they are dusty and dirty again by the afternoon. Although having dirty shoes is a small problem, it reflects a serious problem, namely that our ground cover is so poor that the dry, bare soil sends dust out in every direction. At first glance, it seems like soil erosion results from poor soil, but when wood does not constrain earth; when the roots of plants do not weave their way into the ground, the soil loses its fertility.

Nowadays, soil erosion and water runoff is a popular topic. Vegetation prevents loss of soil. This soil in turn prevents the loss of water. Soil not only nurtures living things, it receives and stores for living things. One of the most important things that the soil and earth store is water. If the soil fails to store the water, then the water will of course be lost.

The soil's ability to store water is not limited simply to the creation of a water reservoir. Those who are a bit older, like me, can remember when periods of rain did not cause such a rapid rise in water. Nowadays, whenever it rains heavily or for a longer period of time, the streets are flooded. And why is this? This is because the quality of our soil is not as good as it used to be; it has lost some of its ability to store water. Unless there is an exceptionally long and hard rain, the soil should be able to absorb this water better than it does today. Nowadays, the soil is no good. When it rains, it cannot absorb the water, rivulets form and become streams, and before long the streets are flooded and the rivers rise. The ability of the earth to absorb water is becoming an increasingly important problem. If we cannot improve this capacity of the soil to take in water, we will be caught in a vicious cycle of increased erosion and loss of vegetation, decreased absorption of water, and further flooding and desertification.

The connection between vegetative ground cover and a decrease in the soil's ability to absorb water is clear. Why does vegetation have such a profound effect on the quality and capacity of the ground? There is an important characteristic of wood that is reflected by the trigram *Kun* Earth. In the *Three Character Classic*, there is a song about the lines of trigrams that goes like this:

Qian Heaven's continuous three,

Kun Earth's broken six,

Zhen Thunder's wide-mouthed jar,

Gen Mountain's bowl overturned,

Li Flame's center is empty,

Kan Water's center is full,

Dui Lake's top is lacking,

Xun Wind's bottom is broken.

Qian Heaven's three yang lines are continuous, without any breaks in them. *Kun* Earth consists solely of broken lines, and its appearance is entirely pervious. It is these six broken lines that make *Kun* Earth so easily permeable, and this is, of course, an important aspect of earth. If the earth is not pervious, if it is not open and loose, what sort of soil is it? It is dead soil, and dead soil cannot perform its usual functions.

Those who come from small villages or who have had an opportunity to see Chinese peasants cultivating crops know this very well. Before the peasants sow their seeds, they first turn and loosen the soil in order to maintain this open, loose aspect of the soil. The soil must be relaxed, not tense. Where there is good vegetation, the soil is loose and malleable. Where the soil is barren, it is hard as a rock, having lost its healthy plasticity and porosity. Having lost its essential nature, it cannot receive and store; being unable to receive and store, it cannot give birth and grow. The looseness of the soil is of great importance; without this quality, it cannot store. If you have no experience in agriculture, perhaps you have grown plants in pots before. If you leave the soil in the pot for a long period of time without turning it, it becomes hard and dry. When you water this soil, the water does not go into the soil, instead it runs off to the side and out of the pot. The Chinese peasants would say that the soil does not "eat" the water. If the soil is hard and solid instead of loose and porous, how can it "eat" the water? When the soil has been dry a long time and become hardened in this way, Chinese peasants will always turn the soil before watering it, in order that the soil can "eat" the water, and store it away.

China's eminent Tsinghua University has a famous school motto: "Constantly Strive to Improve, Great Virtue Can Carry All Things" (自強不息，厚德載物; the official English version is "Self-discipline and Social

Commitment"). Both of these are quotes from the *Classic of Changes*: the first describes the *Qian* Heaven trigram, and the second the *Kun* Earth trigram. These mottoes, often quoted together as a single line and encapsulate the immanent instruction of both heaven and earth, perhaps have played a role in bringing Tsinghua University to its present greatness! We can understand the *Kun* Earth line, "Great virtue can carry all things," from two contexts. The first is the line: "Oh ultimate *Kun* source, all living things emerge from it." Is the essence of *Kun* Earth that from which life stems? It is most certainly the source of life. Everything we eat, everything that sustains us, comes from this *Kun* Earth source. This is the aspect of *Kun* that births, grows, and nourishes living things. But this function of *Kun* as the source and sustenance of life is not without a certain cost. There is another aspect to *Kun*: "*Kun*'s greatness carries all living things." This aspect relates to the one we discussed earlier: the capacity of *Kun* Earth to store all things. To store within requires entering, whereas providing sustenance involves exiting. This entering and exiting are very different. At present, everything we no longer want we bury in the earth. Our excrement and urine, our garbage, our trash and waste, we put underground. The earth seems not to resent us for this; it quietly accepts what we fold into her. She encloses and holds our refuse, and after a time she brings forth that which we need to live. *Kun* Earth returns insults with kindness. Confucius referred to *Kun* as "boundless virtue."

In order for *Kun* Earth to support all living things, there is one prerequisite that the nature of *Kun* remain soft and supple, easygoing and slow, relaxed and flexible. Besides the modern problems related to vegetative ground cover, there are also problems related to this requirement of suppleness. This is especially true in China, with what seems to be a perpetual booming of construction and urbanization, the building of cities full of high-rises, the widening and lengthening of roads and highways, the paving of parking lots, the whole host of construction projects that result in the impervious hardening of the ground. Through this sort of building and construction, the earth has lost its softness and suppleness, its receptive nature. Once the rebar-reinforced concrete has been whitewashed, the surface of the earth has all of the gentle receptivity of a battleship's hull. Without the receptive nature of *Kun*, how can it receive and store? And, from a five-element perspective, how can it control water? As soon as rainwater strikes its surface, it rolls away. This is what is meant by "water loss." When the rainwater comes down and is stored within the earth, this is of great use. What does the wood element depend upon for its growth? What does vegetation depend upon for its sustenance? They depend upon the nourishment of water.

Another aspect of this problem is the agricultural use of chemical fertilizers. Over the past few decades, the agricultural yields have increased beyond what was previously achieved with traditional fertilizer. In the coming decades, however, our soil will be hardpan. The nature and quality of our soil is changing significantly. Soil should have a high constituency of organic material. If you use inorganic fertilizer for a long period of time, the soil will gradually accumulate this inorganic matter. The *Kun* Earth is organic, so if it gradually shifts toward an inorganic nature, it will lose its original quality. It can no longer take things down inside it, and can no longer receive and store. It used to be that when we had a heavy rain, the soil would soak it all up, but now it has lost much of its previous ability. It is extremely important that the soil be able to absorb water, and there is a significant difference between the water going into the ground and running off to the river. You may recall our earlier discussion of the "dragon veins," the presence of water flowing below the ground. There is a crucial connection between the dragon veins and ecology. The absorption of rainwater by the soil helps to conserve these dragon veins. As long as the dragon veins are conserved, the landscape will remain lush and verdant.

The softness and permeability of the *Kun* Earth is affected by a multitude of influences, and once so influenced, a vicious cycle of deterioration in our water and our wood ensues. The influences we have listed above are related to nature, but in Chinese cosmology, human beings and the heavens also reciprocate and empathize with one another. This particular function of nature can also influence human beings. Once the *Kun* Earth has received these influences, what influence does it exert on human beings? *Qian* Heaven is male, and *Kun* Earth is female, and so this influence of nature is primarily exerted on women. In recent years, in China, we have seen many changes in our women. It is the nature of *Kun* Earth to contain and conceal. If you take a look at the sort of clothing women used to wear, then you will know what is meant by this containing and concealing. Their long garments touched the ground and no one glimpsed their bound feet. Even when laughing, they covered their teeth. We need not speak of other areas of the body. And nowadays? One may do a survey oneself and go out on the street and take a look around. Compare the amount of surface area of the female and the male body that is revealed by passers-by. This calculation makes my point clear. Do the women of China still contain and conceal? Men wear long sleeves and long pants, whereas women wear short-sleeved shirts and short skirts, or sleeveless shirts and shorts. They let everything be seen, and what they do not wholly reveal is still dimly visible through their scanty garments. Although this choice of clothing is related to current fashion trends, we cannot ignore the close link between human beings and the natural world, and the changes in *Kun* Earth, and in the vegetation that covers it, is a variable we should also consider.

Long ago in our history, the first persons of China were divided into tribes. These tribes lived in a particular area for a period of time and then moved on. They were nomadic rather than sedentary. They moved about in order to ensure that the natural world around them would have a chance to recuperate after their harvests of meat and vegetable foodstuffs began to decline. Nowadays, we humans remain in one place year after year, century after century, and, in China at least, millennium after millennium. Therefore, if people do not pay close attention to their behaviors, it will have a wide-reaching influence on the natural world, and eventually the natural world will return in kind. We mentioned nature's indirect influence on women's clothing. What effect does it have on our biology? This hardly needs mention. To provide a simple example, look at the rapidly increasing morbidity of atrophic gastritis throughout the civilized world. Do you think that this has perhaps a relationship with environmental changes? Of course. Among the five elements, the stomach is earth, and more specifically, it is yang earth. It is the relatively superficial earth, the topsoil. The topsoil must be loose and porous. The stomach is the yang earth, so the health of the mucous membranes and glands of the stomach depends upon their likewise possessing such a loose and supple porosity. The incessant development and urbanization of China has resulted in an ever-increasing atrophy of the *Kun* Earth. Human life is the result of the convergence of the terrestrial and celestial *qi*, and so when these influences are exerted on the human body, is it any wonder that the incidence of atrophic gastritis is constantly increasing? The *qi* of human beings and nature are intertwined. If the city is going up in flames, can humans expect to be unaffected?

To be a Chinese Medicine physician, especially in the twenty-first century, I think one must do more than simply look at physiological disease. We should widen our view a bit. We possess a set of theories, and if the Chinese Medicine physician applies these theories to the problems currently besetting our globe, their source and solution may become clear. If you, as a Chinese Medicine physician, apply these theories to understand and regulate the environment, this will be treating the root rather than the branch. Currently, there are a whole host of regulations aimed at protecting the environment, but these regulations are aimed at merely alleviating the symptoms. They provide superficial improvements and do not treat the source of the problem. For instance, if the United States does not reduce its greenhouse gas emissions, how can it possibly speak of "protecting the environment"? If we attempt to propose a strategy of sustainable development without consulting the wisdom of tradition, and without applying the philosophical tenets of traditional Chinese Medicine in the construction of such a strategy, then I fear such a strategy, however earnestly implemented, will not produce the desired result. Chinese Medicine physicians should expand their horizons. Why shouldn't Chinese Medicine physicians use their knowledge to elucidate the many challenges we, as citizens of this earth, are facing?

These are my thoughts concerning the relationship between the union of water and earth, and the current problems of soil erosion and water runoff.

I.2. The Meaning of the Taiyin Channels

The meaning and significance of the Taiyin channel is relatively easy to explain. There are the hand and the foot Taiyin channels, but in the Taiyin chapter of the *Treatise on Cold Damage*, it clearly discusses the foot Taiyin. The chief points concerning the hand Taiyin are addressed in the previous chapters of the *Treatise on Cold Damage* regarding Taiyang and Yangming.

The Taiyin foot channel begins on the tip of the big toe with the point Yinbai (SP 1). It proceeds from this point along the medial aspect of the foot and leg until it enters the abdomen where it joins with the spleen and intertwines with the stomach; it then traverses the diaphragm to the root of the tongue and spreads out beneath the tongue. Why does the spleen open

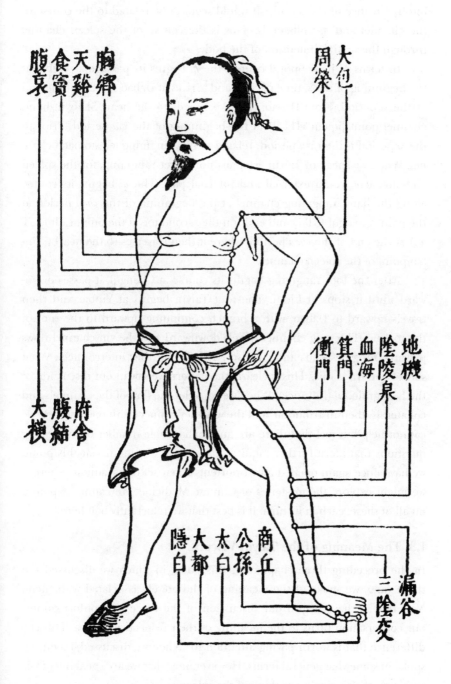

into the orifice of the mouth? It would seem to be related to the course of the channel and its collaterals. This is the course of the spleen channel through the spatial dimension of the body.

In terms of its temporal course, the *qi* begins its passage at Yinbai at the beginning of the *si* time period, and arrives at Dabao (SP 21) at the end of the *si* period. From Dabao, the *qi* proceeds to the heart Shaoyin hand channel point Jiquan (HT 1) at the beginning of the *wu* period. Prior to the *si* period is the *chen* period, related to the Yangming leg stomach channel. When we speak of Taiyin, we must not forget Yangming, for the spleen and stomach are an external and internal pair. The *qi* begins its course along the hand Yangming channel at the beginning of the *chen* period at the point Chengqi (ST 1) and ends on the second toe at the point Lidui (ST 45) at the end of the *chen* period, where it then traverses to the nearby Yinbai point of the spleen channel.

After the foot Yangming begins its course at Chengqi, it passes downward until it stops at Lidui. The foot Taiyin begins at Yinbai and then travels upward to Dabao, with a branch continuing upward to the root of the tongue. The yang channel travels downward and the yin channel flows upward. Yang descends and yin rises. This is how they interconnect. What sort of pattern is this? This is clearly the pattern we saw in our discussion of the hexagram *tai* (Advance). When we consider the flow of the channels and collaterals, their distribution, and the way they connect with one another, we cannot help but feel that there are an inexhaustible number of interesting questions that merit further inquiry. If we begin our inquiry at this point, we have once again opened a vast portent, a new set of paradigms whereby we might explore the mysteries of Chinese Medicine. We cannot expound on all of these, each in its turn. It is best that we reluctantly halt here.

I.3. The Meaning of the Taiyin Viscera

In the preceding three chapters of this book, in which we discussed the three yang, we spoke of the meaning of the bowels associated with them. Now that we have begun our discussion of the three yin conformations, our conversation turns to the meaning of their respective viscera. This is a difference that is worth paying attention to. When we discussed Taiyin, we spoke in somewhat general terms. However, now that we are speaking of viscera, we are principally speaking of the spleen.

I.3.a. The Chinese Character Pi

If we wish to thoroughly investigate the deeper meaning and significance of the spleen, we might as well begin with an examination of the Chinese character used to represent that organ, and analyze its construction. The construction of characters, for example liver, lung, and kidney, is well worth looking into; if you have earnestly pondered these concepts, then you probably sensed the richness of this topic. Like all the other characters representing the viscera, with the notable exception of the character for "heart," the character for spleen (*pi* 脾) is composed of the radical *yue* 月 ("moon" or "flesh") on the left. When we reference the character that forms this radical, as we did in the previous section, we must think of it containing both four and six simultaneously, the coincidence of both the moon (*yue* 月) and flesh (*rou* 肉). Earlier in this work, when we examined the concept of the pulse, we pointed out an error in the *Kangxi Dictionary*, but I believe our point was not complete and would like to take this opportunity to round it out. When we discuss the character *yue*, we must always keep in mind its dual nature. If we speak only of "the moon," our treatment will be incomplete, and if our discourse focuses only on "flesh," our discourse will likewise be slanted. Only if we discuss the two as one can we adequately convey the meaning of this character. Ultimately, this is in accord with the maxim that heaven and human are one.

When we speak of the moon, we are referring to the celestial realm. When we speak of flesh, our frame of reference is the human sphere. Those who wish to discuss the cosmos must ultimately anchor their findings in humanity. If we discuss that which is celestial and neglect that which is human, we entirely forsake the notion that "heaven and man are one." The fact that all four of the viscera besides the heart contain this *yue* radical on the left indicates their common foundation in both the moon and flesh. To understand the differences in these organs, we should look at the right side of each character. The right side of the character *pi* (脾) is the character *bei* (卑). What does *bei* represent? We can understand it from the following quote from the *Great Commentary of the Classic of Changes*:

> Heaven is exalted and earth is modest (*bei* 卑), and thus the positions of *Qian* Heaven and *Kun* Earth are determined. The lowly (*bei* 卑) and the lofty are thereby displayed, the eminent and the humble given their

respective positions. Stillness and movement have their intervals, hard and soft interrupt one another.

And so, what is *bei*? *Bei* is *Kun*, it is earth, and it is the soil. And so, the character *pi* (脾) clearly indicates the attributes and the orientation of the spleen.

The position of the spleen is earth, and its nature and function is also one with this element. If we wish to examine the spleen's capacities, we can do so entirely by relating it to the earth, to the soil. In Chinese Medicine, we say that the spleen governs generation and transformation, and is the root of the postnatal *qi*. Does spleen really govern birth and transformation? It is said that from the *Kun* Earth trigram "the myriad living things emerge." The fruits we eat—apples, longan fruit, lychees—all come from the soil. Wheat and rice are also products of the soil. Unless you are one of the immortals, you still have to eat food, and you cannot do without the soil's produce. The soil is absolutely the master of birth and transformation and the source of postnatal vitality. Another aspect of the spleen is its governance of the blood's circulation and the movement and transformation of dampness and water. In Chinese Medicine, it is said that blood is water, and prior to this section we thoroughly discussed the relationship between water and earth, and the union between these two. Now that we understand this union, understanding the connection between the spleen and the blood is easy. Our examination of the construction of the character *pi* reveals its orientation, its function, and almost everything about the organ. But writing is for revealing the truth, and we should not waste words once a point is made.

I.3.b. Spleen Does Not Rule a Season

The composition of the characters referring to the five viscera is worthy of our earnest study, especially the right-hand side of the character that indicates the individual character of the particular viscera.

When we look at the character for the liver *gan* (肝), we should look to the character *gan* (干) to understand the individual characteristics of this organ. When we look at the character for kidney *shen* (腎), we should look to the radical *jian* (臤). Likewise, when investigating the character for lung *fei* (肺), we should look to the radical *fu* (巿). Among the five viscera, the lungs govern autumn, the kidneys winter, the liver spring, and the heart rules summer. Since the four seasons of spring, summer, fall, and winter are ruled respectively by the liver, the heart, the lungs, and the kidneys, the spleen finds itself without a season of its own. Hence, when discussing the spleen earth, the *Plain Questions* chapter "Treatise on Taiyin and Yangming" says that it "does not have a season that it governs." This means that it does not govern any of the four principal seasons. Not obtaining a regular position ruling any of the four seasons, the spleen assumes an irregular position. Thus, according to the *Plain Questions's* "Treatise on Taiyin and Yangming": "The spleen is earth, it rules the central region, it holds fast to the four seasons, and extends the four viscera. Eighteen days from each season are entrusted to it, but it does not have a season all its own." From this, we know that the spleen does not have a season of its own, but it constantly abides with the other four seasons and aids in the growth of the four remaining viscera. Furthermore, it is conferred with eighteen days from each season, but which eighteen days are these? They are the last eighteen days of spring, summer, fall and winter. The eighteen days at the end of each season belong to the *ji* month of the season; because each of the four seasons is divided into a *meng* month, a *zhong* month, and a *ji* month, the last eighteen days must fall in the *ji* month. The last eighteen days of the *ji* month of each season are also referred to as the "four nooks," in sharp contrast to the "four orthodox" positions of the year where the heart, liver, lung, and kidney reside. The four orthodox seasons of the year are exalted and noble, and the four nooks are lowly and humble. When we compare the orthodox seasons of the year with these nooks that punctuate each of their passages, we see that the station assumed by the spleen in the course of the calendar is in keeping with the etymology of the Chinese character denoting this organ.

The spleen earth does not reside in a cardinal season all its own, but rather in a nook of time trailing behind; its station is not venerable, it is humble; and yet, Dong Zhongshu's *Luxuriant Dew of the Spring and Autumn Annals* referred to it as "The lord of the five elements." How is it the "lord of the five elements"? It is the ruler of the other elements because metal, wood, water, and fire cannot come into being without earth. Spring, summer, fall, and winter cannot succeed one another without earth. The period in which the spleen prevails at the end of each season is the period in which each orthodox season shifts toward a realization of the coming season. For instance, can spring shift directly to summer, and, in succession, can the seasons pass directly to fall, winter, and back to spring? The transition from one season to the next hangs upon these eighteen days at the end of each. If this eighteen-day transition does not go smoothly, then the normal shift from one season to the next cannot occur. So, although the spleen does not have a season of its own, the other four seasons cannot do without the spleen. The earth does not abide with any of the four orthodox seasons, but none of these cardinal periods can do without the action of the earth. If any of the seasons did neglect the action of the spleen period, they would not be able to transition to the next season in a normal way. The excess would be detrimental. If the four seasons were to stop and linger in summer and not proceed to autumn in the normal fashion, how would this be? If *qi* of summer is obstinate and persists too long, this intransigence would result in harm. Summer, like all the seasons, must relinquish (*chengzhi* 承制). What is meant by *chengzhi*? *Cheng* refers to *chengjie* (承接): "to accept another's mandate." When summer transitions to fall, it means that the heat and stuffiness give way to the crisp, cool air of autumn; the sonorous summer fades into the quiet of fall. To give way is to cease resisting, to accept restraint. Thus, the *Plain Questions's* "Great Treatise on the Six Subtleties" says: "If there is obstinacy harm result, there must be submission (*cheng*) and restraint; once restrained, it can be transformed." The key to restraining this undue persistence is in the concept of *cheng*, this voluntary submission, and this capacity would seem to fall back upon the spleen earth. Why is the spleen so important to the human body? Why is the earth and soil so important in nature? It is because it is related to this submission and restraint. Why, in our present age, are climate changes and weather patterns so volatile and prone to destructive episodes? An important contributor is the decomposition of the mechanism whereby one prevailing atmospheric influence gives way to another: the degradation of the earth and soil.

In the first chapter, we discussed how the lungs govern the regulation of the seasonal nodes and how the lungs govern the *qi*. At the level of the seasonal nodes and the twenty-four calendrical periods, human beings manage to keep pace with the changing weather via the faculties of the lungs. But at the level of the four seasons that entail a larger transformation of heaven and earth and a relinquishing of one seasonal influence to make way for another, it all depends on the spleen earth. The concept of the spleen "not governing a season of its own" allows both human beings and the larger cycle of nature to maintain a harmonious transition from one season to the next.

I.3.c. Spleen Rules the Flesh

The spleen rules the flesh, and this particular function of the organ is well known to anyone who has studied basic Chinese Medicine physiology. I entreat the reader to think a bit more deeply on the subject we are about to explore, for it can be linked with the topic of discussion we just concluded.

Earlier, we discussed how the spleen belongs to the element of earth, and how the earth is able to grow and support the myriad forms of life, aid them through their transformations, and store them in her bosom. The relationship between the earth and living things is extraordinarily close. Our discussion then turned to how the spleen does not govern any of the principal seasons, but none of these seasons can come into being without the aid of the spleen; metal, wood, water, and fire cannot do without earth, and the changing of the seasons cannot occur without the influence of the earth. If we follow this train of thought and think of the concept of the spleen ruling the muscles of the body, we can place this idea within the context of the other four major systems of the body: the epithelial tissue; the muscular system; the connective tissue system, including the skeleton and the adipose tissue; and the nervous system. Among these various systems of the body, the muscular and adipose tissues belong to the category of flesh, and fall under the scope of the spleen. Now let us consider the five viscera and six bowels of the body's interior, as well as the four limbs and the hundred bones of the body's exterior. Do any of these lack flesh or fat? Aren't all of these to a large extent composed of flesh or fat? Even the circulatory system, which seems to have nothing to do with the muscular system, is largely composed of smooth muscle.

I invite the reader to earnestly examine this question and see if there are any real exceptions. If there is an exception, then the exception would be the heart, because it lacks this "moon and flesh" radical. All other parts of the body contain this moon-flesh sign. The lungs (肺) contain this sign; the liver (肝) contains it, too. So too do the characters for large intestine (大腸), small intestine (小腸), the brain (腦), the blood vessels (脈), and the gallbladder (膽). Because they possess this radical as part of their composition, it indicates that these anatomical structures cannot exist without flesh. Is there any part of the body that can do without flesh? They cannot depart from flesh any more than they can depart from earth, or the influence of the spleen. And so, when we say that the spleen rules flesh, we should expand our understanding of this idea; after all, what part of the body is devoid of flesh? The heart has cardiac muscle, and even bones are filled with a sort of flesh. The spleen rules the muscles and flesh, and the characters representing nearly every part of the body contain this "moon and flesh" radical. This connection establishes the close relationship of the spleen with almost every part of the body. Why is the spleen considered to be the "foundation of the postnatal"? The word Chinese word for "root" or "foundation" (*ben* 本) should not be misused. The numerous discussions we have conducted thus far in this book should be enough to demonstrate the usefulness of a careful and exacting, if seemingly pedantic, study of individual Chinese characters. Once the meaning of a character is clearly understood, it opens the way to a deeper understanding.

Moreover, when studying and researching characters, the student must adopt an attitude of earnest conscientiousness. The process of uncovering the meaning of a Chinese character is not a casual process any more than the construction of the character itself is a casual affair. Chinese characters are uncannily exact crystallizations of actual phenomena in two dimensions, and with only a handful of brushstrokes. They are constructed according to specific principles, and these principles are grounded in reality. Principle emerges from phenomena, and matters are completed by means of principle. Principles and worldly matters are inseparable, and this point is made amply evident in Chinese characters. Take, for instance, the character *gu* 骨 (bone) which contains the "moon-flesh" radical. Flesh is soft and supple, but bones are exceptionally hard. In the modern age of microscopy, we know that the bones are filled with fat, connective tissue, and cells that form the blood. Long before the advent of microscopes, the ancients placed the "moon-flesh" radical in the character for bone. How, we should ask, did the ancients apprehend this subtle anatomical fact and furthermore place it so eloquently in the Chinese character? We must regard this question carefully, not casually or carelessly.

I.3.d. People Are the Chief of the "Naked Creatures"

In the *Yellow Emperor's Classic*, all animals are referred to as *chong* 蟲 (worms). Worms form a large category and this category is identical with that of animals. When I was small, I read the popular Chinese martial arts epic *Outlaws of the Water Margin*. When I came across the passage in which the mighty, but recently inebriated Wusong defeats a tiger with his bare hands, the author referred to the tiger as a "furry worm." At the time, I did not understand, and thought it must be some sort of mistake. It was not until much later that I realized it was an allusion of sorts.

The *Yellow Emperor's Classic* divides worms, or creatures, into five types: furred, feathered, naked, shelled, and scaled. Those with fur belong to the element of wood, those with feathers to fire, the naked to earth, the shelled to metal, and those with scales to the water element. The furred creatures are those that are covered with fur, such as tigers, lions, cats, and dogs— all animals that are covered in a coat of fur. The feathered creatures are, of course, those that are covered in feathers and can usually fly, such as birds. The naked creatures are those that have no real covering over their bodies. The muscles and flesh of the naked creatures is immediately visible. It is true that Europeans, on the whole, have more body hair than Chinese people do, but a little bit of hair here and there cannot compare with the furry pelt of a tiger or a leopard. So even the hairiest person belongs to the category of "naked" creatures. The shelled creatures are the crustaceans as well as tortoises and turtles. Finally, the scaled creatures, for the most part, are those that are born in the water, such as fishes.

Dividing all animals into these five classes, there are obviously a great number of different sorts of animal in each particular class. Among these many different animals, there is one that is deemed to be the most representative of its class, and referred to as the "chief." The ancients said, as recounted in the *Plain Questions*: "There are 360 different types of furred animals, and unicorns are their chief; there are 360 feathered beasts, and the phoenix is the chief; 360 different types of naked creatures, and the human is their chief; 360 scaled animals, and the dragon is their chief; and 360 types of animal with shells, and the tortoise is their chief." People are the chief of the naked creatures, and are the most representative of the animals belonging to the earth class. This is of great significance. Any single person has a certain amount of metal, wood, water, fire and earth, just as he or she possesses lungs, a liver, kidneys, a heart, and spleen. However, human beings as a whole belong to the class of naked creatures, to the class of animals related to earth. It is similar to this planet of ours. Although we can find metal, wood, fire, water, and earth, the planet as a whole can be deemed "earth." Why is it that human beings are referred to as the most divine of all creatures? Or, put another way, how is it that humans have achieved this status as the most conscious animal? One important aspect of this lies in the fact that humans are the chief of the earth creatures. The category to which people belong is the same as that to which our planet belongs, thus it is only fitting that humans should have dominion over the earth.

We must be clear on this point: humans belong to the class of animals related to the earth element. If you wish to find wood, fire, metal, or water in a human being, where can you look? You must search among the earth; you must find the wood of earth, fire of earth, the metal of earth, the water of earth. If you learn how to find these things within the earth, the meaning will become of great importance. Therefore, if we study human beings, our starting point must be the earth, and our perceptions must be centered upon the earth: they must be centered upon the spleen and stomach.

During the Jin and Yuan periods, there was a famous physician named Li Dongyuan. One of his most deeply influential works was called the *Discourse on the Spleen and Stomach* (Piweilun). If we examine all of Chinese Medicine history, besides this particular book, are there any works of similar magnitude that are named after any internal organs? No, this is the only one. Why is it called the *Discourse on the Spleen and Stomach*? As a matter of fact, it is because it rests upon the earth element. It seeks all the other elements—metal, wood, water, and fire—within the earth element. Everything it investigates, it does so in the earth element. I think this is a correct way of pursuing Chinese Medicine. Human beings are the chief of the naked creatures; if you do not seek to understand humans via the earth element, where should you search? Now, if you are studying tortoises, or dragons, or phoenixes, then perhaps you should shift your direction. In that case, you might do well to look within metal, water, or fire for the other elements.

When studying the human being, we must base our investigations upon the earth. The entire *Treatise on Cold Damage* makes this point abundantly clear. In the 112 prescriptions in the *Treatise on Cold Damage*, the number of herbs used is not more than 100, and those herbs that are frequently used number in the dozens. If we examine the use of these herbs to see which herb is used most frequently in the *Treatise on Cold Damage*, we find that Gancao is most often prescribed. Gancao is used in more than 70 formulas in the *Treatise on Cold Damage*, more than half the prescriptions in the *Treatise on Cold Damage*. Some formulas even use Gancao as the emperor herb, for instance, Zhigancao Tang, Gancao Tang, Gancao Ganjiang Tang, Gancao Fuzi Tang, Gancao Xiexin Tang. Nowadays, everyone looks down on Gancao and deems it a dispensable ingredient that can either be used in a formula or left out entirely. It is thought to be nothing more than an assistant, unfit to be an emperor herb. Why is Gancao so important in the *Treatise on Cold Damage*? Why do so many formulas make use of this herb? It is because it belongs to the category of earth! Just as we saw how animals can be categorized according to the five elements, so too can herbs. We can also choose a "chief" to represent each class of herb, and Gancao is the chief of the earth herbs. If Gancao is not the chief, then no herb deserves to be chief.

The flavor of Gancao is sweet and its *qi* is neutral; it is yellow in color, the color associated with the earth. Of all medicinal herbs, it best embodies the *qi* of earth. From the fact that this herb is used most frequently in the prescriptions of the *Treatise on Cold Damage*, we can see that Zhang Zhongjing must have known this. People are the chief of naked creatures; therefore, to treat the diseases of human beings, we must use herbs related to earth, and the foremost of these herbs is Gancao. Gancao is not only a "peacemaker," a harmonizing herb. Rather, it represents a very deep principle of Chinese Medicine.

I.3.e. Spleen Rules the Middle Burner

The spleen and stomach rule the middle burner, but what is the purpose of the middle burner? The function of the middle burner is enormous. The middle burner can also be thought of the burner that is neither upper nor lower. When we discussed the larger implications of the hexagrams *pi* (Hindrance) and *tai* (Advance), one of the key points we examined was that the interchange of the *qi* from above and that from below resulted into the life-giving *tai* state, whereas when this interchange is lost, disease and death take hold. The interchange of that which is above with that which is below depends upon the middle, where they meet. Therefore, the function of the middle burner is to allow for the interchange between the upper and lower, to connect the upper with the lower. The *Yellow Emperor's Classic* advises to "Seek the root with regard to heaven and seek the position with regard to earth." And what should we seek with regard to human beings? We should seek the "intercourse of *qi*." What is meant by the intercourse of *qi*? The heavenly *qi* descends, the earthly *qi* rises; this is called the intercourse of *qi*. The *qi* of the upper burner descends and the *qi* of the lower burner rises; this is also called the intercourse of *qi*. Whether it is the interchange between the upper and lower burners or between heaven and earth, we must look for it in the middle. Ultimately, this exchange comes down to the middle burner, to the spleen and stomach, to the earth. The relationship between the spleen and stomach and the exchange of *qi* is huge and as a result, its relationship to human health is also great. This brings us back to the topic we discussed earlier. Confucius said, "all things are unified by the one Dao." If we look back upon the Dao of Chinese Medicine, we can see that it, too, is unified by a single thread.

I.4. The Meaning of Taiyin in *Yunqi*

The Taiyin *yunqi* is clearly defined; in the heavens it is dampness, and on the *terra firma* it is earth. Together, these are referred to as damp earth. I have already written on the topic of earth, and I trust that the reader is sufficiently familiar with the topic. At this point, I would like to emphasize the subject of dampness.

I.4.a. Explaining Dampness

In the Yangming chapter of this book, we discussed the meaning of dampness in relation to the etymology of the Chinese character. However, there were two different characters used to represent dampness in ancient times. The first is the character we discussed in the Yangming chapter, and the second is the form that we will discuss now. The form of the character we discussed in the Yangming chapter is not the original form of the character, but is a form that was borrowed later. Discussing that borrowed form is also useful, for it illustrates the thought process behind its adoption.

Now, let us discuss the second form of the character representing dampness (溼). The pictograph on the left hand side of this character (氵) is just as it is in the form we discussed earlier. It indicates the close relationship between dampness and water. On the right, the phonetic component consists of a horizontal line above, which represents heaven. The lower portion of the phonetic component on the right is the earth or soil radical (土). The earth radical represents the earth. What does the repetition of the *you* (幺) radical between heaven and earth represent? According to *Explaining Writing and Analyzing Characters*, this character, pronounced *you*, means "tiny." *Extensive Rhymes* also defines it as "tiny." So what is this tiny thing between heaven and earth? Within the context of the pictographic component, we know that this tiny thing is water of some kind. What is this "tiny water" that lies between heaven and earth? Clearly, this character represents the tiny particles of water that lie suspended in the atmosphere, the humidity that cannot be seen but can be felt. The beads of moisture on a glass of ice water appear to congeal out of nowhere. In the natural world, when this moisture becomes visible, it does so as rain. Rain and dampness are essentially the same thing, but the one is gross and visible, and the other is tiny and invisible. Thus, the *Plain Questions* regards rain and dampness as the same category of thing, and both are classified with earth.

From our analysis of these two complex characters representing dampness, we can see that the first represents the principle underlying dampness, and the second represents the actual object. Because it represents the actual event, it is a slightly more direct and graphic representation of the concept.

As we discuss the basic significance of dampness, besides understanding character construction, understanding the difference between dampness and water is also of crucial importance. We have already mentioned how the tiny particles of dampness, the humidity, can be felt but cannot be seen. However, if you use a modern dehumidifier, you will find water in the reservoir of the machine when its work is done. Furthermore, when humidity becomes less subtle, it becomes rain, and the difference between it and water becomes less well defined. Thereupon, water and dampness are easily confounded.

Water and dampness have a very close relationship with one another; this we can see from our discussion of "the union of water and earth." However, water and dampness are not synonymous, just as water and earth are not synonymous. After the liberation of China, especially during the time of the Cultural Revolution, everything was thought of in terms of class status and the theory of the unique importance of class origin. Regardless of your other qualities, and regardless of what sort of person you were, if the class you hailed from was wrong, if for instance your family had been wealthy landowners prior to the communist takeover of China, your situation was hopeless! Whenever I filled out a form, the line I feared the most was where I was instructed to indicate my "family class origin." Now, when we research Chinese Medicine, it seems there is a sort of "theory of class origin" at work. Is this medicine, this formula effective or not? How can we research it? It must be researched in terms of the active constituents. Of course, the active constituent is an important aspect of an herb, but it should be only one of many different approaches to understanding the properties of an herb. This process of evaluation cannot be as simplistic as what I witnessed during the Cultural Revolution. It is like water and dampness. If you look at it only from the modern perspective of constituents, how is dampness any different from water? Their molecular formula of both is H_2O, so how can they be any different from one another? If we look at the two from a Chinese Medicine perspective, the two are very different. The one is earth and the other water, the two are in a mutually restraining relationship with one another—the difference is obvious. Therefore, the perspective from which we contemplate and evaluate the issue is of crucial importance to Chinese Medicine.

At times, Chinese Medicine emphasizes physical state and their process of change. When in the state of a river or lake or sea, it is water, but when it spreads everywhere, filling the air, it is dampness. When its state changes, so too does its nature and its orientation. This is because its yin and yang have changed as well. If yin and yang do not change, how can its state possibly change? If you examine the chemical composition of a substance and ignore its apportionment of yin and yang, or, to put it another way, if you cannot understand the constituent in terms of yin yang, then this research is not really pertinent to Chinese Medicine; it is merely wishful thinking that fails to address the basic requirements of Chinese Medicine. Therefore, if you wish to evaluate whether a scientific study adheres to particular standards, or whether it can genuinely benefit Chinese Medicine, you must see whether it pays heed to yin and yang. If it does not pay close attention to the play of yin and yang, then it is merely an intellectual exercise. Even if it costs thousands, or hundreds of thousands, or even millions of dollars, as far as Chinese Medicine goes, it is an intellectual exercise with no real bearing, and a waste of money rather than an investment.

In addition, when researching the meaning of dampness, besides clarifying the connection between water and dampness, the relationship between rain and dampness must also be elucidated. Rain belongs to the category of dampness and to the category of earth. This categorization of rain is abundantly emphasized in the seven Great Treatises on the five movements and six *qi* (*wuyun liuqi*) in the *Plain Questions*. For instance, in these chapters we read: "When it rains heavily, the *qi* of dampness is at play"; and "In a year with earth emerging early in a *taiguo* ('overstepping') pattern, heavy rain and dampness spread." Despite this, a great number of my colleagues consider rain to belong to the category of water. For instance, when it is a *xinsi* year, characterized in large part by *buji* ("falling behind") movement of water, some of my friends may ask me: "This is supposed to be a dry year, isn't it? Why has it been raining so much? And why have there been so many floods in the south?" If this is how you understand the *yunqi*, the cyclical transformation of universal *qi*, then you are mistaken. Water is the north, it is cold, and it is ice and snow. It is not rain. If water is falling behind, then it is these particular factors, ice and snow, that are also deficient. Why is it so warm in the north this year (2000)? Why is there an increase in the melting of the icecaps and glaciers relative to previous years? It is because the water *yunqi* is falling behind.

I.4.b. Why Is Dampness Paired with Earth?

Why is dampness paired with earth? Why does earth accompany dampness? The answer to this question is probably clear to someone who hails from rural China. The earth brings forth the myriad creatures, but upon what does it rely in order to bear and rear its offspring? As the reader may be aware, the year in which I write this it has been especially dry in the north of China. This drought has affected agricultural fields and wild grasslands alike. As soon as earth loses its quotient of water, everything upon it withers. Earth cannot go without water, and so dampness and earth are paired with one another. However, the earth cannot become too damp. If it does, its productivity is equally hampered. In the *Fundamentals of Chinese Medicine* textbooks, in their discussion of the disposition of the spleen, it emphasizes that the spleen is fond of dryness and dislikes dampness. This statement refers, in fact, to this aspect of the earth. In point of fact, the earth cannot do without dampness, nor can it perform its normal function when overly damp. It must be neither too dry nor too damp. Why is this? In his commentary on the *Plain Questions*, Wang Bing makes a point that causes us to thump the table in admiration:

> Only if its interior is damp is the soil truly whole. When it is damp, the soil is alive, and when it is dry, the soil dies. When it dies, the multitudes of living things die, and when it lives, the myriad things flourish. In order for the damp *qi* to bring about transformation, it must settle into the earth, the clouds must course across the sky, and the rain must fall. If it becomes too extreme, then there will be landslides.

In the *Plain Questions's* "Great Treatise on the Progression of the Five Movements," we learn: "The central region produces dampness, dampness creates earth, earth creates sweetness, sweetness generates the spleen, the spleen creates flesh, and flesh gives rise to the lungs. In the heavens it is dampness, on earth it is the soil, in the body it is flesh, among *qi* it is the *qi* that fills, and among viscera it is the spleen." This treatise on the five elements, or elements of Chinese Medicine theory, discusses dampness, earth, sweetness, the spleen, flesh, the lungs; if we contemplate this chain of occurrences clearly, we arrive at a definite explanation. In a preceding portion of this chapter, we explored the concept of humans as the chief of the "naked" creatures, and our discussion led us to a number of interesting assertions upon which we now can rely. When brought together, dampness and earth form a single body; separated, they constitute the difference between heaven and earth. Dampness refers to the *qi* and earth to the physical form. What is the relationship between form and *qi*? The *Yellow Emperor's Classic* is very clear on this: "*Qi* gathers together and then form comes into being." In light of this, what is earth? How is earth formed? Do we know how this ground of ours assumed form? It came into being as the *qi* of dampness gathered. Thus, the *Plain Questions* says that the central region produces dampness, and this dampness produces earth. It does not say that the central region produces earth, and the earth produces dampness. This is a matter of root and branch, a matter of the proper sequence. We should understand this clearly. As *Great Learning* tells us: "Things have their root and their branch, and affairs have their ends and their beginnings. If one knows what one thing leads to, then it will bring the person nearer to the Dao." If one does not know the root from the branch, or how one thing leads to another, how can one come closer to the Dao?

I.4.c. Chen, Xu, Chou, *and* Wei

In the above discussion, when we discussed Taiyin and damp earth, we discussed it from the perspective of *qi*. The *Plain Questions's* "Great Treatise on the Six Subtleties" says: "when a time period begins, the respective *qi* spreads"; and "if you do not know what each year contributes, the abundance and weakness of the *qi*, and how deficiency and excess arise, then you cannot be a practitioner." Once one knows the connotations of different *qi*, one must also understand the particular timing of these *qi*. With regard to Taiyin damp earth, the time of year that corresponds to Taiyin damp is the period related to the earthly branches in the heading of this section of the book: *chen, xu, chou,* and *wei*. To be more exact, the period spanning the earthly branches *chen* and *xu* is the period in which Taiyang cold water holds dominion in the heavens, and Taiyin damp earth is welling up. That which holds dominion over the heavens is augmented during the first half of the year, whereas that which is welling up is augmented during the second half of the year. The *chou* and *wei* years are exactly the opposite; during these periods, Taiyin damp earth commands the heavens, and Taiyang cold water is welling up.

When Taiyin damp earth is augmented, or when Taiyin *qi* pattern has arrived, what sort of changes take place? Regarding this point, the *Plain Questions* chapter "Great Treatise on the Policies and Arrangements of the Six Principal *Qi*" describes the constants related to the seasons, the constants of the transformation of the commanding energies, of *qi* transformation, of virtue, the spreading of governance, the constants of the changes of *qi* and of inducing the phases, as well as the constants of disease, and so on, from eight different angles, namely: (1) The seasonal change related to Taiyin is dust and humidity. (2) The dominant quality related to Taiyin is the palace of rain associated with volume and abundance. (3) The transformation of *qi* related to Taiyin is transformation and clouds and rain. (4) When Taiyin arrives, the virtue of its change is that dampness emerges and concludes with pouring rain, and when Taiyin arrives, it denudes.

(5) It moistens. (6) Thunder peals, rain billows, and the wind gales. (7) The Taiyin sky is dark and gloomy, or white with haze, or dark with gloom. (8) When Taiyin dominates, rheum accumulates, and there is glomus and distention; when Taiyin dominates, it becomes bloating and fullness; when Taiyin dominates, the abdomen is bloated, and there is a general tendency to epidemic episodes of vomiting and diarrhea; there is heaviness, and swelling.

The year 2000 was a *gengchen* year, the seventeenth year in the Chinese sexagenary cycle. *Chen* years are characterized by Taiyang cold water ruling the heavens and Taiyin damp earth residing at the source. As we saw, in the second half of previous year there was a great deal of dampness and rain, especially in Taiwan, where there was flooding and landslides like nothing seen in the last 50 years, destroying a large amount of farmland and property. Typically, flooding occurs in the first half of the year, usually in summer. Why were the previous year's floods during the second half of the year? This is clearly related to the arrival of Taiyin. Taiyin damp earth is welling up, and so the Taiyin mechanism was increasingly dominant in the second half of the year, and so the Taiyin influence could "end in pouring rain," or could take the form of "pealing thunder, billowing rain, and strong gales of wind." It is not unusual for floods to occur during such a period.

The study of the five movements and six *qi* (*wuyun liuqi*, abbreviated as *yunqi*) is a complex subject. There are not only constants in this study, but also permutations; there is domination and submission of particular energies. It is not easy to grasp this subject. In the above example, we see the *yunqi* expressed in Taiwan's meteorological disasters last year, but it has already passed, and we are simply reviewing the course of the year according to our understanding of *yunqi*. Such an exercise is somewhat belated, but serves to aid us in understanding *yunqi*, and we should not avoid doing such parenthetical analyses. If one looks at the meteorological changes as well as the epidemiological patterns of past years and correlates them with the *yunqi* of that year, analyzing and evaluating them for their regularities, their permutations, their dominant and submissive influences, then one will gain skill in understanding the relationship of the *yunqi* to these phenomena. Once this skill is achieved, these parenthetical efforts might lead to prediction and prognosis of what is to come. Then the practitioner can "first establish the year, and thereby understand the *qi*."

I.4.d. Outward Sign of the Communication between Heaven and Earth

In the above section, we discussed a constant related to the sort of changes wrought by the prevalence of Taiyin *qi*. This constant was the transformations that become clouds and rain. When the Taiyin *qi* is set in motion, it produces transformation and subsequently clouds and rain. What does transformation (*hua* 化) mean? The *Plain Questions* says: "When things come into being, this is transformation (*hua*). When things reach their extremes, this is called change (*bian* 變)." The *Gathered Rhymes* (Yunhui) therefore says: "The Revolutions of the yin and yang between heaven and earth are such that things exist and then they do not exist; they do not exist and then they exist. The myriad living things are born and die; this is what is meant by transformation (*hua*)." Thus, the most important thing indicated by transformation is the birth and death of living things. "Great Treatise on the Policies and Arrangements of the Six Principal *Qi*" says that both "transformation" and "clouds and rain" are the constant of Taiyin *qi* transformation. What does this mean? We are all familiar with the clouds and rain; however, if we wish to explain the secret relationship these have with *hua*, with the birth and death of the myriad things, then we must contemplate the question thoroughly.

The production of clouds and rain is explained with complete clarity by the "Great Treatise on the Correspondences of Yin and Yang": "The terrestrial *qi* rises as clouds, the celestial *qi* descends as rain. Rain brings forth the terrestrial *qi* and clouds bring forth the celestial *qi*." Clouds and rain are produced by heaven and earth. More precisely, the earth *qi* rises, the heavenly *qi* descends and the intermingling of the *qi* of heaven and earth produces clouds and rain. When we discussed the hexagrams *pi* and *tai*, we discussed this same process of *qi* intermingling as the earth *qi* rises and the heavenly *qi* descends. As a result, we know the importance of the exchange of celestial and terrestrial *qi*. If heaven and earth do not exchange with one another, the myriad living things are obstructed and die. If the *qi* of heaven and earth is exchanged, the myriad things are connected and can be born and die. However, in spite of our previous discussion, the process of this interchange of *qi* still seems somewhat murky and unclear. Is there some method with which we might be able to better grasp the mystery of this exchange of *qi*? There is, indeed! This method, this technique, is embodied by clouds and rain.

Clouds and rain are products of the exchange between heaven and earth, outward and obvious signs of the process of intermingling earthly and heavenly *qi*. Only when the *qi* of heaven and earth interplay can the myriad things live on. By exploring this outward sign, we can better understand the mystery of this exchange of *qi* between heaven and earth, and of this life and death of the myriad things. Therefore, if you thoroughly understand clouds and rain, then you have arrived at an excellent method of understanding the play of yin and yang among living things.

If you wish to examine the nature of the life and death of living things, or the state of the interchange of celestial and terrestrial *qi*, you need only observe the clouds and rain. Let us pull back a bit: Is there life on Mars? Is there life on the moon? Must we go there to find out for ourselves? I do not think that is necessary. We need only look to see if there are clouds and rain to know. If there are no clouds, then there is no exchange of *qi* between heaven and earth. If there is no intermingling of the earth and the firmament, then we will not find any life there, and searching would be a waste of time. Modern satellite technology is excellent, and although determining whether or not a planet in our solar system possesses life presents certain difficulties, these satellites have no problem determining whether or not these planets have clouds and rain. If we ever determine that there are clouds and rain on another planet, then we have made a large stride toward discovering extraterrestrial life.

To be more exact, on this planet of ours, due to differences in region and season, there are differences in the degree of exchange between heavenly and earthly *qi*. Regarding particular regions, some regions have a great deal of clouds and rain, and others few clouds and little rain. There are parts of the earth where neither clouds nor rain can be seen all year long. In places where clouds and rain are abundant, where they are evenly distributed, the exchange of celestial and terrestrial *qi* is very good. If you go to these parts of the world, you will find that plant and animal life are plentiful, and it is more than likely that the area is densely populated. Take a look at the provinces of Yunnan and Sichuan, or the area south of the Yangzi River, and you will know that I am not simply making this up. The regions where there are few clouds and little rain, where it may not rain at all in the course of the year, are almost invariably deserts, remote and barren tracts of desolation. Why is this? It is because the interchange of heavenly and earthly *qi* is so lacking. If heaven and earth do not intermingle, then the myriad living things will be obstructed, and there is no life, and no signs of habitation. With regard to the time of the year, this difference is even more salient. In most parts of China, there is abundant rain during the two seasons of spring and summer, and little rain during fall and winter. During the seasons of spring and summer, the myriad living things cast off age and flourish, prosper, and blossom. During the autumn and winter, the many living things hole up, wither, and accord their behavior with the bleak scenery. Spring and summer are set in motion by the scenario represented in the hexagram *tai* (Advance). *Tai* represents the exchange between yin and yang, and because heaven and earth exchange *qi*, there are clouds and rain. Autumn and winter are instigated by the pattern of the hexagram *pi* (Hindrance) in which heaven and earth do not intermingle, and so there are few clouds and little rain.

From the arrival of Taiyin there are clouds and rain, and from the clouds and the rain we know of the exchange between heaven and earth, and we ascertain the presence of life. Thus, deducing the presence of Taiyin is crucial in this chain of logic. Now, let us shift from the macrocosm of the sky and the earth to the microcosm of the human body. How does the "arrival of Taiyin becomes transformation and then clouds and rain" in the human body? By "transformation" (*hua*), we are still referring to life and death, to creation and transformation. The Taiyin spleen (stomach) earth is the root of postnatal *qi*, the source of creation and transformation of *qi* and blood. This tallies well with the transformation that comes from the arrival of Taiyin. The Taiyin spleen and its bowel, the stomach, are the central hub of rising and falling in the body. How does the microcosm of the human body intermingle with *qi*? It relies upon the hub at the center of the rising and falling. To what do the clouds and rain, the outward sign of the exchange of heavenly and earthly *qi*, correspond in the human body? Can we find something that makes the exchange of *qi* within the human organism obvious in the way that clouds and rain make obvious the intermingling of celestial and terrestrial *qi*? Yes, saliva. Saliva should not be disregarded! It is the outward sign of the exchange of *qi* in the human body and is also the mark of living things. The classics say: "To speak of people, we must investigate the exchange of *qi*." If the exchange of *qi* is the root of human life, then we cannot afford to underestimate its importance.

If, in the larger macrocosm of the natural world, we can use clouds and rain to evaluate the state of *qi* exchange, and of life in general, then we have discovered a very simple method indeed. Is it not equally simple, if not still simpler, to assess the state of the saliva in your own mouth? We talk about the state desired by living things in terms of "life" (*shengxi* 生息), or "transformation" (*hua* 化). Besides these two, there is a different Chinese term that would seem to express this state desired by living things: *huo* (活), meaning "alive" or "lively." Look at the construction of the character *huo*. On the left we have water (氵) and on the right the tongue (舌). The fluid on the tongue, or the fluid that surrounds the tongue, what is this fluid? It is saliva, is it not? This saliva is our liveliness, the outward sign of vitality. Why not use this tongue-water, this saliva, this "drool and spittle," this fluid that is so simple and straightforward to assess, to infer the person's inner vitality, to investigate the hidden physiological processes in the human frame?

Whether we are referring to the larger world of nature or the microcosm of the human body, there are, in fact, a great many outward signs on the order of "clouds and rain" that are remarkably easy to obtain, that can reveal very secret, very esoteric phenomena. But it is precisely this obviousness and easily perceived quality, this easy obtainment, which makes it hard for us to perceive its meaning, to understand what is thereby revealed. This is a common failing among us humans: when something is too easily obtained, we do not cherish it. It is for this reason that Confucius said: "The Dao consists of one yin and one yang. It is good to continue this, and completing it is our very nature. The benevolent see it and say that it is benevolence, the wise see it and say that it is wisdom, while the common people use it every day and do not even know it, thus the path of the person of noble character is a rare way indeed."

"When Taiyin arrives, it becomes transformation, becomes the clouds and rain," and Taiyin refers to the spleen; the orifice or opening related to the spleen is the mouth, and the lips are the splendor of the spleen. All five of the viscera have a fluid associated with them, and the fluid of the spleen is the saliva. Regarding the fluids, Wang Bing commented: "They overflow at the mouth and lips." So then, why not consider saliva, this fluid that overflows at the mouth and lips, to be the equivalent of clouds and rain? Why not begin your inquiry into the state of health of the patient before you by examining the saliva, the "clouds and rain" of the human body? In truth, can the saliva of the spleen correspond to the exchange of *qi*? Does it reflect the body's overall state of health? We need only examine our own experience to know. When you are energetic, when you feel your body is at its best, pay attention to what goes on in your mouth: see whether there is a fine, aromatic, almost fragrantly sweet saliva in your mouth. If you do, then you have found what you are looking for. If your saliva is sweet and fragrant in this way, then the exchange of *qi* is optimal, and so too is your vitality. Your entire being is in a state of "Heaven and earth exchanging and the myriad things being connected," so of course you have great vitality! Conversely, when you are exhausted, or when you are sick, check to see if this sweet, fragrant flavor is still in your mouth. I can assure you it will not be. Your mouth will probably taste bitter, or feel dry or sticky, or malodorous. In any case, it will not feel clear and fresh. Why is this? Because there is a problem with the exchange of *qi*, and the postnatal source of *qi* has a problem. Why not use such a simple and convenient method? Therefore, if you wish to know your state of health, you need not rush for a CT; first taste and feel the sensation of saliva in your mouth, and you will have a general idea.

Earlier, we discussed an important Daoist practice, that of opening the microcosmic orbit. This is no easy task; the practitioner must practice assiduously to build basic skills in this method. Just a few years ago, China was full of so-called *qigong* masters claiming to be Buddhists or Daoists and who offered to teach *qigong* methods that would allow the practitioner to circulate the microcosmic orbit in less than a week. Is it so easy? There were far too many people who thought so, and they were taken in accordingly. There must be a way of knowing whether or not someone has really opened the microcosmic orbit. To use modern scientific parlance, we must have an objective measure of the ability to circulate the microcosmic orbit. It is not so simple a thing that one needs merely think about it to achieve the opening and circulation of the microcosmic orbit. An important testament to achievement of this ability is an abundant, sweet, and fragrant aspect to the saliva of the mouth. Some call his sort of saliva "sweet dew," and by others it is referred to as "golden fluid, jade elixir." Whatever we choose to call it, it is none other than the "clouds and rain," the saliva of the spleen, and of course this includes the saliva of the kidneys, which also flows into the mouth. From this perspective, is circulation of the microcosmic orbit not simply a way to increase the exchange of *qi* between the celestial and the terrestrial, and raise this exchange to a new level? One should fully grasp the significance of saliva, and see it for what it really is; one should truly see it as the "living water" (*huo shui* 活水) at the fountainhead of vitality. In China, those in the medical profession know of the medicinal use of edible bird nests, and it is generally known that these are a treasured delicacy. These nests are made from saliva out of the mouth of the esculent swift, are they not? If even the saliva from these little birds has such a salubrious effect, then what about our own saliva? Contemplation will reveal the answer. The classics say that good advice should resonate with the advisee. If you sincerely explore the ideas I have just presented, I believe that you will find your study to be a process of discovering sound advice.

I.4.e. Dragons Contend in the Open, Their Blood Is Black and Yellow

I have discussed the *Classic of Changes* on a number of occasions already. Ultimately, what sort of book is the *Classic of Changes*? In his *Commentaries on the Appended Judgments of the Classic of Changes*, Confucius wrote an authoritative and classic account of this work. "The *Classic of Changes*," he writes, "is comprehensive and wide in its scope; the way of heaven, human, and earth are all contained within it. These three basic constituents of the cosmos are coupled, and so there are six altogether. These six lines show the way of these three—heaven, earth, and man." Confucius is not alone in his assessment. The *Yellow Emperor's Classic* states: "Understanding of the Dao requires knowledge of the pattern of the Heavens above, the earth below, and the affairs of humanity in between; this way it will last forever." The *Classic of Changes* simultaneously considers heaven, earth, and human, and it is comprehensive and broad in scope. Physicians, by knowing heaven, earth, and human affairs, open the way to longevity. From this perspective, the ancient claim of *yi yi tong yuan* (醫易同源), that there is a close correspondence between medicine (*yi* 醫) and the changes (*yi* 易), and that they share a common origin, seems quite reasonable.

Do Chinese Medicine and the *Classic of Changes* correspond to one another? Let us look at the text corresponding to the last, uppermost line of the *kun* (Responding) hexagram, when it consists of a "six" or "changing" line: "Dragons battle in the wild, their blood is black and yellow." What are these dragons? If dragons battle in the wild, why is their blood black and yellow? A cursory examination of this passage might suggest that there were really two dragons fighting in the wild, inflicting injury on each other, such that black and yellow blood flowed forth. Since ancient times, a great number of experts in the *Classic of Changes* have held this very view. For instance, a well-known expert in the *Classic of Changes* of our current era argues: "According to the understanding of the ancients, dragons were cold-blooded and did not possess red blood. The blood of black dragons was black, and that of yellow dragons was yellow, which is why it says that 'Dragons battle in the wild, their blood is black and yellow,' providing the image of these two dragons fighting one another and both sides suffering injury." The dragon is the symbol of China, and the Chinese people are descendants of the dragon. If we regard the dragons described by the *Classic of Changes* in this light, then we will not find these dragons in real life, lest we belittle the people of China. How could the hot-blooded men of China possibly descend from a cold-blooded reptile? This view is not only improper and unreasonable; it does not jibe with reality.

What then do these "dragons" really refer to? If these dragons battle in the wild, why is their blood black and yellow? At this point, I would like to cite *Master Shang's Study of the Zhou Yi* regarding the six in the uppermost line of the *kun* (Responding) hexagram:

> A yin six in the uppermost line completes the virtue of the hexagram *kun*. Thus, the myriad living creatures come into being, for if this line were not changing and were merely a yin line, it would not give birth. Xun Shuang says: "Vacillation in this last line indicates that *kun* in the position of the earthly branch *hai* proceeds to the hexagram *qian*. Yin and yang moderate one another, thus it says that the dragons battle in the wild open." *Kun* is the wild open space and *qian* the dragon. Under the entry *ren* (壬) in *Explaining Writing and Analyzing Characters*, it says: "When the *Classic of Changes* says that the dragons battle in the wild open, their battling is how they receive one another." Qian Zaodu says: "the joining of the *qi* of *qian* and *kun* is during the periods *xu* and *hai*, their *qi* merges and so they are receiving one another." The *Jiujia* commentary says: "black and yellow are the colors of heaven and earth, and describe the cohabitation of *qian* and *kun*." Thus, if it is mutual joining, if it is a merging of *qi*, if they reside together, then their battling is clearly a harmonious union. All of the above definitions of the word "battle" are in accord with one another. Furthermore, the root of life for all

living things is blood and the dense mixture of yin and yang it inherits from heaven and earth. Heaven is black and earth is yellow, and so if we regard the flowing of this blood to be the merging of heaven and earth, then it is this merging that brings forth the myriad things. The Yilin says: "the left part of the tally fits the right one, and they come together as one; *qian* and *kun* are beneficial for a wish to come true, and together they generate the sixth son." Thus, when it says they contact one another and describes them joining as one, it means that *qian* and *kun* receive one another, and the dragons battle in the wild. When the six is at the bottom of the hexagram, *kun* becomes *zhen*. Thus, it says that they bring forth the sixth son. The *Commentary on the Judgments* says: "reaching the end there is occasion to celebrate." Only the *Xun* and *Jiujia* commentaries regard blood as yin, but this is contrary to what is written. The *Classic of Changes* clearly indicates that heaven and earth are mixed, and so the blood cannot be purely yin. If it were pure yin, this would mean it leaves its category; how could it produce life? Even Hou Guo says overabundant yin is like yang. Wang Bi and Gan Bao say that excessive yin forces yang, and yang cannot take anymore and so it struggles, and they understood this to mean "makes war." Later Kong Yingda and Zhu Zi, on account of the fact that the classic refers to both war and blood, suspected that yin and yang were harming each other. Pure nonsense. Of the Qing Dynasty Confucian scholars, only Hui Shiqi went so far as to say that perhaps this battling was, in fact, their way of receiving one another. Yin and yang intermingle and receive one another, and the hexagrams are devoid of injuring. This is what our predecessors have thought on this topic.

The *Classic of Changes* uses imagery to imply principles, and uses language to speak about the images. Thus, the image cannot be separated from the language, and the language is inseparable from the image. Without the explanation, the image would be incomprehensible, and the principle pertaining to that image would remain obscure. If we treat the image as unessential and pontificate only about the principles, it is like Cui Hao's Tang dynasty poem about trying to talk about the cranes seen from the "Yellow Crane Tower," where cranes have not been seen for centuries; rarely does it result in much more than rambling nonsense. So it is with the discussion of dragons as cold-blooded animals, a perfect example of the above. Dragons are most certainly not cold-blooded animals, and their struggling is not a form of fighting; it is not contention. The phrase "dragons contend in the wild," if taken as a whole, in its actual context, discusses the harmonization of *qian* and *kun* and a state of mutual reception between yin and yang. *Qian* and *kun* at their essence have the separate distinctions of nobility and humility, and are "male and female who do not directly exchange gifts with one another," as described by Mencius. They are different, separate, but now they merge together and harmonize with one another. And why? It is once again a case of yin rising and yang descending, the intermingling of heavenly and earthly *qi*. When the *qi* of heaven and earth intertwine, clouds and rain are produced. One minute the sky is high and clear with only a wisp or two of pale cloud; and the next, lightning is flashing and the sound of thunder fills the air, black thunderclouds fill the sky, heaven and earth join and the ground is covered with water made yellow by the earth. Is this not the very picture of "their blood is black and yellow"?

Thus, "Dragons contend in the open, their blood is black and yellow" is actually describing the occurrence of thunder and lightning, rain and clouds in nature. Actually, such a description of this natural phenomenon is not at all strange, but it *is* quite strange that such an image be used to describe the last line in the *kun* hexagram. This just shows that if you wish to explain the meaning of these words, you must include the image of this unique hexagram line in your analysis. Through this image, the true significance of the *Classic of Changes* is revealed. Neglecting the image and proceeding to discuss the meaning of the *Classic of Changes* results in nothing but nonsensical rambling. Taking, for instance, the dragon to be a cold-blooded animal, or their contention to be battling, aptly illustrates the sort of nonsense to which I am referring.

Earlier, we explored the implied meaning of the dragon, which is in charge of arousing the clouds and distributing rain. Those who have read *Journey to the West* surely find this very clear. When Sun Wukong, the Monkey King and protagonist of the *Journey to the West*, wishes to cause rain, how does he do it? He entreats the Dragon King. As soon as the Dragon King appears, the sky fills with clouds and rain begins to fall. If we were novelists, we would not have to go any further into the connection between the Dragon King and clouds and rain, but as physicians or students of the *Classic of Changes*, we must delve deeper. We must keep in mind that these clouds and raindrops are "the earth *qi* rising to form clouds, and the celestial *qi* descending to become rain." From the interplay of heavenly and earthly *qi*, clouds and rain emerge. In this way, we know that the dragon actually represents the exchange of *qi* between heaven and earth.

Why are dragons associated with the east? Why is the thunder associated with the calendrical period *Jingzhe* (Awakening of Insects) in the spring? Why is spring the time of year in which the myriad living creatures emerge? All of these ultimately relate to the mutual exchange of earthly with heavenly *qi*, do they not? The *Great Commentary of the Classic of Changes* says: "Heaven and earth's misty union; all living things are transformed by it and develop. Male and female commingle their essence, and all living things thereby procreate." When heaven and earth are thick with mists and vapors, it is then that living creatures develop their unique properties. Why are heaven and earth shrouded in mist? Confucius must have been afraid that the faculties of his descendants might be lacking, for he appends this slightly difficult metaphor with more specific detail: "Male and female commingle their essence, and all living things thereby procreate." At the very least, we should catch the drift of "male and female merge their essence." The mist that enshrouds heaven and earth is used to express the intercourse between heaven and earth, or put more coarsely, the lovemaking of heaven and earth. The fermentation of the many different living creatures is the direct result of the coitus between heaven and earth. But rather than using the language of sex to describe the union between the two primary poles of ancient Chinese cosmology, let's go back to the term *yinyun* (氤氲), literally, "dense mist."

The term *yinyun* is very interesting. Its meaning can be sensed but it is difficult to express, and it remains doubly ineffable when attempting to explain its meaning on paper. We will have to make do with our own understanding of the term. When heaven and earth are engaged in the act of *yinyun*, they do not wish to be seen, for this is a secret and intimate affair. How do they maintain their privacy? They sound thunder and drop rain. When thunder and lightning split the sky and rain buckets down from the sky, living things retreat to take cover, and heaven and earth can engage in *yinyun*. We can see what a discreet and respectful term this is.

We see that both "dragons contend in the open, their blood is black and yellow," and "heaven and earth's misty union; all living things are transformed by it and develop" mean the same thing, for "dragons contending" is another way of saying that heaven and earth are shrouded in mist.

People are unique among living creatures, first and foremost among them, and as the descendants of dragons, there is nothing they cannot do. If we look at old dramatic novels, such as those by the Ming dynasty authors Feng Menglong and Ling Mengchu, how did the authors of old refer to sexual relations, to the interplay of yin and yang? They used martial terms, and the language of clouds and rain. This only serves to show that man and the natural cosmos are one, and that the words of Master Shang (whom we quoted above) and myself are not mere whimsical musings.

Why is the phrase "dragons contend in the open, their blood is yellow and black" the adage for a changing sixth line in the hexagram *kun* (Responding)? When the uppermost line of *kun* is changing, its virtue is complete. When the full virtue of *kun* is complete, it is identical to Taiyin. In the final analysis, is there any real difference between the meaning of "dragons contend in the open, their blood is black and yellow," "heaven and earth's misty union; all living things are transformed by it and develop," and "the arrival of Taiyin signals change and transformation, clouds and rain"? If there is no real difference, then the study of Chinese Medicine and the study of the *Classic of Changes* are interlinked, from the same source, and this is beyond all doubt.

The significance of Taiyin damp earth is broad and far-reaching, but the ideas conveyed by "transformation" and "clouds and rain" are clearly crucial to understanding the specific meaning of this concept. My advisor for my master's degree, Professor Chen Zhiheng, believed that the most important problem in Chinese Medicine was the "two roots and the three pivots." Which two roots? The roots of the prenatal and the postnatal. The root, the foundation of the prenatal are the kidneys, and the roots of the postnatal lie in the Taiyin spleen and stomach. What are the three pivots? One is the Shaoyang pivot, one is the Shaoyin pivot, and the third is the rising and falling pivot of the spleen. Among these two roots and the three pivots, Taiyin embraces one root and one pivot. The importance of Taiyin to Chinese Medicine is obvious. There are those who, seeing the brevity of Taiyin chapter, mistakenly think it is enough to skim over it. On the contrary, we must go further afield and explore concepts, such as the "naked creatures" and human beings as the chief of these creatures and the descendants of dragons, in order to fully understand Taiyin.

II. An Outline of Taiyin Disease

Our outline of Taiyin disease will be based upon line 273 of the *Treatise on Cold Damage*: "When Taiyin is diseased, there is abdominal fullness and vomiting, inability to eat, severe spontaneous diarrhea, intermittent spontaneous abdominal pain, and downward purging results in a hard bind below the chest." Below, we will discuss these lines from various perspectives.

II.1. The Taiyin Disease Trigger

Line 273 provides us with an outline of Taiyin disease. This same line informs us of the Taiyin disease trigger, and so our discussion of the trigger is also centered upon this line. Accordingly, we could rephrase this line in the style of the nineteen disease triggers from *Plain Questions* as: "All abdominal fullness and vomiting, inability to eat, severe spontaneous diarrhea, and intermittent spontaneous abdominal pain belong to Taiyin."

II.2. Characteristics of the Taiyin Position and Nature

Earlier in this book, we discussed how Taiyin belongs to *Kun* Earth. The *Classic of Changes* says: "*Kun* is the most soft." What is the softest area of the human body? The softest part of our body is clearly the abdomen. No other area of the body is as soft as the abdomen. Everywhere else there are bony prominences and projections, but the abdomen is devoid of these. So the position of *Kun* Earth, of Taiyin in the body is the abdomen. The *Explanation of the Trigrams* (Shuogua) of the *Classic of Changes* says: "*Kun* is the abdomen." Taiyin pathology will tend to appear in this particular part of the body, as we saw in line 273, where both abdominal fullness and abdominal pain are mentioned. This is a matter of the position of Taiyin disease.

What about the nature of the Taiyin *Kun* Earth? *Kun* is associated with the qualities of thick, deep and wide. In the *Commentary on the Judgments of the Classic of Changes*, it says: "*Kun* greatness carries all things, its virtue is boundless." Many of the characteristics of Taiyin are related to this "great" or "thick" nature of *Kun*. First of all, *Explaining Writing and Analyzing Characters* as well as the *Erya* dictionary say that "The abdomen is thick," and this once more ties together the abdomen position with *Kun*, which is also thick. There is no doubt now that the abdomen is the region of the body specifically related to Taiyin and to Taiyin disease. This issue warrants our attention, as any disease involving the abdomen requires us to understand its connection to Taiyin.

Besides the above points, Taiyin chapter primarily discusses the *Kun* Earth, and focuses on the spleen and stomach. The "Treatise on the Spiritual Orchid Secret Canon" in the *Plain Questions* says: "The spleen and stomach hold the office of the granaries. The five flavors originate from them." By mentioning the granaries and the five flavors, this passage raises two important questions. First of all, because they are the granaries, this means that they are loaded with things, and as a result, they are "thick." Thus, it says that *Kun* is thick and carries things. Therefore, when we inspect the *Kun* Earth, or Taiyin, or the spleen and stomach, it is important that we examine their thickness. If they are thick, then they can carry things and act as a granary. If they are too thin, then they will not be able to carry things or perform their function as a granary.

We can see the thickness of Taiyin by examining its position: the abdomen. If the abdomen is too thin, perhaps even to the point of being concave, then Taiyin's basic nature definitely has a problem, and the spleen and stomach are weak. If *Kun* is thin instead of thick, then it does not possess its essential quality. How then could it act as a granary and store things? When looking at the thickness of the abdomen, there is something else that we need to pay attention to, especially when examining children. The thickness we are examining is also the thickness of the musculature. There are children with protruding bellies whose abdominal muscles are very thin; we cannot regard the abdomen of these children as being "thick" in such a case. Another place we can examine the "thickness" is at the navel. Whether the navel is shallow or deep, thick or thin, reflects the corresponding strength or weakness of Taiyin, of the spleen and stomach. This is a very direct and convenient method whereby we can make an immediate correlation between the patient's physique and the state of their Taiyin spleen and stomach. Of course, although it is fitting for Taiyin *Kun* Earth to be thick, for if it is thin, it indicates that there is some failure in the nature of the *Kun* Earth; if it is too thick, this is also not good. If the *Kun* Earth is too thick, then the person will be obese. In the *Plain Questions*, this sort of rotundity was also deemed pernicious. This question of "granaries" is the first issue.

The second issue is that as it says in the judgment of *Kun* Earth in the

Classic of Changes, that "Oh ultimate *Kun* source, all living things emerge from it, for it obeys heaven." This is, in fact, the same issue presented by the line from the "Treatise of the Spiritual Orchid Secret Canon" in the *Plain Questions*," which says ". . . the five flavors emerge from them." In nature, the *Kun* source brings forth the myriad living things; what is its role in the human body? In the human body, it brings forth the five flavors. The issue of the five flavors is an important one in Chinese Medicine. In the *Plain Questions*, it is written: "Heaven nourishes human beings with the five *qi*, and the earth nourishes human beings with the five flavors." In practical terms, if we wish to preserve life, what should we depend upon to do so? For one, we must breathe. We cannot go more than a moment or two without breathing. Respiration provides us with the five flavors of heaven. Besides this, we also rely on the five flavors of the earth. And so, besides breathing, we also must eat. That which we ingest is nothing more than the five flavors bestowed by earth.

Modern medicine regards foods according to their nutritional content: proteins, fats, carbohydrates, vitamins, mineral contents, etc. Chinese Medicine categorizes foods according to two words: "five flavors." Besides breathing the *qi* of heaven, we can describe all our other nourishment in terms of these two words. Regardless of whether we are talking about protein or fat content, or the vitamins and minerals it contains, all of these can be expressed in terms of the five flavors. When a Western physician encounters a patient with dry skin, it is assumed that there is some sort of vitamin deficiency. If the patient is suffering from hair loss, it is also deemed to be a deficiency of particular vitamins or minerals and the patient is supplemented accordingly. If, as a Chinese Medicine practitioner, you adopt a similar methodology and, in light of a mineral deficiency revealed by Western lab tests, prescribe Longgu (fossilized bones) or Muli (oyster shell), you will run into trouble.

This is not to say that a Chinese Medicine practitioner cannot draw lessons from Western Medicine. The Chinese Medicine practitioner can take in and borrow from anywhere and anything. As the Chinese saying goes: "There are other hills whose stones are good for working jade." However, the Chinese Medicine physician must do so in accord the basic principles of Chinese Medicine; she cannot mistake the slave for the master. This would be a disservice to both Chinese Medicine and to other disciplines. Recently,

I visited a renowned physician in Yunnan province, Mr. Wu Rongzu, the eldest grandson of the famous Chinese Medicine doctor Wu Peiheng. In the course of our conversation, Mr. Wu made an interesting point: when we attempt to integrate the knowledge of outside disciplines into Chinese Medicine, we must be certain that our efforts at addition ensure that one plus one is greater than one. If, by adding one thing and another, we arrive at something less than what we began with, we should avoid such integration. Mr. Wu raised this point in response to what he himself had seen resulting from efforts at integrating Western medical knowledge into the framework of Chinese Medicine, which was that more often than not he saw a net decrease rather than a net increase. For instance, if sufficient antibiotics are used to treat an infection and, in addition, herbs that clear heat and resolve toxin are given adjunctively in the name of "Integrated Western and Chinese Medicine," the result is a reduction in the efficacy of the antibiotics! Not only does such adjunctive therapy not augment the effect of the treatment, but it actually increases the cost of such treatment. This is a problem in many Chinese Medicine hospitals today. When discussing this topic, it was clear that Mr. Wu felt helpless and pained.

So what are the guiding principles of Chinese Medicine? If, as we illustrated in the above example, we just follow Western Medicine and supplement a deficiency in this vitamin or that mineral, then your thinking lacks a guiding principle, in the Chinese Medicine sense. As a Chinese Medicine physician, you must think in terms of the five flavors. There are five external flavors and five internal flavors. The five external flavors are those referred to in the judgment of the trigram *Kun* Earth: "Oh ultimate *Kun* source, all living things emerge from it, for it obeys heaven." The five flavors are generated by the *Kun* Earth of the cosmos around us. The five internal flavors are those that are mentioned in the passage from the "Treatise of the Spiritual Orchid Secret Canon": "The spleen and stomach hold the office of the granaries. The five flavors originate from them." They are the five flavors that emerge from the microcosm of the spleen and stomach *Kun* Earth. In the clinical setting, we see many patients whose diets are more or less the same—they eat rice from the same pot, and eat the very same dishes—but why then is the one patient deficient in a particular vitamin or mineral, and the other not? Clearly, this patient is not deficient in terms of the external five flavors. He is deficient in terms of the internal five flavors.

If the patient's Taiyin, if their spleen and stomach, their office of the granaries, cannot bring forth the five internal flavors, then they will naturally be deficient. If this is the case, and the physician attempts to supplement externally, how helpful can it be? Such efforts are a stopgap measure, and they do not constitute a method that is in accord with the fundamentals of Chinese Medicine. In order to exercise such a method, the physician must examine the patient's Taiyin, their spleen and stomach, their internal *Kun* Earth source. The patient must thicken, fortify, and regulate accordingly. If this aspect of the patient is able to have "all living things emerge from it" and "originate the five flavors," then the patient's vitamin or mineral deficiency will be resolved. Such a method is in accord with the guiding principles of Chinese Medicine, and such guiding principles must never be neglected.

II.3. Characteristics of Taiyin Disease Signs and Symptoms

II.3.a. It Has Two Functions, and Also Two Diseases

Above we discussed the nature and function of Taiyin spleen and stomach network. First, the thickness of the *Kun* Earth carries all living things. Secondly, the myriad living things are born from it. By "carrying," it is meant that all living things are loaded into it and stored inside it. The birth of the myriad living things involves their transport, change, and transformation. This nature and function of Taiyin are amply expressed in the description of Taiyin pathology. The outline of Taiyin disease that opens the *Treatise on Cold Damage* chapter on such pathology tells us that "vomiting, inability to eat, and spontaneous diarrhea" all demonstrate an inability to "carry" things. If the Taiyin *Kun* Earth cannot carry things, then, of course, there will be lack of appetite, diarrhea, and vomiting. An inability to eat, spontaneous diarrhea, and vomiting are therefore characteristics of Taiyin being unable to carry things. On the other hand, if there is a problem generating life, if this second aspect of Taiyin is hindered, then the "origination of the five flavors" will be affected. If this hindrance is not corrected in a timely fashion, then it will begin to affect the spleen and stomach as the source of postnatal vitality. The loss of this vitality is gradual; it does not happen from one day to the next. Nevertheless, its impact on our patient's health is so great that it warrants our vigilance. The opening line of the Taiyin chapter in the *Treatise on Cold Damage* mentions "abdominal fullness, intermittent spontaneous abdominal pain," and these are signs that the normal ability of Taiyin to transport has been negatively impacted.

II.3.b. Characteristics of Taiyin Diarrhea

Diarrhea is a characteristic sign of Taiyin disease, and shows that the *Kun* Earth is not able to store. At this juncture, I would like to point out to the reader that Zhang Zhongjing uses the two characters: *zi li* (自痢). The use of these characters requires that we clearly differentiate the meaning of this particular phrase. What is *zi li*, translated thus far in our discussion of Taiyin as "spontaneous diarrhea"? Let us suppose we prescribe Da Chengqi Tang, and after the patient takes the formula, they have diarrhea up to ten times in the course of a day. Can we say that this is *zi li*? Obviously, this is not spontaneous, self-induced diarrhea; it is the result of the physician's prescription. Or suppose that a group of friends goes out to eat at a restaurant, and afterward everyone comes down with a bout of diarrhea. These loose stools also cannot be called *zi li*, as they have clearly been induced by an external factor. *Zi li* has a narrower definition than simply "diarrhea." *Zi li* is diarrhea that is not caused by an evident outside influence. This is an important characteristic of Taiyin disease.

Taiyin diarrhea, besides being spontaneous, is also characterized by accompanying lack of thirst. This thirstless aspect to Taiyin diarrhea is indicated in line 277 of the *Treatise on Cold Damage*: "Spontaneous diarrhea with no thirst belongs to Taiyin." Why is a lack of thirst such a key characteristic in Taiyin diarrhea, and why is this peculiar? Normally, diarrhea is accompanied by thirst because of the concomitant loss of fluids. We should expect thirst when one has diarrhea. Only the diarrhea of Taiyin disease exhibits no thirst. It is a peculiar idiosyncrasy of Taiyin disease and can be quite useful in differential diagnosis.

II.3.c. Cold in the Viscera

Many of the pathological changes associated with Taiyin disease are related to cold afflicting the viscera. Thus, in line 277, it clearly points out that "Spontaneous diarrhea without thirst belongs to Taiyin and is induced by cold afflicting the viscera. It is appropriate to warm the patient, and prescribing a Sini type of formula is suitable." Cold afflicting the viscera can adversely affect the functions of Taiyin; its ability to store all living things and to bring forth life becomes hampered. All of the signs and symptoms referred to in the opening line of the Taiyin passage are related to cold in the viscera. The *Yellow Emperor's Classic* says that "Cold of the viscera produces illnesses characterized by fullness," and the first of the signs of Taiyin illness mentioned in the opening line of the chapter is "abdominal fullness." This explains the close relationship between cold of the viscera and Taiyin disease, and also demonstrates that the sequence of signs and symptoms in the opening outline of Taiyin disease conform to a strict, logical pattern. Nowadays, those who research the *Treatise on Cold Damage* pay little heed to the original order of the lines in the text. They gladly rearrange the sequence of the lines or elements within a line according to their own understanding, thereby obscuring Zhang Zhongjing's superb logic. Why are the viscera afflicted by cold in Taiyin disease? We discussed this topic at some length in the third chapter of this book. I invite the reader to review that material if questions persist.

Why are the viscera cold? It is, of course, because there is a deficiency of yang *qi*. Yang governs warmth and warming. If the yang is lessened, then warmth is lessened too, resulting in coldness of the viscera. Any discussion of the factors causing coldness of the viscera must revolve around yang *qi*.

II.3.c.1. Relationship to the Constitution

The factors that influence the constitution are identical to the prenatal influences; if, when your parents joined in sexual union, a deficiency of yang *qi* was transmitted, then your yang *qi* will naturally be deficient after birth. If the yang *qi* is weak, then the viscera will be cold. This sort of viscera coldness is especially difficult to remedy because there is no way to directly modify the prenatal endowment, and all we can do is adjust the postnatal influences. The postnatal is Taiyin; it is the spleen and stomach. This is why addressing viscera cold in the Taiyin chapter is especially pertinent.

II.3.c.2. A Preference for Cold Foods

This is a postnatal factor, and this particular point is extremely important, especially to those of us who live in the south of China. The people of China's south have a tendency to ascribe their symptoms to the effect of "rising fire," and in the clinic nine out of ten patients will tell you that they have excessive fire *qi*. These people will say that this dish and that dish contain too much hot *qi*, and that they cannot eat any standard fare. So what do they do? They limit themselves to eating foods that are cold, and drink herbal teas that clear fire. Nowadays, it is easy to get cold foods; all one has to do is open the refrigerator. This is why I consider the fridge to be both a blessing and a curse. It is difficult to cultivate even a bit of yang *qi*, and then we go and waste it with cold foods. As a clinician, this particular issue has made a deep impression on me. I have observed that upward of 80 to 90 percent of patients native to the south drink cooling herbal tea on a regular basis. I have even seen some patients who were so cold and deficient that I feared even Fuzi would not be enough to warm them, but that were still drinking cooling herbal tea, and taking formulas to clear heat prescribed by their doctors. It really pains me to see this.

It was clear to me that there were two different factors afflicting these particular patients. One aspect was the deficient knowledge and understanding of the physician. This can be addressed by raising our overall standards of knowledge and practice. The other factor was the physician's inability to clearly apprehend the patient's problem. The physician, unable to differentiate yin from yang in the patient's pathology, only increased the patient's suffering. The patient complains of heat, and the physician obliges by prescribing herbs to clear heat, regardless of whether there really was a problem with heat. Whether it is heat or cold, excess or deficiency, must be clearly established prior to administering treatment. As physicians, we cannot simply defer to the patient's complaints. Even if the patient suffers from a sore throat or even a bloody nose after eating fried food, signs that most people ascribe to "rising fire," does the patient necessarily suffer from fire and heat? We must still examine their tongue and their pulse to determine whether they truly suffer from fire and heat. Earlier, I gave the example of watering a potted plant and described how, when the soil in that pot became too dry, it could not absorb the water that was poured onto it, and the water would simply run off. In such a case, it seems like there is so much water that it is overflowing, but in point of fact the soil is dry and hard as a bone, and no water is able to soak into it. This is a situation that farmers in China are very familiar with. When the soil has been dry and hard for a long period of time, it must first be loosened up before irrigating it. First loosen up the "channels and collaterals" of the soil, and then pour water on it; then the soil will be able to absorb all of the water and none of it will run off.

The patient's situation is the same: they eat a little bit of fried food, or even smell a bit of food cooking in an oily wok, and fire stirs up in them. But is it because they have too much fire, or because their yang *qi* is too vigorous? As a matter of fact, this is rarely the case. It is because their channels are obstructed, and their *qi* and blood cannot move unobstructed. Because the channels are obstructed, the addition of even a small amount of yang causes it to overflow. This is why eating just a bit of fried food can cause the throat of such a patient to feel sore. When your average patient experiences this, they will feel they are afflicted by heat, and the physician also thinks that it is heat that is causing the trouble and prescribes cooling formulas and antibiotics. They never suspect that it is actually cold that is congealing and obstructing the channels, and that the cooling herbs and antibiotics, which are also very cold in nature, further obstruct these channels. And so it goes for a few years, or several years, or even a whole decade. The physician continues to prescribe cold medications and fails to see the true reason for the "fire" that blazes up. To use a Chinese expression, they are truly "lost in a sea without shores."

In how many instances of such "rising fire" has this particular disease state been established? Only a small minority. The majority of these patients exhibit tongue and pulse pictures that indicate deficiency cold syndrome. In cases like these, the physician should boldly use the warming herbs Fuzi, Ganjiang, and Rougui. Once these herbs have had a chance to warm the congealed cold and free up the channels, then they are able to absorb the fire from "hot *qi*" foods with ease. Additionally, when true water is no longer cold, then quicksilver fire (*gong huo* 汞火) will no longer fly. Then if the patient eats fried foods or other spicy dishes, there is no problem.

The famous late Qing dynasty physician Zheng Qin'an said, "On the path of the physician, the challenge is not using medicinals, but rather understanding patterns. At the same time, one could also say that the challenge is not understanding patterns, but rather understanding yin and yang." The practitioner of Chinese Medicine must devote considerable effort to develop skill in differentiating yin from yang and cold from hot. If the physician cannot clearly differentiate between yin and yang or cold and heat, and the physician mistakenly uses heat-clearing herbs when there is no heat to clear, the patient's yang *qi* will suffer. The function of the yang *qi* should be known to any Chinese Medicine practitioner. The *Plain Questions's* "Treatise on the Vital *Qi* Connecting to Heaven" says: "The yang *qi* is like the sun in the sky. If it is lost, the lifespan is shortened and obscured." To damage one's yang *qi* on account of a sore throat is a grievous error.

Why do so many people like Chinese Medicine at present? It is because they believe that Chinese Medicine does not induce side effects like those of Western medications. Many of those who practice Chinese Medicine also see it this way. I adamantly oppose this point of view. I think that the side effects of Chinese Medicine may be even more injurious than those of Western Medicine. And why is this? It is because the side effects of Western pharmaceuticals are easy to recognize. Each and every medication has a clear list of possible side effects, and these are listed for the patient to read. Penicillin can easily induce an allergic response, and patients are reminded to test the medication topically first. Rifampicin can easily cause kidney or liver damage, and the patient is admonished to do baseline and regular follow-up tests to assess renal and hepatic function so that any changes can be detected early in treatment. But Chinese Medicine? Chinese Medicine masquerades as a therapy with no side effects whatsoever, as if anything can be prescribed and anyone can take it. This is blatant disregard for human health. If damage is done to the yang *qi*, this is more than just a matter of a loss of renal or hepatic function; it can shorten a patient's life. Chinese Medicine treats disease with bias: it uses cold to treat heat and heat to treat cold. To treat heat with cold, it must first be determined that the patient suffers from a condition that is too hot; only then can cold medicines safely be prescribed. If there is no heat but the person uses cold medications, what will come of this? It will be as described in the *Yellow Emperor's Classic*: "Over time the *qi* will accumulate, and an early death results." Can we, as Chinese Medicine practitioners, say that Chinese Medicine does not have side effects? The side effects of Chinese Medicine are terrible indeed! Otherwise, why would the ancients have said that "A quack can kill a person without using a knife"? If you wish to practice Chinese Medicine, especially if you wish to be a true practitioner of the art, then you must never be confused about this. This section on the significance of cold deserves the attention of both the patient and the doctor.

II.3.c.3. Excessive Vexation and Worry

The *Yellow Emperor's Classic* says: "The yang *qi* is spread (*zhang*) by vexation and worry." What is meant by the Chinese term *zhang* (張) exactly? *Zhang* here means to spread or stretch; to direct outward; to release. At an earlier point in this book, we discussed how an important aspect of Taiyin is its ability to open internally. When Taiyin opens, the yang *qi* enters the interior. After entering the interior, the yang *qi* not only warms and nourishes the viscera and bowels, but it itself is replenished. If the person is troubled by vexation and worry, then the yang *qi* is spread out on the exterior and is unable to enter the interior of the body. As a result, the yang is not stored and nourished, and over time it becomes deficient and the viscera become cold. Excessive worries and troubles cause a loss of yang *qi* and a subsequent hindrance of the opening mechanism of Taiyin.

II.3.c.4. Irregular Rest

The loss of yang *qi* can result from a number of causes. Even if the person does not eat cold, raw food, or takes cooling herbs, he or she can experience undue loss of yang *qi*. For instance, if our periods of rest are irregular, this can result in a loss of yang *qi*. In an earlier part of this book, we discussed how the "three months of winter is called closing and storing." During this period of shutting and storing, our rest should correspond with the energy of the time period, which is to say we should "retire early and rise late, waiting for the sunlight." If, during the three months of winter when heaven and earth are closed and stored, you yourself are not, and instead you go to sleep very late, then your yang *qi* will not have an opportunity to rest and recuperate, and it will be lost. If the yang *qi* is lost, then there will naturally be cold of the viscera. This viscera coldness will lead to "abdominal fullness and vomiting, inability to eat, severe spontaneous diarrhea, intermittent spontaneous abdominal pain."

We should be clear: Upon what does our digestion depend? It depends upon the yang *qi*. Physicians nowadays, when they encounter a patient with "an inability to eat," will prescribe Shanzha, Maiya, Shenqu, and other such herbs. Are these herbs useful? Yes, of course. When the patient is definitely suffering from food stasis, the application of these medicines demonstrates good effect. But if the loss of appetite is not due to food stasis, if the tongue and pulse picture do not correspond with those of a food stasis condition, but instead correspond with a picture of deficient yang and coldness of the viscera, then the use of these herbs that can resolve food stasis is not indicated and will not be effective. In such a case, the physician should warm and nourish the yang *qi*, and should use a Lizhong Tang type of formula. When the patient ingests Lizhong Tang, the yang *qi* will resurge and the patient's appetite will naturally return.

II.3.d. The Official of Remonstration

The concept of an "office of remonstration" stems from a passage from the *Plain Questions*, which was remarkably preserved within the lost chapter entitled "Treatise on the Methods of Needling." The *Plain Questions's* "Treatise of the Secret Library of the Miraculous Orchid" discusses twelve organs, but only eleven officials: "The heart holds the office of the sovereign and ruler"; "The lungs hold the office of chancellor and mentor"; "The liver holds the office of the general"; "The gallbladder holds the office of centered righteousness"; "The pericardium holds the office of minister and envoy"; "The spleen and stomach hold the office of the granaries"; "The large intestine holds the office of transmitting along the way"; "The small intestine holds the office of receiving sacrifices"; "The kidneys hold the office of making strong"; "The triple burner holds the office of clearing the canals"; and "The urinary bladder holds the office of regional rectifier." Of these eleven officials, with the exception of the spleen and stomach, all of the organs are assigned their own posts singly. It is only when we get to the "official of the granaries" that the spleen and stomach are listed together. Sharing a single office, it is difficult to discriminate between the individual functions of the spleen and stomach. Therefore, in the "Treatise on the Methods of Needling" in the *Plain Questions*, it gives the spleen and stomach their own official posts. The original "official of the granaries, the five flavors emerge from it" was assigned solely to the stomach, and the spleen received its own line: "The spleen holds the office of remonstration. Understanding the complete cycle originates from it."

The importance of distinguishing the spleen as the "official of remonstration" cannot be overestimated. By conveying this distinction alone, we see the importance of the "Treatise on the Methods of Needling." We should by no means dismiss this chapter as a mere postscript. To do so would be an error. Remonstration (*jian* 諫) was an official position in ancient times, and later it was referred to as the "senior official of remonstration." What is meant by *jian*? The Xu Kai commentary to *Explaining Writing and Analyzing Characters* says: "*Jian* means to differentiate between good and evil, and present these findings to the ruler." It follows that this official was very important: he enjoyed a special privilege. It was this official who could expound upon any good or evil deed to the face of the monarch. It was on account of this official that the sovereign could not be kept in the dark, or make poor judgments based on hearing only one side of an issue. It was also because of this official that the ruler was able to make his spirit bright, and could not become fatuous and self-indulgent. This is what was meant by the "understanding the complete cycle emerges from it." This "understanding of the cycle" was directed at the "office of the sovereign and ruler." In the *Great Commentary of the Classic of Changes*, it says: "By knowing the complete cycle of the myriad things, the Dao can transform everything under Heaven, so that nothing is overstepped"; this line also refers to this particular office of the spleen. In order for the monarch to avoid making mistakes, in order that he might understand the complete cycle of everything and every situation and the way in which the myriad things are transformed from one realm to another, the monarch relies upon this official of remonstration.

Now that we have discussed the topic to some extent, we probably hold a particular view of the "official of remonstration." A person's life, even the rise and fall of a nation, are tied to the "office of the sovereign and ruler," but this ruler can only be made bright and see the big picture through "remonstration." As a result, the Dao can then transform everything in the world without fail. We can see that the office of "remonstration" is unusual. It is not an office that can be taken lightly, nor is it one that any sort of individual could fill. In order to hold such a position, the individual must meet three requirements. First, the person must be honest. If the person is not honest, then they will not know the difference between right and wrong and will not be able to distinguish between good and evil. Thus, the *Guangya* defines *jian* as "rectitude." Secondly, the person must be righteous. If the person in this post does not possess a spirit of lofty morality and instead is overcautious and indecisive, afraid of his own shadow and always seeking cover for his own backside, then any "remonstration" will be in name only. The *History of the Early Tang* says:

There are five types of remonstration:
the first is called mocking remonstration;
the second is called obeisant remonstration;
the third is called exhorting remonstration;
the fourth is called detailed remonstration;
the fifth is called direct remonstration.

Without this righteousness, carrying out even just one of the above would be difficult. Third, the admonisher must be magnanimous, a great person without personal interest. If the remonstrator is your kith and kin, or someone whom you owe a favor to, then even if they perform an evil act, you will not remonstrate against them. If it is your enemy, you will easily make accusations against him, and the basic meaning of *jian* will be lost.

When we consider the three requisite virtues of the official of remonstration, we see that, as the "Treatise on the Methods of Needling" of the *Plain Questions* stated, no organ is better suited than the spleen to fill this office. Only the spleen possesses all of these virtues. The spleen belongs to *Kun* Earth, and shares the characteristics of the *kun* (Responding) hexagram. If we open the *Classic of Changes* and read what it says about a changing line in the second position of the *kun* hexagram, we read: "Straight, square and great." What is meant by "straight, square, and great"? The description of the image that follows reads: "Straighten his rectitude, square his selflessness. A noble person is respectful and thereby straightens his inner workings; he is selfless and thereby squares his outer conduct. Respectfulness and selflessness, once firmly established, result in great virtue. With straightness, squareness, and greatness, everything can be accomplished." Reading this passage from the *Classic of Changes* and remembering that the spleen possesses the qualities of *kun*, it is clear that the spleen possesses all of the qualities required of the official of remonstration. Furthermore, according to the discussion of the *kun* hexagram: "A family that accumulates goodness will be happy and fortunate. A family that accumulates bad deeds will come to ruin. If the subject kills his ruler, or if a son murders the father, it is not something that comes about in the span of a single morning and night. Such events come about gradually; they were not criticized and debated early enough." "Accumulation" refers to the way in which *Kun* Earth's thickness stores all things. Without *Kun*, there can be no discussion of accumulation. Furthermore, this accumulation can be differentiated into the accumulation of good and the accumulation of that which is not good. Accumulation of good results in good fortune, and accumulation of bad results in calamity. When a subject kills his ruler, or a son his father, such actions are abominable, but crimes like these do not come to pass in short order. Events like these may seem sudden and unexpected, but they are the result of a gradual process of accumulation. Why was such a process, doomed for misfortune, not detected earlier? It is because "they were not criticized and debated early enough." Here, it is clear that "debate and criticism" refers to the process of remonstration.

It is in the discussion of the hexagram *kun* that we read of "a subject killing his ruler and a son murdering his father," and it is also in the discussion of *kun* that we read of the ill consequences when bad behavior does not meet with reprimand early in its inception. Raising this connection, we find excellent testimony to the statement made in the *Plain Questions's* "Treatise on the Methods of Needling," that "The spleen holds the office of remonstration. Understanding the complete cycle originates from it." Any country, or any family, if they wish to avoid such calamity, must ensure that remonstration can take place freely. What about our bodies? Regicide or fratricide is analogous to those diseases that are violent and sudden, and illnesses that resist all treatment, malignant diseases. They are like cancer or malignant tumors. Such pathologies are discovered suddenly, as if they appeared overnight, but this is not the case. They come about as described in the discussion of the hexagram *kun*: "It is not something that comes about in the span of a single morning and a single night. Such events come about gradually." And why is it, during the gradual course of development of such disease, that the organism does not recognize what is happening? Why does it fail to discover the cancer and seek to correct it on its own, but instead waits until disaster is inevitable? This is because the "office of remonstration" has lost its normal function.

A malignant tumor is the result of the uncontrolled division of an aberrant human cell line. How can such a disease come about? Modern science views the advent of such a cell line to be the result of a failure in the immune system. The human immune system has three main functions: defense against pathogens, maintaining immunity, and the third is to constantly monitor and keep watch on tissues. If the aspect of the immune system that monitors the health of tissues is functioning properly, then it will detect these aberrant cell lines and, through a complex series of immune responses, terminate the cell line and correct the problem, preventing the possibility of a malignancy. The function of this aspect of human immunity and the function of the "office of remonstration" are remarkably similar. The "Treatise on the Methods of Needling" describes the particular orientation of the spleen, and we find a very detailed and concrete discussion of this orientation in the discussion of the *kun* hexagram. When we parallel this discussion with modern scientific understanding of human immunity, it seems that there is much that could be explored at length. At present, the rate of cancerous malignancies is rising steadily. Despite the advent of numerous cancer treatments, the specter of relapse hovers over every cancer survivor. How do we prevent the recurrence of cancer? In Western Medicine, the answer is sought in the immune system, and great effort is applied to discovering this answer. I believe that properly understanding the "office of remonstration" is crucial to finding the answer to this same question within the halls of Chinese Medicine theory and understanding.

If we study the Chinese Medicine classics, such as the *Treatise on Cold Damage*, in this new century, could it be that we might be in store for a new crop of breakthroughs and discoveries? Our current discussion of Taiyin probably influences your opinion on this possibility. Earlier, we discussed the perennial nature of the classics, which is to say that the content of the classics never loses its pertinence. If you are researching a new topic, if you are at the summit of a fascinating, new field of research, you can always find a point of reference in the classics. It all depends upon whether or not you have the power of intuition to discover this connection, whether you dare to undertake such an endeavor. If you do not dare to do so, then you will certainly miss the opportunity. Neither the modern nor the ancient understandings are perfect. In fact, the two depend upon each other. The ancient cannot be separated from the modern. We are now in the twenty-first century. The ancient, the traditional, must adapt to modernity, serve modernity, and to the utmost of its ability, influence and guide modernity. This is something that those who study the traditional arts and the classics must keep firmly in their minds. This is, after all, the very reason for the existence of tradition. If the purpose of traditional understanding is not clearly recognized, then the classics will remain archaic and outmoded. In such a case, the classics have no real significance. By the same token, the modern cannot do without the traditional. It is our first and probably shallow impression of the classics that leads us to a low regard for the classics and for traditional studies in general. It is as Confucius said: "Everyone uses it daily but does not know what it is. Thus, the Dao of the noble person is rare."

III. The Timing of Taiyin Disease

Our discussion of the time that corresponds with Taiyin disease has its basis in the text concerning the resolution of Taiyin disease, line 275: "Taiyin disease tends to resolve in the time from *hai* to *chou*." We will expound upon this point from several angles in the following section.

III.1. From *Hai* to *Chou*

The period of the daily cycle that corresponds to *hai*, *zi*, and *chou* spans from nine in the evening to three in the morning. In the cycle of the month, based on the lunar cycle, each of these three time periods comprises about two and a half days. The entire period comprises the seven and a half days straddling the new moon. During this period of the lunar cycle, the face of the moon is at its darkest, and the light of the moon most hidden. The period when the moon is new, when its bright face is hidden, corresponds with the time when the yang is being received and stored. This conforms with our understanding of Taiyin. In the cycle of a year, these three periods correspond to months of the same name, which are the tenth, eleventh, and twelfth months of the Chinese lunar calendar. These three months are paired with the hexagrams *kun* (Responding), *fu* (Falling Back), and *lin* (Approaching). The six lines of the *kun* hexagram are yin, and many people mistakenly assume that this indicates that yin is abundant and yang is weak, that the yang *qi* is debilitated and extinguished. This is a misunderstanding of the hexagram. The six yin lines do not indicate that there is no yang *qi*, it indicates that the yang has been received and stored. It is this storage that results in the accumulation and recuperation of yang *qi*, and it is this that leads to the re-emergence of yang in the first and then the second positions of the hexagram.

Besides their temporal placement, these three earthly branches, *hai*, *zi*, and *chou*, also have a spatial orientation: the northern direction. Earlier, we discussed the prenatal and postnatal trigrams. Among the prenatal trigrams, the north is occupied by *Kun* Earth. The prenatal constitutes the form, the postnatal the function. Thus, the form or body of *Kun* is in the north, but its function is in the southwest. The *Kun* Earth form occupies the north together with the trigram *Kan* Water, and earlier we described this cohabitation in terms of the union of water and earth. The fact that the time period when Taiyin disease tends to resolve is also the time period in which Taiyang disease tends to become exacerbated merits further contemplation and discussion.

III.2. The Essentials of the Time It Tends to Resolve

Nowadays, most modern editions of *Treatise on Cold Damage*, books such as *Commentary on the Treatise on Cold Damage*, have been edited and revised, and cuts were made. However, in the ancient *Treatise on Cold Damage* edition compiled and arranged by Wang Shuhe, there are four other chapters before the chapter on Taiyang, namely: "Chapter 1, Differentiation of the Pulse"; "Chapter 2, The Normal Pulse"; "Chapter 3, Guide to Cold Damage"; and "Chapter 4, Differentiating Spasms, Dampness, and Sunstroke." In "Chapter 1, Differentiation of the Pulse," there is an interesting passage:

> During the time of the fifth month of the lunar cycle, the yang *qi* is on the exterior, the stomach center is deficient and cold. The attenuated yang *qi* in the interior of the body cannot overcome the cold, and so the patient has a tendency to wear extra clothing. During the eleventh month, the yang *qi* is in the interior, and the stomach center is vexingly hot. Because the yin *qi* is weak in the interior, and cannot overcome the heat, the patient desires to remove clothing.

This passage discusses both physiology and pathology. Although it is discussing a different matter, this piece of writing helps us to understand the time in which Taiyin disease tends to resolve.

The fifth month is the month in which summer arrives; it is the month that corresponds with the earthly branch *wu*. This month conveys the meaning of the entire summer, and is shorthand for the three earthly branches: *si*, *wu*, and *wei*. What are the special characteristics of the fifth month? Zhang Zhongjing says: "The yang *qi* is on the exterior, the stomach center is deficient and cold." Why is the yang *qi* on the exterior at this time? It is because all of the yang *qi* of spring and summer is steaming upward and outward toward the exterior. Because of this inclination toward the exterior during this time, the yang of the interior becomes scanty. When yang *qi* is deficient internally, cold will result. Thus it says: "The yang *qi* is on the exterior, the stomach center is deficient and cold." But when winter comes around, when we are in the eleventh lunar month, the situation is reversed. At this time, the yang *qi* moves toward the interior of the body, and is in a state of receiving and storing. During the wintertime, the yang *qi* in the exterior gradually becomes scanty, and the yang *qi* in the interior gradually becomes excessive, resulting in heat. Thus it says: "The yang *qi* is in the interior, the stomach center is vexed by heat." There is a popular folk rhyme about this: "In winter eat radishes, in summer eat ginger, the doctor needs not lift a finger." Why is this? Those who study Chinese Medicine understand the reason for this: radishes are cool in nature and ginger is warm in nature. The weather is warm in summer, so why eat warm ginger? Because the yang *qi* is on the exterior, and the stomach center becomes deficient and cold, we should eat warm things to warm the interior, to warm the stomach. Winter is, of course, cold, so why should we eat cool radishes? Because in winter, the yang *qi* is in the interior of the body, and the stomach and center are afflicted with heat; eating cool radishes cools the interior and restores balance to the body, avoiding the advent of accumulated heat.

In the wintertime, the yang *qi* inclines toward the interior, so the interior tends to become warm. If the patient suffers from Taiyin disease, then it can take advantage of this yang *qi* to warm the cold viscera, and the deficient cold syndrome that characterizes Taiyin disease will take a turn for the better. That is why Taiyin disease tends to improve during *hai*, *zi*, and *chou*. When we fully understand *hai*, *zi*, and *chou*, we will naturally be able to grasp what guides the curing of Taiyin disease. Zhang Zhongjing's description of the diseases of the six conformations has two facets. One facet is the textual outline of the disease. This part of his discussion often has physical description of the disease, and provides cases for our review. This is also the facet that most people pay attention to. Another facet is the text related to when the disease has a tendency to resolve. This aspect does not provide a physical description of the disease, nor does it provide any case studies. It is this facet that, from ancient times up until the present day, very few physicians have paid close attention to. As a matter of fact, this portion of Zhang Zhongjing's writings lacks concrete physical description yet there is no disease that is excluded; it does not contain cases yet there is no case that is not referred to. Its contents are deeper and more profound, more penetrating than those of the former facet. The *Yellow Emperor's Classic* says: "Understanding of the Dao requires knowledge of the pattern of the heavens above, the earth below, and the affairs of humanity in between; this way it will last forever." From the two aspects we have introduced above, the textual outline of the disease is essentially a discussion of the affairs of human beings, whereas the text that discusses the time in which the disease has a tendency to resolve, expounds upon the patterns of heaven and earth. If only the outline of disease is studied, and Chinese Medicine limits itself solely to the affairs of human beings, can Chinese Medicine live long?

III.3. The Time When It Tends to Act

The time in which a particular conformation of disease tends to worsen or erupt is a topic we have already discussed in the course of this book. This time is exactly opposite to the time in which it tends to resolve. Taiyin disease is of course better during the time in which it tends to resolve, and the patient feels more comfortable. It is reflexive that there would be a different time in which Taiyin disease is notably worse, during which the patient's suffering increases. If this were not the case, if there were only times in which the disease improved and none in which it worsened, then the natural balance, a principle of the way of heaven and earth, would be lost.

Taiyin disease tends to resolve during the periods of *hai, zi,* and *chou*; it is during this period that the yang is in the interior of the body where, as far as the internal deficiency cold of Taiyin is concerned, this is a situation of "achieving the Dao and thus enjoying much support." So then, during what time does Taiyin disease tend to worsen? It must be the three earthly branches of *si, wu,* and *wei*. During this time, the yang *qi* is at the exterior, and the interior is deficient and cold. As far as Taiyin is concerned, this is "losing the Dao and finding little support." Thus, these three earthly branches are the time that corresponds with an exacerbation of Taiyin disease.

During *si, wu,* and *wei,* the yang *qi* hastens to the exterior of the body, predisposing the patient to internal deficiency and coldness of the viscera organs, Taiyin disease. This is an analysis based on theory. Now, let us pursue a more concrete discussion. The weather in summer is very hot, so the yang *qi* steams outward. During this time of year, because the weather is so hot, people crave cold and raw food and drinks. Everything they eat, they wish to eat cold. The stomach and digestive center are already suffering from a state of deficient cold, and in comes a large amount of cold food. It is like a hard frost descending on a snow mountain. Thus, people easily contract Taiyin disease during this time. We should not think that winter is the time of year when it is easy to contract Taiyin disease. The truth is just the contrary: it is during the summer when we are most likely to develop Taiyin disease. There are plenty of opportunities to prescribe Lizhong Tang in the summer. It is a shame that so many people do not realize this simple fact. It is not just the patients who are ignorant of this simple truth, many practitioners of Chinese Medicine do not even know. They only know that the summer is hot and humid, they never consider that summer also contains coolness and cold. During the summer, the sky is hot and the earth is cold. The difference between heaven and earth must be clear. It falls especially to those of us who have studied Taiyin chapter to make this truth known.

Taiyin is divided into the leg Taiyin and arm Taiyin. The lungs of the arm Taiyin refer to heaven, and the foot Taiyin spleen refers to earth. Thus, the summer pattern of hot heaven and cold earth is a pattern in which the lungs are hot and the spleen is cold. If we as Chinese Medicine practitioners only keep heat pathogens in mind, if we think only as Ye Tianshi did that "When warmth pathogens afflict the upper part, they attack the lungs first," and the only medicines we think to apply are cold and cool ones, it is not enough. At most, such a physician will only know and understand the heavenly aspect. Among physicians who used cold and cool medicines during the summer, one of the most famous was Liu Wansu. In his *Formulas from the Discussion Illuminating the Yellow Emperor's Plain Questions,* the formula Yiyuan San is also referred to as Liuyi San, and as Taibai San. What is meant by *taibai* ("supremely white")? If we read the *Journey to the West,* then we know that there is a Supremely White Metal Star, and so "supremely white" refers to metal, and thus to the lungs. We thereby know that Taibai San is directed at the state of the celestial *qi,* of the lungs, during summer.

But should we not also pay attention to the earth aspect? And is not the earth aspect Taiyin? If we do not take care of Taiyin, then it can easily influence Shaoyin. Once the Taiyin door is open, the other three yin follow suit. We must thoroughly grasp the pattern of heaven and earth, and besides formulas such as Yiyuan San, we should also keep in mind such formulas as Lizhong Tang, for it is equally useful.

From a temporal perspective, the period spanned by the three earthly branches *si*, *wu*, and *wei* is the period of time in which Taiyin disease tends to flare up. Earlier in this book, we repeatedly emphasized how time and space (i.e. direction) are interwoven in Chinese cosmology, and how they can express the same energy. We must complete our discussion of the time in which a disease tends to resolve or become exacerbated with a discussion of how the particular period of time relates to the spatial dimension. When we plot *si*, *wu*, and *wei* on the compass, we see that they represent the southern direction. The south, then, is the direction in which Taiyin disease tends to become exacerbated. This would then indicate that people who live in the south would have a greater tendency to contract Taiyin disease, and that, relative to northerners, have weaker spleen and stomach function. Let us think for a moment: Is this really the case? If we compare the southerners of China with the northerners, it becomes clear. Northerners tend to be taller and burlier than southerners. Why is this? It is because the earth *qi* of northerners is strong and that of southerners is weak. If the earth *qi* is weak, then the flesh of the four limbs does not develop, and the body will be smaller. We should understand this difference between northerners and southerners: southerners have an increased tendency to be afflicted by Taiyin disease. Southerners and those physicians who treat them should be conscious of the importance of warming and protecting the spleen and stomach, and should avoid cooling herbal teas.

The above discussion was actually an exposition upon a passage in the "Differentiation of the Pulse" chapter in *Treatise on Cold Damage*. There is another passage, a dialogue, from that particular piece of writing that is brilliant:

Question: Regarding disease, I wish to know when one will contract it and when it will improve.

Answer: If one contracts disease in the middle of the night, then it will get better at midday; if it is contracted at midday, then it will get better in the middle of the night. Why do I say this? If one becomes ill at midday, and improves at midnight, it is yang obtaining yin that causes the disease to resolve. If one becomes sick in the middle of the night, but recovers when the bright midday sun shines, then it is yin obtaining yang that causes the disease to resolve.

Which earthly stem corresponds to midnight? It is the *zi* earthly stem. To speak more broadly, it is the time constituted by *hai, zi,* and *chou.* Midday is the time of *wu,* the time of *si, wu,* and *wei.* Contracting a disease at midday that improves at midnight corresponds perfectly with Taiyin disease, which resolved with *hai, zi,* and *chou,* and worsens with the pattern represented by *si, wu,* and *wei.* Once this basic pattern is apprehended, it is easy to determine the times in which each of the six conformation diseases will tend to resolve. From this, we see that the content of the "Differentiation of the Pulse" and the three other chapters in Wang Shuhe's edition of *Treatise on Cold Damage* are closely related to the content of the other six conformation chapters. This is not something we can neglect. Currently, those who study the *Treatise on Cold Damage* attach little importance to these chapters. There are some who seem completely unaware of these pieces of writing. Reading the *Treatise on Cold Damage* without the benefit of these chapters makes the meaning of the book very difficult to penetrate.

Si, wu, and *wei* make up the period of time in which Taiyin disease tends to worsen, and these three branches can signify the three corresponding two-hour periods, the three two-and-a-half-day periods around the full moon, or the fourth, fifth, and sixth months of the Chinese lunar calendar. In any case, these three earthly branches correspond with relatively fixed periods of time. These are the times when the yang *qi* steams outward and upward, the yang *qi* of the interior is thereby made deficient, and deficiency cold of the stomach center easily comes about. After recognizing that it is tendency that the yang *qi* adopts during the temporal periods related to *si, wu,* and *wei,* that affects Taiyin disease, we must deduce that, in addition to these fixed time periods related to *si, wu,* and *wei,* there is also an indeterminate and variable "*si, wu,* and *wei.*" This is namely whenever the yang *qi* of an organism steams outward, or whenever the stomach center suffers from deficiency cold, any such time is indeed *si, wu,* and *wei,* and should be regarded as times in which Taiyin disease will tend to be contracted or worsen. For instance, if we engage in strenuous exercise, or are troubled, the yang *qi* will be at the exterior, and the stomach center will experience a period of deficiency cold. At such a time, one is more likely to contract Taiyin disease. Therefore, during these times, we must be very careful not to just open the fridge and eat something cold. If one wishes to drink, drink warm water or hot beverages to quench your thirst. If you absolutely have to drink iced beverages, wait until the yang *qi* settles down and slowly returns to the interior of the body, then you can drink a bit. These are the times in which Taiyin disease acts up.

III.4. The Essentials of Treating the Taiyin Orientation

The Taiyin curative method can be summarized by a single sentence in line 277 of the *Treatise on Cold Damage*: "One should warm it; it is suitable to use a Sini type of decoction." What does "warm it" mean? It means to warm the viscera, to warm the interior. This curative strategy is obviously in accord with our understanding of what happens during the time in which the disease tends to resolve, the periods of *hai*, *zi*, and *chou*.

III.4.a. The Meaning of Sini

Taiyin disease is disease in which the viscera are deficient and cold. Most Chinese Medicine practitioners should be familiar with the use of Lizhong Tang to remedy such a situation. However, in the Taiyin chapter, Zhang Zhongjing recommends the Sini type of decoction. This points to a close relationship between this sort of decoction and Taiyin.

Why is the governing formula of Taiyin referred to as *sini* ("four counterflow")? What is the relationship between Taiyin and "four counterflow"? Let's start with the word "four." The word "four" primarily refers to the four limbs of the body. The four limbs are endowed with *qi* from the stomach, and the spleen rules the four limbs, so these four have a very close relationship with the spleen and stomach. Now, let us look at the term "counterflow." Often, this term is mentioned in the compound "counterflow cold" and together with the full meaning of "four," we can understand four counterflow as "counterflow cold of the four limbs." What does counterflow cold refer to? The opposite of counterflow is to move in the direction of the flow: to flow, as it were. To flow means to move in a downward direction, from near to far, from the center to the four sides. Counterflow indicates precisely the opposite. Counterflow moves in an upward direction, from far to near. Counterflow cold refers to cold that moves like this. It begins in the distant tips of the extremities, and gradually moves upward, past the elbows and knees. How is counterflow cold produced? From an absence of fire, of course; from deficient and attenuated yang *qi*.

The *Treatise on Cold Damage* divides diseases into two main types: yin and yang. The yang diseases are Taiyang, Yangming, and Shaoyang. The yin types of disease are Taiyin, Shaoyin, and Jueyin. When a disease enters yin, yang *qi* begins to be deficient. This insufficiency of yang *qi* is primarily a deficiency of the interior, and leads to interior deficiency cold. Therefore, a basic characteristic of the three yin diseases is that the interior is deficient and cold. Furthermore, this interior deficiency cold of the three yin diseases begins with Taiyin. When Taiyin is deficient and cold, when the yang *qi* is insufficient, where does this problem first appear? It manifests first in the areas that it governs, in the four limbs which receive their *qi* from Taiyin. The four limbs are not warmed, and the pattern of four counterflow emerges. This lack of warmth in the four limbs begins at the furthest extreme of the limbs, from their very tips. Although this coldness of the four limbs is mild in Taiyin disease, it is still a clear signal. It indicates that the disease has begun to develop in the three yin, and the constitution of the patient is already leaning toward deficiency cold. At this point, the physician must act quickly to warm the interior. If the interior is promptly warmed, the constitution of the patient can be shifted quite easily, and the disease will not progress to the Shaoyin stage. Therefore, raising the issue of four counterflow in the Taiyin chapter brings up a crucial warning sign, and using Sini Tang at the Taiyin stage nips the trouble in the bud.

Furthermore, there is another meaning to the word "counterflow" in traditional Chinese culture. We find this meaning in the *Plain Questions's* "Treatise on Phenomena Reflecting the Status of *Qi* in a Normal Person": "In a balanced person, the mainstay of *qi* is in the stomach. Those who do not have stomach *qi* are referred to as suffering from counterflow. Those with counterflow die." What is counterflow? It refers to those patients who do not have stomach *qi*. Those without stomach *qi* are said to suffer from counterflow and are en route to death. The counterflow syndrome, also called four counterflow syndrome, is a dangerous syndrome, a foreboding syndrome, and even a fatal syndrome. The syndromes in the *Treatise on Cold Damage* for which Sini Tang is prescribed are also dangerous, foreboding, and fatal conditions. In the *Treatise on Cold Damage*, Sini Tang is used when the condition requires caution, when there is the need to pay attention to the situation at hand, and when the strategic pass occupied by Taiyin needs to be brought under control. If this pass is left open, then the disease can move to the Shaoyin and Jueyin layers from a state that could have been controlled by Sini Tang. Thus, in the treatment of Taiyin disease, we should pay close attention to the notion that we should "Warm it and it is suitable to use a Sini type of decoction." The implications of this statement are far-reaching, and we should by no means skim over this line as if it were trivial.

III.4.b. An Explanation of Sini Tang

Sini Tang is used with all three diseases of the yin conformations. It is a formula that warms, that enlivens the fire, and that stems counterflow. Of the three ingredients in Sini Tang, Fuzi and Ganjiang are both very warm and hot, and using both to warm the interior and build the inner fire seems a natural choice. Where there is debate is with question to the role of the third ingredient, Zhigancao. Zhigancao is listed as the first ingredient in Sini Tang. As we have already discussed, in the *Treatise on Cold Damage*, the order in which the ingredients of a decoction are listed is related to their role in the formula. They are not in random order. This is similar to the order in which our leaders come on stage during a public appearance here in China. Who follows whom is strictly choreographed, as their order is indicative of their relative rank. In the classics, the first herb in the list of ingredients is usually the emperor herb, the main herb. Those that are arranged afterward are the helper herbs, the minister and courier herbs. Zhigancao, the king of herbs with regard to the central earth element, is neutral and harmonizing. These neutral, harmonizing qualities seem to have little to do with the main effects of Sini Tang. However, the fact that this seemingly dispensable herb is seated in the king's throne of Sini Tang has sparked a great number of debates throughout history. Some physicians hold that, based on the listed order of the herbs, Zhigancao is the emperor of the formula. For instance, Cheng Wuji in the Jin dynasty wrote: "It is yin that supports yang, and so the sweet flavor must be paramount, and so Zhigancao is the emperor." The Qing dynasty physician Wu Qian, in his *Golden Mirror of the Medical Tradition* (Yizong Jinjian) also states: "The sweetness and warmth of the emperor herb, Zhigancao, warms and nourishes the yang *qi*. The pungent heat of the minister herbs Ganjiang and Fuzi assist the yang to triumph over cold." But the majority of physicians, on account of the neutral *qi* and harmonizing action of licorice, assign it the position of minister or courier in the formula, harmonizing the actions of ginger and aconite, and do not regard it as playing any other important role.

Is Zhigancao an assistant or courier herb, or is it the emperor herb? In my opinion, it is the emperor herb, and I will tell you why I think so, for it is worthwhile relating it to you here. Sini Tang is a prescription to warm the yang, stoke the fire, expel cold, and relieve counterflow. This much is definite. And as we mentioned in our discussion of the Taiyin chapter, Sini Tang is used to head off the pass constituted by Taiyin, to nip the disease process in the bud. However, the orthodox use of Sini Tang is in the treatment of Shaoyin and Jueyin. At these stages of disease, yin cold is even more exuberant. Not only are the upper and middle burners deficient, the yang of the lower burner is also on the point of death. When yin cold is overabundant, and the yang *qi* is deficient and under duress, a peculiar phenomenon can occur. This phenomenon is referred to as "cold water being unable to store the dragon." If the dragon cannot be stored inside, then the fire of the dragon's thunder, the source of *qi*, the root of life, can fly off. When the dragon's fire flies off, what do we see? Despite the fact that the patient has been very cold for some time, and their yang is sorely deficient, we see a state described in the Shaoyin chapter of the *Treatise on Cold Damage* in connection with Tongmai Sini Tang: "The body, contrary to its prior condition, is not averse to cold, and the face becomes red." When the dragon fire flies, the situation is critical. At this time, the patient has only a slim chance of surviving and it depends upon the physician's ability to escort the dragon back to its original dwelling place. Why do books on Chinese formulas regard formulas like Sini Tang and Tongmai Sini Tang to be able to restore yang and stem counterflow? "Restore the yang" means to return the dragon to its proper place, and to "stem counterflow" means to prevent the dragon fire from flying off again.

For those whose yang *qi* has become deficient and weak, with yin and cold flourishing on the interior, we must warm the interior, strengthen the fire, and dispel cold; in essence, we must use warm and hot medicines, fire medicine. But in this case, because the water is cold, the dragon cannot rest. The dragon fire is already leaping upward more and more. In this situation, it is as the ancient Daoist alchemists described: if the medicine is mercury rather than true alchemical quicksilver, when it encounters fire it will blaze upward. If the patient ingests only warm and hot herbs, such as Ganjiang and Fuzi, as soon as this "fire" medicine enters the body, the dragon fire, already ready to escape, will blaze upward with greater intensity. This is why so many people who clearly suffer from a yang deficiency syndrome actually experience fire blazing upward, with sore and swollen throat and sores on their tongue, as soon as they take in Ganjiang and Fuzi. If we use solely use warm and hot herbs to treat patients that are suffering from yang deficiency, it will not have the effect we are seeking. Is there a technique to induce the fire in these warm and hot medicines to go straight to the root of life and warm and nourish it there, and produce a persistent warming effect? What is this technique? Probing after this technique, our minds naturally return to the Zhigancao in Sini Tang. Does the Gancao in Sini Tang resolve this issue?

I remember when I was a child and lived in the countryside how far we would have to go to graze cattle or collect firewood. Often, there was no way of returning home for lunch, so I would bring with me some yams or sweet potatoes. While the cows grazed, I would take clods of earth and make a small oven and then pick up pieces of wood and kindling to make a fire in the little kiln. I would wait until my little earthen oven was almost glowing red, and then take out the remaining pieces of kindling, put my yams or sweet potatoes in and stamp the oven flat with my foot. When the noon hour came round and I was hungry for lunch, I would return to the little oven that had received my sweet potatoes. I would dig in the flattened oven to find it piping hot and fragrant inside, offering up the most delicious feast. Yams or sweet potatoes roasted in this way were baked all the way through but not burnt in the least. They were even sweeter and more flavorsome than if they had been baked in an oven. My childhood is now long past, but when I think back on these events, my mouth still waters.

This childhood experience proves very helpful to understanding the use of Zhigancao in Sini Tang. If we try to use fire alone to roast a yam, the skin on the outside may turn to charcoal, while the inside of the tuber remains cold and raw. If we use the technique I just finished describing and use the fire to "cook" the earth, and then use this earth to cook the sweet potato, not only will it be cooked all the way through, but the skin will not be in the least bit burnt, either. This is the magical effect of earth. The storing nature of earth can take the burning, scorching intensity of fire and turn it into persistent, tempered warmth. Thus, when earth acts as the intermediary for fire, it can warm things, heat things, but it will not burn or scorch them. With this said, it should be clear why licorice is used in Sini Tang. It is used to bring to bear this particular characteristic of earth. Although earth contains no fire of its own, it can turn the potency of fire toward its intended goal. By means of earth, fire can heat without burning and warm without scorching. When the yin cold flourishes in the interior and the yang *qi* is enfeebled, the dragon fire, just like mercury, will blaze upward when it encounters fire. But, through the use of Zhigancao (i.e. the use of earth), this problem is resolved. The Zhigancao, by storing and slowly releasing the heat of the fiery Ganjiang and Fuzi, induces the dragon to return to its proper abode. From this we can see that, in order for Sini Tang to be able to warm and nourish, to restore yang and stem counterflow, Zhigancao is absolutely crucial. As it says in the renowned Qing dynasty physician Chen Xiuyuan's *Changsha Collection of Formula Verses* (Changsha Fanggekuo): "Perfecting the powers of Ganjiang and Fuzi like a brilliant general, Gancao slowly and unhurriedly holds them like a basket." Gancao is compared to a brilliant general, in complete accord with its station as emperor in Sini Tang. The Zhigancao in Sini Tang should not be disregarded or taken lightly; it is absolutely crucial to the efficacy of the formula.

Many Chinese Medicine physicians do not dare to give herbs that are hot in nature, for as soon as they do, their patients complain of "rising fire." This is because they have not yet grasped the importance the relationship between earth and fire. As my years in the clinic progress, my admiration for the genius of using Zhigancao together with the hot natured Ganjiang and Fuzi grows deeper and deeper. There are many physicians who begin by using warm and hot herbs to treat an illness, but as soon as signs of rising fire present in their patient, they stop and, more often than not, switch to giving these same patients cool and cold herbs instead. There are many patients who get a sore throat or sores as soon as they eat anything fried or oily, and only eat raw and cold foods or self-prescribe cooling herbs.

The physicians in such cases are all too often ready to change tack when they encounter such adversity. It is little wonder that the *Yellow Emperor's Classic* says: "As long as you are completely familiar with yin and yang, you do not need more sophisticated schemes." If the physician thoroughly comprehends yin and yang, there is no fear if fire temporarily blazes upward. If your understanding of yin and yang is fuzzy, then your footing will be uncertain, and you will be easily confused.

Recently, I treated a patient who had suffered from an intense sore throat for more than a month. The patient had been taking antibiotics for more than a month, and was also taking Niuhuang Jiedu Pian types of formulas, but they provided no relief of her painful symptoms. Examining her, I found her tonsils swollen and covered with little dots of what looked like pus. Her tongue was pale, and I could see the impression of her tongue on its soft sides. The tongue coat was thin and white, and both sides of her pulse were deep, fine, and fragile. She experienced a bitter taste in her mouth. Observing her pulse, I found it to be the spitting image of yin cold. That is why the antibiotics and heat clearing herbs barely had any effect. Her swollen throat was not the result of heat toxins. Rather, the only explanation was that her "dragon fire" was seething. This case required a formula that was able to warm the utmost depths of the patient. On account of the bitter taste in her mouth she experienced, I hesitated for a long time with the prescription. I pondered her condition for a long time, and gradually resolved to use Xiao Chaihu Tang together with Zheng Qin'an's favorite remedy, Qianyang Dan. I used the herbs Chaihu, Huangqin, Dangshen, Banxia, Zhigancao, Dazao, Shengjiang, Fupian, Sharen, Guiban, and Jiegeng. I prescribed five doses of this medicine, without any doubt of its efficacy. But wouldn't you know it: the patient came back five days later for a checkup without the slightest sign of improvement! I felt the patient's pulse again, and once more noted how deficient and cold it was, void of yang. I decided to set aside Xiao Chaihu Tang entirely, and use a prescription that was solely warming and heating. The medicine contained Fupian, Sharen, Guiban, Zhigancao, Jiegeng, and Shudihuang. I used 60 grams of Fupian and 24 grams of Zhigancao. After just five doses her sore throat went away, the exudate disappeared, and her tonsils decreased in size. As this case demonstrates, painful swelling is not necessarily induced by heat, nor is suppuration or a bitter taste in the mouth. The important thing is to use the four diagnostic methods, look at the tongue and take the pulse, and clearly differentiate yin from yang. Once yin and yang are understood, the battle is almost won, and even if we are off a bit, we are headed in the right direction.

It is my sincere hope the reader of this book will have faith in this simple principle, and adhere to it morning and night, both when things go smoothly and when setbacks are encountered. If you do, then you will glimpse the true power of Chinese Medicine. I can furthermore assure you that you will do justice to the legacy of Zhang Zhongjing.

At present, many people only know how to descend fire with cold, bitter herbs or by nourishing the yin. If the fire does not descend after that, then they have no idea how to proceed. They should know that there is more than one way to descend fire. This is especially true of those of us who study the Taiyin chapter of the *Treatise on Cold Damage*: the opening of that chapter is devoted to explaining how to induce the fire to go inward, to store the fire, to induce the fire to descend. Why is it that the sweet and warm together can produce such heat? We know from reading the opening passage of the Taiyin chapter carefully. If we recognize the meaning of this opening passage, we can understand Sini Tang and the significance of Zhigancao's importance in that formula, as well as the meaning of the chapter as a whole. That is as far as I will discuss Taiyin for now.

CHAPTER NINE

THE ESSENTIALS OF SHAOYIN DISEASE

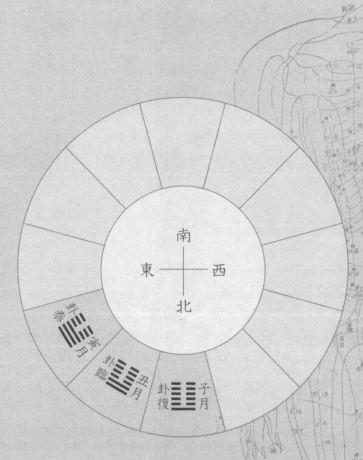

Shaoyin disease tends to
resolve in the time from *zi* to *yin*.

I. An Explanation of Shaoyin

Shaoyin is the pivot of the three yin. When a disease progresses to the Shaoyin stage, the pathological process is at a crucial point. Why? The answer is directly related to the meaning of Shaoyin. The following sections explore the meaning of Shaoyin from four different perspectives.

I.1. The Meaning of Shaoyin

The meaning of Shaoyin is the same as that of fire and water. It is common knowledge that fire and water are inimical to one another. In Shaoyin, however, water and fire are not only compatible, they are interdependent.

I.1.a. The Meaning of Kan Water

First, let us examine water. In the trigrams of the *Classic of Changes*, water belongs to *Kan*. This trigram is commonly referred to as *Kan* Water. Zheng Qin'an's *True Transmission of Medical Principles* contains a poem devoted to the *Kan* trigram. Its beautiful summary goes like this:

Heaven emits and the earth conceives, only then does water pass

One *qi* contains three workers of the Creation

The roots of myriad start right here

Life and change are bathed in time

I.1.a.1. The Formation of Kan Water

The *Classic of Changes* says that the *Qian* Heaven trigram and the *Kun* Earth trigram gave birth to six offspring, three female and three male. Which are the three male offspring? They are *Zhen* Thunder, the eldest; *Kan* Water, the middle child; and *Gen* Mountain, the youngest. *Kan* Water is one of the six children of *Qian* Heaven and *Kun* Earth. The lines from Zheng Qin'an's poem which read: "Heaven emits and the earth conceives, only then does water pass," stem from this point.

Qian is heaven and *Kun* is earth, *Qian* is the father and *Kun* is the mother. Thus, the intercourse of *Qian* and *Kun* brings forth six children. So how did this middle child *Kan* Water come about? It comes from the intercourse of the middle line of *Qian* and *Kun*. If *Qian* Heaven has intercourse with *Kun* Earth, the *Kan* Water trigram emerges, consisting of two yin lines with a yang line between the two. If *Kun* Earth exchanges with *Qian*

Heaven, then we would find a yin line between two yang ones, and we would have the trigram *Li* Flame.

In the first case, the central line of *Qian* Heaven is given to *Kun* Earth and the trigram *Kan* Water emerges, and although *Kun* has changed to *Kan*, her body still exists. Thus, *Kun* and *Kan* dwell together, as water and earth are united. The virtue of *Kun* Earth is in its storing ability, and this is also the virtue of *Kan* Water. And what is stored? It is the yang line in the center of the *Kan* trigram. The yang in *Kan* comes from heaven; it is the true yang, the prenatal yang, and is also referred to as life gate fire, as dragon fire. We mentioned this yang as the dragon fire in our discussion of Sini Tang in the Taiyin chapter. This yang, this fire, should be drawn down and stored, and it is not suitable for it to fly about. What can be used to store it? Besides *Kan* Water, it can also be stored by *Kun* Earth. Thus, the union of water and earth is not only important to the understanding of the Taiyin chapter; it cannot be overlooked if we are to understand Shaoyin either.

I.1.a.2. The Life Fire of the True Yang

The yang within *Kan* Water is referred to as the true yang, the original or prenatal yang, the dragon fire, or the life or destiny fire. These names reveal its paramount importance within the human body. As long as this fire persists, there is life; without it, there is no life. This most important fire has a very prominent characteristic: it is fit to be subdued and stored but should not be let fly loose. In China, there is a saying that a real man does not flaunt his true worth, and those who do are not real men. Why is the true yang put in hiding? It is because it is when it is stored and concealed that it is able to warm and nourish the life-giving *qi*, and in turn allows it to gradually bring forth life and graciously nourish it. This is how longevity is brought about. If the true yang is not stored away, or if the true yang is used to perform some other function, then the life-giving *qi* is not warmed and nourished. If this important force is not warmed and nourished, can you imagine what a crisis for the body this would be?

The life fire is vitally important to life. If it is not contained, and true yang flies upward and outward, then external syndromes indicating dangerous crises will arise accordingly. If we look at the Shaoyin or the Jueyin chapters, we see a disproportionate amount of discussion related to this issue. Why, in the discussion of Shaoyin disease, are upcast yang syndrome (*daiyangzheng* 戴陽證) and repelled yang syndrome (*geyangzheng* 格陽證) both mentioned? Why do so many fatally ill persons, just before they pass away, become reinvigorated? This is a sign that the true yang is departing.

In human physiology, this true yang, this life fire, is used to warm and nourish the life *qi*, and allow life to persist. Humans correspond to heaven and earth, to the macrocosm. In this living world of ours, is there something that is analogous to the true yang, to the life fire, that causes the life *qi* of our earth to persist on and on? There is! It is stored away in the *Kan* Water and buried in the *Kun* Earth: it is the natural energy sources.

At present, the most important energy sources are petroleum, coal, and natural gas. Some of these fossil fuels are found under the seabed, and others are found deep inside the earth, in exact parallel to the true yang of the body. Furthermore, petroleum is a liquid, and is similar to water in its appearance. Coal is a solid, but it is black in color, making it akin to the color of the water element. The petroleum, coal, and natural gas reserves are not limitless. At the rate that we are extracting them from the earth, they will soon be gone. When these are gone, what energy source will be used in their place? The October 28, 2000 issue of *Reference News* featured an article titled "The Future Energy Source on the Sea Floor." This article proposed that perhaps the future source of clean energy will be pure, white crystalline hydrate of methane from the sea floor. There is little doubt that fossil fuels, our current source of energy, as well as future potential sources of energy are analogous to the true fire that is stored in the earth of *Kun* or in the water of *Kan*. This reminds us of a very important issue. Why is there life on earth? An important prerequisite for life is life *qi*. Without this life *qi*, there could be no life, neither plant nor animal. Without this life *qi*, all life would disappear. No life would be possible. This life *qi* stems from the "true yang, the life fire." From this, we can see that the energy sources that we extract from the depths of the earth or from the sea bottom are there for a reason! The life of this planet depends upon these for warmth and nourishment, for our safekeeping. These energy sources are the earth's "true yang," they are the earth's "life fire." They should be left hidden. Only if they are left hidden in the earth will they serve to warm and nourish life *qi* on earth. This "true yang" and "life fire" that we extract from within the earth is for the large part used up in our everyday life. What kind of process is this? It is the process of externalizing the "true yang," the "life fire." I invite the reader to contemplate whether or not this is the case. As the earth's "true yang" and "life fire" is largely consumed, the source of earth's warmth and nourishment is gradually lessened. The emerging life decreases daily and is not conserved. This living world of ours is encountering a crisis.

The way we treat this planet is how we treat ourselves. At present, although modern science knows nothing of this "true yang" or of the "life fire," it is eminently aware that the unlimited extraction of fossil fuels will not end well for humankind. The *Yellow Emperor's Classic* has told us long ago that we should cultivate a state of calmness and emptiness, for "Those who are able to maintain a state of tranquility and lightheartedness, without ambitions or preconceptions, will always stay connected to the source of true *qi*, their spirit and essence will be contained and preserved, and no illnesses will develop." The fact of the matter is that many persons know of this principle and of the benefit of this sort of "emptiness," but they persist in their own self-corruption, constantly brimming with desire for gain. In the words of the *Yellow Emperor's Classic*, they drink alcohol as if it were juice, and make impulsive actions their routine behavior. Take for instance smoking. There are very few who smoke who do not know the evil of this habit. Still more interesting are the cigarette advertisements. All other advertisements make every effort to convince you that their product is the best. Cigarette advertisements, on the other hand, tell you directly that "cigarette smoking is hazardous to your health." But in spite of this, cigarette consumption in China is steadily increasing. This reminds us that the problems currently confronting humanity cannot all be solved by science. They also require philosophy and religion. The world is pluralistic and by the same token, culture should be pluralistic and diverse.

Every day, we see the "true yang," the "life fire" discharging outward. Why is the earth's temperature rising every year? Why are the glaciers gradually melting? This is a sign of the earth's "true yang," its "life fire" externalizing. It is a form of "upcast yang" syndrome or "repelled yang" syndrome. If we apply our understanding of cold damage and the six conformations to diagnose the current state of the world, we can see that it is currently at the Shaoyin stage of disease. How can we induce the yang to return back to the depths, to rescue it from counterflow? This is a question of great magnitude that humanity, as a whole, must seek to answer.

I.1.b. The Meaning of Li Flame

The earth births, heaven completes, its name is fire king,

The intercourse of yin and yang, the hidden, obscure emperor,

The emerging and entering of the spirit's light is truly undefinable;

Each lies concealed within the organism.

Regarding the significance of *Li* Flame, we might well begin our conversation with the above poem by Zheng Qin'an.

I.1.b.1. The Formation of Li Flame

The formation of *Li* Flame in Zheng Qin'an's poem on the *Li* trigram, depicted in the opening line: "The earth births, heaven completes, its name is fire king," is once again the picture of the intercourse of *Kun* Earth with *Qian* Heaven. When heaven and earth have intercourse, the center line of *Qian* is delivered to *Kun*, the center line of *Kun* turns into a yang line, and we have the trigram *Kan* Water. If the center line of *Kun* is transmitted to *Qian*, we have *Li* Flame. So, *Li* Flame is exactly opposite in form to *Kan* Water, and the *Li* Flame trigram assumes the body of *Qian* Heaven.

We have already discussed that from the *Qian* and *Kun* trigrams the six children are born, three male and three female. *Kan* is water, it is yin, yet it is labeled male. *Li* is fire, it is yang, but it is labeled female. The reason for this is related to form and function, and to interdependence, and it has a still deeper and more pertinent meaning. Yang refers to birth and transformation, and yin refers to subsiding and storing, as is commonly understood. But if we read Zheng Qin'an's poem, we see that *Kan* Water is related to birth and transformation, whereas *Li* Flame is connected to subsiding and storing. This is different from the middle son and middle female names given to *Kan* and *Li*, but ingeniously achieves the same result. If one can thoroughly understand the purport of this apparent contradiction, the principle of yin and yang will be more firmly in his grasp. That concludes our discussion of the creation of *Li* Flame.

I.1.b.2. The Nature and Function of Li Flame

The preceding discussion of *Kan* Water began with a discussion of the human body. With this conversation concerning *Li* Flame, we will turn this around and start with nature. Regarding the nature and its particular characteristics of *Li* Flame, we can summarize them in the following six points.

First, fire is hot.

Second, fire is bright. These two qualities, the heat and luminosity of fire, are probably the most obvious ones.

Third, fire has power. The power of fire is a major contributor to modern technological achievements. Modern industrial civilization began with our understanding of the power of fire. The steam engine is a classic example of this.

Fourth, fire cooks things; in a sense, it ripens them. Things that are raw are cooked by fire. The rich variety of cuisines is a direct result of our ability to cook with fire. Without fire, we would be like other animals, eating only raw foods.

Fifth, fire transforms things. The ability of fire to change things is obvious. Ice is a solid, but if we apply fire to the ice, it soon turns into liquid water. If we continue to apply this heat to the water, it will turn into gaseous steam. Those who have studied chemistry are fully aware of the transformative power of fire. Why do most chemical reactions in the laboratory require the application of fire? It is done in order to accelerate change.

Sixth, we can clearly see the function or effect of fire, but it has no clear form. We have already mentioned that the biggest difference between humans and animals is the ability to use fire. The implications of our ability to use fire are twofold. First, if there is no fire at hand, we can actively find materials to make fire. Our current extraction of petroleum and other fossil fuels is the result of this search for fire. Secondly, humans can actively discover the above uses and applications of fire. No other animal is able to do this. What is it that has transformed the course of human civilization? What allows human societies to develop at such blinding speed? In the final analysis, it is fire that fuels the growth and development of human society and civilization. The function of fire is evident everywhere in the modern human world, but fire maintains this special quality, that "its effects are evident but it is without a tangible form."

Among the five elements, all of them, except for fire, possess a visible, tangible form. Wood, for instance, has a tangible form that can be shaped and fashioned into useful objects. We can take wood and turn it into a desk or a round table. Both metal and wood exhibit this sort of pliability.

Although water does not possess this same sort of pliability, it still has a physical form that we can touch and see. Only fire does not possess this common characteristic: we can only have an intense appreciation of its effects, but cannot see a form that we can shape or hold.

Among the five elements, only fire is formless. In the *Classic of the Dao and Its Virtue* of Laozi, there is also mention of the formless: the "Great image is without form." What function does the formlessness of the "great image" serve? Laozi goes on to say: "The great image, all under heaven flock to it." Why fire is able to transform every aspect of human existence, why it possesses such important uses, are essentially inseparable from its being formless, and being the "great image."

I.1.b.3. The Function of Fire in the Human Body

The nature of fire in nature is as we described above. This function corresponds with its role in the human body. It says in the *Yellow Emperor's Classic*: "Those that know to speak of heaven must also find its reflection in humans." Thus, in the human body the functions of fire, that is, of yang *qi*, should be analogous to the six aspects we listed above.

First, fire warms the human body. The living human body is always warm. Where does this warmth come from? It comes from this warming characteristic of fire. We can understand the fire in a person's body by observing how they grow warm or cold, or how their extremities change temperature. From this alone, we can determine whether the person's fire is ample or insufficient.

Second, fire allows us to see clearly. How are we able to see the world around us with our eyes? Our eyesight depends upon fire, yang *qi*. Most Chinese Medicine practitioners know that the liver opens into the orifice of the eyes, the eyes receive the blood and thereby possess vision, but this is not enough. We must also make it clear that the form of the liver is yin but its function is yang. The ability of the eyes to see is just as closely related to the southern brightness of the *Li* Flame. As a person ages, the eyesight tends to grow dim, and various obstructions to our eyesight, such as cataracts, tend to occur. This decrease in our ability to see is related to the weakening of yang fire with age.

Third, physiological activity. Upon what does the mental and physical energy of the human body depend? It mainly depends upon the yang fire. This is closely related to the ability of fire to move, its power as a driving force. Why is somnolence a hallmark of Shaoyin disease? Why does the Shaoyin patient hardly want to move? Why is the beating force of the heart gradually diminished? It is because the fire is weakening each day.

Fourth, the decomposing and ripening function of the stomach is closely related to fire's ability to cook things. The stomach depends upon fire in order to decompose things. If the stomach fire is weak, then that which is eaten will not decompose, and it will come out of the body in much the same form that it went in. If the stomach fire is excessive, then the food will be digested swiftly, but the person will be hungry no matter how much they eat.

Fifth, all of the changes and transformations that are occurring throughout the course of a person's life (their metabolism, to use a modern term) are dependent upon fire. This is almost identical to the role that fire plays in the natural world.

Sixth, we discussed before how "The effect of fire can be seen, but it has no clear form." This is one of the most important and peculiar characteristics of fire. What does this particular aspect of fire correspond to in the human body? It is clear that this corresponds with the spirit brightness, the light of consciousness. The light of consciousness, the "spirit brightness," is paramount to human existence: it is formless and does not reside in any one location, and there is no aspect of human life or existence that is not immediately impacted by this feature of the human body. Thus, it says in the "Treatise on the Spiritual Orchid Secret Canon" of the *Plain Questions*: "The heart holds the office of the sovereign and ruler; spirit brightness originates from it." If the function of the spirit brightness is lost, what sort of situation arises? The situation that arises is as Zhang Zhongjing describes in the preface to the *Treatise on Cold Damage*: "The body falls unconscious and dies, the spirit brightness is extinguished, they becoming something else, and descend deep into the underworld, crying and sobbing as they roam about." The function of the spirit brightness is so important that we might say that life can only exist as long as the spirit brightness exists, and without it, there is no life. What form does this spirit brightness, this consciousness take? What does it look like? It is hard to say, and harder still to make certain of. Thus, the *Doctrine of the Mean* says: "We look for it but cannot see it, we listen for it but cannot hear it, living things possess it but it cannot be left behind. It is the light within all of us." In the *Classic of Poetry* we read: "Where and when the spirit goes, no one on earth ever knows; that's why our veneration grows." This is spirit!

Among the five elements, fire is the one element whose function and effects are unmistakable but whose form cannot be discerned. In the human body, the spirit brightness, the consciousness, is ruled by the heart. How is the heart different from the four other viscera organs? This is a point that we discussed earlier in this book. Besides the heart, all the other viscera are indicated by Chinese characters that possess the moon or flesh radical (肉). Things that are indicated by characters containing this radical have a tangible, physical form, a form that can be examined and appraised. Thus, the liver, spleen, lungs, and kidneys all have a physical form. Only the Chinese character for heart (心) lacks this radical, and without this must not possess a physical form that can be seen or assessed. When we consider the particular characteristics of fire as one of the five elements, the character for heart among the five viscera, and the particular characteristics of consciousness, all of these should give us a strong impression of the basic concepts that this medicine was constructed upon. It would seem that the object of study in Chinese Medicine is primarily humans, so why, then, does the *Yellow Emperor's Classic* emphasize that the practice of Chinese Medicine requires discussion of heaven and earth? Because if you do not discuss heaven and consider earth, you cannot understand humans. And if you do not understand human beings, how can you possibly grasp Chinese Medicine?

I.1.c. Two That Share the Name Shaoyin

Earlier, we discussed *Kan* Water and *Li* Flame. How do we classify *Kan* Water and *Li* Flame in the human body? They are referred to as Shaoyin. Water and fire are basically incompatible, but in the human body, they must not only be compatible with one another but furthermore, they both share the same name. Below, we will discuss why this is the case.

I.1.c.1. Water and Fire Are the Male and Female of Qi and Blood

Water and fire are together referred to as Shaoyin. In one way, this emphasizes the importance of water and fire to the human body. From another perspective, it stresses the desirability of joining water and fire. Water and fire must remain conjoined and interdependent in the body. They should never separate from one another. If they do separate, problems arise. Why is this? The "Great Treatise on the Correspondences of Yin and Yang" in the *Plain Questions* explains what water and fire are in clear terms. Water and fire are yin and yang. And what, in turn, are yin and yang? Yin and yang are male and female. The water and fire of the human body are its yin and yang, they are its male and female. When a male and female live together in the same residence, we have husband and wife. If they are husband and wife, then of course they depend on each other and want marital harmony. In China, it used to be the custom that the bride would go and live in the house of the husband's family, and take his family name. Thus, water and fire are both called Shaoyin, and this has profound implications.

Yin and yang, male and female, water and fire—it is suitable that these are harmonized with one another and that they remain interdependent. Earlier, when we discussed Taiyin, we cited a passage from the *Great Commentary of the Classic of Changes*: "Heaven and earth's misty union; all living things are transformed by it and develop. Male and female commingle their essence, and all living things thereby procreate." If they are not in accord with one another, if they are not mutually dependent, how will they "roil in harmony"? How will they pool their essences? Therefore, the *Plain Questions's* "Treatise on Heavenly Truth in Remote Antiquity" says: "Yin and yang are harmonized, and thus children can be born."

The roiling in harmony and commingling of essence described above exhibit differences in their internal and external aspects. From the external perspective, this harmonization and joining refers to the descent of the celestial *qi* and the ascent of the terrestrial *qi*. From this roiling, this misty tryst, the myriad things emerge from the development and fermenting of essence. All of the plant and animal life on earth is the result of this harmonious merger. The "commingling of essences" refers to the exchange and joining of essence between the male and female, husband and wife. From this joining, the myriad things are reborn, and new males and females emerge.

Today, a polite and civilized way to refer to the commingling of essences described above is "innate behavior" (*xing xingwei* 性行為) and in Confucius's time, everything relating to sexual intercourse was referred to as "color" (*se* 色). Confucius said, "Appetite for food and sex (*se*) is innate," and "the principal desires of human beings are for food, drink, and sexual relations." The character 性 (*xing*) refers to natural things, i.e. basic human needs. This natural thing had two aspects. The first aspect is desire for food. Humans cannot live without food. Humans must eat to survive. Thus, the ancients often said: "the people value food above all else." The literal translation of this would be: "the common people regard food as heaven." The importance of food is illustrated by equating it with heaven. What is the other aspect of our natural appetites? It is for "color" (*se*), which is the customary way of referring to the affairs of men and women: their sexual intercourse. This aspect is equally important, for without sex, human beings could not procreate. The meaning of "color" exceeds that of mere procreation. It has other meanings as well. We can glimpse this larger meaning by looking at the "Treatise on the Vital *Qi* Connecting to Heaven" in the *Plain Questions*: "It is most essential to know this about the relationship of yin and yang: as long as yang remains sealed in, the entire system is stable. When the two are not harmonized, it will be like a spring without autumn, or a winter without summer. Consequently, the harmonization of these two aspects is referred to as the measure of the sage." Thus, the essentials of yin and yang consist in "harmonization." If they are not harmonized, it is tantamount to spring without fall, or winter without summer. What sort of world or system would consist of spring without fall or winter without summer? However, the harmonization of yin and yang is not wanton, for if it were it would be mere licentiousness. This harmonization is formalized and steeped in ritual propriety. If it were not, why would Qi Bo refer to it as the "measure of the sage"?

The aforementioned misty union, pooling of essences, and harmonization of yin and yang, besides the development of living things and the procreation of life, have another important purpose: arousing internal harmonization through exterior harmonization. By harmonizing the exterior, internal harmonization is also brought about, and the yin and yang, the water and fire, of the interior is able to harmonize. Thus, internal yin yang, internal water and fire become interdependent rather than separating. This means that "as long as yin stays at an even level and the yang is safeguarded, essence and spirit remain in a balanced state." This is how the changes associated with life can occur ceaselessly. Thus, the intercourse of male and female, the harmonization of yin and yang, besides allowing for the procreation of future generations, also has profound implications for the health of body and mind. The crucial thing is that this process achieves the "measure of the sage"; it must not be a careless process. In ancient times, there was a branch of learning referred to as "art of the bedchamber" that was particularly devoted to this issue. Human life requires that we eat. Without food, we cannot continue. Besides food, there is something of equal importance, and this is the relation between male and female. Thus, regulation of the diet and of our sexual behavior makes a strong impact on the health of both our bodies and minds. Food and sex are basic necessities of human life that are worthy starting points from which to consider human life. These two fundamental aspects of humankind are summarized with two Chinese characters by Confucius: *shise* 食色 ("food and color"), thereby demonstrating Confucius's incomparable scholarship.

To summarize the above discussion, the human body has two basic needs, and these are food and drink, and the relationship between male and female. Food and drink supply the sustenance for the yin and yang of the human body. The relationship between male and female realizes the harmonization of the yin and yang, and water and fire of the human form. This begs the question: The layperson might easily satisfy this basic need, but what of the monk or nun who renounces sexual intercourse? In their case, this necessity is resolved through spiritual practice. In Daoist spiritual practices, we come across methods with titles such as "The Beautiful Maiden," the "Copulation of the Dragon and the Tiger," "Reciprocation of Water and Fire," and "Obtaining the *Kan* Water and Filling the *Li* Flame." In truth, these are all methods of harmonizing the interior. These are direct methods of harmonizing the fire and water, the yin and yang by means of a sort of internal sexual intercourse.

I.1.c.2. How the Fire and Water of Yin and Yang Are United with One Another

The fire and water of the human body must be closely united with one another. They cannot separate from one another even for an instant. However, in accord with common sense, water is yin, it is heavy and turbid and sinks downward; whereas fire is yang, it is light and clear and tends to float upward. If what tends to sink sinks and what tends to float floats, the two will separate further and further from one another. How can they be induced to harmonize and have intercourse with one another? The copulation of water and fire is a truly marvelous process.

The *Classic of Changes* says: "The relations of that which is rooted in heaven has relations above and of that which is rooted in earth has relations below." Earlier, when we discussed the form of *Kan* Water and *Li* Flame, we also mentioned that *Li* is fire, and the broken line in the middle of *Li* comes from the trigram *Kun* Earth. *Kan* is water, and the solid line in the trigram *Kan* comes from the trigram *Qian* Heaven. Thus, the solid center line in *Kan* Water roots it in heaven, and "That which is rooted in heaven has relations above"; *Li* Flame with its central yin line is rooted in earth, and "That which is rooted in earth has relations below." It is precisely this factor that allows that which is above to descend and that which is below to ascend. Thus, water and fire can exchange with one another, and *Kan* and *Li* can have intercourse.

From this, we can see that in order to deeply understand Chinese Medicine, one must have a firm grasp of the *Classic of Changes*. At the ordinary level of study, it appears as if knowledge of the *Classic of Changes* is hardly necessary, but once one begins to understand Chinese Medicine at a deeper level, one finds it impossible without a clear understanding of this work. Why is it that Sun Simiao said that "If one does not understand the *Changes*, one cannot become a great physician"? If your ambition is only to be a lesser physician, then you can be indifferent to the *Classic of Changes*. The barefoot doctor of bygone years had no need of the *Classic of Changes*. However, if you wish to become a great physician, if you would like to attain deep understanding in the field of Chinese Medicine, then you must know the "changes."

I.1.c.3. Qian *and* Kun *Are the Form, Water and Fire Are the Function*

If you wish to understand the "changes," you must first grasp the eight trigrams. In order to comprehend these, you must first be clear about the prenatal and the postnatal. The relationship between the prenatal and the postnatal is the relationship between form and function. The prenatal is the form, and the postnatal is the function. Among the prenatal trigrams, *Qian* Heaven and *Kun* Earth occupy south and north. Once we get to the postnatal trigrams, the pattern changes, the positions originally occupied by *Qian* and *Kun* are occupied by *Kan* Water and *Li* Flame. *Li* Flame occupies the position of *Qian* Heaven, and thus orchestrates the union of heaven and fire into the hexagram *tongren* (Seeking Harmony); *Kan* Water occupies the

Kun Earth position, and thus orchestrates the union of earth and water into the hexagram *shi* (Multitude). When we discussed the form of water and fire, why did we state that the body of *Kan* Water was *Kun* Earth, and the body of *Li* Flame was *Qian* Heaven? It was because of the particular prenatal and postnatal positions of each.

Of the eight directions of the eight trigrams, there are four orthodox directions and four nooks or angles. The prenatal trigrams place *Qian* Heaven and *Kun* Earth at south and north respectively, and *Kan* Water and *Li* Flame at the east and west points. In the postnatal pattern of the eight trigrams, *Qian* and *Kun* retire to the angles from their cardinal positions, but *Kan* and *Li* vault from east and west to south and north. If we take in this transition from prenatal to postnatal configurations, then we can clearly see that, although the compass is divided by the eight trigrams, the two trigrams that are most prominent in the *Classic of Changes* are *Kan* and *Li*, water and fire. This is because, among the eight trigrams, only *Kan* and *Li* perpetually occupy cardinal positions. In the prenatal pattern, *Kan* and *Li* occupy the latitudinal poles, and in the postnatal pattern, *Kan* and *Li* occupy the longitudinal apices.

The *Classic of Changes* state that the prenatal is the form and the postnatal is the function. However, *Qian* Heaven and *Kun* Earth are the form within the form, and *Kan* Water and *Li* Flame are the function within the function. Based on the fact that in both the prenatal and postnatal patterns, *Kan* and *Li* occupy cardinal positions, we know that the *Classic of Changes* emphasize function over form. Why is this the case? Because the prenatal does not change but the postnatal does. The character "changes" (*yi* 易) carries three meanings. One of these meanings is "to alter." Therefore, the *Classic of Changes* emphasizes transformation, it emphasizes the present state of consciousness; in this instance, it is abundantly clear.

The *Classic of Changes* emphasizes *Kan* Water and *Li* Fire, and it is clear that water and fire refer also to *Qian* Heaven and *Kun* Earth, and when we speak of water and fire, we are also speaking of male and female, as well as yin and yang. In any case, the name Shaoyin and the channel belonging to Shaoyin refer directly to water and fire. Thus, we know the emphasis placed on the Shaoyin conformation. And so, when the disease reaches the Shaoyin layer, we often see *Qian* and *Kun*, the *qi* and the blood, water and fire, and yin and yang thrown into chaos, such that yin and yang separate from one another. That is why, when a disease reaches the Shaoyin layer, the disease is often fatal.

I.1.c.4. The Water and Fire of Kan and Li, the Root of Establishing Life

How can the function of *Kan* Water and *Li* Flame be so important that these two, alone, occupy the four cardinal points of the compass? This question was elucidated by Zheng Qin'an in his book *True Transmission of Medical Principles*: "Of *Qian* Heaven and *Kun* Earth's six children, the youngest and oldest are all imbued with biases of *Qian* and *Kun*. Only the middle male and female have received their natural disposition from *Qian* and *Kun*. People receive the cardinal *qi* of their original nature from heaven and earth and thereby come to life. *Kan* Water and *Li* Flame therefore act as the root of establishing life." From the principle expressed in "People receive the cardinal *qi* of their original nature from heaven and earth and thereby come to life," we can easily see why it is that *Kan* and *Li* are able to act as the root of establishing life. The classics say that wisdom regarding heaven must resonate with on a human level. On the other hand, a wisdom regarding humans must resonate with society. This undoubtedly causes us to think of the two thousand years of feudalism, how each generation of emperors and kings passed its power on to the eldest child, rather than the middle child. This was indeed a serious error!

The name Shaoyin implies both water and fire aspects. Above, we discussed this from the four perspectives of water and fire, yin and yang, male and female, and *Qian* and *Kun*. If we open the *Classic of Changes*, we will be completely clear on this point. How are the trigrams in the *Changes of Zhou* (Zhouyi) organized? They are organized with *Qian* Heaven and *Kun* Earth as their head. *Qian* is the first trigram and *Kun* is the second. And what makes up the tail of this sequence? There are two different tails in the classical *Classic of Changes* and in both, the end of the sequence consists of *Kan* Water and *Li* Flame, though in the second tail they are represented within the hexagrams *jiji* (Already Fulfilled) and *weiji* (Not Yet Fulfilled). Thus, we can see that the entire structure of the *Classic of Changes* places *Qian* and *Kun* at the head, *Kan* and *Li* at the tail, and throughout, *Qian* and *Kun* perform the role of form, and *Kan* and *Li* that of function. Therefore, although it is merely Shaoyin, it embodies *Qian* and *Kun*, heaven and earth, yin and yang, and water and fire.

The *Classic of Changes* use *Qian* and *Kun* as their head, and *Kan* and *Li* as their tail. When we speak of diseases of the six conformations, we must be clear that although Jueyin is regarded as the last conformation, the most important outcome is determined by Shaoyin. If this one crucial area is completely understood, then there will not be any major problems. But if this crucial point is not well understood, then there will be trouble. For this reason alone, among the three yin conformation chapters, we should focus our energies on the Shaoyin chapter.

I.1.d. Qian *and* Kun *Produce the Six Children*

In the past, I did not attach much importance to the saying: "*Qian* Heaven and *Kun* Earth produce the six children," and it was not until after contemplating the question of Shaoyin that I realized its importance. Many principles of the play between heaven and earth are conveyed by this sentence. *Qian* and *Kun* produce the six children, not the singular child, and this reveals a distinguishing feature. Confucius, in the *Great Commentary of the Classic of Changes*, says: "Heaven and earth's misty union; all living things are transformed by it and develop. Male and female commingle their essence, and all living things thereby procreate." If we look at the living things of this world, we are struck by their variety. There are stark differences from one plant to the next, and still more extreme differences in animal life. When we say "the six children" born of men and women, this also indicates there is a vast variety. Some children will become emperor, others a beggar; some are as rich as whole nations, some are destitute and frustrated. It is truly as the poet Du Fu wrote: "From the lacquered gates the air is rife with meat and booze, on the road are frozen bones." The correspondence between humans and the natural world, between person and nature, is visible everywhere to those who look for it.

Qian Heaven and *Kun* Earth make love and give birth to the six children; yin and yang have intercourse and create the five elements. Most Chinese Medicine books of the present era often lump yin and yang and the five elements together, but what is the nature of the relationship between yin and yang and the five elements? Rarely do the authors seem to know. After the preceding discussion, I trust that the reader is able to be clear as to whether the five elements are the final word or whether we should seek them within yin and yang.

Qian Heaven and *Kun* Earth give birth to the six children, and occupy the cardinal directions of south and north respectively. In the postnatal configuration, once we have transitioned from form to function, where do *Qian* and *Kun* move? They move to the "four nooks," the oblique corners. The oblique corners—northwest, southeast, etc.—are a step down in rank from the cardinal directions. Confucius said, "The *Classic of Changes*, as a book, is both wide-reaching and detailed. In it, we find the way of heaven, of humans, and of earth." *Qian* and *Kun* step down from their position at the cardinal directions, just as Laozi proposed we should "retire after achieving our goal." The ninth chapter of Laozi's *Classic of the Dao and Its Virtue* says: "Having achieved to one's satisfaction and then to retreat is the way of heaven." And according to Chapter 10 of the *Classic of the Dao and Its Virtue*: "Bringing forth and nourishing it, creating without possessing, laboring without claiming credit, being great without oppressing: this is hidden virtue." The workings of heaven and earth are great indeed! The six children, the "myriad things," all emerge from them. However, as soon as the six children emerge, as soon as Water and Fire take over, they retire from their lofty positions. This is what Laozi referred to as "hidden virtue" (*xuan de* 玄德). This is an important point, and, at the bottom, is the very reason why heaven and earth are able to persist indefinitely. Thus, in Chapter 7 of the *Classic of the Dao and Its Virtue*, we read: "Heaven and earth are everlasting; it is their selflessness that allows heaven and earth to remain unchanging, and to gain eternal life."

There is an interesting example of this from ancient Chinese history. Liu Bang, the founder of the Han Dynasty, had two outstanding subjects: one was named Zhang Liang, and the other Han Xin. Zhang Liang was a devout disciple of Huang Shigong, a Daoist hermit, and truly understood the *Classic of Changes*. As soon as the Han territory was captured, he went into seclusion. Han Xin, however, was not like Zhang Liang. He gained great success but did not retire, and in the end he ended up decapitated. If we look at more recent history, we find it riddled with such situations. Everyone claims that they have learned from history, but it is hard to put that learning into practice. No one who gains great success wants to retire into seclusion. Instead, they take credit for their achievements, then seek to enjoy the fruits of their victory. They cannot do as Laozi instructed: "create without possessing, labor without claiming credit, be great without oppressing." They live for themselves and so they do not live long. The vast majority meets an undesirable end. The *Classic of Changes* is far-reaching and deeply profound. In it, there is natural science and social science, as well as the humanities. Once one penetrates the meanings of the *Classic of Changes*, one discovers the logic behind human behavior.

I.2. The Meaning of the Shaoyin Channels

The meaning of the Shaoyin channel includes both the hand and leg Shaoyin channels. The foot Shaoyin channel begins with the Yongquan (KI 1) acupuncture point at the time interval *you* (酉). Yongquan is the well point of the leg Shaoyin channel. This is an unusual place in the human anatomy. All of the other well points of the leg channels are on the tips of the toes; only the Shaoyin leg channel has a well point on the sole of the foot. As the name Yongquan ("bubbling well") suggests, Shaoyin rules water. The spring water bubbles up from this point. The foot Shaoyin begins at Yongquan point at 5 pm, and at 7 pm, when the *you* period is at a close, the energy is at Shufu (KI 27) on the upper chest. In the *wu* time period, at 11 am, the *qi* begins flowing through the hand Shaoyin channel from the point Jiquan (HT 1) in the armpit, and at the end of *wu* concludes its course at Shaochong (HT 9) on the tip of the little finger.

I.3. The Meaning of the Shaoyin Viscera

I.3.a. The Heart

Shaoyin and the heart have already served as the topic of a number of discussions in this book. At this point, I would like to address certain points that easily lead to confusion.

I.3.a.1. "The Myriad Creatures of the World Emerge from Being, and Being Emerges from Non-being"

How is the heart different from the four other viscera? In the first place, as we discussed earlier, unlike all the other internal organs, the Chinese character for "heart" does not contain the flesh radical. This signifies that all the other internal organs are physical; they are "being." Without this particular radical, the heart is "non-being." In Daoist philosophy, "being" (*you* 有) and "non-being" (無) are central concepts. In the *Classic of the Dao and Its Virtue*, we read: "The myriad living things emerge from being, and being

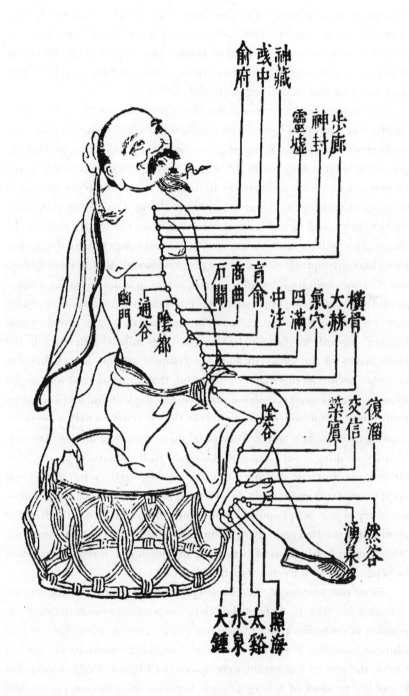

emerges from non-being." The importance of "being" is undeniable. Our existence, everything about us, cannot depart from "being," but this being derives from non-being. And so the Daoists place heavy emphasis on the importance of *wuwei* (無為) or non-striving. Thus it is said: "The Dao never does anything and yet nothing is left undone."

The concept of *wuwei* is as useful as it is praiseworthy. It can be used to further one's study, to better one's conduct in society. It can even be used to govern a country and bring peace to the world. It is regrettable that the people of today cannot attain this virtue; individuals cannot attain it, and nations as a whole are incapable of attaining it. We are all in the practice of stopping at nothing, but cannot do without doing. The minute something starts to grow, and we cut it down. We fall far short of Laozi's ability to let things grow without our oppression. The United States is a good example. Its technology flourishes, its military prowess exceeds that of its neighbors and it cannot help itself but to scatter its troops in other countries, engage in conflicts, and create oppression. It is ignorant of the old Chinese adages that "an army is a bad omen," and "in the wake of a large army, we find famine." Instead, it relies on the strength of its military extending to the four corners of the globe, its ability to conquer anyone. Does it hope to overcome terrorism this way? I do not think that it can succeed with such a strategy. In the end, it is merely a matter of playing with fire and ending up badly burnt. It is my sincere hope that the United States, as well as any other country that attempts to use force of might to dominate another country, learns something from Laozi and does away with militaristic means. Militarism cannot persist, and once this fact is recognized, countries that rely upon martial influence would do well to do away with it. What, then, allows a country to rule with popular support and consensus? This is the result of manifesting the Dao and relying upon real virtue. This is as Confucius said: "One must rule by means of virtue, like the north star: it remains constant in its place and all the other stars revolve around it."

From our analysis of the characters referring to the five viscera, the character for "heart," without the "flesh" radical, also holds the supreme position of sovereign ruler. Examining this arrangement, we can see that Chinese Medicine is steeped in Daoist thought. In previous decades in China, the official line on the development of Chinese Medicine was that it was the product of a long struggle between the common people and disease. The political flavor of such an analysis is too strong to swallow. It has no real meaning. So then, where did Chinese Medicine originate? There are those who say that Chinese Medicine originated with the *Classic of Changes,* and there are those who say that it originated from Daoism. I believe that both of these are possible sources. From a certain perspective, we might say that Chinese Medicine, the *Classic of Changes,* and Daoism form a sort of trinity. In the *Yellow Emperor's Classic,* we come across much that derives from the *Classic of Changes* and also much from Daoism. The first person to provide commentary to the *Yellow Emperor's Classic* was the Tang Dynasty scholar Wang Bing. His commentary remains authoritative up until the present day. Interestingly, his commentary is thick with Daoist overtones. Still more interesting is the fact that Wang Bing's pen name was Enlightened Master of the Profound: this is an authentic Daoist appellation. Here we can see that there is a sort of perfect harmony between Daoism and Chinese Medicine.

I.3.a.2. The Heart Holds the Office of the Sovereign and Ruler; Spirit Brightness Originates From It

Among the nineteen disease triggers described in the *Plain Questions* chapter titled "Great Treatise on the Essentials of Ultimate Truth," there are five lines directed at the five viscera. The line related to the heart reads: "All pain with itch and sores belongs to the heart." This line, defining the disease trigger of the heart, the most crucial manifestation of illness related to the heart, indicates that its core manifestations broadly encompasses all "pain with itch and sores" and that all of these are directly related to problems with that particular organ. Both pain and itching are a sort of sensation or feeling. Feelings, sensations, and perceptions are complex. Besides pain and itching, there are distention and tingling, misery and suffering, and a great number of other things felt only in the psyche. Pain and itching, however, are the most basic sensations, and perhaps the most easily perceived. Qi Bo, in his response to Huangdi's question, uses these two to represent the rest. It is not only pain and itching that belong to the heart; all sensations belong to the heart.

This close rapport between the heart and pain reminds us of how pain and itching as well as the whole host of uncomfortable sensations can cause a wide range of discomforts and sufferings, even preventing us from being able to sit still. We must keep in mind that pain and itching are not always a bad thing. If the body is afflicted with disease, or if any organ of the body is out of tune, then pain, itching, or some other discomfort allows the patient to perceive that disharmony. The heart, as sovereign ruler, is preeminent. The sovereign is clear and perceptive. If there is any movement in the kingdom, the sovereign knows it. If abnormality occurs within the body, the heart is able to reflect this flaw with sensations of suffering. Disaster can be averted if the patient changes course in time. Are pain and suffering good or bad? From this perspective, they might be seen as a blessing. If the sovereign ruler is clear and bright, it is able to bring all affairs to light.

Consider the consequences of remaining unaware of illness or even serious disease. Would it be desirable to remain oblivious to such disharmony? To remain ignorant of a disease process at work in one's own body reveals that the sovereign ruler—what the Chinese refer to as the heart—in the person is failing. Rather than being clear and bright, the ruler is becoming confused and insensible. The heart rules pain and itching. If you are suffering from a condition that should cause you discomfort and you fail to feel it, then the seat of cognizance, the "sovereign ruler," is surely in shambles. In such an instance, the sovereign is akin to Nawaz Sharif, the former president of Pakistan who suffered a coup d'état in 1999, while he remained seemingly unaware. Can such a ruler be considered "clear and bright"? If he were truly clear and bright, he would have known everything that was happening in his domain, and not be caught unawares by a coup.

Nowadays in the clinic, we often come across patients with advanced, serious diseases, such as late-stage cancer or renal failure, who are almost totally unaware of their plight. They felt no pain or itching, despite their dire situation. Why do such serious diseases remain unbeknownst? It is because the sovereign is obscure. If the sovereign is confused, he cannot perceive subtle changes. And what is the result of this befuddlement? The result is as described in Chapter 8 of the *Plain Questions*: "If the ruler is not bright and clear, the twelve offices are all imperiled. The Dao will be closed off and obstructed, and the physical form will be greatly harmed. To nourish life on the basis of this results in disaster. To rule the world in this way will greatly endanger the ancestral temple. Beware! Beware!"

The heart ruler is conscious and bright. If the spirit is bright, there is nothing it does not see and scrutinize. Only then may the role of remonstrator, as described in the Taiyin chapter, be given full play. If the remonstrator is operating properly, then the person will have a long life of health free from danger of a sudden fatality. Likewise, when this role is adequately filled in the larger schema of society, there is great peace and prosperity. As it says in the *Plain Questions*: "If the ruler is bright and clear, there is peace below. To nourish life on the basis of this results in longevity. There will be no risk of failure till the end of all generations. To rule the world in this way results in great abundance." What allows for this to happen? The cognizance of the sovereign ruler, the heart, makes it possible. Any change that takes place is known to the heart, and the heart can make subtle adjustments to deal with those changes. Every day, potentially cancerous cells in the human body begin their abnormal replication, but cancer does not ensue. This is because the body is able to recognize this abnormal cell division and address it by killing off the potentially cancerous cell lines. All other diseases are similar. As long as the lord and ruler of the body is bright and clear, able to detect and address subtle imbalances and abnormalities at their inception, disasters in health are avoided.

Lines from the *Yellow Emperor's Classic* like "The heart holds the office of the sovereign and ruler; spirit brightness originates from it," and "All pain with itch and sores belongs to the heart," reveal the importance of the heart. If the heart and its associated physiology and pathology are clearly understood, medicine will have gained much. Many fatal organic diseases, such as cancer, may then be eradicated. Chinese Medicine is full of valuable riddles, but it depends upon your ability to delve deeply after them and contemplate their implications.

I.3.a.3. Pain

We have already discussed the intrinsic relationship between the heart and the sensation of pain, and expanded upon this to include other related subjects.

Actually, when we pay a bit more attention to the construction of these characters that we use every day, as we did above, relationships like the one between heart and pain become obvious. For instance, in Chinese, we use the word for pain (*tong* 痛) together with the word for heart: *tongxin* (痛 心), meaning "to be pained or heartbroken," or *xintong* (心痛), "to feel distressed." *Tong* is used with equal frequency together with the word for bitterness (*ku* 苦), the flavor associated with the heart and with fire, such as we find in the compound word *tongku* (痛苦), a general term for pain or suffering. These compound words point to the close relationship between the heart and pain and suffering in Chinese thought. The Chinese, as a people, as evidenced by their everyday colloquial use of language, associated bitterness with the heart, and the two together with the concept of suffering. We cannot overlook the significance of this ingrained habit of language, for it has persisted precisely because it resonates with a deeper understanding of the association. These deeper resonances have both philosophical and medical implications. If we read the *Classic of Changes* or the works of Laozi or Confucius, we find they are constructed of very ordinary, common language. Wielding this common language, the authors were nonetheless able to convey profound insights. This is the work of great masters, sages even!

Another word that is often used together with the Chinese word for pain (*tong* 痛) is *teng* (疼). I doubt that most Chinese persons have considered the deeper meaning of these two characters, so commonly used together. Why are these two characters so often found together, and why are they in most instances interchangeable with one another? Inside the character *teng*, we find the character *dong* (冬), meaning "winter." The *qi* of winter is cold. What do *teng* and *tong* have to do with cold? *Plain Questions* has a chapter devoted to the issue of pain, called the "Treatise on Pain." In it, more than ten examples of pain are given, and except for one, all of them point to cold as the cause of pain. Furthermore, in the "Treatise on Blocks," it says: "Pain is the product of a surplus of cold *qi*; the presence of cold causes pain." The explanation of pain in the *Plain Questions* is very clear: "The presence of cold causes pain." From this, we understand why the characters *tong* and *teng* are so interchangeable in Chinese thought and speech. If we are speaking of pain, we are speaking of the presence of cold.

The construction and etymology of the character for *tong* (痛) itself also merits examination. The character *yong* (甬) together with the "disease" radical (疒) forms the character *tong*. What then, does *yong* signify? *Yong* refers to a way, path, or corridor. When the disease radical is placed together with this character signifying a thoroughfare or path, it points to the disease being the result of a problem with the thoroughfares or passageways of the body. The passageways and paths are used for transportation and communication. When the passageways and paths of the body have a problem, they will not be "open and unobstructed" (*tong* 通) and then, of course, there will be pain. This is in accord with the Chinese Medicine concept that "Because there is obstruction, there is pain; obstruction causes pain." The Chinese character for pain *tong* as well as the compound word *tengtong*, as well as the interchangeable nature of the two characters *teng* and *tong*, all serve to reveal both pain's cause and the mechanism underlying pain.

Pain is a common feature of countless diseases, and is one of the most unpleasant aspects of sickness. Many diseases, such as late stage cancer, are so painful that some patients would prefer euthanasia to end the ordeal. It is clear then that the physician's responsibility to understand and thereby alleviate pain is of urgent importance. At present, our understanding falls far short of completion. I would offer that the preceding discussion may provide crucial help in making the understanding and alleviation of pain possible.

I.3.b. The Kidney

I.3.b.1. "The Highest Virtue Is Like Water"

Regarding the "Dao" of the kidney, we should begin with an examination of the character for kidney, *shen* (simplified: 肾; traditional: 腎). The character *shen* is composed of *qian* (臤) above and the moon (*yue* 月) below. What is signified by *qian*? In ancient times, *qian* was written as *xian* (賢), which denotes ability or virtue. As for *yue* (月), we have already discussed the significance of the character at some length: it indicates the moon, the *qi* essence of water. When we speak of the moon, we also speak of water. When we combine the top and bottom portions of the Chinese character for kidney, it confirms what was said by Laozi long ago: "The highest virtue is like water." The higher portion is virtue, and the lower water, so we have a symbolic representation of Laozi's statement.

I.3.b.2. The Kidneys Hold the Office of Making Strong; Technique and Skill Originate from Them

In Chapter 8 of the *Plain Questions*, the "Treatise on the Spiritual Orchid Secret Canon," it says: "The kidneys hold the office of making strong; technique and skill originate from them." I have contemplated the kidneys for many years, and it is only in the last several years that I felt have begun to understand them. Examining the etymology of the characters in the original Chinese of this line from the *Plain Questions* reveals much of its meaning. First, we have the phrase "making strong" (*zuoqiang* 作強). The character *zuo* means to make or do, to produce an effect. More important to our discussion here is the character *qiang*. In this instance, *qiang* has two layers of meaning. The first layer, the basic meaning of the character, is that of an insect, the rice weevil. As it says in the *Jade Discourse*: "A grub inside the rice." And as the *Erya* says in its "Explanation of Insects": "*Qiang* is the name of an insect." The first layer of meaning in the character *qiang* is that of a vermin in the rice. Most Chinese have seen this particular insect, the rice weevil, and might have noted that it resembles a particular feature of human anatomy, namely the male reproductive organ. This organ is referred to as *qiang*. And why is it the kidney that is associated with *qiang*? Because the kidney rules the two yin. From the first layer of meaning, we can see the close connection between the kidneys and the genitals. Since the kidneys hold the office of *zuoqiang*, it is little wonder that they are related to the reproductive faculties. If we think for a moment of all the "skills and techniques" in the world, is not life's ability to reproduce and multiply the most wondrous? This kind of great skill and technique is also known as "creation." Wang Bing explained that "Creation manifests takes form; it is called technique and skill."

The second layer is the extended meaning of *qiang*, which is "strong and firm," or "staunch, unyielding, tough, or hard." If we search the human body for what in it accords with such a description, we find that only the bones fit the bill. The bones are the hardest, firmest part of the body. They are the best able to resist the pull of gravity and exert brute force. Thus, there are two implied meanings of the character *qiang*: the first is that of the reproductive organs, and the second is that of the bones. Furthermore, in Chinese Medicine theory, the kidneys rule the bones, just as they rule the external genitalia. The kidneys are indeed the officials of making strength.

The kidneys rule water, and water is the softest and gentlest of the five elements. Why is water, contrary to its own nature, able to make things strong? Let us look at the *Classic of the Dao and Its Virtue*, where the profound reason for this seeming contradiction is discussed. According to Chapter 43: "The softest thing in the world is intermingled with the hardest thing in the world." And in Chapter 78 where this point is expounded upon:

There is nothing softer or weaker than water, but in its ability to assail the hard and the strong, nothing surpasses it, for its emptiness is able to change things. The weak triumph over the strong and the soft over the hard. There is no one in the world who does not know this, and also no one who can put it into practice.

The kidneys rule water and also rule the bones. Water and the bones would appear to be completely unrelated, but they are joined by this aspect of the body. Thus, the softest and the hardest in the body are both collected in the Chinese conception of the kidney. Combining the hardest and the softest together in one place certainly requires skill and technique! Thus, the office of the kidney truly embodies what Laozi referred to when he wrote: "the softest thing in the world is intermingled with the hardest." Chinese Medicine and Daoism share the same origins.

In deeper terms, the "techniques and skills" are life's ability to reproduce and multiply. In more general terms, this ability is a sort of technical skill or craftsmanship. When we speak of the deeper meaning, we must think in terms of hard and soft, and what better example of such a skill than the ability of two human beings to reproduce? When we speak of the general meaning, we are also speaking of the combining of hard and soft, for this is also part of any art or craft. Thus, if we wish to summarize the functions of the kidneys in a single line, we can do no better than the line from *Yellow Emperor's Classic*: "The kidneys hold the office of making strong; technique and skill originate from them."

I.3.b.3. The Kidneys Rule Hibernation; They Are the Root of Sealing and Storing, the Dwelling Place of the Essence

The following discussion is in response to the following line in Chapter 9 of the *Plain Questions*, the "Treatise on the Six Nodes and the Visceral Manifestations: "The kidneys rule hibernation; they are the root of sealing and storing, the dwelling place of the essence." The kidneys rule hibernation (*zhe* 蟄), but what did the ancients mean by *zhe*? Here, "hibernation" is synonymous with "sealing and storing" (*fengcang* 封藏). "Sealing and storing" refers to sealing and storing the yang *qi*, just as we discussed earlier in this book. In addition to this, we can also think of it in terms of our discussion of *Kan* Water, for the kidneys are the water organ, the *Kan* organ. What is the trigram that represents *Kan*? It is two broken yin lines with a solid yang between. By extension, that which is stored by the two yin lines is yang. Now, what is meant by "the dwelling place of essence"? The "essence" (*jing* 精) is the yang *qi* in its stored form. Thus, where the yang *qi* is stored is, by definition, the dwelling place of essence. Knowing this, we can see that the quotes "the basis of sealing and storing" and "the dwelling place of the essence" from *Plain Questions* Chapter 9 serve to clarify the deeper meaning of "essence."

At present, many physicians in China treat patients with steroids. I feel compelled to comment on this practice. The effects of steroid treatments on a wide range of diseases are simply astonishing. Steroids can be used with remarkable efficacy to reduce swelling and albuminuria in the patient suffering from nephritis; the patient suffering from an asthmatic attack is rescued almost immediately; high fever that resists all other treatments comes crashing down when steroids are applied. The Nobel Prize in Medicine in the 1950s was won with the discovery of the clinical applications of steroid treatment.

From a Chinese Medicine perspective, why do steroids have such marked effects on human physiology? In accord with our current discussion, we can see that the action of steroids is on what the ancient Chinese referred to as the kidneys, and primarily depends upon the release of yang *qi* from its storage place in the kidneys. This yang *qi* stored in the kidneys is nothing less than the person's essence! This incomparable substance is enormously powerful, like an atomic bomb. It can handle many different problems, and has extraordinary efficacy with a wide variety of diseases. We should be clear, however, that the yang sealed and stored up in the kidneys is needed to nourish the life *qi*, and is used to extend the life. If the stored yang *qi* is put to use for another purpose, although an almost miraculous effect may be brought about almost immediately, if used in this way for a period of time, the yang *qi* that has been sealed and stored will be depleted; the essence will be depleted. Along with this depletion, the source of the creation of *qi* will lessen, and the material used to nourish and extend the life will also be reduced. The result of long-term steroid treatment is predictable. Presently, clinicians in the west are aware of the dangers of steroid treatment, and use it only as a last resort. However, here in China, especially in rural areas, there is a sort of reckless enthusiasm regarding the use of steroids to treat disease. When even ailments as harmless and commonplace as a cold and fever are being treated with steroids, one can see what kind of situation we have come to: "A quack does not need a knife to kill." This is true in both Chinese and Western Medicine.

Steroids act upon the kidneys, and so abuse of steroid treatments will inevitably cause damage to the kidneys. It damages the kidney's ability to rule hibernation, and its ability to seal and store. If hibernation is not maintained and sealing and storing are lost, is there still a "dwelling place of the essence"? Therefore, in the case of excessive use of steroids, it is the kidneys that need to be the focus of our rescue efforts. However, a much preferable option to having to rescue the kidneys is to focus on preventing this kind of disaster in the first place! This is an issue that the entire medical community needs to acknowledge and address together.

I.3.b.4. All Cold with Contraction and Pulling In Belongs to the Kidney

Above, we discussed the normal physiology of the kidney, and now we will follow up by discussing the disease trigger associated with the kidney from "Great Treatise on the Essentials of Ultimate Truth" in the *Plain Questions*. The disease trigger of the kidneys is this: "All cold with contraction and pulling in belongs to the kidney." Earlier in this chapter, we discussed how pain and aching are primarily caused by cold. Here, where it says that "all cold . . . belongs to the kidney" helps us understand this. Furthermore, as we discussed earlier, pain can result even more directly from obstruction. Why is there an obstruction in the first place? Because there is contraction and pulling in. When the channels or the blood vessels are contracted, they become smaller, and there is a tendency for obstruction. This contraction belongs to the kidney.

Knowing that pain is readily induced by cold and by contraction and spasm allows us to recognize the close connection between the kidneys and pain. We might even say that pain has its origin in the kidneys and displays its effects by way of the heart. Pain can be readily understood as the cause-and-effect relationship of the two Shaoyin organs, the kidney and the heart. The issue of the cause and effect of pain is a profound one, nevertheless we can house it within our current discussion. How should we, as physicians, manage pain? Should we treat its cause or its effect? If we wish to resolve pain thoroughly, then we must treat both its cause and its effect. There are times, of course, when the specific cause of pain eludes us, and in cases such as this, we are best served by focusing our efforts on the pain's effect rather than its cause. For this reason, to relieve pain, and especially severe pain, we should emphasize treating the heart.

Earlier, when we discussed the disease trigger line from Chapter 34 of the *Plain Questions* related to the heart ("All pain with itch and sores belongs to the heart"), we also pointed out that the functions of the heart are just as they are described in Chapter 8 of the *Plain Questions*. It is important to understand the function of the heart, as described in Chapter 8: "The heart holds the office of the sovereign and ruler; spirit brightness originates from it," for as soon as disease begins in the organism, as soon as there is abnormal functioning, the spiritual brightness brings this abnormality to light, allowing it to be eradicated in a timely fashion. This is a very natural process in the human body. In fact, this is the reason why common illnesses such as a cold or diarrhea almost invariably resolve without any medication.

When a person becomes ill, the first thing is to experience that illness. This creates a certain manifestation, certain signs and symptoms. This is actually a process of recognition. Once the disease is recognized, the organism can make adjustments to itself, and after readjustment, the disease will be resolved without the assistance of a physician. This is not to say that the disease has not been treated, for without treatment it would not resolve. The treatment is devised and administered within the patient's own body, rather than from without. This self-regulation of disease is carried out by through the regulation of yin and yang; "Cooling that which is hot and heating that which is cold"; "Carefully examining yin and yang, making note of what is soft and what is hard. The yang diseases are treated with yin and the yin diseases with yang, determining the state of the blood and *qi* of the patient, being watchful that each pertains to its own domain; if the blood is excessive, it should be opened; if the *qi* is deficient, it should be pulled." It is not only the physician who applies these methods to the patient; the true master of these techniques is the patient's own body. If there is excessive fire in the body, the body will activate its water system to "cool that which is hot." If the fire is insufficient, another system of the body might be employed to "heat that which is cold." Within the body, there is a consummate system whereby pathological qualities and processes are resolved. It is only when this function of this faculty within the human body is decreased or hindered in some way that the patient comes before the physician, in need of external help. In any case, the methods employed by the physician are mere imitations of those employed by the body itself. In Chinese Medicine, we say: "the highest physician treats diseases before they manifest." What is a disease before it manifests? I believe one implied meaning of this statement is that such a physician frequently adjusts the patient, helping the patient's body to recover its ability to treat disease internally.

The body's own system of self-regulation is highly complex. It involves recognizing the abnormality, addressing the particular quality of the abnormality, and appropriately dealing with it. The guide and leader of recognition is the heart, as we discussed earlier. Under normal circumstances, this body's ability to recognize functional abnormalities is extremely sensitive, and it is able to detect even the slightest changes. It is only when this system no longer functions, when it is paralyzed for whatever reason and fails to recognize problems when they arise, that calamity befalls the body.

When I was living in rural China, I often heard the people use a particular idiom: "A broken-down wall withstands wind and rain." In the countryside where I resided, we often came across old, broken-down houses. Sometimes, all that remained of them was a ragged wall or two that received the brunt of sun, wind, and rain. Decades went by, but the walls remained the same, seemingly impervious to the passage of the seasons and the abuse of the elements. In contrast, some other houses that seemed sturdy and well-fashioned would simply collapse when assailed by wind and rain. If we apply this same metaphor to human constitutions, there are those who are constantly suffering from some complaint or other, one day their throat feels scratchy and the next their head aches, but these people rarely suffer from serious diseases and, on the contrary, tend to be long-lived. Then there are those who never even get a cold, but when one day they do fall ill, it is with a serious, perhaps even life-threatening illness. How do we explain this? I think this is related to the sensitivity with which the body is able to recognize abnormal processes at work. It is not that those who never get colds are without illness; it is just that the body does not detect and set about trying to correct these minor imbalances. As physicians, we must be able to differentiate those who are truly healthy and those whose bodies are simply unaware of trouble brewing. If the person is truly healthy, that is of course good. But if it is simply a deficiency in the person's ability to detect and respond to minor aberrations in normal physiological processes, then a dangerous situation is at hand. It is dangerous precisely because the ability to recognize disease has been dulled, and we are dealing with a sovereign who is largely oblivious and unable to uncover danger lurking in the body. Is this not a dangerous situation?

From the above discussion, the importance of Chapter 8 of the *Plain Questions*, "Treatise on the Spiritual Orchid Secret Canon," should be clearer than ever. Now, more than ever, we are impacted by society and social constructs. In Chapter 8, a social framework is used as a metaphor for the human body. In this metaphor, the sovereign rules over its subjects, holding each to its appropriate share of the work, the performance of its designated function. This is an important point. Whether we are discussing the five elements or the functions of the individual organs, it is still a matter of each performing its duty.

When we discuss the organs related to Shaoyin, we are primarily referring to the heart and kidneys. It might be said that it is impossible to overstate the importance of the relationship between the heart and kidneys. This relationship is none other than the relationship between fire and water, yin and yang, male and female, and essence (*jing*) and spirit (*shen*). In the Chinese language, the term *jingshen* (精神) is used every day to refer to consciousness or vigor, but what is *jingshen* exactly? It is none other than the heart and the kidney. Chapter 9 of the *Plain Questions*, the "Treatise on the Six Nodes and Visceral Manifestation," tells us: "The heart is the root of life, the manifestation of the spirit . . . the kidneys rule hibernation, they are the root of sealing and storing, the dwelling place of the essence." One is the dwelling place of the essence (*jing*), the other the manifestation of the spirit (*shen*). The kidneys store the *jing* and the heart stores the *shen*. From the essence and spirit (*jingshen*) of the person, we can perceive a complete picture of the state of the heart and kidney. Furthermore, we can see the state of fire and water, and yin and yang in the person. The heart belongs to Fire, to *Li*, and the kidneys belong to Water, to *Kan*. Under normal circumstances, the fire and water should complement each other, and the heart and kidneys should communicate with one another. The heart fire descends in order to warm the kidney water, that is, the yang within *Kan* Water. The kidney water ascends to nourish the heart yin, which is none other than the yin line within the *Li* trigram. *Kan* and *Li* intermingle, each in its proper place.

I.4. The Meaning of Shaoyin in *Yunqi*

Let us now discuss the meaning of Shaoyin from a fourth perspective, that of the meaning of Shaoyin in the five movements and six *qi* (*wuyun liuqi*, abbreviated as *yunqi*), the cyclical transformation of universal *qi*. To what does Shaoyin belong in the *yunqi*? It is the imperial fire. As we discussed in the Shaoyang chapter of this book, the imperial fire is associated with brightness, and the ministerial fire is associated with position. We will not recount that discussion here in this chapter. In the previous section of this chapter, we cited Chapter 8 of the *Plain Questions* on a number of occasions. In this chapter, titled the "Treatise of the Spiritual Orchid Secret Canon," we read: "If the ruler is bright and clear, there is peace below. [. . .] If the ruler is not bright and clear, the twelve offices are all imperiled." To a large extent, Shaoyin refers to the ruler or sovereign. If the ruler is not bright, then the entire organism is imperiled. The reason the Shaoyin chapter contains so many references to signs and symptoms that portend danger stems from the fact that the chapter explores the issue of the "ruler not being bright and clear."

From what does the brightness of the ruler stem? When we discussed the characteristic uses of fire, the brightness of fire was listed as one of its most useful qualities. There is nothing that can illuminate objects like yang fire. In order for the sovereign ruler to be bright, it is crucial that the yang fire be sufficient. The heart belongs to fire and rules the spirit, the imperial fire provides brightness; these reinforce the close association between fire and brightness. Only if the yang fire is in force will the sovereign ruler be blessed with brightness of spirit. When the ruler or sovereign is not bright, it is because the yang fire is weak. If we examine the signs and symptoms in the Shaoyin chapter of the *Treatise on Cold Damage* that foreshadow a health crisis or even death, we find that each and every one of them arises from weakness and insufficiency of the yang fire.

In general terms, Shaoyin disease can be divided into cold-induced and heat-induced syndromes. Of the syndromes induced by heat, none are dangerous or deadly. All of these foreboding signs and symptoms are associated with the cold-induced syndromes. Cold-induced syndromes are nothing more than syndromes brought about by weakness and deficiency of yang fire. This is the case throughout the *Treatise on Cold Damage*. Dangerous signs and symptoms caused by heat, in other words an overabundance of yang endangering life, are very infrequent, and only a few lines in the Yangming chapter of the book are devoted to them. The overwhelming majority of signs and symptoms that foretell a critical turn in the course of health are found in the Shaoyin and Jueyin chapters of the *Treatise on Cold Damage*. From this, we realize that regardless of the Western diagnosis of the disease, whether it be cardiovascular disease, cancer, cardiopulmonary disease, etc., when these diseases become critical and the patient's life is on the line, the primary reason is insufficiency of the yang fire. If we take a wide view, we see that it was not only at the end of the Eastern Han dynasty that seven out of ten deaths were due to cold damage, as described in Zhang Zhongjing's preface; even today, the majority of fatal illnesses result from cold damage. Why is this? It is because when the yang fire is attenuated, the sovereign ruler is not bright, and all twelve of the officials are in danger.

Let us look back at the nineteen disease triggers found in *Plain Questions*. In the description of these triggers, there are nine lines devoted to fire and heat, but only one line each for wind, cold, and damp. This emphasizes the close connection between fire and heat with a great number of diseases. This correlation does not necessarily indicate that fire and heat are overabundant in the patient. These diseases can be brought about whether or not the fire and heat pathogens are present, whether fire and heat are excessive or deficient. Qi Bo clarifies this point in a passage following the text on the nineteen disease triggers. Later scholar-physicians only read the passage directly related to the nineteen disease triggers and neglect this other crucial part of the text. As a result, they mistakenly believe that diseases resulting from fire and heat are more abundant in the world, and that most dangerous and deadly diseases are the result of an excess of yang fire. They know that when yang fire is overabundant, it can lead to a clouding of the spirit and unconsciousness or delusion; but they are seemingly unaware of the fact that when the yang fire is deficient and weak, the sovereign ruler is not bright, and because the ruler is not bright, all twelve of the officials are endangered, and unconsciousness and delusion readily come about. Today, clinicians know how to rescue a patient from counterflow with the "three treasures" (Angong Niuhuang Wan, Zixue Dan, and Zhibao Dan), but they fail to recognize that the right way to correct counterflow in the patient is with a Sini type of formula.

Among the writings of Dou Cai of the Song Dynasty, there is a book called *Bian Que's Heart Book*. This book is primarily an acupuncture and moxibustion text, but one of its main ideas is especially deserving of our attention. Dou Cai believed that yang syndromes are relatively easy to treat because they are easily detected. Excess yang fire in the body is like a fire within a paper bag: it will quickly burn its way out. Excess yang syndromes do not lie concealed, and will be able to be detected and treated in time. Yin syndromes, on the other hand, are not as obtrusive. Yin syndromes easily hide in wait, eluding our view. It is only in the end when there is little room left to maneuver that they come out of hiding, presenting as a dangerous and possibly fatal disease, that we realize the lurking threat. This ability to lurk and hide while developing is a direct result of a weakness of the yang fire, and with it an attenuation of the ability to perceive, recognize, and thereby respond to pathological changes. In a word, the sovereign is not clear and bright. Dou Cai's understanding of the difference between yin and yang is well worth investigating further.

Generally speaking, the imperial fire is above, and the kidney water is below. The *Classic of the Dao and Its Virtue* says: "The high uses what is below for its foundation, and the noble uses the common as a foundation." The imperial fire is high up above, noble as the sovereign ruler, but its foundation, its basis, is below, in the water of the kidney. When a disease reaches the Shaoyin layer, it is often the case that functions very high up and very low down no longer work properly. If the foundation down below is not addressed, it is difficult to have an effect on the ruler on high. Thus, when disease progresses to Shaoyin, we physicians are confronted with a thorny problem.

II. An Outline of Shaoyin Disease

The outline of Shaoyin disease presented here is in accord with Zhang Zhongjing's outline of Shaoyin disease summarized in line 281 of the *Treatise on Cold Damage*: "When Shaoyin is diseased, the pulse is faint and fine, and there is only desire to sleep." If we rewrite this line in the same style of the nineteen disease triggers, we might say: "All fine, faint pulses with desire to sleep belongs to Shaoyin." We will discuss the guiding principles of Shaoyin disease from three different angles.

II.1. The Subtlety of the Pulse

From the fact that the title of each and every one of the six conformation chapters in *Treatise on Cold Damage* includes the pulse, we can tell that Zhang Zhongjing laid a heavy emphasis on the importance of the pulse. However, the pulse is not described for all of the six conformations in their initial outline. For instance, at the beginning of the Yangming chapter, we read: "When Yangming is diseased, the stomach family is full." We do not read: "When Yangming is diseased, the pulse is big and the stomach family is full." Likewise, the opening line of the Shaoyang chapter is: "When Shaoyang is diseased, there is a bitter taste in the mouth, the throat is dry, and the eyesight is blurry"; it does not say: "When Shaoyang is diseased, the pulse is wiry and fine, there is a bitter taste in the mouth, the throat is dry, and the eyesight is blurry." Despite an obvious emphasis on the importance of the pulse, the only conformation outlines that touch upon the pulse are the Taiyang and Shaoyin chapters. This tells us that there is a special relationship between the pulse and the Taiyang and Shaoyin levels of disease.

The significance of the pulse is very subtle. It is just as it says in Chapter 17 of the *Plain Questions*, the "Treatise on the Essentials of Vessels and the Subtleties of the Essence": "There is wonderful subtlety in the pulse, it must always be examined. There is a method to examining the pulse, and that originates from yin and yang." From this passage alone, we know that when taking the pulse, the most important thing is to observe its yin and yang qualities. As we discussed before, it is yang combining with yin that makes the pulse. The physics of the pulse are easily correlated with the tides of the oceans. The pulse is formed by the rising and falling pressure of blood, initiated by the unceasing beating of the heart. This rise and fall of pressure is akin to the pulsating ebb and flow of the tides. Blood is yin and so it is essentially still and quiet. Why then is it so lively in the blood vessels, forming the pulsating changes we describe as the pulse? This is a function of the yang. This is why the pulse is described as being a combination of the quiet, yin blood together with the dynamic, moving yang. From this perspective, when we palpate the pulse, we are examining the yin and the yang of the body, its water and fire, and by extension, the heart and the kidneys. The heart and the kidneys, fire and water, yin and yang, all belong to Shaoyin. Shaoyin is the storehouse of the fire and water, of the heart and kidneys. The relationship between the pulse and Shaoyin is unique. Shaoyin and Taiyang have "root and branch" and internal-external relationships with one another, which is why only the outlines for Taiyang and Shaoyin disease mention the pulse directly.

Regarding the internal-external relationship of Taiyang and Shaoyin, Taiyang, on the exterior, emphasizes water and fire, just as Shaoyin does on the more interior level. Taiyang is linked together with cold water, emphasizing the yin yang pair, water and fire. When fire rises, water rises, and when fire descends, so too does water; this constitutes the water cycle. Shaoyin refers to the yin and yang, the fire and water, of the interior. The external Taiyang is related to the function of yin and yang, water and fire. The internal Shaoyin relates to the form of this same yin and yang, water and fire. The relationship between Taiyang and Shaoyin is one of form and function, of material body and implemented use. When the disease reaches the Shaoyin stage, it becomes evident that both the form and the function are impaired. Debilitation of the function causes the pulse to appear faint and weak. An insufficiency of the form causes the pulse to become fine and delicate. A "faint and fine" pulse indicates that both the form and the function are incapacitated.

In the *Treatise on Cold Damage*, a faint and fine pulse is described more than once in the Shaoyin chapter. The only other place we find mention of a faint, fine pulse is in the Taiyang chapter. In line 60 of the Taiyang chapter, we read: "After downward purgation, if sweating is promoted, the patient shivers, and the pulse is faint and fine; it is because both the interior and exterior of the body are deficient." This vivid description of the syndrome at hand, with its underlying rationale, the dual deficiency of both the internal and external aspects of the patient, summarizes our current discussion perfectly.

The patient, who suffers from an exterior Taiyang syndrome, has been mistreated with sweating and downward purging, resulting in shivering and a faint and fine pulse. This pulse appears because now both interior and exterior are deficient. By "interior," we are referring to Shaoyin and to form; by "exterior," we are referring to Taiyang and function. The function is deficient, and so the pulse is faint and weak. The form is deficient and so the pulse is fine. Thus, a pulse that is "faint and fine" unquestionably reveals that the water and fire, the heart and the kidney, the interior and the exterior, the form and the function are all implicated in the current pathological state. The pulse is indeed subtle and wondrous!

II.2. There Is Only Desire to Sleep

II.2.a. Sleep and Waking

Let us first look at human sleep and waking. What factors lead to sleep and waking? We have discussed this topic previously in this book. We compared waking and sleep to the bright sky of day and the darkness of night respectively. Thus, in the *Yellow Emperor's Classic*, it says: "the sky has day and night, people have waking and sleeping." A key characteristic of Chinese Medicine is the concept that human beings and nature are one with one another and correspond to one another. It is my opinion that "the sky has day and night, people have waking and sleeping" is the greatest example of this correspondence. If there are people who are unable to see the correspondence between humans and nature inherent in this example, and if they continue to think that the conceptual foundations of Chinese Medicine are illusory and abstruse, then I can only say that differences are so great that we cannot work together.

Since night and day are no different from sleep and waking, the two are of course deeply interconnected. Most people do not realize this point. They mistakenly think that only the amount of sleep is important, not what part of the day they sleep in. However, when there is daylight and the sky is bright, we should be awake, and when the night sky is dark, we should sleep and rest. Only then can we say that there is a close correspondence and harmony between human beings and nature. To correspond with nature, to be one with nature, was also referred to as "obtaining the Dao." This is the Dao of heaven, and obtaining it is incredibly helpful, while if one loses this same Dao, one gains little support. For this reason, if we wish to nourish our life and preserve our strength, we would be greatly benefited by thoroughly comprehending the appropriate times for sleep and wakefulness.

Why is it light during the day? The sun seems to rise from under the earth and the sky brightens. Why is the night dark? The sun goes back below the rim of the horizon, seemingly descending back into the earth, and the sky darkens. Because the cycle of day and night corresponds with human wakefulness and sleep, we know that there is a process parallel to the emergence and submergence of the sun below the earth in the human physiology of waking from slumber and falling asleep.

When the sun emerges from the earth, it is bright, and so we have the image of the hexagram *jin* (Proceeding Forward, ䷢). In this hexagram, the upper trigram is *Li* Flame and the lower is *Kun* Earth. The *Li* trigram represents the sun, and *Kun* represents the earth. When the fiery sun emerges from the earth, brightening every corner, nothing in the open remains unilluminated. Thus, *Explaining Writing and Analyzing Characters* says: "*Jin* represents progress. When the sun emerges, the myriad things progress." The *Miscellaneous Hexagrams* (Zagua) commentary of the *Classic of Changes* says: "*Jin* means daytime." In the *Commentary on the Judgments*, it is written: "*Jin* is progress. When the light emerges from the exterior of the earth, what follows is the splendor of great illumination."

When the sun goes back into the earth, there is darkness, and we have the image of the hexagram *mingyi* (Brilliance Injured). This hexagram is exactly the opposite of *jin*; if we take the previous hexagram and turn it upside down, so that earth is above and fire below, we have the hexagram *mingyi* (䷣). The character *ming* (明) refers to bright light, and the character *yi* (夷) literally means "to wound" or "injure." When the light is injured, we have darkness. Only when the sun emerges from the earth is there light; this is *jin* (Proceeding Forward), and is also the state of wakefulness. When the sun goes back into the earth, the light is injured, and we have the *mingyi* (Brilliance Injured), night, and sleep.

According to the *Great Commentary of the Classic of Changes*,

> In ancient times, the kings made sacrifices. They looked upward and observed the heavens, looked downward and observed the earth. They observed the language of beasts and birds, so fitting to the earth. They looked at their own bodies and at things far away and thereby created the eight trigrams, and were thus able to penetrate into the virtue of the spiritual light and the compassion of the myriad creatures.

Thus, the hexagrams *jin* and *mingyi* can be used to describe the world at large as day and night, and at closer range, human waking and sleep. That they describe day and night in the macrocosm of the world is clearly explained in the classics. We need look no further than our eyes to perceive the way in which these hexagrams pertain to sleep and waking.

In the Chinese Medicine understanding of the body, the upper eyelid belongs to the spleen, and the lower to the stomach. Their closing together is governed by these two organs together. Thus, our eyelids belong to the category of the earth element, to the ground beneath our feet, to the trigram *Kun* Earth. When the eyelids part, allowing us to perceive light, there is brightness (*ming*). The *Explanation of the Trigrams* says: "*Li* Flame governs the eyes." When the eyelids part to reveal the eyes, it is like the *Li* Flame of the sun emerging from the earth. When the sun emerges from the earth, we have the hexagram *jin*, and we see the image of that hexagram again when a person opens their eyes and stirs from sleep.

When the sun goes back beneath the earth, just as when our eyes close with slumber, we have the image of *mingyi* (Brilliance Injured). If we wish to sleep, the first thing we must do is close our eyelids. The bringing together of the two eyelids, each of which belongs to the earth element, severing the beam of light that enters our eyes, is a fitting representation of Brilliance Injured.

The close correlation between the two hexagrams *jin* and *mingyi* with human sleep and waking once again illustrates the close connection between the *Classic of Changes* and Chinese Medicine. At the outset of our discussion, the process of sleeping and waking seemed obscure and confounding. However, once we examine them in light of the hexagrams *jin* and *mingyi*, these same processes become perfectly clear and obvious in terms of Chinese Medicine theory.

The physiological process of sleeping is important for the health of both the body and the mind. In the present day, more and more people suffer from sleep disorders or insomnia. To treat insomnia, Western physicians usually prescribe sedative drugs, with their side effects and complications. The method the Chinese Medicine physician employs can be intuited from the hexagrams *jin* and *mingyi*. To go from waking to sleep, the patient must undergo a transition parallel to *jin* changing to *mingyi*. If we can actualize the state represented by *mingyi* in the patient, the patient's insomnia will be resolved.

How then, do we create the *mingyi* state in the patient? In a manner of speaking, we must place *Kun* Earth above and *Li* Flame below. We must understand how to handle both the *Kun* and *Li* of the patient in this way. For many years, I have been successfully treating insomnia with Banxia Xiexin Tang, a formula from the Taiyang chapter. We discussed this formula when talking about *pi* and *tai*. It is primarily designed to treat epigastric focal distention, and is most often used today to treat disorders of the stomach and intestines. How is it that a formula originally designed to treat gastrointestinal disorders can be used to treat insomnia? It is because it can create a scenario in which *Kun* Earth is above and *Li* Flame is below. The emperor herb in the formula, Banxia, is able to open up binds and obstructions, allowing the upper and lower to connect and communicate with one another. Once this passageway is open, movement between the upper and the lower is facilitated. Huanglian and Huangqin help to descend the *Li* Flame, while Renshen, Ganjiang, Zhigancao, and Dazao assist the *Kun* Earth to rise. When the *Li* Flame can descend and the *Kun* Earth can rise, the patient naturally regains the ability to sleep soundly. In this way, without sedating the patient, her ability to sleep naturally returns. Imagine if we did not understand the *Classic of Changes*, how could we understand this method of treating insomnia?

When studying the *Classic of Changes*, we must never forget the fundamental importance of the trigrams. The ancients referred to the *Classic of Changes* as "the study of images and words," "the study of images and numbers," and as "the study of images and divining." When studying a hexagram of the *Classic of Changes*, we must consider its underlying principle, its numerical implications, and the image associated with it, as well as what it predicts. If one ignores the image, it will be difficult to make sense of the written commentary. The hexagrams we have just discussed, *jin* and *mingyi*, though relatively simple, would be unintelligible if we did not know what they were an image of. As soon as the image is perceived, the meaning of the hexagram becomes eminently clear, and the student of Chinese Medicine understands its implications.

II.2.b. When the Sun Enters the Earth, This is Taiyin; When It Emerges from the Earth, this is Jueyin

When the sun "enters" the earth, when it disappears below the rim of the horizon, this is an action of Taiyin, for it is Taiyin which opens, allowing the sun to enter. This accords with Chinese Medicine principles, at the very least. Of course, the opening of Taiyin also relies upon the cooperation of Yangming. When the sun emerges from the earth, it does so as a result of Jueyin, but this process is assisted by Taiyang. Taiyin opens and Jueyin closes. Once this opening and closing are understood, *jin* and *mingyi* are easy to understand. And what does the opening and closing of Taiyin and Jueyin rely upon? It is the Shaoyin hinge or pivot. So we can see that in the opening line of the Shaoyin chapter, the line "there is only desire to sleep" is rife with meaning.

What precisely is meant by "only desire to sleep"? It means that the patient wants to sleep all day. If the patient desires to sleep all day, is she able to sleep? Of course not. If she could, she would not want for sleep. Desiring to sleep all day means the patient wishes to sleep, but cannot fall asleep. The patient cannot sleep, she is awake and conscious, but because of the lack of sleep, her mind is foggy and her consciousness impaired. "Only desire to sleep" indicates that both the ability to sleep and the ability to be wakeful are impaired. If we were to describe this deficit in terms of the hexagrams, we could say that the patient is incapable of both the *jin* and *mingyi*. This is because the seat of disease is in the Shaoyin layer, Shaoyin governs the hinge, and so both opening and closing are hobbled. "There is only desire to sleep" reveals the way in which Shaoyin pathology affects the hinge governed by Shaoyin.

In addition, we can discuss difficulty with sleep and wakefulness from the perspective of the heart and kidneys. The state of wakefulness is a state in which yang *qi* is being set free, where the sun is emerging from the earth. The heart rules this state. Sleep is a state in which the sun (the yang *qi*) is being collected and stored and the sun is going back into the earth. This state is ruled by the kidneys. Sleep and waking are indubitably a matter of the heart and kidneys. Let us say that the patient before us is constantly somnolent, desires to sleep but cannot, is also unable to be fully awake, and is beset with listlessness and depression. Such a state indicates that both the heart and kidney are malfunctioning, and both are tending toward debility. If, during the course of an illness, a patient "only desires to sleep" and exhibits a fine, weak pulse, it is a sign that the patient has entered a dangerous place in the course of his pathology. The signs and symptoms listed in the opening outline of the Shaoyin chapter, along with the inherent danger of Shaoyin syndromes generally, are representative characteristics of Shaoyin disease.

II.3. The Form of Shaoyin Disease

Line 281 of the *Treatise on Cold Damage* is very simple. It is easy to miss its full meaning, and Zhang Zhongjing rounds it out with the following line.

Line 282 reads: "Shaoyin disease: the patient wishes to vomit but does not, he is vexed and only desires to sleep. If for five or six days there is spontaneous diarrhea and thirst, this is Shaoyin disease. Because the patient is deficient, he keeps drinking water and the symptoms improve. The urine appears clear. These are the signs of Shaoyin disease. The urine is clear because the lower burner is deficient and cold and unable to control water; this is what causes it to lose its color." I would like to examine line 282 further, and supplement two aspects of the opening outline of the chapter.

II.3.a. Vexation with the Desire to Sleep

There is something that, with even a cursory reading, stands out in line 282 of the *Treatise on Cold Damage*. In the *Treatise on Cold Damage*, vexation (*xinfan* 心煩) is consistently connected with insomnia. For instance, in line 61: "During the day, the patient is vexed and agitated and cannot sleep"; in line 71: "There is dryness in the stomach, the patient is vexed and agitated and cannot sleep"; in line 76: "There is vexation from deficiency and the patient cannot sleep"; in line 303: "The heart is vexed, the patient cannot recline"; and in line 319: "The heart is vexed, the patient cannot sleep." The examples go on and on. Vexation is very closely related to insomnia, and in fact, might be in a cause-and-effect relationship with one another. However, contrary to the trend, this situation is reversed in line 282. Instead, vexation is accompanied by a desire to sleep. In my opinion, this change in the trend must indicate a change in the underlying cause, so here we will explore the connection between vexation and a desire to sleep to better understand this cause.

II.3.a.1. What Is Vexation?

What sort of thing is vexation (*fan* 煩)? When the person is vexed, they feel disquieted but, as this is an internal feeling, exhibit no sign of this disquiet; this is why vexation is also known as "heart vexation" (*xinfan* 心煩). However, as soon as this internal unrest extends to the external body, and the body itself becomes restless, we refer to this as "vexation and restlessness" (*fanzao* 煩躁). Vexation means that the heart and spirit are unsettled; there is disorder in the heart and spirit. What causes vexation? If we look at the construction of the Chinese character *fan* (煩), we see the fire radical (火) on the left, and *ye* (頁), a character meaning "head," on the right.

Explaining Writing and Analyzing Characters explains *fan* as a "hot head-ache." The construction of the character might lead us to guess as much. This is not, however, the way in which we interpret the meaning of this character in our current discussion, but it is not terribly different. The head represents the top of the body, and together with the radical for fire, it indicates that fire is afflicting the uppermost portion of the body. Fire is floating upward, and this is what is causing the affliction.

The *jin* hexagram we just discussed has fire in the superior position. *Jin* is waking, just as the *mingyi* hexagram is sleeping. *Jin* does not sleep. This explains why *fan* is so strongly associated with insomnia.

II.3.a.2. Return to the Root: Stillness

When the fire reaches upward, vexation easily arises. To remedy this malady, the fire must return to the root. Why is the interaction of the heart and kidney emphasized so strongly in Chinese Medicine? The interaction of the kidneys and the heart, their mutual dependence, depends upon the kidney water to calm the heart fire, to prevent it from flaring too high and return it to the root (*guigen* 歸根). This is one aspect of it.

From another perspective, as we know from our discussion of the hexagram *mingyi*, that to restrain fire from flaring upward, the action of Taiyin spleen earth is of equally great importance. When the fire flares upward, the person becomes vexed. To be without vexation is to be quiet and still (*jing* 靜). In the case of *fan* and *jing*, we once again see the union of water and earth.

Chapter 16 of Laozi's *Classic of the Dao and Its Virtue* reads: "Creatures teem and multiply, and each returns to its root. Return to the root means stillness; to be still means to return to life endowment; to return to life endowment means constancy; to know constancy means to be illuminated. If one does not know constancy, one becomes reckless and fiendish." To return to the root, to become still, is of utmost importance. If we examine human beings, indeed all living things, how do they "return to the root"? How do they restore themselves? "Return to the root means stillness." If we look at the twenty-four hours of the day, what time of the day is quiet and still? The quiet time is when we are sleeping. When a person sleeps, it is a sort of return to the root, a type of quieting. It is this quiet that allows us to return to our life endowment. For this reason, every day we have an opportunity to replenish ourselves. Otherwise, how would we be able to go on living?

The topic of a scientific article in the *Reference News* published on November 8, 2000 was "Insufficient Sleep Decreases Longevity." In that article, we read: "Recent research has demonstrated that insufficient sleep is as much a menace to health as improper nutrition and lack of exercise. Both insufficient sleep and lack of sufficient sleep during the night can seriously damage your health." This article based its findings on experiments performed on monkeys. The monkeys were deprived of sleep during the times that they tend to sleep. The health of these deprived monkeys quickly declined, and the monkeys perished. Of course, this research says nothing new to the Chinese Medicine physician.

Earlier, when we discussed the working mechanism of yin and yang, it was clear that sleep is when the yang *qi* is retrieved and stored, and renewed in the process. Although sleeping is not like eating, where the material provisions of the body are clearly being ingested, sleep hygiene may be even more important than that of food. When we eat, we can wolf an entire meal down in just a few minutes if we want, but sleep is not consumed like food or drink. Its quantity is measured in time and when we take sleep; it takes hours, not minutes.

Sleep is a means of restoring the life force, life's natural vigor. Without this reinvigoration, life cannot continue. Both Chinese and Western Medicine recognize sleep as a key to longevity. When we sleep, the yang *qi* is being retrieved and stored in the yin regions, where the root is located. Sleep is the process whereby the yang returns to the root. When we raise the quality of our sleep, we also raise the degree to which the yang returns to the root. If the return to the root is good, then longevity is ensured. Quality sleep improves not only the quality of our life, but also its length. The *Yellow Emperor's Classic* says: "As for the yang *qi*, if it is quieted it will be stored in the spirit, if it is restless it is frittered away." This tells us that the process of returning to one's life endowment is the process of storing the spirit. The Daoists say: "To return to life endowment means constancy; to know constancy means to be illuminated." In Chinese Medicine, it is said: "The spirit is stored and so the ruler is bright. If the ruler is bright and clear, there is peace below. To nourish life on the basis of this results in longevity." Daoism and Chinese Medicine are one in their view of the world.

II.3.a.3. Sleeping Is the Great Return to the Root, Inhalation Is the Small Return to the Root

Sleep is the great or large return to the root, but there is also a small return to the root, and this is the inhalation of breath. The breath is a very mysterious process, but this process is ultimately one of yin and yang. Humans are constantly breathing, every minute in every hour. Long ago, Ananda, the most learned disciple of the Buddha, asked the Buddha Siddhartha to conceptualize life and death. The Buddha responded by saying that the time between life and death is like a moment between exhalation and inhalation. We can also frame the question of life and death in terms of yin and yang, and it may be a more apt way to describe life and death, for inhalation and exhalation are also yin and yang.

When we exhale, this is a yang process, and when we inhale, it is a yin one. Yin is form and yang function. If we inhale deeply, our exhalation will be long, and if we exhale completely, our inhalation becomes deep. This embodies the form and function of yin and yang, their mutually engendering relationship, and also clearly embodies the concept of "Yang births and yin grows, yang kills and yin stores." Exhalation is yang, yang is release; it is the functional aspect. Inhalation is yin, yin is receiving and storing; it is saving up. Those who have practiced Chinese martial arts know that when exerting great force, it is fitting to exhale. It is almost impossible to exert such force while inhaling. Prior to such exertion, however, a deep breath is almost always necessary. Even if we have never practiced Chinese martial arts, the relationship of exhalation to an act of great exertion is familiar to anyone. In any case, categorizing inhalation and exhalation in terms of yin and yang, form and function is profoundly revealing.

Both Daoist and yogic exercises focus on the importance of the breath. In *Zhuangzi*, we learn of "heel breathing" (*zhongxi* 踵息) which refers to the practice of very deep breathing. This sort of long, deep breathing is also given the technical term "breathing to return to the root." If this technique is mastered and the student attains a strong foundation, he will be able to stand firmly. Mastering breath is the foundation of Daoist practices. Breathing practices are in fact a way of returning to the root. Returning to the root is a means of attaining quietude. For this reason, deep breathing allows us to enter into a state of greater calm. If we take the inverse as an example, how deep is our breathing when we are running about, troubled, or confused? At such times, our breathing is not deep at all; it is fast and shallow. Breathing long and deep has a powerful calming effect. Those who suffer from insomnia would benefit from deep breathing exercises before bed, to quiet their minds and return to the root.

Deep breathing quiets us; it returns us to the root and preserves our bodies. When the form is made substantial, the function becomes strong. After quietude, our vigor is renewed. The "return to life endowment" is a functional process. Deep breathing affects not only the form but also increases the functional capacity. It is an excellent method for restoring both the form and the function, the body and its utilization, yin and yang. The ancients said: "The great Dao is not complicated." Taking a deep breath is not complicated, but the great Dao can be found within it. The way we breathe should not be regarded as inconsequential.

Among the common people of China, a very graphic way of referring to a person's longevity is "the number of breaths." If you have not used up all of your breaths, you may yet live for a time. If you have used up all your breaths, your life is near its end. What is meant by the "number of breaths"? It is very simple: it is the number of times a person inhales and exhales in the course of their life. The number of breaths allotted to an individual is commensurate to the length of his or her life. Of course, not all persons are bestowed with the same number of breaths. This concept is a little bit like the longevity of an electrical switch. When you purchase an electrical switch and look in its accompanying manual, there you may find that the manufacturer gives a standard number of times that the switch can be turned on and off before failing, perhaps 30,000 times. Such a number may be accompanied by a guarantee for replacement of the switch should it fail before being flipped 30,000 times. If the switch has already been used more than 30,000 times, the manufacturer will not replace it, for it has outlived its intended period of use. Let us assume the average lifespan of a human being to be 72 years. If the average frequency of breaths per minute is fifteen, then we breath 21,600 times per day; and if we calculate one year as having 360 days, then we get 7,776,000 times a year. If we multiply this number by 72, we arrive at an average number of breaths per human life: 559,872,000. This is the average "number of breaths" bestowed upon a person.

There is more than meets the eye with this number. Let us say that each breath takes half the time of a normal breath. In that case, the person would live only thirty-six years, half the average. Why is it that athletes that participate in vigorous sports, such as soccer, tend to live shorter lives than average? For the very same reason: they breathe faster while playing. If, on the other hand, we can be like Laozi and return to the root with each breath, so that we breathe only at half the normal rate, say seven or eight times a minute, then we can greatly extend our lives. We may not be able to double the average life span, but we can certainly extend our life. If it were not so, how would Daoists dare to utter the words: "My fate lies with me, not with heaven"?

"Heel breathing" is the small return to the root; to return to the root means to quiet, to not be vexed. Without vexation, we can retire into sleep. Sleep is the great return to the root, and thus the great quiet is attained whereby we renew our life force. We can see that this is a process of the small return guiding the large return. It is as the Buddha said: life and death are like a moment between inhaling and exhaling. If life and death are a matter of breath, then we might as well start with the breath in our attempt to comprehend life and death. As the Chinese proverb says: "If the noble person recognizes the importance of breath, he will be able to swim through the sea of life and death." I believe this proverb to be true.

II.3.a.4. With Vexation, Desire to Sleep Is Unexpected

As we discussed, vexation is the result of fire not returning to the root; it is the fire *qi* floating upward. When the fire *qi* rises up in this way, and vexation occurs, we expect the patient to be unable to sleep, and would not expect the patient to desire to sleep. In the preceding discussion, several lines were quoted to illustrate the connection between vexation and insomnia. Vexation is the cause, and insomnia the result. However, here in the Shaoyin chapter, vexation and a desire to sleep occur together. This contradictory presentation indicates that the disease is unusual; it is not an ordinary illness. The desire to sleep that accompanies vexation in this instance is not ordinary fatigue, nor is it simple insomnia. Vexation indicates that the true yang is on the loose and ascending upward. A desire to sleep, on the other hand, indicates that the heart fire is weakened and deficient, and the consciousness is therefore clouded; this is a sign of the impending debilitation of both the kidney and the heart. The occurrence of these seemingly contradictory symptoms together is an important indicator of Shaoyin disease. These contradictory symptoms allow the physician to differentiate this from the more common presentation of vexation with insomnia.

II.3.b. Thirsty but the Urine Is Pale in Color

In the *Treatise on Cold Damage*, there are many lines devoted to thirst. Generally speaking, this thirst is the result of heat having damaged the fluids. The typical sign that presents in relation to this damage to the fluids and subsequent thirst is concentrated yellow urine or even short voiding of reddish urine. In line 282, however, the patient is thirsty but, rather than having yellow urine, the urine is pale in color. In other words, the patient has both thirst and copious clear urine. How is this so? As it explains in line 282, this is a case when "The urine is clear because the lower burner is deficient and cold and unable to control water; this is what causes it to lose its color." Here we have another contradictory presentation, one that is also an important indicator of Shaoyin disease.

If we examine earlier chapters in the book, we find instances of thirst. For instance, in the Taiyang chapter, there is a discussion of thirst in relation to Wuling San. For instance, in line 71 it says: "If the pulse is floating, the urine inhibited, and the patient suffers from slight heat and dispersion-thirst, Wuling San governs the treatment." In Taiyang disease, thirst is accompanied by scanty urination and a floating pulse. Thirst is an even more salient symptom in the Yangming chapter. Thirst is an important part of both Baihu Tang and Baihu Jia Renshen Tang syndromes. This is severe thirst, and the patient will drink liters of water in an effort to slake it. Despite this copious ingestion of fluids, the voiding of urine is short and yellow. Thirst also appears in Shaoyang disease, and some of the modifications to Xiao Chaihu Tang specifically mention thirst. In line 147, thirst is mentioned in relation to Chaihu Guizhi Ganjiang Tang syndrome. In this instance of thirst, the urine is also scanty. All three of the yang diseases exhibit thirst, but in each, thirst is accompanied by other symptoms, and the mechanism that causes the thirst is different in each case. Once we arrive at three yin disease, the situation is different. In the discussion of Taiyin disease, there is a line devoted to the discussion of this particular topic. Line 277 reads: "When there is spontaneous diarrhea but no thirst, this is a sign of Taiyin disease." In the Shaoyin chapter, the discussion of thirst begins again in line 282: "When after five or six days there is spontaneous diarrhea and thirst, this is Shaoyin disease." The presence of thirst clearly distinguishes between the "spontaneous diarrhea" of Taiyin and the same in Shaoyin disease. In the Jueyin disease chapter, thirst is the chief feature of the opening line, the outline of Jueyin disease. If we take all six of the conformations of disease into account, we see that only Taiyin disease is without thirst, and this lack of thirst is a key feature of Taiyin disease. Today most clinicians, when presented with thirst, immediately prescribe Huafen, Maidong, or other herbs that similarly benefit the yin and nourish the fluids. Is this a good habit? Of course not! If the patient's thirst is the advent of Yangming disease, then nourishing the yin and generating fluids would be in fitting with the presenting syndrome. If, however, the disease is Shaoyin, then nourishing the yin and generating fluids is a complete mistake!

III. The Timing of Shaoyin Disease

The time that corresponds with Shaoyin is indicated by line 291 of the *Treatise on Cold Damage*: "Shaoyin disease tends to resolve in the time from *zi* to *yin*." This time period is composed of *zi*, *chou*, and *yin*. In terms of our modern clock, this period of time is from 11 pm until 5 am of the following day. In the lunar cycle, it is the seven-and-a-half days from the reappearance of the moon until its first quarter. In the lunar calendar, it is the three months from the eleventh month of one year through the first month of the following year. Below, I will discuss the time correspondence of Shaoyin from two different perspectives.

III.1. *Zi* Is *Fu* (Turning Back)

III.1.a. In Seven Days Comes the Return

There is an important difference between the time periods that correspond with the three yin disease conformations and those that correspond with the three yang disease conformations. Among the three yin conformations, each time span that is correlated with the resolution of the yin disease in question shares two of its two-hour time periods with one of the other conformations. Taiyin disease corresponds with *hai*, *zi*, and *chou*, and both the *zi* and *chou* periods are shared with the time in which Shaoyin disease tends to resolve. Likewise, the time in which Shaoyin disease tends to resolve is the time period consisting of *zi*, *chou*, and *yin*; both *chou* and *yin* are shared with the time period in which Jueyin disease tends to resolve. This arrangement makes the first two-hour period of the time when the disease tends to resolve seem especially significant. Taiyin begins with *hai*, Shaoyin with *zi*, and Jueyin with the earthly branch *chou*.

With regard to the twelve tidal hexagrams, the *zi* earthly branch corresponds with the hexagram *fu* (Turning Back). The description of the *fu* hexagram reads: "*Fu*: Returning. Pushing through. Coming and going without haste. When a friend comes, there is no fault. The Dao of falling away and turning back, in seven days comes the return. It is beneficial to have somewhere to go." The hexagram *fu* indicates the return of the yang *qi*, its recuperation and renewal. The recuperation of the yang requires seven days, thus it says: "The Dao of falling away and turning back, in seven days comes the return." Why does it require seven days? An examination of the twelve tidal hexagrams makes the answer clear. According to the *qimen dunjia* method of divination, the twelve tidal hexagrams divide up into yin and yang categories. The hexagrams *fu*, *lin*, *tai*, *dazhuang*, *guai*, and *qian* belong to the category of yang, for in these hexagrams, yang is in the process of increasing. On the other hand, the hexagrams *gou*, *dun*, *pi*, *guan*, *bo*, and *kun* are yin in nature, and in the progression of these hexagrams, we witness the steady increase of yin. After the yang progression is complete, the yin progression begins with the hexagram *gou*. If we regard each hexagram in this succession as a single day, the entire course of yin's increase takes exactly six days. When this yin progression concludes, the cycle returns to the beginning of yang's increase at the hexagram *fu*. From the last of the yin hexagrams to the first of the yang hexagrams takes seven days, just as it says in the explanation of the hexagram *fu*: "The Dao of falling away and turning back, in seven days comes the return." In the same way, it takes seven days for the yin to recover. Thus, seven is the number of repeating processes. The seven-day week is not purely a custom imported from the West. Seven was also the number of the cycle in the *Classic of Changes*. If we look at the passage and transmutation of the six disease conformations according to the chapter "Treatise on Heat" in the *Yellow Emperor's Classic*, we see that on the first day the disease enters Taiyang, the second it enters Yangming, the third it enters Shaoyang, the fourth Taiyin, the fifth Shaoyin, and the sixth Jueyin. After the sixth day, the seventh day the disease returns to Taiyang. In the *Treatise on Cold Damage*, the periodicity of the cycle in which disease moves from one conformation to the next is also seven.

III.1.b. At the Winter Solstice, the One Yang Emerges

The part of the lunar calendar ruled by the hexagram *fu* contains within it a very important node *qi* (*jieqi*), the *dongzhi* (winter solstice). Although the *fu* hexagram is associated with the eleventh month of the lunar calendar, strictly speaking the *qi* of the *fu* hexagram does not find expression until the winter solstice. The "one yang" of the winter solstice is also the "one yang" of the hexagram *fu*.

The hexagram *fu* consists of the trigram *Kun* Earth above and *Zhen* Thunder below. In other words, the earth's thunder returns. On the image of the hexagram, we read: "Thunder within the earth is *fu*. The kings of old closed their borders when the solstice arrived, and traveling merchants could not move about." Here, "solstice" refers to the winter solstice. The former sovereigns closed their borders during this time precisely because this was when the "one yang" was nascent; it was the return of the yang *qi*, the time when the yang *qi* returned to the root, when yin transformed into yang. If this return of the cycle, this transition from yin to yang is successful, the next turn of the cycle will be smooth. Closing the borders, closing off the outside world and closing in that which is internal is an excellent method for ensuring the success of this transition. When the borders are closed, the domain is quieted. When the borders are closed, a whole host of vexing issues disappear, allowing the transition from one cycle to the next to proceed smoothly. In fact, it is not only during the winter solstice that we should close the borders, but also during the summer solstice. Thus, according to the *Book of the Later Han* section titled "Account of Lu Gong": "According to the *Classic of Changes*, in the fifth month when the forces exemplified by the tidal hexagram *gou* are in power, the kings of old ordered that movement in every corner of the kingdom should cease." During the fifth month, when the summer solstice takes place, it is the time of the hexagram *gou* (Encountering). The order to cease all movement in the four corners of the kingdom is identical in its implications to "The kings of old closed their borders when the solstice arrived, and traveling merchants could not move about." Every seventh period marks the return. Thus, it is not only during the winter solstice that the borders should be closed, but also at the summer solstice. In this way, the transition from yin to yang and from yang back to yin can proceed with grace and care.

The earthly branches *zi* and *wu* are the eleventh and the fifth months respectively. In the course of the day, these earthly branches correspond to the two two-hour periods: between eleven and one in the middle of the day, and eleven to one in the middle of the night. During these two time periods, it is advisable to "close the borders" as well. How do we close off the outside world in the middle of the day? We can take a little rest, or sit quietly, or take a nap. The Chinese custom of taking a nap at midday stretches all the way back to the Zhou dynasty. Those who mistakenly think that taking a nap at midday has no health benefits clearly have little understanding of the *Classic of Changes*.

III.1.c. The Essentials of the Time in Which Shaoyin Disease Tends to Resolve

The earthly branch *zi* resides in the north; it is the place of water and form. The yang function returns to the root in order to return to the interior of the form, the body. This return to the interior allows the body to recuperate. The *zi* period marks the return, when the yang *qi* begins to slowly increase. In Shaoyin disease, the yang *qi* is weakened and deficient and the yang does not return to the root. When the time period of *zi*, *chou*, and *yin* is entered, it precisely the time when yang *qi* has returned to the root and begins to recuperate. This time period contains the process of the gradual recovery of the yang *qi*; it is little wonder that the deficiency and weakness of yang *qi* in Shaoyin disease will therefore tend to recover. This is the effect of the larger cosmic trend assisting the human organism to overcome a pathological process. This is evidence that "Humans are born of the *qi* of heaven and earth."

An important formula for treating Shaoyin disease is Sini Tang. As we discussed in the Taiyin chapter, the "emperor herb" in this formula is Zhigancao. Zhigancao is sweet and neutral, and best embodies the *qi* of earth. Therefore, it is associated with the trigram *Kun* Earth. Ganjiang and Fuzi are warm, pungent, and hot. Their *qi* is that of thunder, the trigram associated with them is the *Zhen* Thunder trigram. In Sini Tang, dried ginger and aconite act as the minister and emissary herbs. The emperor is above and the minister below, the trigram *Kun* Earth is above and the trigram *Zhen*

Thunder below, so we have the hexagram *fu*, consisting of earth above and thunder below. In this way, Sini Tang and its derivatives correlate perfectly with the time in which Shaoyin disease tends to resolve.

III.2. Why Resolving Covers Three Two-Hour Periods

Above, our discussion emphasized the *zi* time period, in which Shaoyin disease tends to resolve. It is not only this one period in which Shaoyin disease tends to resolve, but all three of the time periods *zi, yin,* and *chou*. Although the *zi* time period is especially significant to the resolution of Shaoyin disease, we must still pay attention to the fact that there are three time periods associated with its resolution. Why three? This invites a look at Chinese numerology.

Three has its own unique qualities and characteristics. In the third chapter of the *Plain Questions*, "Treatise on the Vital *Qi* Connecting to Heaven," it says: "its nature is five, its *qi* is three." In Chapter 9 of the *Plain Questions*, the "Treatise on the Six Nodes and Visceral Manifestations," we read: "Five days make up a *hou*, three *hou* make up a *qi*." Thus, *qi* consists of three. The year is made up of four seasons, and each season consists of three months. Three is also the number of the seasons. The trigrams of the *Classic of Changes* consist of three lines each. There are three Dao, the Dao of heaven, of earth, and of man. In the *Classic of the Dao and Its Virtue*, Laozi says: "The Dao produces the one, the one produces two, the two produce three, and the three generate the myriad things." We have already discussed how seasons and directions are one and the same. If seasons are tripartite, so too are directions. *Hai, zi,* and *chou* make up the northern direction; *yin, mao,* and *chen* make up the eastern direction; *si, wu,* and *wei* the south; and *shen, you,* and *xu* the west. Each direction is made up of three parts. Why did Chinese Medicine develop from single-herb formulas into compound ones? It is because each direction (*fang* 方, the same character meaning formula) cannot be summed up by a single flavor, but rather requires several herbs to form an entire direction; for the same reason, each time period in which disease has a tendency to resolve consists of three parts. One time period on its own does not make for a direction; only three times, combined, constitutes a complete direction. If the direction is complete, the *qi* is also complete. Only if the *qi* is complete can it resolve the disease.

Another important aspect of the number three is the concept of three combinations. The five elements can be used to categorize the earthly branches: *yin* and *mao* are wood; *si* and *wu* are fire; *shen* and *you* are metal; *hai* and *zi* are water; and *chen, xu, chou,* and *wei* are earth. Besides these pairings, they can also be organized according to the three unities (*sanhe* 三合). What are the three unities? *Hai, mao,* and *wei* are united with wood; *yin, wu,* and *xu* are united with fire, *si, you,* and *chou* are joined with metal; and *shen, zi,* and *chen* are joined with water. In this way, three earthly branches are joined with a single element, and these combinations of three branches act as one of the five elements. The concept of the three unions is extremely important. As we can see, within wood, fire, metal, and water, we find the earthly branches *chen, xu, chou,* and *wei.* These four branches actually constitute the earth element. Earlier when we discussed the five elements, we talked about how metal, wood, water, and fire cannot be complete without earth. When discussing how the spleen does not rule a season of its own, we also talked about how the transition from one of the four seasons to the next cannot occur without earth. The reason for this should be clear from the perspective of the combinations of three.

The implications of these unities of three are many. For instance, in the clinic, we can speak of water being deficient or fire deficient, but we may hesitate to tonify the patient's water or fire. As soon as we tonify water, the patient's spleen and stomach suffer. As soon as an effort to rebuild the patient's fire is undertaken, the patient may suffer from mouth sores. The reason for these thwarted efforts may lie in the time at which the effort to tonify is undertaken. If we keep the three two-hour time periods and their pertinent element in mind, I do not believe that we will encounter this problem. For instance, water should be tonified during the period of *shen, zi,* and *chen;* fire during *yin, wu,* and *xu;* wood during *hai, mao,* and *wei;* and metal during *si, you,* and *chou.*

IV. Contemplating Alzheimer's Disease

Alzheimer's disease is the most common form of senile dementia. Among the elderly, Alzheimer's disease is the most prevalent disease of the central nervous system. In North America and Australia, there is a morbidity between 6.6 and 15.8 percent. In the past, it was believed that morbidity of Alzheimer's in China was lower than that of the West, but a comprehensive study in 1995 revealed that the prevalence of the disease is roughly the same in China and the West. This survey revealed that, in Beijing, the rate of Alzheimer's morbidity among those above 56 years old was 2.3 percent. Every increase in five years of age was accompanied by a doubling in the rate of morbidity. Among those over 70, the rate of Alzheimer's was 5.3 percent. In those over 75, the rate was 11.9 percent, and in those over 80, 22 percent. According to the *Health Report* of November 6, 2000, by the same year, there were 80 million people in China over the age of 65, so there were at least 5 million persons in China suffering from Alzheimer's.

Modern science considers Alzheimer's to be a chronic, irreversible disease. At the present, no effective method of curing or preventing the disease has been found. Once the disease is present, the disease progresses inexorably, until the patient is dead. The twenty-first century is the century of modernization in China, but it is also the century of the elderly. In the metropolitan areas of China, there has been a one-child policy in place since 1978. This policy will inevitably result in a situation where two children are responsible for four parents. If one of the elderly parents develops Alzheimer's, the situation for the entire family will be unbearable. The negative impact Alzheimer's disease exerts on Chinese society increases day-by-day; so too does the importance of finding effective medical methods to treat and prevent the disease.

As Chinese Medicine physicians, how do we view Alzheimer's disease? Can Alzheimer's disease be cured? I am optimistic about the answer to that last question. Alzheimer's disease, from the perspective of the six conformations, is a Shaoyin disease. In the initial stages, Alzheimer's disease is characterized by loss of memory, which progresses to loss of consciousness. As we discussed earlier, memory is a function of the heart and kidney. The kidneys rule hibernation, and so the storing of memory is ruled by the kidney. Recalling memory is a process of drawing up. This sort of process is a release of what has been stored, and is akin to the release of *qi* we witness in summer. Impediments to memory and recall represent impediments to the function of the heart and kidney, and impediment to the normal functioning of Shaoyin. The loss of spirit (*shen*) and will (*zhi*) are even more closely related to the heart and kidney, for they are ruled by the heart and kidney respectively.

The earmark of Shaoyin disease is a fine, faint pulse and desire to sleep (*mei* 寐). We have already discussed *mei* in terms of sleep, opposite to wakefulness. This is only one facet of *mei*. There is another facet to the meaning of this Chinese character, as illustrated in *Kangxi Dictionary's* definition: "*Mei* means to be lost; not bright." What mental state is characterized by senile dementia? It might best be characterized as "lost and dark." If this were not the case, how could explain the inability to name one's own children, or remember the home in which one has lived for many years? Since senile dementia is undoubtedly a state of *mei*, we must consider it from the perspective of Shaoyin disease. Shaoyin disease is certainly grave, but there are ways to reverse or counteract this grave disease. It would be well worthwhile to research and explore the Alzheimer's disease from the perspective of Shaoyin disease.

CHAPTER TEN

THE ESSENTIALS OF JUEYIN DISEASE

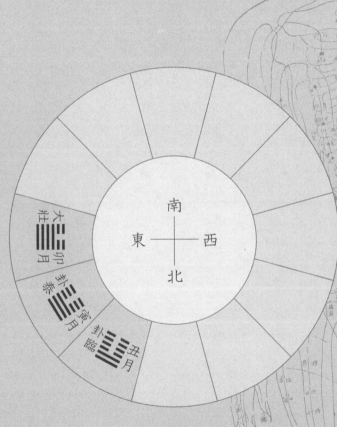

Jueyin disease tends to
resolve in the time from *chou* to *mao*.

I. An Explanation of Jueyin

I.1. The Meaning of Jueyin

Jueyin is the last of the six conformations in *Treatise on Cold Damage*. What does Jueyin mean? Let us first examine this problem from the perspective of its basic meaning. In the "Great Treatise on the Essentials of Ultimate Truth" in the *Plain Questions*, we have this exchange: "The Emperor said: What is Jueyin? Qi Bo replied: The two yin exchange completely." What is meant by the "two yin"? The "two yin" refers to Taiyin and Shaoyin. The arrangement of the *Treatise on Cold Damage*, placing Jueyin after Taiyin and Shaoyin chapters, also indicates what is meant by "The two yin exchange completely."

Furthermore, in that same chapter of the *Plain Questions*, it says: "The two yin exchange completely, thus it is called *you* (幽)." In the previous line, the completion of the exchange of the two yin is Jueyin, and in this line, the same is referred to as *you*. What does you mean? In *Correct Rhymes* (Zhengyun) it says: "*You* means confinement." Jueyin is *you*, which means that it "confines." What is confined? Earlier, when we discussed the opening and closing, or separation and union of yin and yang, we discussed how Jueyin represents union, or closing. What does it rejoin with or enclose? The yin *qi*. By closing up the yin *qi*, the yang *qi* can rise and emit properly. Thus, *you* refers to the confinement of the yin *qi*.

Third, the *tai* and *shao* of Taiyin and Shaoyin refer to greater and lesser, old and young, numerous and scanty, respectively. What is meant by the *jue* (厥) in Jueyin? In the *Jade Discourse*, it says: "*Jue* means short." In the *Kangxi Dictionary*, it quotes the *Book of the Later Han* as saying: "*Jue* means to pause or stop." Thus, Jueyin is the short yin, it is the paused yin. If we consider Jueyin to be the conformation in which the yin is completed and the yang emerges, in which the yin pauses and the yang grows, then it is fitting to think of Jueyin as the short yin or paused yin. In the *Spiritual Pivot* chapter titled "Yin and Yang as related to the Sun and Moon" (Yinyang xi ri yue), it says that "The tenth month *hai* is Jueyin of the left leg, and the ninth month *xu* is Jueyin of the right leg. Here the two yin exchange completely, so it is referred to as Jueyin." *Xu* and *hai* are the last two of the twelve earthly branches. After *hai* we return to *zi*, the first earthly branch and the return of yang, so this is called Jueyin. That is the basic meaning of Jueyin.

I.2. The Meaning of the Jueyin Channels

The Jueyin channel refers to the hand and foot Jueyin channels. The Jueyin channel of the hand begins at the time of *xu* behind the breast at the acupuncture point Tianchi (PC 1) and terminates when the *xu* period ends at the tip of the middle finger, where the acupuncture point Zhongchong (PC 9) resides. The foot Jueyin channel emerges from the acupuncture point Dadun (LV 1) at the time of *chou* and ends on the ribcage below the breast at Qimen (LV 14) when this same time period concludes. From this point on the chest, it branches up the nape of the neck to join with the Baihui (DU 20) point at the vertex of the head.

Every student of Chinese Medicine should be completely clear about the movements of the six channels and the areas of the body they traverse. When we speak of differentiating a syndrome from the perspective of the six conformations, an important aspect of this differentiation is the differentiation of the course of the channels and their collaterals, as well as the areas of the body into which they penetrate. Why is a headache at the vertex of the head so often thought of as a Jueyin headache? The reason for this is related to the course of the channel.

I.3. The Meaning of the Jueyin Viscera

I.3.a. The Liver

Already in this book, we have looked at the functions and special characteristics of the heart, spleen, lung, and kidney. From this discussion, I hope that all readers have gained a deep appreciation of the relationship between the characteristics of each organ and the construction and etymology of the Chinese characters used to represent them. Now let us look at the liver. What is the relationship between the construction of the character for liver (*gan* 肝) and the particular characteristics and functions of the liver? On the right side of the character for liver, there is the character *gan* (干). *Explaining Writing and Analyzing Characters* says: "*Gan* (干) means to offend or violate." The *Erya* says: "*Gan* means to ward off or protect." The *Kangxi Dictionary* says: "*Gan* is a shield." Thus, in the *Classic of Poetry*, we find the sentence: "*Gan*, halberds and battle-axes," which encompasses all weapons of war. If we look at all of these definitions: "to offend," "to protect or defend," "a shield," "a weapon of war," we see that all the terms are

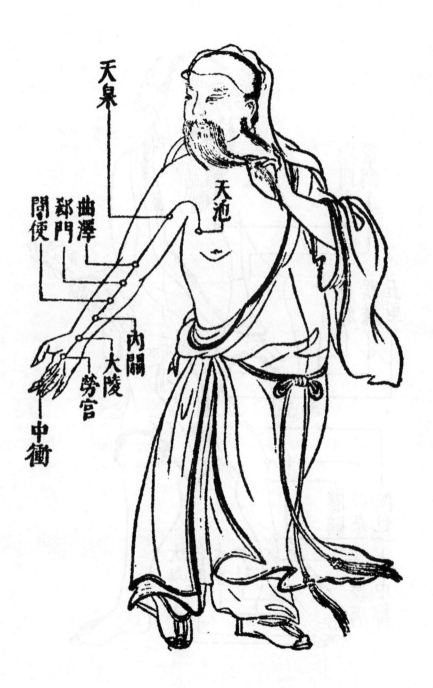

天泉

天池

曲澤
郄門
間使

內關
大陵
勞宮

中衝

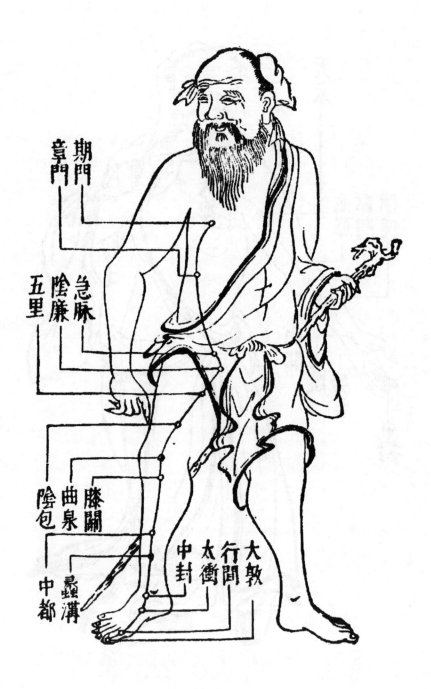

related to warfare. This reminds us of the line in the "Treatise of the Spiritual Orchid Secret Canon" in the *Plain Questions,* where it says: "The liver holds the office of the general. Planning and deliberation originate from it." When it comes to warfare, as was indicated by the character *gan* (干), we look to the general to handle it. The etymology of the character for liver (*gan* 肝) is therefore perfectly fitting to its role as the marshal of the armies, the general, in the body.

I have emphasized several times how important Chapters 8 and 9 of the *Yellow Emperor's Classic* are for the understanding of Chinese Medicine. The former discusses organ network function by utilizing metaphors drawn from society, while the other discusses them from a more directly physiological perspective. In Chapter 8, the "Treatise of the Spiritual Orchid Secret Canon," the liver is called: "The liver holds the office of the general. Planning and deliberation originate from it"; and in Chapter 9, the "Treatise on the Six Nodes and Visceral Manifestations," it says the liver is "The root of dismissal of the ultimate (*baji* 罷極), and the domain of the *hun* soul." Here, what is meant by *ba* is "to cease" or "to end," as we find it referred to in the *Jade Discourse.* Thus, in the *Analects,* we find the phrase: "want to stop but cannot," a phrase which is used even today by modern Chinese speakers. The character *ji* means "ultimate" or "extreme." Military means are used in conflicts between polarized parties; it is polarization that gives rise to the chaos of war. Thus, by getting rid of polarities, the liver also does away with conflicts and chaos. Once war and chaos arise, how are they dismissed? Martial means must be used to subdue war. This is the reason for providing for an army and implementing military means. We can see then that the "general" and the "root of dismissal of the ultimate" are two different ways of saying the same thing.

Extremes are the source of all disorder and chaos. Thus, the ancients spoke of the "six extremes." The *Kangxi Dictionary* says: "The six extremes are evils." In the *Classic of Documents,* we read: "The imposing uses the six extremes. These six are: violent death, disease, despair, poverty, hatred, and weakness." In the Shaoyin chapter, we discussed how the human body has a complex system for dealing with disease and in this system, the spleen, as the official of remonstration, detects if anything is amiss and then warns the heart. The heart, as the sovereign ruler, then determines if the disturbance should be dealt with by softer means or by military means. The liver is the general, the root of dismissing of the ultimate. The liver can employ extreme means, the "six extremes," to calm chaos. This role of the liver in preventing and resolving disease in the body is in agreement with the modern scientific understanding of its function and merits further investigation.

I.3.b. The Pericardium

The Jueyin channel of the foot corresponds with the liver, and that of the hand corresponds with the pericardium. The pericardium is that which encircles the heart. It is a structure that is wound around the heart ruler, and was referred to as the "residence of the heart ruler." The ancient Chinese believed that the heart was the sovereign and ruler, and could not be afflicted by evil influences directly; afflictions directed at the heart were intercepted by the pericardium. The primary purpose of the pericardium was to protect the function of the heart. The liver is the general of the armies that uses the six extremes to settle all disturbances, and also guards the sovereign ruler. We can see that there is a very close relationship between the functions of both the Jueyin organs, the liver and the pericardium.

I.4. The Meaning of the Jueyin in *Yunqi*

In terms of the *yunqi* (the cyclical transformation of universal *qi*), Jueyin is wind in the heavens and wood on earth. Thus, the two are commonly referred to as Jueyin wind and wood. In the following discussion, we will look at the Jueyin *yunqi* in terms of wind and wood.

I.4.a. The Meaning of Wind
I.4.a.1. Wind Is the Envoy of Heaven and Earth

Wind is peculiar among the six *qi* in that it arises not only from the direction with which it has the strongest affinity, namely the east, but can also arise from any of the eight directions, each of which has its own wind. The *Spiritual Pivot* has a chapter titled "Nine Mansions and Eight Winds" (Jiugong bafeng). The main topic of this chapter is the eight types of wind from the eight different directions. The wind from the south is called the "Great Gentle Wind"; from the southwest, it is called the "Scheming Wind"; from the west, it is called the "Strong Wind"; from the northwest, it is called the "Swirling Wind"; from the north, it is called the "Great Strong Wind"; from the northeast, it is called the "Ferocious Wind"; from the east, it is called the "Infant Wind"; and from the southeast, it is called the "Gentle Wind." There are descriptions of various divisions: four winds, or eight winds, or twelve winds, and we can speak of the east wind, or the west wind, or the south wind, but note that Chinese Medicine does not speak of the "east damp" or the "south damp." Nor do we speak of the "eastern cold" or the "northern cold." In this way, wind is different from the other five pathological *qi*.

Another important characteristic of wind can be found in the *River Chart*, where it says: "Wind is the envoy of heaven and earth." What is meant by the "envoy" of heaven and earth? Here, the meaning of envoy is similar to our modern understanding of an ambassador. An ambassador acts as a representative of his or her country. When the *River Chart* says that wind is the envoy of heaven and earth, it means that wind acts as the representative of heaven and earth. Any change in the *qi* of heaven or earth can first be reflected in the wind. For instance, when the weather is about to turn cold, the north wind might blow. When the north wind blows, we know that cold weather is on its way. On the other hand, when the south wind blows, it brings with it warmth and dampness. When the south wind begins to blow, we know that warmth and moisture are on their way. As complex as weather can be, once the forewarnings of the winds are understood, we can begin to glimpse its underpinnings. In the *Rites of Zhou*, we read: "Through examining the harmony of the twelve winds with heaven and earth, one can know signs of good or ill."

According to the *Plain Questions's* "Great Treatise on the Essentials of Ultimate Truth": "The Yellow Emperor said: Praise! As for the advent of the hundred diseases, the all emerge from wind, cold, summer-heat, damp, dryness, and fire and from these they change and transform." This is a key point: it is not simply a small handful of diseases that are caused by these six pathogenic influences, but rather all diseases (here referred to as the "hundred diseases") arise from wind, cold, summer-heat, damp, dryness, and fire. This is true of diseases that are acquired from without as well as those that develop from within, as well as conditions that result from neither external nor internal injury. Why is it that a bout of indigestion resolves without incident on one occasion, but results in vomiting and diarrhea the next? Why does one recover so quickly from a back strain one time, but the next time the same mild strain results in near immobility? The answer lies in our understanding of the six *qi* and their relationship to the changes and transformations of heaven and earth. This alone should incite us to consider the role of the six pathogenic *qi* whenever we are diagnosing a patient. This is why in this passage of the *Plain Questions*, we are entreated to "carefully attend to the appropriate *qi*, and do not miss the disease trigger," and to "Carefully investigate the disease trigger, and do not miss the appropriate *qi*." Here, the "appropriate *qi*" (*qiyi*) are none other than the six *qi*: wind, cold, summer-heat, damp, dryness, and fire. How do we pay close attention to and grasp the appropriate *qi*? If we fully comprehend the implications of wind, it will be possible. If we understand wind, then the six *qi* will be clear to us. Wind is the envoy of heaven and earth, and so it is also the envoy of the six *qi*. Why does the *Yellow Emperor's Classic* reiterate the role of wind in disease in lines such as: "Wind is the chief of the hundred diseases," and "Wind is the inception of the hundred diseases"? It is because all disease results from the six pathogenic *qi*, and wind is the envoy of these six *qi*.

I.4.a.2. How Wind Produces Wood

In a number of chapters of the *Plain Questions*, we find the adage: "The east produces wind and the wind produces wood." Although wind is the envoy of heaven and earth as well as the envoy of the six *qi*, although it can come from any of the eight directions, we should keep in mind that the original position of wind is in the east. How does wind produce wood? What is the relationship between wind and wood? Why is the *yunqi* of Jueyin described in terms of wind and wood? I do not know if the reader has spent time contemplating these questions before.

Let us begin by looking at five-element classification, and identify what things belong to the category of wood. In the *Classic of Documents*, we read that "Wood refers to that which bends and straightens," but this explanation is too theoretical. In more concrete terms, all plants can be referred to as "wood," all belong to the category of wood. What then is the relationship between wind and wood? This relationship is very close. First, let us consider how it is that plants are able to reproduce and propagate, and how, in short, they are able to persist. Animals reproduce through the copulation of males with females. When animals are in heat, they can run long distances to find a mate. People are no different. They may travel great distances to encounter their beloved, and often the result is not merely the sharing of affection, but also reproduction. Animals, including humans, move about to find their mates.

What about plants? Plants are fixed in place by their roots. They cannot traipse about courting, nor can they cross the ocean to marry. Plants depend upon the wind to find their "beloved," to mix male with female. It is the wind that carries the pollen from plant to plant, allowing for copulation and reproduction. It is for this reason that wind is the most important factor in the ability of plants to reproduce and multiply. We might go so far as to say that without wind, plants could not reproduce and persist in the world. The close connection between wind and wood is one of necessity. The sentence in the *Plain Questions* that reads: "The east produces wind and wind produces wood," expresses the closeness of this relationship perfectly.

I.4.a.3. Wind and Animals

Wind's relationship to plants and to wood is undeniable. But what is the relationship between wind and animals? If we look at the traditional character for wind (*feng* 風), we see that the character contains the radical *chong* (虫). In classical Chinese, there are three different ways of writing the character *chong*, but each of them represents an animal. Any creature belonging to the category of animals could be called a *chong*. The use of this radical in the character for wind (*feng*) indicates a close relationship between animals and wind. In *Explaining Writing and Analyzing Characters*, it says: "The wind moves, the creatures (*chong*) are born, thus creatures change every eight days." The wind is also clearly connected to the reproduction of animals as well as plants. In the simplified Chinese, the character for wind (风) is written without the *chong* radical. This radical is replaced with the simple radical *yi* (メ). The richness of the original etymology is lost with this simplification.

The mutual love, attraction, and arousal of the sexes is referred to as "wind," thus when "The wind moves, the creatures are born." The Chinese phrase indicating that two things will have nothing to do with one another, "the wind between a horse and a cow" (*feng ma niu* 風馬牛) derives its meaning from the fact that a cow and a horse, regardless of whether either is in heat, share no attraction for one another. In the phrase "The wind moves, the creatures are born," the term for "creatures" (*chong*), physiologically speaking, refers to the spermatozoa of the male animal. In the rural areas of China, you can sometimes hear the cries of a cat in heat. These howling cats are sometimes referred to by the peasants as "spring cats," or it is said that the cats are "yelling spring." Why is the word "spring" used? The east produces wind, integral with the *qi* of spring. During the three months of spring, heaven and earth and the myriad creatures produce and spread and are filled with vitality. Hopefully, this look at the Chinese concept of wind will provide some clinical insight.

I.4.b. The Meaning of Wood

I.4.b.1. Wood Refers to That Which Bends and Straightens

The first meaning of wood can be considered in light of the phrase from the *Classic of Documents*: "Wood refers to that which bends and straightens." Bent and straight, or bending and straightening, are characteristics of wood; none of the other elements, such as metal or water, possess the bending and straightening properties of wood. In the *Plain Questions's* "Great Treatise on the Correspondences of Yin and Yang," we read: "The east produces wind, wind produces wood, wood produces sourness, sourness creates the liver, the liver generates the tendons." It also says: "In the sky, the spirit is wind, on earth it is wood, in the body it is the tendons, among the viscera it is the liver." Thus, in the body, both the tendons and the liver are characterized by "bending and straightening." This is clear in the case of the tendons, they orchestrate the bending and straightening of the joints of the body. Without tendons, our bodies would not be able to move as they do. The tendons animate the joints and we find the tendons on or around the joints of the body. The tendons are largest and most prominent at the knee, and the knee is referred to in the *Yellow Emperor's Classic* as the "palace of the tendons." Wood is straightening and bending; in the body, wood is the tendons. The function of the tendons is beautifully resonant with this definition of wood.

Another aspect worth looking at is the "ancestral tendon" referred to in many chapters of the *Plain Questions*. The term "ancestral tendon" (*zongjin* 宗筋) is rich in meaning. One of its meanings is the external genitalia, or more specifically, the penis. The *Spiritual Pivot* chapter "Five Sounds and Five Flavors" (Wuyin wuwei) can shed light on the significance of the ancestral tendon: "When a eunuch loses his ancestral tendon, his penetrating vessel is damaged." The palace eunuchs of the past were castrated prior to entering the palace. It is this castration that is referred to as losing his "ancestral tendon." This implied meaning of "ancestral tendon" brings us back to our former discussion of wind. Wind is that which induces the bull and the cow to copulate, wind brings about the reproduction and multiplication of animals, and the ancestral tendon is the most salient reproductive organ. From the wind of heaven to the wood of earth to the tendons of the body to organ of the liver, we see that it is as Laozi said: "Humans take the earth as model; the earth takes the heavens as model; the heavens take the Dao as model; the Dao takes nature as model." This discussion provides clear evidence of the holistic relationship between heaven and humans.

According to the *Record of Rites*: "Spring acts as birth; the birthing and abundant virtue of heaven is in the position of wood." This brilliant line reveals that the life and overflowing virtue bestowed upon us by heaven are located in the wood element. Wood rules the ancestral tendon, and this is in keeping with the location of "abundant virtue." In order for the ancestral tendon to function properly, it is crucial that it is able to straighten from a bent position. Nowadays, erectile dysfunction is an increasing problem. Erectile dysfunction is a case of the ancestral tendon being bent and unable to straighten. Why is it unable to straighten? There are many reasons. One important reason is linked to moral or ethical principles. A prescription for Viagra is not enough to resolve such problems. As physicians of Chinese Medicine, we should contemplate this malady in light of Jueyin wind and wood.

I.4.b.2. The Sequence of the Five Elements

In earlier chapters, we focused on water, fire, earth, and metal. Now, we will discuss the wood element. In order to have a basic understanding of the five elements, it is not enough to discuss each of the elements in isolation; we should also explore the significance of the sequence of the elements. Regarding the sequence of the five elements, the *Classic of Documents* is clear: "One refers to water, two to fire, three to wood, four to metal, and five to earth." The sequence of the five elements is the same in the *River*

Chart: "The one of heaven produces water, the six of earth completes it; the two of earth produces fire, the seven of heaven completes it; the three of heaven produces wood, the eight of earth completes it; the four of earth produces metal, the nine of heaven completes it; the five of heaven produces earth, the ten of earth completes it." Why do the five elements follow this sequence? Why does one refer to water, two to fire, and three to wood, and not "one to wood, two to fire, three to water," etc.?

This is a crucial question, since the sequence of the five elements corresponds to the sequence of the genesis of all life as well as the sequence of all material phenomena in the world. This sequence reveals that water was the first element of our world, is the most basic prerequisite of all life, which also distinguishes our planet from the rest of the objects in our solar system. After water comes fire. Water and fire are first, and this corresponds with what is said in the "Great Treatise on the Correspondences of Yin and Yang": "Water and fire signify yin and yang." When water and fire arise, it means that yin and yang have emerged. Furthermore, as it says elsewhere in the *Yellow Emperor's Classic*: "Yin and yang are the way of heaven and earth, the guiding principle of the myriad things, the father and mother of change and transformation, the origin of life and death." Therefore, after water and fire have appeared, the rest of the five elements easily come into being, and all the myriad forms of life on the earth can gradually emerge. Naturally, the first living things to emerge are the plants, and after them come the animals. Plants refer to wood and animals to earth. Correspondingly, after water and fire come wood and then earth.

Additionally, regarding the advent and evolution of animal life, the sequence of the five elements reveals the stepwise progression of that evolution. From the five elements, we know that the earliest animals to emerge on the earth were aquatic, and after them came the animals living on the borders between land and water, and then finally the land animals. As we discussed earlier in this book, scaled creatures belong to water, feathered creatures to fire, hairy creatures to wood, shelled creatures to metal, and lastly, naked creatures to earth. What is a "naked creature"? The best example is humans! From this progression, we can see that humans the last of all animals to have evolved. This sequence of evolution agrees in its most important aspects with the modern scientific timeline of evolution. The classics are indeed worthy of our respect and veneration!

I.4.b.3. The Significance of Wood Producing Fire

Earlier, when we discussed wind and wood, we did so primarily from a medical perspective. Now, let us broaden our perspective to include a look at the role of wood in the five-element system of mutual engenderment from other angles, such as social, environmental, and even global frames of reference. First, let us look at the significance of how water produces wood and wood produces fire. I believe its significance is akin to the principles of sustainable development. We might say that the role of wood in producing fire is the most crucial link in sustainable development. Sustainable development is essentially a problem of energy resources. If the energy resources are sufficient, then development will be sustainable. If the energy resources are unrenewable, then how can we speak of sustainable development?

The term "energy source" is a broad one, but in terms of the existence and development of people, energy sources are primarily fuel. From a five-element perspective, fuels are fire. Fire is produced by wood. The ancients used wood as fuel. The use of wood as fuel is in complete keeping with the five-element theory and by extension with nature. As it is in keeping with nature, the use of wood as fuel is sustainable. Those of us who have spent time in China's rural areas would attest to this. Rural peasants used to collect their firewood in the mountains, and the trees that were felled in one year were replaced by the next year's growth. Year after year, there was no shortage. There are several tens of households in each village, but surrounded by a few mountains, the denizens of such a hamlet have enjoyed thousands of years of firewood, without diminishing the supply. This is because wood replenishes itself, and this ability to replenish itself is extremely important. The United Nations Environmental Program gives two conditions for determining whether a resource is sustainable. The first is whether the resource being used can be replenished. The second is whether the materials that are used can be recycled and reused. By this reckoning, wood is a source of sustainable energy.

Modern fuels are primarily coal and petroleum and, as we discussed earlier, these belong to the water element. In this sense, we of the modern age use water to produce fire. How is it that water can produce fire? The fire in water is true yang, the dragon fire. Thus, the fuels we burn today are the fire of the true yang within the water of *Kan*. The true yang of *Kan* Water is as we already discussed; its function is to warm and nourish the earth and produce *qi*. The lifeblood of the earth stems from this true yang within water. Now we are extracting it and burning it as an ordinary source of fire, but unlike wood, this fire source cannot be replenished. Wood can be cut down only to grow back the following year. When the true yang of the *Kan* Water is extracted, life on earth will no longer be nourished and restored. When this happens, the earth will become senile and life will perish from its face.

Traditionally, wood was used to generate fire, but in the modern age, it is water that is used to create fire. In the past, wood was used to create fire and wood was the primary energy source, but wood was still the product of water. Water produced wood and wood produced fire. From this perspective, water is still the ultimate origin of fire. Why does the sequence of the five elements begin with water? I believe that the reason for this is related to this point. If water was effectively the origin of fire both traditionally and in modern reliance on fossil fuels, then what real difference is there between the fire of modern times and the fire of the past? An important difference is that the process of fire generating wood is a natural process and one that accords with the natural scheme of things. This distinction may seem contrived, and one might argue that the collection of wood from nature in order to produce fire is as artificial a process as any other, and requires that a person intentionally go about collecting wood and setting it afire. However, the production of wood is not a contrived process. It rains or the water flows along or under the ground and the wood is nourished. The extent to which water nourishes the wood results in the extent of wood production, and thus the extent of fire production; the production of wood is the result of natural processes, not human ones. Humans cannot cut down more wood than nature produces. Our best bet to increase yields of wood is to simply close off the mountainsides, so that they can reforest on their own. The process of water producing wood and wood producing fire is, at the very least, a very interesting one.

When we burn fossil fuels, robbing the true yang from the *Kan* Water, there is a very different sort of process at work. This is not a process that naturally occurs in nature, nor is it tied to the rhythms and vicissitudes of nature. It is a process that is dependent upon the plans and intentions of people. Oil production is related to the decisions of OPEC, not to annual rainfall. OPEC decides how many barrels of oil to fill based on the price those barrels will fetch, with no regard for the true yang within water. It is not a process over which nature has any control. The two defining characteristics of a renewable resource, as laid out by the United Nations, are not completely perfect. A more basic, and more perfect, definition of a renewable resource might be any resource that is produced and controlled by entirely natural forces. Only when the resource is controlled and developed by the processes of nature can it be said to be renewable. Why did Laozi place the idea that the Dao is patterned after nature to be one of the highest edicts of Daoism? One reason is that Laozi recognized that man had separated himself from nature, but the other lies in the recognition that it is by heeding nature that the enduring Dao can be obtained.

II. An Outline of Jueyin Disease

The essential features of Jueyin disease are those listed in the first line of the Jueyin chapter of the *Treatise on Cold Damage*: "When Jueyin is diseased, there is dispersion-thirst, the *qi* rises and collides with the heart, within the heart are pain and heat, there is hunger with no desire to eat, eating induces vomiting of worms, and downward purging results in unceasing diarrhea." Line 326 also reveals the disease trigger related to Jueyin disease, and is the longest opening line of a six conformation chapter in the *Treatise on Cold Damage*. The following section will discuss each of the signs of disease mentioned in this line.

II.1. Dispersion-Thirst

II.1.a. The General Meaning of Thirst

The first sign mentioned in the outline of Jueyin disease is dispersion-thirst (*xiaoke* 消渴). In some syndromes, people are thirsty but do not necessarily want to drink, or they drink a bit just to moisten their mouths; these are examples of syndromes in which there is thirst without desire to drink. That is thirst (*ke*) without dispersion (*xiao*). On the other hand, if the patient is afflicted with dispersion-thirst as in Jueyin disease, they thirst and drink to quench that thirst, but after drinking there is dispersion and they quickly become thirsty again. This is basically what is meant by dispersion-thirst.

Why does disease of Jueyin result in dispersion-thirst? A great number of past generations of Chinese Medicine physicians believed that dispersion-thirst was caused by the heat of the liver and stomach consuming and damaging the fluids of the body. This idea is still held by the authors of most modern Chinese Medicine textbooks. If we contemplate this matter carefully, however, it appears that heat damaging the fluids is not an entirely adequate explanation for Jueyin thirst. If we explain that dispersion-thirst is the result of exuberant heat consuming fluids, then how do we compare this with the great heat of Yangming disease? In Yangming disease, the Baihu Renshen Tang syndrome patient presents with a dry tongue, vexation, and thirst, and drinks liter after liter of water. If we are to use the explanation of excessive heat damaging the fluids to describe dispersion-thirst, then perhaps this term belongs in the Yangming chapter of the *Treatise on Cold Damage*! If that were the case, the opening line of the Yangming chapter should read: "When Yangming is diseased, there is dispersion-thirst, and the stomach family is full." However, that is not the case. Zhang Zhongjing clearly places dispersion-thirst (*xiaoke*) at the start of the opening line of the Jueyin chapter, indicating that it is caused by a different factor and, for the same reason, indicating that dispersion-thirst is an important sign of Jueyin disease.

II.1.b. How Jueyin Thirsts

Why is dispersion-thirst an important characteristic of Jueyin disease? Why does Jueyin disease so readily predispose the patient to thirst? When a person thirsts, it is because the mouth and tongue lack fluids. This is why, when thirst is described in relation to Yangming disease, it is referred to as dryness of the surface of the tongue. From these descriptions, we can see that the organs used to sense thirst are the mouth and tongue. The mouth is the orifice of the spleen, and the tongue is the sprout of the heart, so when we refer to the mouth and tongue, we are actually referring to the heart and spleen, to fire and earth. Thirst results from the mouth and tongue, from the heart and spleen, and from fire and earth. This indicates that it is Jueyin that most readily affects the mouth and tongue, the heart and spleen, and the fire and earth of the body.

Thirst and drought are analogous. Out in the macrocosm, there is drought, and in the human body, there is thirst. Both are the result of insufficient fluids moisturizing and nourishing the environment. As we said before, the water found in rivers, streams, lakes, and seas is by nature quiet, and it cannot moisten the myriad creatures on its own. It requires the action of a mediator in order to do so. One of the most important mediators is Jueyin wood. Wood is generated by water; it is the child of water, so there is nothing closer to water from a five-element perspective. The ancients described this relationship as: "*Yi* and *gui* stem from the same source." The second and tenth of the heavenly stems, *yi* and *gui*, refer to water and wood, and so the above statement means that water and wood come from the same source. The heart is the fire of the five elements, and is the child of wood, and is generated by wood. In order for the sprout of the heart—the tongue—to receive moisture, wood must first draw this nourishment upward, and thus fire is dependent upon the mediator of wood. This is one aspect of the importance of Jueyin.

Another aspect is the relationship between wood and earth, the way in which wood can help to maintain the moisture in the soil. Looking at it another way, we can ask how Jueyin maintains moisture in the mouth, the orifice of the spleen. This is a point that nature has made very clear. In the natural world, plants are able to maintain the moisture in the soil around them. This is especially true in old-growth forests where, throughout the year, the vegetation keeps the soil soft and moist. Where there is no vegetative ground cover, for instance, on the Loess Plateau or in the desert, we find the opposite situation; the soil in these areas is usually arid. Although Taiyin is referred to as "damp earth," without wood we can see that the earth does not remain moist. Earlier, we discussed the hexagram description: "Dragons contend in the open, their blood is black and yellow." Dragons are those that excite the clouds and distribute rain, and these are of course important in ensuring that the world does not become too dry. Dragons also belong to the east and to wood. These correspondences are key to understanding the process whereby wood moistens all living things. Under normal circumstances, Jueyin can moisten the mouth and tongue, the orifice and sprout of the spleen and heart respectively, and prevent thirst from occurring. As soon as Jueyin is afflicted, the mouth and tongue no longer receive their appropriate moisture, and dispersion-thirst easily occurs.

II.1.c. Differentiating Thirst in the Six Conformations
As we discussed in the previous passage, there is a special relationship

between Jueyin and thirst, and despite the fact that Jueyin disease easily leads to thirst, it is not the only cause of thirst. With the exception of the Taiyin conformation, all of the *Treatise on Cold Damage* chapters include this symptom, so we are obliged to take the time to distinguish the way that thirst presents in each of the other conformations.

First, let us examine thirst among the three yang. Taiyang thirst is described in relation to Taiyang bowel syndrome, and is caused by the inhibition of the Taiyang transformation of *qi*. Thus, Taiyang thirst is accompanied by a floating pulse, heat effusion, and inhibited urination. Yangming thirst is brought about by overabundant heat damaging the fluids. Yangming thirst is part of the "four great symptoms" of Yangming disease: high fever, copious sweating, intense vexation and thirst, and a flooding pulse. Shaoyang thirst results from inhibition of the pivot, and affects the opening and closing mechanisms as well as the three burners. Thus, Shaoyang thirst is typically accompanied by maladies of the pivot, such as alternating chills and fever, unpleasant fullness of the chest and rib-sides, a fine, wiry pulse, a bitter taste in the mouth, dry throat, blurry vision, and so on. The thirst of each of the yang configurations is accompanied by distinctive symptoms; distinguishing one conformation from the other is not too difficult. The thirst of each conformation requires its own particular treatment. We can use Wuling San to treat Taiyang thirst, Baihu Tang to treat Yangming thirst, and a modified Xiao Chaihu Tang or Chaihu Guizhi Ganjiang Tang to treat Shaoyang thirst.

Among the three yin diseases, Taiyin disease is not characterized by thirst, and even if thirst is present, there is no desire to drink. We can really only speak of thirst with relation to the Shaoyin and Jueyin disease conformations. Shaoyin disease is as we have described earlier: the urine is clear, and there is a whole set of yin-cold signs, so Shaoyin thirst is easily distinguished from the other conformations, especially thirst of the three yang. To treat Shaoyin thirst, it is necessary to use a Sini Tang type of formula.

The thirsts of the three yang confirmations described above, including the thirst of Shaoyin disease, are easily distinguished from one another. Any other type of thirst besides those that we have just described belongs to Jueyin. The scope of Jueyin thirst is thus very broad, and includes any atypical thirst that does not fit the four categories described above. From this, we can see that thirst is as indicative of Jueyin disease as a floating pulse is of

Taiyang disease. When the patient has a floating pulse, eight or even nine times out of ten, that patient is suffering from Taiyang disease. Except for a tiny minority of cases where a floating pulse is indicative of deficient yang that is crossing to the exterior, the majority of floating pulses are related to Taiyang disease. Likewise with thirst: unless the thirst is accompanied by any of the four specific symptoms of the other four disease conformations that exhibit thirst, we can assume that the patient is suffering from Jueyin disease. Thus thirst, especially thirst with the ability to drink, or in other words thirst with the ability to disperse, is of premiere importance in determining Jueyin disease.

II.1.d. Formulas to Treat Jueyin Thirst

In the above passage, we discussed the thirst of the three yang and the formulas specifically used to treat each. In the *Treatise on Cold Damage*, no specific formulas are indicated for the thirst of either Jueyin or Shaoyin disease. Regarding the thirst of Shaoyin, we can chalk this omission up to the fact that thirst is not an important sign of Shaoyin disease, and in Shaoyin disease thirst can be treated through modifications to the primary formula. In Jueyin disease, where thirst is a preeminent indicator of the type of pathology at work, it is difficult not to expect a formula specific to treating the thirst of Jueyin disease. I believe that this formula is none other than the chief formula of the Jueyin chapter, Wumei Wan.

Recently, I treated a colon cancer patient who had had a colon resection in order to stave off metastasis. It had already been a year since the surgery, but his bowel movements were still abnormal. He had diarrhea five to eight times a day, which initially consisted of loose stools and then became clear fluid. Besides the liquid feces, the patient also suffered from serious thirst, and drank almost incessantly. Each day, the patient drank two large thermoses (approximately five liters) of water. Six months before I saw him, he began receiving adjunct Chinese Medicine treatment, but its effects were not significant. Looking over the formulas that had been used by previous physicians, I saw that most were formulas to strengthen the spleen and dry dampness or formulas to consolidate the kidneys and astringe: Shen Ling Baizhu San, Xiang Sha Liujun Tang, Bupi Yichang Wan, etc. I can understand the thought process behind the use of these formulas, and we should be thankful that previous physicians had not prescribed bitter cold "anti-cancer" herbs. The patient suffered from chronic diarrhea, so from the perspective of modern viscera-bowel (*zangfu*) diagnosis methods, it is quite natural to focus on the spleen. However, if one has studied the *Treatise on Cold Damage* and learned to differentiate the six conformations of disease, then I believe there is absolutely no way that one could focus their treatment on the spleen and Taiyin. Why? Because of line 277 from *Treatise on Cold Damage*: "Spontaneous diarrhea without thirst belongs to Taiyin." Here we have a patient that drinks two large thermoses of water a day. How could this possibly be Taiyin disease?

So how does one approach a condition such as I have described above? The patient's bowel movements were disinhibited, but loose stools can occur in any of the six conformations. The patient was thirsty and drank copious amounts, meaning that he suffered from dispersion-thirst (*xiaoke*). Diarrhea together with thirst is unique to the Jueyin conformation of disease. Thus, there is no doubt that the treatment for this illness must be determined from the perspective of Jueyin disease; Wumei Wan must be used.

Based on this, I prescribed to this patient the original Wumei Wan, without adding or subtracting a single ingredient. I prescribed three or four days worth of this medication at each visit, and by the third time I saw him, the patient's thirst and the amount he drank were reduced considerably. Instead of drinking two thermoses of water a day, he drank just one, and his watery diarrhea improved significantly as well.

From the example of this patient, the simplicity and practicality of the six conformation diagnostic method must be becoming clear to the reader. As long as we have a firm grasp of the outlines of each type of disease, determining the conformation of the patient's disease should be relatively easy. If we take this case as an example, we can imagine the path the Chinese Medicine physician might take if there were no knowledge of the six conformations: treatment aimed at the Taiyin spleen and stomach would most probably be selected. However, basic knowledge of the differences between the six conformations of disease completely precludes selecting Taiyin as the focus of treatment. Six conformation differentiation of disease is not only convenient, it is also very reliable. If there is such a convenient and reliable method at hand, we physicians of Chinese Medicine would be wise to grasp it!

II.1.e. Contemplating Diabetes

In our discussion of "dispersion-thirst" (*xiaoke*), or "wasting thirst" as it can also be translated, it would be unsurprising if the reader associated this disease with the modern conception of diabetes, which is also characterized by dramatically increased thirst, a commensurate increase in urination, and wasting of the body. If we review the literature, we see that already by the close of the Sui dynasty (AD 581–618), the same name *xiaoke* (here translated as "wasting thirst") was used to refer to a disease that is equivalent to what we now call diabetes. What, then, is the connection between the disease described in the outline of Jueyin disease and our modern conception of diabetes? When I was in college, when we discussed the outline of Jueyin disease in the *Treatise on Cold Damage*, I remember the professor specifically saying that it would be a mistake to confuse the "dispersion-thirst" of the Jueyin chapter with the more modern conception of "wasting thirst" (diabetes), and our textbooks reiterated this point. However, a key feature of Jueyin disease is dispersion-thirst, and this is also a key sign in diabetes. The symptom of dispersion-thirst referred to by the opening line of the Jueyin chapter is not identical to diabetes, but does this mean that diabetes and Jueyin disease are completely unrelated? This question circled around in my head for ages, and would not give me peace.

As we all know, a directly observable change in diabetes is a rise in blood glucose levels. When the concentration of glucose in the blood of the diabetic patient reaches a certain point, the kidneys are no longer able to prevent it from being lost in the urine. This is why, in order to diagnose diabetes, the ancients primarily examined the urine to see if it contained sugar. How did they determine if it contained sugar? With the help of ants. Ants have an excellent sense of smell, especially for sugar. Normally, urine does not attract ants, and the smell of urine can even ward off ants. The urine of the diabetic patient, if left on the ground, attracts ants in large numbers. Thus, the ancient Chinese physician used ants to diagnose diabetes.

In the body, glucose serves as the energy source, supplying all the tissues with fuel. Why is the blood glucose elevated in diabetics? From a modern perspective, the crucial factor is an insufficiency of insulin. As a result, the past method of treatment depended either upon supplementing insulin or stimulating insulin secretion. However, the most recent research has revealed that insulin insufficiency is only one aspect of diabetic pathology. Another, perhaps more important factor in the development of diabetes is an obstruction to glucose metabolism at a cellular level. At first glance, it appears that the patient's glucose is overly abundant, but on the cellular level the patient is starving for glucose. It is this cellular dearth that induces the blood to be flooded with glucose. Furthermore, it causes the patient to become extremely hungry and to increase their intake of food. From a biomedical perspective, the problem is still that the blood sugar is too high. We must keep in mind that from the human body's perspective, it is not that the blood sugar is too high, but that it is too low. Thus, the crucial problem in treating diabetes is devising a way to resolve the obstacles to glucose metabolism at the cellular level; once these impediments in the process of glucose metabolism have been resolved, the linchpin of diabetic pathology is removed.

We have already sketched out the basic picture of diabetic pathology from the perspective of modern science. How is diabetes explained by Chinese Medicine, and more specifically, how is it is explained by the six conformation theory of the *Treatise on Cold Damage*? Diabetes is the result of obstacles in the metabolism of blood sugar. What class of things does sugar belong to, from a Chinese Medicine perspective? Sugar is sweet, and of the five elements, sweet flavor belongs to earth. Thus, sugar belongs to the earth element. From a Chinese Medicine perspective, the diabetic hindrances in the metabolism and utilization of glucose are hindrances in the earth element of the human body. How is the earth element hindered or obstructed? From the perspective of our previous observations, we know that diabetes is the result of an excess of sugar in the blood. What is the correlate of the blood in nature? The blood flowing through the vessels is like the rivers and streams. Thus, the ancients said: people have blood vessels, and the land has rivers and streams. If the sugar in the blood is too high, it is analogous to an overabundance of soil in the rivers and streams.

In the past, the waters in the western reaches of the Yangzi river were bluish green, and the hills and mountains through which these clear waters wound westward were decked in verdant vegetation, creating a scene that was almost too beautiful to behold. Now, if we return to the Yangzi, we now find the hills denuded of their forests and lush foliage, and find that the formerly aquamarine water of the river itself has turned a turbid yellow color.

How does clear green water become turbid and yellow? It contains too much earth. Soil should remain where it is, not be borne off by the river. Why then does it end up in the Yangzi? We discussed the cause in the Taiyin chapter: erosion causes soil to migrate to the waterways. Once the forests are cut down and the fabric of vegetation decimated, soil has a hard time staying put. The wind blows, the rains fall, and soon the soil ends up in the churning waters of the river. From this, we can see that the excess of soil in the water, which causes the water to be muddy and turbid, is ultimately caused by the scarcity of trees and other vegetation. At first glance, it seems as if the soil in the water is the problem. Here it is in the water making things mucky and ruining the formerly cyan clarity. If we trace the problem back to its source, however, the problem lies with the wood, not with the earth.

If we follow Laozi's adage that "Dao accords with nature," then we know that although the central pathologic agent in diabetes is the blood sugar, which belongs to the earth system, the real culprit is wood, Jueyin. Why is the first sign of Jueyin disease dispersion-thirst (*xiaoke*)? Is there a relationship between this dispersion-thirst and the "wasting thirst" that from the Sui dynasty onward referred to diabetes? It is clear that, if we place diabetes within the context of Jueyin disease, it frees us from the conceptual constraints of the "doctrine of the three dispersions," as first proposed in the early Qing dynasty and now included in modern textbooks. This same perspective provides us with a real source treatment method for diabetes. By understanding and treating diabetes from the perspective of Jueyin pathology, we raise the discussion up to a higher level, that of the natural world. Up until the present day, modern medicine has regarded diabetes as an incurable disease, and one that requires lifelong medical treatment. Is it possible that we, from the Jueyin perspective, might be able to find a permanent cure for diabetes? I am confident that such a cure is possible. Using Chinese Medicine methods and thought to cure a disease that Western Medicine considers incurable is not just "modernization"—it surpasses "modernization." For the sake of humanity, I hope that Chinese Medicine is able to supply the crucial strategies whereby modern medicine will make new breakthroughs in the treatment and cure of disease. We are not limited to arming ourselves with modern medical technology and equipment in our exercise of Chinese Medicine principles. More important than modern technological devices is "arming ourselves" with our own thorough understanding of Chinese Medicine, and gaining the ability to exercise that understanding through traditional technique. Only in this way will the path of Chinese Medicine be long and prosperous.

II.2. The *Qi* Rises and Collides with the Heart, within the Heart Are Pain and Heat

At this juncture, I would like to discuss an important issue, namely what precisely is meant by "heart" (*xin* 心) in the *Treatise on Cold Damage*. Of course, one of the most direct meanings of *xin* is the heart of the five viscera of the body. However, in the *Treatise on Cold Damage*, we find that in the majority of instances the term *xin* does not refer to viscera, but rather to a part of the body that is defined relative to a certain area of the body's surface. We can divide the usages of *xin* in the *Treatise on Cold Damage* into three categories. In the first category, the character *xin* does not appear with another character indicating location. For instance, the *Treatise on Cold Damage* refers to "palpitations of the heart" (*xinji* 心悸), "vexation of the heart" (*xinfan* 心煩), "chaotic movement of the heart" (*xinluan* 心亂), and so on. In these examples, it is often very difficult to determine the exact location of the sensation in question.

Secondly, there is the term "below the heart" (*xinxia* 心下). There are a great number of references to *xinxia* in the *Treatise on Cold Damage*, such as "palpitations below the heart," "vexation below the heart," "pain below the heart," and so on. The area of the body referred to by *xinxia* is relatively clear: it is the area above the belly and below the xiphoid process of the sternum.

Third, we have the term "within the heart" (*xinzhong* 心中). For instance, we read of: "palpitations and vexation within the heart," "knotting and pain within the heart," "pain and heat within the heart," and so on. So where in the body is the region described by "within the heart" actually located? There are two possibilities. First, as it says in the *Treatise on Cold Damage Dictionary*, it is possible that "within the heart" refers to the heart itself or the area directly surrounding it: the chest. A second possibility stems from the fact that when the ancients spoke of the heart, they were often not referring directly to the organ itself, but rather to the central portion of the torso. This central region is located right at the center of the chest below the xiphoid process of the sternum, what the ancients referred to as the "heart's nest" (*xinwo* 心窩). The common Chinese expression of "heart pain" is used to refer to pain in the entire midsection of the torso, and so in this second meaning of "within the heart" in fact refers to the epigastrium.

In the outline of Jueyin disease, it says: "The *qi* rises and collides with the heart, within the heart are pain and heat." This section refers to two of the different aspects we discussed above. The first indicates the precordium and behind the breast bone, the area of the Jueyin channel of the hand. The second refers to the area below the xiphoid process, a region governed by the central earth of the body. Thus, the phrase "the *qi* rises and collides with the heart, within the heart are pain and heat" on the one hand refers to pain and heat in the organ that we know of as the heart, and in another sense includes pain and heat in the epigastric region and its surrounding organs. The first sense refers to what we now think of as the circulatory system, and the second to the digestive system. The pain of the circulatory aspect is pain of the pericardium network, which belongs to the hand Jueyin channel. The pain of the digestive aspect is the result of pathological changes in the earth system of the body. How does the earth become sick? Wood makes it sick, Jueyin brings about sickness in the earth element. Thus, the *Essentials from the Golden Cabinet* states: "When seeing disease of the liver, know it will transmit to the spleen." The phrase "the *qi* rises and collides with the heart, within the heart are pain and heat" from the opening line of the Jueyin chapter in the *Treatise on Cold Damage* should, at the very least, be considered from both the above perspectives.

"The *qi* rises and collides with the heart." Here, the meaning of "collides" (*zhuang* 撞) is as both *Explaining Writing and Analyzing Characters* ("to beat") and *Extensive Rhymes* ("to strike") have explained. Both "beating" and "striking" cause pain, characterized by stabbing, compressing, and gripping. As for the "pain and heat within the heart," the implication of heat paired with pain is that the patient suffers from a sensation that is equally painful and burning. If we combine the above definitions, then we have the stinging, pressing, and gripping pain of angina pectoris, a disease of the circulatory system, combined with a sensation of burning, scorching heat, which indicates a disease of the digestive system. Of course, disease of the gallbladder is similar in quality to angina, but as the position of the gallbladder is close to the "within the heart" area as described above, this requires that we categorize it as Jueyin. In addition, an important topic in the Jueyin chapter is "reversal" (*jue* 厥), and in the Jueyin chapter, *jue* is mentioned 52 times. *Jue* in this context means "counterflow cold of the hands and feet." Pain easily brings about the pathological state referred to by *jue*, and the pain of angina pectoris or a gallbladder attack is especially effective at producing *jue* in the person.

These are issues that must be contemplated when discussing the Jueyin chapter of the *Treatise on Cold Damage*.

II.3. Hunger with No Desire to Eat

There are a number of instances in which the *Treatise on Cold Damage* discusses issues related to eating and drinking. For instance, one of the four great signs and symptoms for the use of Xiao Chaihu Tang is "taciturn and reticent, the patient has no desire to eat"; in the opening line of the Taiyin chapter, it says: "there is abdominal fullness and vomiting, and inability to eat"; and in the opening line of the Jueyin chapter, we read that the Jueyin patient has "hunger with no desire to eat." Each of these instances has to do with food, but each is different. The patient who is described as "taciturn and reticent, with no desire to eat" in relation to Xiao Chaihu Tang has lost all desire to eat, and thinks nothing of food. This passage emphasizes that the patient lacks desire, thinks nothing of food, and stresses the subjective aspect of the desire for food. In Jueyin disease, the patient has "no desire to eat," and in this lack of desire, the patient resembles the Xiao Chaihu Tang patient. However, at the same time that the Jueyin patient does not desire to eat, he suffers from a feeling of ravenous hunger. He is just as hungry and starving as he is without want for food. This is a salient difference between the Jueyin and the Shaoyang patient. The description of the Taiyin patient emphasizes that the patient cannot get food down because the abdomen is distended and full, and therefore it is uncomfortable to eat. This inability to ingest food emphasizes that the inability is an objective fact, and that forced eating produces abdominal discomfort and distention. The descriptions of the inability of Jueyin and Shaoyang patients to eat emphasize their subjective lack of desire to eat. Taiyin is earth, and Shaoyang and Jueyin are wood. It is clear, then, that the ability to eat is related to earth (spleen and stomach), while the desire to eat is related to wood (liver and gallbladder).

When in the clinic we encounter a patient who has problems eating, we cannot simply prescribe Shenqu, Shanzha, or Maiya. We must first carefully interview the patient in order to grasp the root cause of their inability to eat. Is it that they have no desire to eat? Or is it the case that ingesting food makes them uncomfortable? Do they spend the entire day devoid of any desire to eat, and are indifferent to whether they eat or not? Or are they starving but have no desire to eat? To the clinician differentiating one syndrome from another, these are important factors. Recently, I treated a student that had great difficulty with eating. When food was in front of her, she did not have even the slightest desire to eat, and it took her more than an hour to eat a single meal, but paradoxically, she would get hungry very easily. This was a classic case of "hunger with no desire to eat," and a classic instance of Jueyin disease. I prescribed three doses of Wumei Wan, and after the third dose, her appetite greatly improved and she was able to eat an entire meal quickly.

In addition, when discussing the outlines of the six conformations, we must pay attention to the fact that each chapter outline contains elements that are closely related to one another but that can also be understood singly. If we take the opening line of the Jueyin chapter as an example, we see that it is not necessary for all of the signs that are listed in its opening outline to be present for it to be called Jueyin disease. We discussed this phenomenon in the section on the opening line of the Taiyang chapter. It is only necessary for the patient to exhibit one or two of the signs or symptoms indicated by the outline of Jueyin disease for us to establish a diagnosis. This is a point that those who study the *Treatise on Cold Damage* must heed: the first sign of Jueyin disease that Zhang Zhongjing mentions is "dispersion-thirst" (*xiaoke*), but later generations of Chinese Medicine practitioners did not dare to equate this with the "wasting thirst disease" (*xiaokebing*), now known as diabetes. And why is this? It is because the opening line also contains the sign "hunger with no desire to eat." In diabetes, the patient is hungry and eats large amounts of food, a sign that is incompatible with "hunger with no desire to eat." The problem lies in viewing all of the signs and symptoms listed in the opening line as being completely interdependent parts rather than distinct wholes warranting independent consideration. Is it possible for Jueyin disease to have hunger with a strong desire to eat as in diabetes, and also have starving with no desire whatsoever to eat? Of course, this is entirely possible. This is no different from what we see in the case of Taiyang disease, where patients afflicted by wind-strike perspire, and others afflicted by cold damage have no perspiration.

We cannot say that those who suffer from wind-strike suffer from Taiyang disease, while those who suffer from cold damage do not!

II.4. Eating Induces Vomiting of Worms

In the *Treatise on Cold Damage*, there are three instances in which vomiting worms is mentioned. One instance is in line 89 of the Taiyang chapter: "The patient that has cold but is made to perspire will have cold within the stomach and vomit worms." Another mention of vomiting worms is in line 338 where the syndrome suitable for treatment with Wumei Wan is described, and the other instance is the opening line of the Jueyin chapter. Vomiting of worms is not a commonly encountered symptom. The placement of this sign in the basic outline of Jueyin disease should not be understood to mean that Jueyin disease necessarily involves the vomiting of worms. Rather, it is included in order to highlight an important characteristic of Jueyin disease.

Worms lurk within the interior of the body, eluding detection, and can be referred to as "hibernating worms" (*zhechong* 蟄蟲). There are worms that hibernate out in nature as well, and these are creatures that go underground to sleep during the winter. These creatures reanimate and emerge from their underground burrows during the period known as *Jingzhe* (Awakening of Insects), one of the twenty-four node *qi*. This is when the insects that have been sleeping through the winter awake. They are awakened by the stirring of the wood *qi* of spring that invigorates all living things. Hibernating insects emerge from their slumber when Jueyin wind and wood dominate the season, and the insects that hibernate inside the human body are the same way; they are easily roused by the Jueyin *qi* and when roused have a tendency to run helter-skelter. Their chaotic activity can cause "worm reversal" (counterflow cold of the hands and feet induced by the painful movement of intestinal worms) or cause them to be vomited up. The vomiting of worms mentioned in line 326 is significant because it reveals the dynamic between the Jueyin *qi* and the hibernating insects.

II.5. Jueyin Prohibitions

The last item mentioned in the outline of Jueyin disease is "downward purging results in unceasing diarrhea." Why is downward purging prohibited in the treatment of Jueyin disease, and why does downward purging cause unceasing diarrhea? This question can easily be answered if we turn to the *Yellow Emperor's Classic*.

In the "Great Treatise on the Four *Qi* and the Tuning of the Spirit," we read:

> During the three months of spring, the old is cast out, heaven and earth all are reborn, and the myriad creatures flourish. At night one should retire and then rise early, stride about the courtyard, let down one's hair and loosen one's clothing, thus allowing one's resolve to emerge. One should bring forth life and not kill, yield and not force, reward but not punish. This is the mandate of the *qi* of spring, and the way to cultivate life.

Jueyin is wind and wood. Among seasons, it is the spring, and it is responsible for creating life. Thus, as far as Jueyin is concerned, it is fitting to birth but not to kill, to yield but not to force, to reward but not to punish. The use of downward purging techniques is like killing, or forcing, or punishing. If such methods are employed, the *qi* of Jueyin is harmed, and the mandate to nourish life is violated. Thus, when there is Jueyin disease, it is not fitting to use forceful downward purging methods, for when these methods are used, the patient will have unceasing diarrhea.

III. The Timing of Jueyin Disease

An outline of the temporal correspondence with Jueyin disease is provided by line 328 of the *Treatise on Cold Damage*, where it says: "Jueyin disease tends to resolve in the time from *chou* to *mao*." In the course of a day, the period from *chou* to *mao* is from 1 am to 7 am. In the course of a month, this same period is the seven and a half days beginning on the third day of the lunar month. In the traditional Chinese lunar calendar, the time from *chou* to *mao* is the twelfth to the second month. I will divide my discourse regarding the significance of the time period spanned by *chou*, *yin*, and *mao* into two parts.

III.1. The Meaning of the *Chou* Time

III.1.a. The Two Yin Exchange Completely

The tendency for Jueyin disease to resolve begins with the time period *chou* (1–3 am). This time period is particularly significant for Jueyin. From the perspective of the seasons, *chou* is the time of year when winter is at an end. Spring and summer are yang, fall and winter are yin; two yin, two yang. *Chou* is at the very end of the two yin, and thus corresponds with the characteristic of Jueyin disease as described in the *Yellow Emperor's Classic*: "The two yin exchange completely." The tendency of Jueyin disease to recover beginning at this time reveals the fidelity between Zhang Zhongjing's writings and the *Yellow Emperor's Classic*.

III.1.b. Chou *and* Lin *(Approaching)*

Among the twelve tidal hexagrams, *chou* corresponds with the hexagram *lin* (Approaching), which is a yang or growing hexagram. Here, this has two layers of meaning. The first layer of meaning is indicated by the definition of the character *lin* (臨) in *Master Shang's Study of the Zhou Yi*: "*Lin* means 'to see.'" "To see" (*shi* 視) means to look with our eyes. In Chinese, the phrase meaning "to look at things" (*shi wu* 視物) can also be expressed by saying *lin wu* (臨物). How is "looking at" things related to the *chou* time period? First of all, when we discussed the implications of the Jueyin channel, we saw that *qi* begins its course along the Jueyin channel at the outset of the *chou* period at the point Dadun (LV 1), and concludes when the *chou* time period concludes at Qimen (LV 14). This is, of course, the very time period in which Jueyin disease tends to resolve. This reiterates the very close relationship between *chou* and Jueyin, especially the liver. The orifice of the liver is the eyes, and it is through the eyes that we see. Eyesight and problems with our eyesight are closely related to both the liver and Jueyin. The liver, the Jueyin, the *chou* time period, and the hexagram *Lin* are all intimately connected. Such consistency and interconnection between medicine, the *Classic of Changes*, and the workings of Chinese language and culture cause us to ask which of these fields of study preceded the other. At times, they are so intertwined that it is impossible to say. The student of Chinese Medicine must carefully study medicine, the changes, as well as Chinese language and culture, and cannot afford to neglect a single one of these aspects.

The second level of meaning of *lin* is "boundary" (*linjie* 臨界), or "phase boundary" as it is known as in physics. A phase transition is when matter transitions from one state, such as liquid, gas, or solid, to another and the phase boundary is the narrow band of conditions in which one state is on the verge of becoming another. Why is the time period *chou* related to this concept of a phase boundary? In the period of *chou*, at the point when the exchange of the two yin has completed, we are at the end of winter. *Chou* is the time when winter transitions to spring, when yin turns to yang. *Chou* is like a doorway; once we pass through this doorway, we enter an entirely different state.

Regarding the Jueyin channel, the ancients often used the phrase: "Yin is completed, yang is born." Consistent with the significance of the Jueyin, *chou* is the end of winter and the end of a year, when yin is completed. In the *Plain Questions's* "Treatise on the Six Nodes and Visceral Manifestations," it says: "The liver is the root of dismissal of the ultimate (*baji*) and domain of the soul (*hun*)." Earlier, we discussed this "dismissal of the ultimate" (*baji*) in relation to the liver as the general of the armies. In fact, "dismissing the ultimate" has another level of meaning that corresponds with *chou*. The meaning of "ultimate" (*ji*) is as we have discussed: the maximum or farthest point. The end of a traditional Chinese year, coinciding with the end of winter, is the most extreme point in that year, and corresponds with the *chou* period. As the cycle comes to a close, the crucial question is whether another cycle can begin. *Chou* is like a doorway: if we pass through it, we are in a new year; if we do not, we are still in the old year. Why does Chinese Medicine regard excesses and insufficiencies to be undesirable? From the perspective of our current discussion, we can see that if the time is not yet ripe but you proceed prematurely, this is excessive. If on the other hand, the time is nigh but one is tardy, this is insufficiency. The function of "dismissal of the ultimate" is to keep us in step with the procession of the natural cosmos around us, to make sure that we go through the door when we are supposed to.

III.1.c. Chou *and Reversal*

Chou is the time when the yin is completed and the yang is born. It is also the time when yin transitions to yang and the old gives way to the new. This reveals an important facet of the function of Jueyin. If this crucial transition fails in the patient, a grave syndrome presents: reversal (*jue* 厥). There are only 56 lines in the Jueyin chapter of the *Treatise on Cold Damage*, and those lines contain 52 mentions of *jue*. Almost every line in the Jueyin chapter discusses reversal. This tells us that the most important piece of information to understand Jueyin lies with the concept of reversal. Why is reversal the most important topic in the Jueyin chapter? Why is Jueyin disease so prone to producing reversal? What factors contribute to the development of reversal? This problem is discussed very clearly in line 337 of the *Treatise on Cold Damage*: "In all reversal, the *qi* of yin and yang do not mutually flow and connect, instead they reverse. In reversal, there is counterflow cold of the hands and feet." What is meant by "The *qi* of yin and yang do not mutually flow and connect"? This is referring to the inability of the process of the completion of yin and birth of yang to transition smoothly, preventing the shift from yin to yang and from old to new from completion. As we have already mentioned, the function of Jueyin is to ensure the smooth and successful completion of this crucial transition. If Jueyin becomes diseased, how can the *qi* of yin and yang mutually flow and connect? A reversal syndrome will naturally present instead. This is why the Jueyin chapter devotes so much of its text to reversal.

From the meaning of reversal, from the relationship between Jueyin and the *chou* time period, from *chou* and its relationship to the hexagram *Lin*, we can see that Chinese Medicine theory is in fact a medical theory grounded in the pattern of the passage of time. If we mistakenly think that this aspect of Chinese Medicine is related to time and that another aspect has no relation to time, our understanding is incomplete. Time is omnipresent in Chinese Medicine. When we study Chinese Medicine, we cannot depart from the temporal framework even for a moment.

The most important factor contributing to the development of *jue* reversal is the one listed in line 337: "The *qi* of yin and yang do not mutually flow and connect." What are the most salient clinical signs that reversal induced by the failure of the *qi* of yin and yang is failing to connect? The very signs are listed in line 337: "In reversal, there is counterflow cold of the hands and feet." The hands and feet are equivalent to the four extremities. How do the four extremities fit with a conception of the physical human body in accord with a temporal cosmos? What do the hands and feet, as a distinct part of the human microcosm, correlate to in the patterns of time's passage? They must correspond with the earthly branches *chen*, *xu*, *chou*, and *wei*.

The elements relate to the twelve earthly branches in the following way: *hai* and *zi* belong to water (winter); *yin* and *mao* belong to wood (spring); *si* and *wu* belong to fire (summer); *shen* and *you* belong to metal (autumn);

and *chen, xu, chou,* and *wei* belong to the earth element. The earth element occupies the last month of each of the four seasons. According to the "Treatise on Taiyin and Yangming" in the *Plain Questions*: "The spleen does not rule a season, it flourishes in the four *ji* (季)." What does *ji* mean? The *ji* month is the last month of each of the four seasons. Each of these months overlooks or approaches (another meaning of the character *lin*) the next season, and so they are also called the four *lin*. *Chou* overlooks spring, *chen* overlooks summer, *wei* overlooks autumn, and *xu* overlooks winter. We know from our previous discussion that when we are talking about *lin* that we are talking about transitions or connections, the smooth flow and connection from one season to the next mentioned in line 337 of *Treatise on Cold Damage*. *Chou* is when winter flows into spring, *chen* is when spring flows into summer, *wei* is when summer flows into autumn, and *xu* is when fall flows into winter. Spring and summer are yang, fall and winter are yin. Spring is the yin within yang, summer is the yang within yang. Fall is the yang within yin, winter is the yin within yin. When we speak of the smooth flow from one season to the next, we are talking about the flow between yin and yang, and these transitions are primarily during the months indicated by the earthly branches *chen, xu, chou,* and *wei*. These four months belong to the earth element and correspond with the four extremities. With regard to time, whether we are discussing heaven, earth, or human beings, their transitions between yin and yang occur during these four time periods. In the larger macrocosm of the directions of the compass, we see that these four occupy the northeast, southeast, southwest, and northwest directions. In the human body, they are the four extremities of the body. The hands and feet are in fact important areas in which the yin and yang of the body transition from one to the other. Thus, if the transitions between yin and yang *qi* do not proceed smoothly, it is no wonder that this will first be noticed in the hands and feet. This is why line 337 states that "In reversal, there is counterflow cold of the hands and feet."

It is very important to recognize that the hands and feet act as the arena in which the smooth transition or flow of yin and yang occurs. Cold hands from the reversal of *qi* are the most basic sign allowing us to know that the patient is suffering from reversal (*jue*). Because *chen, xu, chou,* and *wei* are all transitional points between yin and yang, when problems arise during these four transitional periods, it easily results in counterflow. I have waited until we came to the earthly branch *chou* to discuss the *chen*, *xu, chou*, and *wei* as the transitional periods between yin and yang, because there is a qualitative difference between the transitional period of the earthly branch *chou* and the other three. The other three earthly stems are responsible for the transitions from one season to the next, but the *chou* earthly branch is responsible for the transition from one year to the next. *Chou* represents the most important transition period. If we look at all of the times in which disease tends to resolve in the six conformation theory of the *Treatise on Cold Damage*, we see that *chen* is the time period in which Shaoyang disease tends to resolve; *wei* is the period in which Taiyang disease tends to resolve; *xu* is the time in Yangming disease tends to resolve; and *chou* is the time in which all three yin, together, tend to resolve; *chou* prognosticates for the three yin. Among the twelve earthly branches, only *chou* has such extensive influence. From the perspective of the temporal correspondences with the six conformations, we can see that *chou* is far more potent than any of the other earthly branches. The salience of reversal (*jue*) syndromes in Jueyin disease, and the prevalence of reversal symptoms in Jueyin disease are easily understood when we recognize the importance of the *chou* earthly branch as a transition between the yin of the previous year and the yang of the next.

III.1.d. Prevalence of Reversal or Return of Heat

"Prevalence of reversal or return of heat" (*jue re shengfu* 厥熱勝復), also known as "reversal of heat" (*jue re* 厥熱), is an important topic in the Jueyin chapter. From our previous conversation, we know that once we pass the time period of *chou*, we enter into spring. In the spring, the yang *qi* increases every day, and every day more is released. If this critical juncture is not traversed, then the yin and yang *qi* do not flow as they should, then the yang *qi* does not increase, nor does it recover. Reversal syndrome means that the yin and yang *qi* do not flow into and connect with each other, but the core problem is that the yang *qi* does not increase and is unable to recover; the yang *qi* cannot emerge from the yin. If the yang *qi* cannot recover, and yang cannot emerge from the yin, then of course the hands and feet will suffer from counterflow cold. If this problem is not corrected and the reversal syndrome is permitted to persist, then eventually the person's survival will be threatened. If the above-mentioned state is corrected, and the yin and yang *qi* allowed to flow properly, then the yang *qi* is able to increase, and the yang is able to emerge from the yin, and the hands and feet will naturally shift from counterflow cold to warmth. This return of normal warmth, relative to the reversal cold, is referred to as "heat." In the Jueyin chapter, "prevalence of reversal or return of heat," or "reversal of heat," refers directly to the state of the hands or feet as exhibiting either counterflow cold or normal warmth. If the *jue* state predominates, and the counterflow cold is prevalent, then the challenge to the transition between yin and yang *qi* is serious. If this is the case, the yin is completed but the yang cannot emerge, the yang cannot recover, and the patient's case may be fatal. If, on the other hand, warmth and heat is more prevalent than counterflow cold, then this indicates that the difficulty transitioning from yin to yang is gradually resolving, the yang *qi* is gradually emerging, and recovering, and the disease will resolve with relative ease. When we observe the relative condition of reversal and heat in the patient, we are in fact observing the transition from yin to yang, and the mutual flow of yin and yang *qi*. This same sign also reveals whether the disease is becoming more threatening or if it is tending toward resolution.

III.2. The Meaning of the Jueyin Orientation

III.2.a. Principles for Establishment of the Jueyin Formula

All of the issues of Jueyin disease are caused by a loss of the original nature of Jueyin, and the treatment of Jueyin disease and the resolution of its consequences naturally revolve around restoring this original nature. What is the original nature of Jueyin? In the above passage, we touched upon a number of important issues; these are in fact discussions of the original nature and function of Jueyin. The nature of Jueyin is best revealed by the nature of the time in which Jueyin disease tends to resolve and by the corresponding direction of that particular time. Jueyin disease occurs when Jueyin loses the inherent qualities embodied by the *chou* time period and its corresponding direction on the compass. Thus, the establishment of a formula for Jueyin must be done on the basis of the direction indicated by the time period in which Jueyin disease tends to resolve: the direction corresponding to *chou*, *yin*, and *mao*. This is not only a basic principle for the establishment of formulas for Jueyin, but is also a basic principle for

Chinese Medicine in general! Laozi and Confucius were in agreement: "We cannot depart from the Dao; all that we can depart from is not the Dao." The Dao of Chinese Medicine is nothing more or less than time and space! This is something we must keep in mind every minute of every hour that we practice or contemplate Chinese Medicine.

The time period spanned by *chou*, *yin*, and *mao* is the time in which winter ends and spring arrives, when yin is completed and yang is born. It straddles both winter and spring, and possesses the characteristics of both. The *qi* of winter is cold and cool, and the *qi* of spring is warm and hot. Thus, the *chou*, *yin*, and *mao* time orientation is a complex of cold and warm, exhibiting cold and heat simultaneously. However, only the *qi* of the *chou* earthly branch is cold, whereas the *qi* of *yin* and *mao* is warm. This makes the warmth and heat predominate over the cold and cool *qi*. The establishment of a formula for Jueyin should include this special characteristic of cold and heat. Additionally, Jueyin belongs to the same category as wind and wood. The numbers of wind and wood are three and eight, and the flavor of wind and wood is sour. We must keep the numbers and the flavor of Jueyin in mind when contemplating the establishment of a formula for Jueyin.

III.2.b. An Explanation of Wumei Wan

In accord with the principles underlying the establishment of a formula discussed above, it is easily apparent that Wumei Wan is the governing formula of the Jueyin chapter. First of all, Wumei Wan is discussed in line 338 of the *Treatise on Cold Damage*. Is it just a coincidence that these are the numbers of wind and wood, the numbers of Jueyin? I do not believe that it is. From the number of this particular line, we can see that the ancients took great pain to order the lines in an appropriate way, and thereby convey additional information by means of the numerical sequence. This information lies in the numbers three and eight, conveying wind and wood. If we look back at line 38 of the *Treatise on Cold Damage* to examine the numerological significance of three and eight further, we see that line 38 discusses Da Qinglong Tang. The *qinglong* (blue-green dragon) belongs to the east, to wind and wood, and from this we know that discussing this formula in line 38 is not mere coincidence; it is an expression of the connection between the numerology of three and eight and the deeper significance of the formula. From the fact that Wumei Wan occurs in this particular line, we already know that it is no ordinary formula.

Next, let us continue by looking at the special characteristics of Wumei Wan when it comes to its use of hot and cold *qi*. As far as the general makeup of the formula is concerned, we can see that Wumei Wan is made up of two sets of herbs: hot and cold. The warm and hot herbs in Wumei Wan are Wumei, Xixin, Ganjiang, Danggui, Fuzi, Chuanjiao, and Guizhi. Altogether, there are seven warming herbs in the formula. The three cold and cool herbs in the formula are Huanglian, Huangbai, and Renshen (in the *Divine Farmer's Classic of Materia Medica*, Renshen is described as sweet and slightly cold). The proportion of hot to cold herbs, with heat predominating over cold, matches precisely the formula establishment principle for Jueyin as we previously described: warmth and heat preponderating over cold and coolness.

This leads us to the next question. The name of this formula is Wumei Wan, which means that it is certain that Wumei is the emperor herb. Why is Wumei the emperor of this formula? It is because the eastern direction generates wind, wind generates wood, and wood generates sourness. The flavor of Jueyin is also sour. Since this is the ruling formula of Jueyin, the sour flavor must also rule. Of all the sour herbs, what herb is more sour than Wumei? It is only natural, then, that Wumei should rule the formula that governs Jueyin. The original formula for Wumei Wan indicates that 300 Wumei be used. Why not 200? Once again, this number has significance with regard to the essential character of this particular Jueyin formula.

In the Wumei Wan formula, this herb, already sour, is further subjected to soaking in "bitter wine" (similar to vinegar) overnight. In this way, the sourness of the vinegar compounds the sourness of the plums. In *Treatise on Cold Damage*, we do find other formulas that make use of sour herbs, but when it comes to the degree of sourness, no other formula can compare with this one. These three aspects of Wumei Wan, its *qi*, its flavor, and its number are all in perfect accord with the time and orientation of Jueyin. This unparalleled correspondence with the essential nature of Jueyin leaves no doubt that Wumei Wan is the ruling formula of Jueyin disease.

Having completed our discussion of the three facets of Wumei Wan in the preceding paragraph, the reader may yet raise an important question. If Jueyin is the time in which the yin is completed and the yang is born, and if it represents wind and wood, then the most essential quality of Jueyin ought to be the raising and releasing of yang. But, as is common knowledge, Wumei and vinegar, being very sour medicinals, have an constraining effect. Although the aim of Jueyin is to raise up and release outward, the emperor herb used to achieve this aim is sour and constraining. This would seem to be a great contradiction. If this contradiction cannot be resolved, then our previous insights into the logic underlying the construction of the Wumei Wan formula have failed to produce a solid, thorough, applicable understanding of this formula. If we do not have a thorough understanding of this formula, then there is no way that we can implement it effectively.

The nature of wood is to rise and to release, but the nature of sourness is to constrain; how can we achieve rising and releasing by using constraint? We can find hints of an answer in Chapter 36 of Laozi's *Classic of the Dao and Its Virtue*: "That which is about to breathe easy must have been tense; that which is about to falter must have been strong; that which is about to fall into disuse must have once been prosperous and fortunate; that which is about to be seized must have once been given. This is called insight into the minute." If we take this "insight into the minute" and apply it to Jueyin and to Wumei Wan, then we might say: "That which is about to rise and release must have been constrained."

Why is this the case? If we look at the composition of Wumei Wan, we can see that it contains a total of seven warm and hot herbs, which is a greater number of warm and hot herbs than is found in any other formula in the *Treatise on Cold Damage*. The warm and hot herbs found in Wumei Wan are both copious and varied: the Chuanjiao and Danggui warm Jueyin; Xixin warms Taiyang and Shaoyin; Ganjiang and Fuzi warm the three yin, although Ganjiang has an affinity for Taiyin and Fuzi for Shaoyin; and Guizhi has an affinity for both Taiyang and Jueyin. Wumei Wan contains such a wild array of warm and hot herbs that it seems to be heading in all directions, and is capable of warming all aspects of the body. However, this particular formula needs only warm Jueyin. How is this cacophony of warm and hot herbs focused solely on Jueyin? If we examine this formula closely, we can see Zhang Zhongjing's answer: by using such a seemingly inordinate amount of sour Wumei, this formula is able to gather and concentrate the warming effects of its various warm and hot herbs under a single banner, exerting all of its effect on Jueyin of the body. The use of Wumei in this formula is ingenious and profound.

Wumei Wan provides us with a glimpse into the uncanny workings of classical formulas, and has allowed us to observe the skill involved in creating and establishing them. Wumei Wan uses the Chinese black plum Wumei as a banner, like a flag held high, to concentrate the effect of the other herbs in the formula, allowing the *qi* of Jueyin to break free of the fetters of yin and bring forth yang from yin. This allows for the ascent and release of yang, and allows for a smooth transition from the yin of winter to the yang of spring. Thus, we see the same principle outlined by Laozi at work, namely: "That which is about to rise and release must have been constrained."

Taking a bird's-eye view of Jueyin and Wumei Wan, we can see that a major factor leading to the inability to rise and release is that the *qi* of Jueyin is fettered by yin-cold. Whenever there is a process of fettering, this must lead to constraint and obstruction. Constraint and obstruction, in turn, must lead to the production of heat. So why does Wumei Wan, in addition to its warming herbs, also contain two herbs that are bitter and cold? They serve to restrain heat that has emerged from constraint and obstruction.

The last herb, Renshen, assists right *qi* and augments the effects of the other herbs. In addition, Zhang Zhongjing also takes advantage of another important effect of Renshen: its ability to produce fluids and stop thirst. Dispersion-thirst is, after all, the first sign of Jueyin disease listed in the opening line of the chapter. The ginseng in this formula has the effect of stopping this thirst. Moreover, besides the thirst-quenching properties of Renshen, we should remember the tale from the *Romance of the Three Kingdoms* in which Wumei are sought to slake thirst.

To summarize, Wumei Wan is an extremely important and very commonly used formula in the clinical setting. It not only treats reversal induced by worms, chronic diarrhea, and dispersion-thirst as listed in line 338, but also can be used to treat vertex headaches and conditions involving testicular inflammation and swelling. Wumei Wan can also be used in accord with its underlying principles to treat other ailments of the reproductive system. As long as the principles underlying the efficacy of Wumei Wan are fully understood, there will be no question of its clinical efficacy or how to implement it. In my opinion, not only Wumei Wan but also each and every one of the 112 formulas in the *Treatise on Cold Damage* is like this. As long as the underlying principles of each formula are fully comprehended, the physician will feel at ease using them in the clinical setting. Conveying this knowledge is one of the main aims of this book. Why is this book titled *"Contemplating Chinese Medicine"* in Chinese? What is it that we are contemplating? It is nothing other than these underlying principles, nothing other than the mysteries of nature and life as deciphered through the orientations of time.

Author's Epilogue
to the English Edition

After ten years of sustained effort, Dr. Heiner Fruehauf and his colleagues have produced the English translation of *Classical Chinese Medicine* and passed it on to The Chinese University Press for publication. At this time, besides expressing my heartfelt gratitude to Dr. Fruehauf and to everyone else involved in this effort, I would like to take the opportunity to say a few words about the spirit of Chinese Medicine and Chinese culture.

A core concept in Chinese Medicine is that of yin and yang. Or, to put it another way, Chinese Medicine views and understands the world from the perspective of yin yang. As this is a characteristic shared by Chinese culture in general, gaining a nuanced feeling of this concept is essential for understanding both the culture of China and its medicine. Confucius expressed the importance of this core concept in the *Tradition of the Appended Statements* commentary to the *Classic of Changes*:

> Yin alternating with yang; this is the Dao. That which follows this is good. That which completes this is nature. The benevolent see this and say that it is benevolence, the wise see this and say that it is wisdom, and the common people interact with this every day without recognizing it; thus the Dao of the person of noble character is rare indeed.

Taking this definition of the Dao as set forth by Confucius, it seems quite natural for the *Yellow Emperor's Classic*, a revered repository of ancient medical knowledge, to refer to those who have mastered the art of medicine as "those of the Dao." Yin and yang are manifest forms of the formless Dao, expressed as opposites: Heaven and earth, man and woman, water and fire, front and back, left and right, and as opposites, they contradict and oppose one another at a fundamental level. The practice of medicine is a process of following these embodied contradictions to bring about their harmonious coexistence, which can be understood in Confucius's words: ". . . that which follows this is good."

The most extreme worldly expression of this yin yang contradiction is the phenomenon of birth and death. One could say that birth and death are the most important events in each and every life, and that both are inescapable. Facing these most important of things, these inescapable eventualities, can one still search for a place of "no death"? This may be exactly what is expressed in ". . . that which completes this is nature." This exquisite search for completion, for perfection, has guided threads that are woven throughout every aspect of Chinese culture.

I personally feel that two different approaches to the yin yang contradiction of birth and death are present in Chinese culture and its medicine. One is the pursuit of a long and healthy life, with the "hundred-year lifespan" ideal of longevity practices as its ultimate expression. At the same time, there is also a pervasive interest in penetrating through this contradiction and realizing the perfection of immortality: freedom from the restrictions of birth and death. *Explanation of the Trigrams* from the *Classic of Changes* says of this: "Go search into the deepest for the fundamentality of all things and understand the ultimate nature of human beings, culminating in the perfection of life." The ideal of leading a long and healthy life is a goal that is comfortably within the confines of birth and death; perfection of life, on the other hand, is a description of a fundamental nature beyond worldly manifestation.

The glorious complexity of Chinese culture has arisen from posing and grappling with the above questions, and different levels of understanding, exploring, and perceiving the problem have been proposed. Or, as Confucius put it: ". . . the benevolent see this and say that it is benevolence, the wise see this and say that it is wisdom."

How can one play a role in the worldly harmonization of contradictory manifestations? How can one "follow the Dao" as expressed by Confucius? The essential clue lies in "harmonizing." And in this world of contradictions, how can one perfect life? How can one "complete the Dao"? Here the essence is in the realization of "centering." Confucius's grandson Zisi, in *Doctrine of the Mean* wrote: "Centering: the great origin of all under Heaven. Harmonizing: the achieved way of all under Heaven. With perfection of centering and harmonizing, Heaven and earth each find their place in the great order, and the ten thousand things are nurtured." From this perspective, "centering" and "harmonizing" are no less than the most essential of all aspects of Chinese culture, and likewise of Chinese Medicine!

On the eve of the publication of the English version of *Classical Chinese Medicine*, it is my sincerest wish that this text might serve as an entryway to a deeper and more authentic understanding of the culture of China, and of the spirit of Chinese Medicine. If my dear readers can achieve this, then they will be able to think out over half of the problems in Chinese Medicine!

January 10, 2016
Liu Lihong
Director, Institute for the Clinical Research of Classical Chinese Medicine
Guangxi University of Traditional Chinese Medicine and Pharmacology
Nanning, China

NINE QUESTIONS ON CONTEMPLATING CHINESE MEDICINE

Question One

Q: In the three years since *Classical Chinese Medicine* was published in China, the book has inspired belief in and enthusiasm for Chinese Medicine in the hearts of many who read it. There has also been a corresponding increase in media interest in Chinese Medicine, which I consider to be a positive phenomenon—no matter whether the news is positive or negative. My question is, after these three years of criticism and appreciation of *Classical Chinese Medicine*, do you, as the "contemplator," have any further thoughts on Chinese Medicine? Or to put it another way, what is your own response to the public reaction to your book?

A: I greatly appreciate the questions you have presented here, and the straightforward manner in which you have expressed them. As the early twentieth-century scholar Hu Shi said of himself: "I am merely an innovator, not a teacher." I'm very much aware that I too am unlikely to be considered as a teacher, as my nature is too frank and honest, and I lack even the patience necessary to give systematic guidance, much less the warm and kindhearted nature we see in great teachers.

   It was back in 2003 that I first received word that *Classical Chinese Medicine* had been published. Around that time I had traveled to Guilin for a short period of voluntary seclusion, and it was just when I was ready to emerge that I received a call from Beijing telling me that the book had been published. This being the first time a work of my own had shown its face to the world, the news naturally affected my seclusion.

Before this I had observed to my wife that the publishing of this book would mark the completion of the first half of my life's work. So what was I to do with the second half? My desire at the time was to live a life of seclusion, of simple days where a belly full of food would be enough to satisfy me. And what was the point of this seclusion? It was not just to stay aloof from worldly things, but rather it was to be able to probe deeply into the scholarly questions of traditional culture, for probing into the questions of Chinese Medicine requires a quiet heart and great swaths of time.

Take the *Treatise on Cold Damage* (Shanghanlun) for example. Although this ancient text has been researched deeply for over a thousand years, when it comes to my own understanding of the complete text, problems stand out acutely. I can only say that I fully apprehend the meaning of several dozen lines of the text, and each and every one of these contains profound elements that shock me to my core! Naturally, to deeply apprehend all 398 lines of the text is no simple task, and without time, and without a quiet heart, it becomes nearly impossible.

Today, three years after the book was published, I can look back on my desires for a life of simplicity and seclusion as if it were just yesterday. And where am I now? I find myself in the unenviable state of having my hands full of work and new responsibilities. Trying to understand what led to this, whether I was indulging in my newfound fame, or whether I was prompted by a sense of responsibility, or a combination of both, I know now what it means to feel tugged and drawn by the demands of worldly things. I respect more than ever those ancients who were able to withdraw themselves from society, and understand Confucius's deep yearning for and praise of solitude.

Just as you stated in your question, there has been both positive and negative attention paid to *Classical Chinese Medicine* in the three years since it was first published. Regarding the praise, as the author, I cannot help but feel a sense of gratitude. The book has served to change many people's attitude toward traditional culture, toward

Chinese Medicine, and has brought such solace to the hearts and minds of many. How could I not feel a sense of pleasure and satisfaction at such a state of affairs?

At the same time, this is tempered by an awareness that, as the ancients said, it is the times that give rise to heroes, not the other way round. It is plain to see from the letters I receive that the issues around which this book centers are on the minds of many others as well. I receive praise because I've been able to contemplate these issues on a slightly deeper level than others, and because I was able to express these out loud in these very unique times.

There have been many people who have argued that the Chinese people and Chinese culture are worthy of the world's attention. It is my opinion that one of the most impressive aspects of the Chinese people is their vitality. The world population stands at about 6 billion, 1.3 billion of whom are in China. And this is in spite of the effects of the one-child policy—without which the number would be even higher. If one compares the total amount of available farmland with the total population, the fact that such a limited amount of land can support so many people is quite extraordinary! This point alone points to the vitality of the Chinese people.

The culture of the Chinese people has undergone various calamities over the millennia, starting with the book burning and anti-Confucianism of the first emperor of the Qin dynasty. In spite of these, Chinese culture has not just failed to collapse as so many others have done, but today it is attracting worldwide attention in this, the twenty-first century. If this doesn't speak to the vitality of Chinese culture, then I don't know what else could!

What is it that imparts such vitality to Chinese culture? It is its adaptability, its ability to renew itself in every era. To use an expression from Buddhism, it is able to adapt to the "three ages"—the past, present, and future. At many times it seemed as if this culture had been beaten down, but her spirit was not vanquished, as the roots of her original *qi* are deep and strong. It was in appearance only that she was beaten down.

When it comes to traditional culture, I cannot help but hold an optimistic outlook. Traditional culture cannot be vanquished, and if she cannot be vanquished, then Chinese Medicine cannot be vanquished. Just as an adolescent goes through a period of rebellious behavior, a period of resistance, misunderstanding, or even ridicule, too must pass. And what is it that gives traditional culture this ability to adapt to every era? This I will address in more detail when answering your other questions.

Getting back to the book, in the first six months after *Classical Chinese Medicine* was published, I received many letters, and I was more or less able to answer every letter I received. Slowly the level of correspondence increased, to the point where it was no longer possible to reply to each and every one of these. As the vast majority of these letters were written praising the book, and critical letters were quite rare, I prioritized replying to the criticism. However, I've heard that there is quite a bit of criticism on the internet as well, and recently an article containing some criticism was also published in the *Chinese News of Traditional Chinese Medicine* (Zhongguo Zhongyi-yao bao).

No one is a saint, and no one is free of errors. The ancients said that the prerequisite for writing a book is that one's "chest is free of even a mote of dust." To me this seems a distant ideal, and as someone with a pile of dust and dirt in my chest, my writings will naturally contain problematic areas as well.

My discussion of the limitations of Chinese Medicine in acute illnesses and medical trauma in the book is one of these areas. At the time I was writing the book, my experience was limited and I had little exposure to emergency medicine. Although my hospital had a busy ER ward, as a Chinese Medicine physician I was not allowed to treat these patients. If the patients' lives were saved, it was at the hands of Western Medicine, and if they died, it was also at the hands of Western Medicine. With such a background, it was natural for me to hold the opinions I expressed in the book.

After the book was written, I had the good fortune to be acknowledged as a disciple of Deng Tietao, Li Ke, and Lu Chong-han. Under their instruction and influence, I was able to advance my understanding of the treatment of acute and critical conditions. Li Ke in particular had been practicing primary-care medicine for nearly 50 years, all at the grassroots level in the countryside. His unique experience with treating acute, critical, and serious conditions has taught us that Chinese Medicine also has a special efficacy in the treatment of emergent and acute conditions, and in some aspects, like the treatment of acute heart failure, it is even superior to Western Medicine.

We can further illustrate this point by looking at the 2003 outbreak of severe acute respiratory syndrome (SARS) in China. SARS attacks fiercely, progresses rapidly, and has a high mortality rate. In Guangdong province, where Chinese Medicine was included as one of the interventions, the mortality rate was 3.8 percent. Compare this to Hong Kong, separated by a cultural and political border from Guangdong but not geographically separate, where Chinese Medicine was used sparingly and the mortality rate was 17 percent. This both illustrates the importance of Chinese Medicine in treating medical emergencies, and should also serve as an important lesson for us to learn from.

When it comes to criticism of this and other problematic areas in my book, I welcome it! Of course, some of the criticism I received was not constructive, but seemed to stem from anger and a desire to establish superiority. In martial arts, where one can distinguish between superior and inferior, one can issue a challenge of this sort. But for scholars, for those debating the Dao, there is no reason to issue such a challenge, and in fact it is more likely than not to result in injury to the challenger. As the recipient, there is a direct benefit to accepting constructive criticism. At the same time, being able to accept criticism of an angry or challenging nature can bring even greater benefit! So I have a sense of deep gratitude to all of my critics.

Question Two

Q: Of the many questions regarding the future of Chinese Medicine, there is one assertion in particular which I feel is impossible to get around; that is the assertion that Chinese Medicine is pseudoscience. There are many who use this assertion to reject the value of Chinese

Medicine. Of course, the way I see it, this is a false assertion, but there is no question that in modern times there is a tendency to assert that "science" is the standard by which all fields must be judged, without which a particular practice cannot and will not be widely adopted by society. As such, the relationship between science and Chinese Medicine has become a question that cannot be neglected.

In *Classical Chinese Medicine,* this problem is discussed to a certain degree. Could you now bring those elements together and discuss your take on this problem?

A: Regarding the scientific nature of Chinese Medicine, the 2005 edited volume *Chinese Medicine in the Eye of Philosophy* (Zheyan kan Zhongyi) dealt with this question in a focused manner, and it contains an article I authored contemplating this issue. My recollection of what I wrote is that, as it relates to daily life, "science" is really no more than a custom or habit of modern times. Just as people from Sichuan province customarily eat very spicy and boldly flavored dishes, called "Chuan cuisine." If a dish is not prepared with hot peppers and Sichuan peppercorn, it doesn't matter how well it's prepared, people from Sichuan will not eat it. When it comes to the relationship between Chinese Medicine and "science," this is comparable to a Sichuan native sitting down to a dish of Shanghai cuisine. Shanghai food is as sweet as Sichuan food is spicy, and although a Shanghai native will water at the mouth at the mention of this, a Sichuan native will consider these dishes intolerable.

This is why I have grown less and less interested in the question of the scientific nature of Chinese Medicine. I feel it is really quite meaningless! Let's say Chinese Medicine is scientific. Can it cure disease? Yes! Let's say Chinese Medicine is not scientific, can still cure disease? Yes, nothing has changed! This is like preparing a dish of Shanghai cuisine for a crowd of Sichuan natives, and adding a dash of hot peppers and peppercorns right at the end. What is the result? Not only will the Sichuanese reject it, but if you send it back to Shanghai, they won't touch it either. This can serve as an analogy for the situation in which Chinese Medicine has found itself in recent decades.

Chinese Medicine represents a complete system of theory that can be applied to address many of today's problems. This branch of medicine is sorely needed in today's world. Of course, due to the fact that Chinese Medicine developed in ancient times, many of its methods are quite dissimilar to modern day practices. This is a problem, so how does one resolve it? On the one hand, in order to be able to obtain the services of this medicine, the modern era needs to adapt itself to Chinese Medicine. At the same time, the question of whether Chinese Medicine can adapt its methods in order to make it easier for modern people to accept it needs to be raised as well, as long as it does not involve harm to the medicine itself.

There is another question, of how Chinese Medicine is to be regarded by modern science. It is my opinion that the principles and methods of Chinese Medicine are a worthy subject of research. Nestled within these principles and methods are many secrets, which if made explicit, will be able to encourage the development of modern science. However, if this research is to have any chance of success, it must be carried out by practitioners of modern science themselves. Of course, Chinese Medicine should play a role in this research, but it should absolutely not be carried out solely by individuals in the field itself. If we continue the way we have over the last several decades, where East is not East and West is not West, then neither East nor West will benefit.

Question Three

Q: The issue of how to pass on the Chinese medical body of knowledge from generation to generation, or to put it another way, the issue of education in Chinese Medicine, is discussed at great length in your book. Your depth of feeling is palpable, and it seems that this is an issue that greatly concerns you.

In the time since the book was published, I have also gained an appreciation of the importance of this issue, and recently published an article on this subject. When it came to discussing the recurring historical movements to "discard the physicians and keep the drugs" (*feiyi cunyao*), I wrote the following: "If the physicians are not saved, what will become of the drugs?" The question of "saving the physicians," of safeguarding and developing physicians truly proficient in Chinese Medicine, is a key issue here.

This brings us to the question of education. What possibilities do you feel exist to change the problems inherent in modern Chinese Medicine education?

A: Education is a huge issue. It is also an area where it is extremely difficult to make significant changes.

Essentially, education consists of those that teach and those who are taught, and an organic teacher-student relationship is fundamental to quality education. Since ancient times the importance of the role of the "Teacher" has been recognized, exemplified in phrases such as "the Dao of the Teacher is dignified and honorable." The individual teacher bears primary responsibility in this teacher-student equation, but in modern times the role of the teacher has been deemphasized in favor of the role of the system in education. This is one of the main characteristics of the modern compulsory educational model.

The position of the teacher in modern education has faded, and the "dignity and honor" of the teacher, and the respect that goes with it, has been accorded to the educational system instead. The twentieth-century scholar and educator Mei Yiqi said that "the greatness of a university should be in its faculty, not in its facilities," but it seems that universities these days are judged by how many PhDs and grants they obtain, not how many great teachers they have.

Emphasizing the role of the teacher in education is a way of individualizing education, and as this puts many choices in the hands of the teacher, it naturally gives rise to different styles or schools of thought. When it comes to Chinese Medicine, it is the teacher who provides the link between theory and practice; between foundational knowledge and clinical knowledge, and two thousand years of history have proven that this model of education is best suited for passing on knowledge in the Chinese medical tradition.

In the twentieth century, this particular model of individualized education is nowhere to be found, having been replaced with the standardized common education model. Chinese Medicine education is no exception. A few decades ago, the situation was a bit better, as the surviving remnants of the teacher-disciple generation of physicians were still teaching. In recent years, however, many from the older generation have passed away, and with them their unique knowledge and experience. They have been replaced by a new generation of educators, all of whom are products of the modern professional training system. The previous generation of teachers with the ability to thread together theory and practice have been replaced by subject specialists, each quarantined from their colleagues by the limitations of their specializations.

This is the basic situation that Chinese Medicine finds itself in today, and this is why I feel that the crux of the problem lies firstly in teachers' ability to connect theory and practice, and secondly in the standardized education model, which does not serve the needs of a field requiring individualized education.

Taken together, the paucity of master teachers and the corresponding compartmentalization of specialties add up to a very serious situation. So serious, in fact, that some of the older generation describe themselves as "the last Chinese Medicine physicians." I myself am not so pessimistic about the situation, as these last few decades represent a mere eddy in the long river of history, and this difficult period too will pass. I am confident that before long people will wake up to the truth, and recognize the value of individualized education, and of the Dao of the Teacher. It is as Confucius said: "Only in winter does one realize that pines and cypress do not lose their color." Perhaps our situation is not yet bitter and cold enough for us to recognize the uniqueness of pines and cypress. But this time should not be far off.

Taking this perspective, we should not be surprised that Chinese Medicine has undergone many trials and tribulations in the twentieth century. This period will be known as one that resulted in a complete re-evaluation of Chinese Medicine; one that brought about a new recognition of Chinese Medicine's value. It will be known as a traumatic but essential experience that resulted in Chinese Medicine rediscovering its own path, not just in education, but in all aspects.

After *Classical Chinese Medicine* was published, I received many letters, phone calls, and visits from those who read the book. Many of those who came to visit me wished to be accepted as disciples. Some had never studied or practiced medicine, but still wished to give up their former careers and start anew. One young college student from the far north even trekked from Jinan to Guangxi province by foot in order to study with me. I am deeply touched by their heartfelt enthusiasm, and they have given me new hope for the future of Chinese Medicine.

At the same time, someone at my own level of learning is only fit to be a student, not a teacher. The Dao of the Teacher is a respectful and serious matter! As said in a traditional rhyming couplet: "One who does not respect the Dao of the Teacher will be destroyed by heaven and earth; when a teacher leads the young astray, they will behave like thieves and whores." This is a serious matter indeed! The first couplet describes a student, a disciple. A disciple must respect their teacher and the Dao of the Teacher. It is as important as the old saying: "A teacher for a day is a father for life." If a student does not respect their teacher, not only will heaven punish them, but earth will as well, with results that are easy to imagine.

The second couplet discusses the teacher. As one with the responsibility of guiding the young, if one can truly transmit the Dao, teach a profession, and resolve confusion, then one is indeed passing on the great arts of the ancients; one is creating a peaceful and tranquil environment among the myriad things. In this way, one has truly performed a great service to mankind. However, if one cannot do this, and instead leads the young astray, then the next generation will be composed of thieves and whores, a prospect that makes one shudder with fear.

Modern education is not based on respect for the Dao of the Teacher. Modern education respects the system. It is a simple business transaction; as long as the price is agreed upon, everything is fine. At the same time, as a member of the teaching profession, it is still important to be aware of your position of power and exercise caution. This is something that those of you wishing to follow a master also need to develop an understanding of.

In the time since *Classical Chinese Medicine* was published, I've apprenticed to three different masters. The first, in June 2004, was the renowned physician and professor Deng Tietao (1916–2019). At 90 years old then, Professor Deng was still campaigning vigorously on behalf of Chinese Medicine, sparing no pains. At every moment I feel the influence of Professor Deng's spirit and character encouraging and spurring me on.

On the recommendation of Professor Deng, I traveled to the small county of Lingshi in Shanxi province to follow the locally acclaimed physician Li Ke. Li Ke was a living Bodhisattva. He never ignored a patient in need. To be in the presence of his depth of compassion and his character makes me feel shame at my own failings. I could spend the rest of my lifetime learning from him. I must also point out his eye-opening use of high doses of Fuzi, the prepared root of *aconitum carmichaeli* Debx., in healing even the gravest of diseases!

In the summer of 2005, the heavens smiled on me, and another master quietly became part of my destiny. I had the opportunity to become on intimate terms with someone I had admired for a long time, the lineage holder of the Lu-family medical tradition, known as the Fire Spirit School, Lu Chonghan. After many twists and turns, a year later on New Year's Day I was accepted as his highest inner-door disciple. The Lu-family medical tradition stretches back over two hundred years, and my master's grandfather was no other than Lu Zhuzhi, the highest disciple of the renowned late-Qing dynasty physician Zheng Qin'an. As the highest disciple he received the genuine tradition from Zheng Qin'an, and by combining it with his own family knowledge he created the Lu branch of the Fire Spirit school. In fact, the mysterious figure I described in my book, the legendary physician from Chengdu Tian "Bawei" (i.e. Dr. Tian "Who Never Uses More Than Eight Herbs") was once a student of Lu Zhuzhi.

After being accepted as disciple by Lu Chonghan, my master passed on his oral teachings to me, and with clear strikes and subtle pushes, over the next several months it was as if my body and form had been shaken to the core. I knew then the astonishing wonder of the master-disciple relationship. I knew then the respect and honor inherent in the Dao of the Teacher!

It is clear to me that to resolve the problems in Chinese Medicine education, it is essential to return to the model I've outlined above.

I would also like to take this opportunity to address those readers who are themselves searching for a master to follow. Please take note: the art of medicine is one of benevolence. Wishing to learn such an art requires a benevolent heart, and even though there are many ways of practicing this art of medicine, this is what all great teachers have in common. Conversely, if one searches for a teacher without first filling one's own heart with compassion, then this will prove to be as impossible as climbing a tree to catch a fish. If you seek to follow a renowned teacher, you must first develop a benevolent heart. And what is this benevolent heart? It is one filled with love and mercy. It is one that does not avoid bitter labor, and it is one that is generous to those in need. It is not filled with a desire for fame, for profit, or for selfish gain.

Having a benevolent heart means that your own heart is your true teacher. If this is the case, then finding a teacher is only a matter of time. If this is not the case, then seeking out a teacher will prove to be a great challenge!

Question Four

Q: I always wanted to ask you about a particularly profound sentence in your book, which you ascribe to your first teacher Li Yangbo: "To prescribe a formula is to prescribe time." Could you further elucidate the meaning here? A conception of time is inherent in the idea of the five movements and six *qi* (*wuyun liuqi*), which seems congruent with recent approaches, such as the medical application of chronobiology. Not too long ago, I was reading about a seemingly related story of the Chinese Medicine physician Shi Jinmo and his treatment of an outbreak of epidemic encephalitis B in the mid-twentieth century. Of the more than 100 patients receiving treatment, 98 were treated successfully, and in spite of their shared diagnosis of encephalitis, each and every one of these were treated with a different formula. I feel that the issue of time may be a factor in these cases. Could you give your opinion?

A: "To prescribe a formula is to prescribe time" is indeed a wondrous statement, full of depth and meaning. To understand this sentence, one must first understand the first part: the meaning of "formula" (*fang*). *Fang* does not simply mean a combination of herbs. *Fang* should be better understood as indicating an "orientation" in time and space. The five phases also indicate an orientation, as do the 64 hexagrams. These "orientations" all represent distinct states of yin and yang.

Why is it that disease arises in the human body? Simply put, it is because of the disorder of yin and yang. So, one must create a unique orientation (*fang*) of yin yang that can regulate a particular yin yang disorder. This is expressed in the *Yellow Emperor's Internal Classic* (Huangdi neijing) in the phrase: "Heat that which is cold, cool that which is hot, drain the abundant, and supplement the deficient."

Time is like this as well. In China, time is not just a number; rather it is a mark or indication of a certain state of yin and yang. This is why China has used the heavenly stems and earthly branches (*gan zhi*) to mark time, not Arabic numerals. What underlies the stem and branches is the five phases; that is, different yin yang states. For this reason, whether we use the term "formula" (*fang*) or "time" is inconsequential, as the underlying concept is the same. From this perspective, "to prescribe a formula is to prescribe time" is easy to understand. For the same reason, areas of study such as the five movements and six *qi* can all be discussed in terms of yin and yang.

It is my opinion that the example you raised, of Jin Shimo using 98 different formulas to treat 98 different cases of encephalitis B, is a good example of this. What does it mean that he used a different formula for each patient? It means that the yin yang disorder in each and every case was unique, which naturally required a unique orientation for each formula. A higher-level physician is able to detect such subtleties, while a lower-level physician is only able to observe similarities. Likewise, when most physicians successfully treat one particular condition, they expect the next patient with that condition to be the same, so they simply use the same formula that had worked before. An experienced physician, on the other hand, is able to detect subtle differences, and address them with a different formula.

"Similarities," in fact, are relative, while "differences" are absolute. This recognition of the differences inherent in every situation is one of the most unique aspects of Chinese Medicine, and it is something that we ought to pay close attention to in this modern era!

Question Five

Q: In the book, you discussed the "path of the channels" and "internal experimentation" (see Chapter One, "I.3.c. Rational Thinking and Internal Experimentation"). I feel this is also a key issue to discuss. Often when we hear that Chinese Medicine is "not scientific," one of the key bits of evidence that this rests on is the fact that the type of experimentation as done in modern biomedicine (for example, that done with laboratory mice) is completely absent in Chinese Medicine. In spite of this, it seems that there must be a form of experimentation in Chinese Medicine, one that may even be superior to animal experimentation.

For example, the *Divine Farmer's Classic of Materia Medica* (Shennong bencao jing), the earliest materia medica, contained about 300 or 400 different medicinals. One and a half millennia later, Li Shizhen's *Compendium of Materia Medica* (Bencao gangmu) contained over 1,900 medicinals, representing an increase of approximately one medicinal per year. There must be an experimental process for these additions to the materia medica, though perhaps one performed on humans themselves rather than on animals.

Not long ago, the scholar Lü Jiage mentioned something interesting to me about the herb Badou, the dried mature fruit of *Croton tiglium* L. Badou is a purging medicinal that evacuates the bowels. However, when given to laboratory mice in an experimental setting, it was discovered that the mice did not develop diarrhea. On the contrary, they even seemed to enjoy eating it! The conclusion of this animal experiment was that Badou does not, in fact, have the function of purging. In response, Chinese Medicine practitioners pointed out that Badou is also known as "mouse beans" (*shu dou*), and that mice do not develop diarrhea from eating it, a fact that has long been recognized in Chinese Medicine. This curious example shows us that at the very least the results of laboratory mouse experiments are not as definitive as one might imagine.

What model of experimentation is inherent to Chinese Medicine?

A: The example you gave is quite interesting, as it demonstrates that the objects of inquiry in Chinese Medicine are not restricted to humans, but also include other animals. If this were not the case, how could "mouse beans" have been discovered?

The Chinese Medicine model of experimentation is expressed quite clearly in the *Great Commentary* (Xici) of the *Classic of Changes* (Yijing) where it describes the process of creating the eight trigrams by the ancient ruler Fuxi: "Near at hand, in his own person, he found things for consideration, and the same at a distance, in things in general" (Legge, *The I Ching*). The first half of this is referring to "internal experimentation," as discussed in my book. This aspect of my book received a lot of praise and some criticism, but regardless of people's opinions, it was one of the empirical methods used by the ancients, including Confucian, Buddhist, and Daoist traditions.

The second half of the quote is about "external experimentation." Of course, this external experimentation is different from modern experiments in the sciences, as technological conditions in ancient times did not allow for such experiments. At the same time, the "external experiments" performed by the ancients were quite ingenious.

For example, in your question you brought up the question of herb function. How were the functions of herbs discovered? We say that one particular medicinal can cause sweating, another increases urination. . . . Was it necessary to try each and every one of these? Of course, there is nothing wrong with direct experimentation with herbs, but even before trying an herb, the ancients had a good sense of its function, through a method which would get one quite close to an accurate understanding of the herb.

There is a farmer in Shanxi, an admirable figure called Ren Guangqing, who has been absorbed in herbal medicine research for the past 40 years. He has spent this time visiting every famous mountain and great river, all of the natural areas in the country. He has even traveled four times to the great mountain range in Guangxi where I live. He has spent these decades living in nature in the simplest and most basic of conditions, usually for several months at a time. In this way, he has been able to closely observe how animals and plants live and die, and observe their every aspect, color, and smell.

After spending so many years in this way, if you randomly picked a plant growing by the side of the road, Ren Guangqing would be able to fairly accurately tell you its functions and properties. How is this possible? It is no more and no less than this ancient method of "external experimentation."

Question Six

Q: You make the case in your book that the heart of Chinese Medicine is yin yang. This also happens to be the aspect of Chinese Medicine that has been attacked the most fiercely, as critics feel that this theoretical basis shows that Chinese Medicine is metaphysical rather than scientific medicine.

Those who have been influenced by classical elementalism in the Western tradition mistakenly believe that the five phases or elements (*wuxing*) in Chinese Medicine refer to five different types of material, rather than a model of five different yin yang relationships. They then criticize the model by misunderstanding it as representing different molecular elements. I feel that having an accurate understanding of the *wuxing* is extremely important, especially if we wish to understand the *wuxing* in the context of Chinese Medicine. I would like to know more about your understanding of yin yang and *wuxing*.

A: I have devoted a lot of space to this issue in my book. The study of yin yang is not metaphysics, but is rather a very simple and concrete branch of learning. The ancients have also written about this issue exhaustively. For example, the late Qing scholar-physician Zheng Qin'an wrote in *The Unbroken Circle of Medical Methods* (Yifa yuantong): "The Dao of medicine can determine life or death.

A physician cannot simply be a supplier of formulas or herbs, but rather must put the highest value on recognizing the substantial evidence of patterns. What constitutes substantial evidence? It is naught but yin and yang, vacuity and repletion. These two words, yin and yang, can express infinite variations. On the higher levels, there is evidence of yin yang; on the middle levels, there is evidence of yin yang; on the lower levels, there is evidence of yin yang. [. . .] When one understands both the yin yang evidence of the disease, and the yin yang evidence of medicinals, then the use of merely one or two herbs can be enough to bring about a response."

So if yin yang most highly values substantial evidence, how can it be metaphysics? Of course, we might not be able to define this evidence in terms of atoms or molecules, and it is going to be difficult to communicate what they are in terms of molecular chemistry and physics. This is as if a scholar has come across a soldier—even if both are reasonable, it is no guarantee that they will be able to communicate! Confucius said this evidence is the Dao. We in Chinese Medicine call this evidence yin yang. But remember: "The Dao that can be spoken of is not the eternal Dao!"

I really feel that it is should not be necessary to set things in stone when it comes to traditional ideas. If one is drawn to these ideas, then their own understanding and closeness to the ideas will develop naturally. If one is not drawn to them, that is fine, just lay it aside. It has already been laying there for thousands of years, and is not going to go bad!

In recent years as cities in China have become more and more developed, a corresponding interest in nature has been growing. So many people are traveling to the once-isolated mountainous region of Jiuzhaigou in Sichuan province that an airport has been created there. This is true of Tibet as well. You can get a discounted air ticket to nearly every major city in China, but you'll never see discounts to Lhasa. This phenomenon is worth noting. I feel that traditional fields of study like Chinese Medicine have something in common with these formerly isolated natural areas: if no one is interested in them, and no one makes the effort to develop them, then they just sit there, quiet in their beauty. Thousands of years ago they were beautiful, and if left alone they will hold this beauty for thousands more years. But as they are developed and as more and more people travel there, if these people are not environmentally conscious, this natural beauty could be destroyed.

The five phases (*wuxing*) are a model of yin yang relationships. This is true. Actually, if we look at the process of creating hexagrams, we can get a general sense of this. In the *Classic of Changes*, it states: "Change contains the Supreme Ultimate (*taiji*), which is what produces the two polarities. The two polarities produce the four images. The four images produce the eight trigrams. The eight trigrams determine good fortune and misfortune. Good fortune and misfortune produce great undertakings of life."

The two polarities are yin and yang. When these two again form groups, changing into four different states, we have the four images. The four images are lesser yang (*shaoyang*), greater yang (*laoyang*), lesser yin (*shaoyin*), and greater yin (*laoyin*). These four images are also spring, summer, autumn, and winter; they are also wood, fire, metal, and water. Wood and fire are spring and summer: they are yang. Now, although wood and fire are both yang, their states are distinct from one another, so we have lesser and greater yang. Metal and water are autumn and winter: they are yin. Again, metal and water are both yin, but being distinct from one another, they are called lesser and greater yin. Spring-wood is warm, summer-fire is hot, autumn-metal is cool, and winter-water is cold.

Both yin and yang states are inclined in one direction or another: it is only earth that is a harmonious balance of yin and yang. Not being inclined in any direction, its *qi* is balanced, and it brings about transformation. Why is it not said that metal, wood, water, and fire bring about transformation and the myriad things? Why is this only said about earth? The fundamental reason is in this characteristic of earth, in its harmonious balance of yin and yang. In the *Classic of Changes*, it refers to this harmonious balance as "Heaven and earth's misty union," and "male and female commingling their essence." Thus the line: "Heaven and earth's misty union; all living things are transformed by it and develop. Male and female commingle their essence, and all living things thereby procreate." In *Plain Questions*

(Suwen), metal, wood, water, and fire each rule a season, but not earth. To rule a season is to be partial and inclined. To not rule a certain time is to be impartial and balanced. Only by not ruling a time can it be there at all times, ruling all times.

If we truly comprehend the essence of the five phases (*wuxing*), especially that of earth, then many questions of nature and of life can be made clear.

Question Seven

Q: When you expound upon the relationship between the six channels or conformations, I found myself still having trouble gaining a holistic understanding what you described as "rising and falling" and "opening and closing." Could you run through this again here? Please use simple language for those of us who are not professionals!

A: These terms—rising, falling, opening, closing, etc.—are just a convenient way of expressing a basic principle that applies to all things. As it says in *Plain Questions*: "Rising and falling, coming out and going in pertain to all vessels." These pertain to nature, the human body, all things that can be understood in terms of a process of rising, falling, exiting, and entering. Just as the sun rises in the east and falls in the west, all things in nature rise and fall. The sprouting of plants can be seen as rising, while their wilting can be seen as falling. Growth and decline over the course of the human life, flourishing and dwindling of culture—are these not rising and falling?

Exiting and entering is the same principle as rising and falling: if there is exiting, there must be entering; if there is entering, there must be exiting. Inhaling and exhaling is one example of this, eating and defecating is another. Understanding this principle can help one move through many challenges in life. For example, many in business want to gain money and not spend money, but gaining and spending are just like natural human functions, like breathing and eating. If we only eat and never have a bowel movement, what kind of situation will we find ourselves in? You will be sent to the emergency room! Realistically, if someone is not having bowel movements, they are unlikely to be eating either. This is the Dao, the Way, but as obvious as it may seem, most do not understand it.

These days one can find a large variety of teas that promote easy bowel movements, marketed especially to the elderly. Here we can see that if an individual has trouble passing stool, we will look for medicine to help with "exiting" and make it not only effortless but even joyful. However, when it comes to business, why do we feel that "exiting" is such a painful affair? Some of the very successful and prosperous businessmen are aware that if a lot of "entering" has occurred, that "exiting" must occur as well, and they make great effort to donate money and engage in philanthropy. They are willing and happy to engage in this sort of "exiting," as they know that it must happen at some point, and they would rather have it happen on their own terms.

"Rising and falling, coming out and going in pertain to all vessels." This is an objective reality, and it is one that will not go away just because we want it to. So, how does one get control of this process of entry and exit? This is where opening and closing comes in. This is discussed at length in my book, so I will not waste ink here in repeating it.

Question Eight

Q: During the process of editing your book, I was intrigued by the question of "medical models." Since then I've looked into the question further, and in particular the "Biopsychosocial Model" of George Engel. Do you feel that the Engel model may be helpful for Chinese Medicine?

A: Modern medicine is gradually shifting from pure biomedicine to the biopsychosocial model you mentioned. One may say that this is a great leap, but in reality this shift is more aspirational, as it has not taken place yet. All medicines need to attend to these three aspects of the biopsychosocial model. For a disease to arise, and for the disease to eventually be cured, involves not just the biology of the organism, but also the psychological and societal environments.

Modern medicine seems to be stuck at the biological level, and has not paid much attention to nor developed much knowledge about the role of psychology and society in disease. Chinese Medicine, on the other hand, encompasses biological, psychological, and social aspects. The primary focus is on the heart and body (*xin shen*), or to use a more traditional term, on form and spirit (*xing shen*). This was laid out quite clearly in the *Yellow Emperor's Internal Classic*, that only when "both form and spirit" are attended to can one live to the end of their allotted years. For medicine to only pay attention to the physical body is not enough; attention must also be paid to the spirit and heart!

Moving from this basic principle, the next step is to emphasize the union of heaven, earth, and mankind. This is what is referred to in *Plain Questions*: "Above know the heavenly writing, below know the earthly principles, in the middle know the affairs of man." The "heavenly writing" and "earthly principles" here are our natural environment. Chinese Medicine places great emphasis on this connection between the natural environment and disease. In the "Great Treatise on the Essentials of Ultimate Truth" in the *Plain Questions*, it says: "As for the advent of the hundred diseases, they all emerge from wind, cold, summer-heat, damp, dryness, and fire." Recognition of this connection has not emerged yet in modern medicine, which lays its emphasis on biology and has not paid attention to the influence of the natural environment. The "affairs of man" here refers to interpersonal relationships, namely society.

Besides the biological, psychological, and social factors in disease, Chinese Medicine also emphasizes the natural environment: heavenly and earthly factors. Regarding your question, I feel that it is more that the Chinese Medicine model will be able to help the medicine of the future than vice versa!

Question Nine

Q: My last question: Is there such a thing as Chinese Environmental Medicine? This is piggybacking on the previous question about medical models. I've drawn a somewhat mechanical equivalence between the following environments: natural, psychological, and social. We've discussed this issue before, that is, the question of how treatment in Chinese Medicine emphasizes not only regulating the disease, but also understanding psychology and regulating the natural environment. Is the fundamental goal to establish equilibrium between the internal and external environments? There are many instances in *Classical Chinese Medicine* where this issue is touched upon, but not fully fleshed out. Could you take some time to do that for us now?

A: I recall that during the editing process, you brought up the question of "Chinese Medicine Environmental Studies," and expressed the hope that I would be able to write my next book exclusively about this topic. I am touched by the high expectations you have of me, and I feel also a sense of shame that my understanding of the topic is not up to really explicating and making these questions clear.

The natural, psychological, and social environments can be thought as of expressing different aspects of the internal and external environments. Modern science has focused on making changes in the external environment, and in the process has brought about a great problem: that of the destruction of our natural environment. The contrast between the goals of changing our environment for the better and the reality that our very existence has become endangered is quite striking, but the reality is that any type of development will bring about a certain amount of damage to the environment.

The solution in ancient times was to focus instead on the internal environment. There is a classical saying that sums this up well: "To regulate the environment is inferior to regulating one's heart." All three principles and eight stages of Confucius's *Great Learning* (Daxue) are rooted in regulating the heart. In this context, the "environment" means everything external. Changing that which is external is inferior to changing one's heart. This is both a simple statement of truth, and a method to be applied in life.

What determines the pain and joy in one's life? External material conditions are of course a factor. One must have food, clothing, and a roof over one's head, but the ancients did not pursue these to any great degree. One should "know how much is enough." The key here is in the "knowing." If this is missing, then one can never have enough. One can never have everything; this is a bucket with no bottom. So if one pursues external conditions excessively, not only will one never be satisfied, but this has the potential to bring about disaster!

Not too long ago in Chinese cities, it was common to see three generations under one roof, living together in close quarters. And nowadays? Now we see a family of three living in a three-bedroom apartment, and still worrying that this is not enough. Likewise, in the past there were no private bathrooms, only public ones, and these were shared by dozens or even more than a hundred families. Now even one bathroom per family is not enough, and we even have guest bathrooms and master bathrooms! My goodness! If we continue down this road, there is no end in sight.

Yan Hui, the disciple of Confucius, had a bowl for rice, a ladle for water, and a room for shelter. Others would not be able to tolerate such a life, but Yan Hui was content. It is Yan Hui that made this lifestyle acceptable, not the other way around.

Confucianism, Buddhism, and Daoism all emphasized internal rather than external changes, as it is the internal factors that are the basis for change, while the external factors are the state of change. Conditions only have to be good enough, or as the sages said, "to know what is enough is to find eternal joy." Here they were specifically talking about external conditions.

Marriage is a good example of this. Marriage is an essential part of having a family, and it is part of the external environment. In the past, it was said of marriage that "one lasts a lifetime," meaning that one would only marry once in one's lifetime. Did this mean that marriages in the past were perfect in every way? No, of course not. But it did mean that when there was trouble that the way to fix it was clear: that was to change the internal environment, and that it was through changing oneself that one could adapt to one's partner. It was not to change to a different partner! A change like this is irreparable, and it does not actually mean that the problem has been resolved. In many cases, divorce just "does away with the tiger at the front door, while inviting a wolf in the back door." And what do these divorces do for families and society?

This marriage problem is a problem between men and women, and as such, is a problem with yin and yang. Confucius says: "One yin, one yang, this is the Dao." It is also said that "the Dao of Confucius starts with the husband and wife." If this beginning is taken care of, then the Dao of yin and yang will be cultivated well, and the family will be well as well. Only when this is done can we talk about the last two stages of Confucius's *Great Learning*, to regulate the country and to bring about great peace throughout the entire world.

How does one go about regulating one's family? How does one cultivate the Dao of yin and yang? *Great Learning* has clear instructions: it is through cultivation of the person. This does not mean cultivating others, and trying to change others; this means cultivating oneself. Now, how does one cultivate oneself? By rectifying the heart. How does one rectify the heart? Through sincerity, through not deceiving oneself. All of this work is done on an internal level. Changing one's heart allows for changing one's person. Changes in this internal environment allow one to adapt to the infinite variations in the external environment.

There are some things we may not realize. If one is unsatisfied with one's partner and wishes to change him or her, they may find that their partner is in fact becoming less and less satisfactory, and is growing further and further away. On the other hand, if one does not try to change one's partner, but rather focuses on changing oneself, one is likely to find that their partner is coming closer and closer to them. In *Great Learning* where it discusses cultivating the person, regulating the family, governing the country, and bringing about peace, it is the second aspect, of regulating the family, that is the center around which all else pivots. Likewise, the center around which the family pivots is the husband and wife. That is why this relationship is so important.

We see that in many cases when a young child comes down with some type of cancer that there are also issues in their family, like a frequently missing or absent parent. If the family environment is not healthy, how can good sprouts emerge? Most families in China today have single children, and while their parents may hope the best for them, how is this supposed to come about? A home full of resentment and hatred can no more bring up a healthy child than sprouts can grow in a polluted environment.

Various environments are in trouble these days, and of all of the different kinds in our world, I feel it is the family environment that is most important. This environment concerns one's entire life, from birth to death. There is only one way to create a harmonious family environment, and this is through cultivation of one's self. The Dao of the family has to be cultivated from the inside; this basic principle has been established in the Dao of *Great Learning.* This is: "to regulate the environment is inferior to regulating one's heart." If one wishes to turn one's back on this principle and still bring about change in one's environment, then achieving health in one's life is truly challenging.

The *Plain Questions* chapter titled "Treatise on Heavenly Truth in Remote Antiquity" (Shanggu tianzhen lun) discusses the followers of the Dao in remote antiquity. The first standard by which they lived was to "take yin yang as model." As I described above, yin yang is the same as husband and wife, so to cultivate the Dao of husband and wife is to cultivate the Dao of yin yang. It is only this way that the family environment can be good, and that the health of body and mind can be guaranteed. This is why I feel that the most important topic of Chinese Medicine's study of the environment ought to be this family environment.

At the turn of the twentieth century in northern China, there lived a remarkable peasant by the name of Wang Fengyi. His Dao was referred to by others as the Path of the Real Person (*shanren dao*). The first step on this path is in cultivation of the family. I feel that this path is one that is most appropriate for these modern times. I was first exposed to this path when I was a visiting scholar at Tsinghua University from 2002 to 2003, and as I learned more about it, I was both astonished and struck with a great sense of shame. I was astonished because this path, spoken by an illiterate peasant, is able to strike and penetrate deep into the heart of those who hear it. I was shamed because I myself was not living up to a single one of the principles espoused by it. After three years, with the assistance of this path, I myself have begun to be healed in body and heart. It is thus that I wish to take this opportunity to recommend this path to all, in the hope that all families under heaven may have health and good fortune!

Liu Lihong

Nanning, 2006

GLOSSARY OF HERBS AND FORMULAS

Angong Niuhuang Wan	安宮牛黃丸
Baihu Tang	白虎湯
Baihu Jia Renshen Tang	白虎加人參湯
Baihuasheshecao	白花蛇舌草
Baishao	白芍
Baizhi	白芷
Baizhu	白朮
Banxia	半夏
Banxia Xiexin Tang	半夏瀉心湯
Banzhilian	半枝蓮
Bupi Yichang Wan	補脾益腸丸
Cangzhu	蒼朮
Chaihu Guizhi Tang	柴胡桂枝湯
Chaihu Guizhi Ganjiang Tang	柴胡桂枝乾薑湯
Chaihu Shugan Tang	柴胡疏肝湯
Chenpi	陳皮
Chuanjiao	川椒
Chuanxiong	川芎
Da Chengqi Tang	大承氣湯
Dahuang Huanglian Xiexin Tang	大黃黃蓮瀉心湯
Dazao	大棗
Dandouchi	淡豆豉
Danggui	當歸
Danggui Sini Tang	當歸四逆湯
Dangshen	黨參
Fuling	茯苓
Fupian	附片

Fuzi	附子
Fuzi Lizhong Tang	附子理中湯
Fuzi Xiexin Tang	附子瀉心湯
Gancao	甘草
Gancao Tang	甘草湯
Gancao Fuzi Tang	甘草附子湯
Gancao Ganjiang Tang	甘草乾薑湯
Gancao Xiexin Tang	甘草瀉心湯
Ganjiang	乾薑
Gaozhen Wuyou San	高枕無憂散
Gengmi	粳米
Gouteng	鈎藤
Gualou San	瓜蔞散
Guiban	龜板
Guipi Tang	歸脾湯
Gui Qi Jianzhong Tang	歸芪建中湯
Guizhi	桂枝
Guizhi Tang	桂枝湯
Guizhi Jia Gui Tang	桂枝加桂湯
Huafen	花粉
Huangbo	黃柏
Huanglian	黃蓮
Huangqi Jianzhong Tang	黃芪建中湯
Huangqin	黃芩
Jiaotai Wan	交泰丸
Jiegeng	桔梗
Jing Fang Baidu San	荊防敗毒散
Juanbo	卷柏
Jupi	橘皮
Lipi	梨皮
Lizhong Tang	理中湯
Lingyang Gouteng Tang	羚羊鈎藤湯
Lingyangjiao	羚羊角
Liuyi San	六一散
Longdan Xiegan Tang	龍膽瀉肝湯
Longgu	龍骨
Mahuang	麻黃
Mahuang Tang	麻黃湯

Mahuang Guizhi Ge Ban Tang   麻黃桂枝個半湯
Mahuang Xixin Fuzi Tang   麻黃細辛附子湯
Maziren Wan   麻子仁丸
Maidong   麥冬
Maiya   麥芽
Muli   牡蠣

Niubangzi   牛蒡子
Niuhuang Jiedu Pian   牛黃解毒片

Pingwei San   平胃散

Qianhu   前胡
Qianyang Dan   潛陽丹
Qingjiu   清酒

Renshen   人參
Rougui   肉桂

Sang Xing Tang   桑杏湯
Sangye   桑葉
Sharen   砂仁
Shashen   沙參
Shandougen   山豆根
Shanzha   山楂
Shen Ling Baizhu San   參苓白朮散
Shenqu   神麯
Shengdihuang   生地黃
Shengjiang   生薑
Shengjiang Xiexin Tang   生薑瀉心湯
Shigao   石膏
Shizao Tang   十棗湯
Shudihuang   熟地黃
Si Junzi Tang   四君子湯
Sini San   四逆散
Sini Tang   四逆湯
Sumu   蘇木

Taibai San   太白散
Tiaowei Chengqi Tang   調胃承氣湯
Tongmai Sini Tang   通脈四逆湯

Wendan Tang   溫膽湯

Wuji San	五積散
Wuling San	五苓散
Wumei	烏梅
Wumei Wan	烏梅丸
Wushi San	五石散
Wuzhuyu	吳茱萸
Wuzhuyu Tang	吳茱萸湯
Xixin	細辛
Xiang Sha Liujun Tang	香砂六君湯
Xiao Chaihu Tang	小柴胡湯
Xiao Chaihu Jia Mangxiao Tang	小柴胡加芒硝湯
Xiao Chengqi Tang	小承氣湯
Xiao Qinglong Tang	小青龍湯
Xiaoshi	消石
Xiaoyao San	逍遙散
Xiexin Tang	瀉心湯
Xingren	杏仁
Xing Su San	杏蘇散
Xuan Mai Gan Jie Tang	玄麥甘桔湯
Xuanshen	玄參
Yiyuan San	益元散
Yinyanghuo	淫羊藿
Yuzhu	玉竹
Zanghonghua	藏紅花
Zexie	澤瀉
Zhebeimu	浙貝母
Zhenwu Tang	真武湯
Zhibao Dan	至寶丹
Zhigancao Tang	炙甘草湯
Zhike	枳殼
Zhimu	知母
Zhishi	枳實
Zhizi	梔子
Zhizi Chi Tang	梔子豉湯
Zhuling	豬苓
Zhuling Tang	豬苓湯
Zisuye	紫蘇葉
Zixue Dan	紫雪丹

GLOSSARY OF NAMES
AND TECHNICAL TERMS

bagua	八卦 (eight trigrams)
baji	罷極 (exhaustion of the ultimate)
baihu	白虎 (white tiger)
Baihui	百會 (DU 20)
Bian Que	扁鵲
bingji	病機 (disease mechanism)
bo	剝 (Falling Away, one of the twelve tidal hexagrams in the *Classic of Changes*)
Bo Gao	伯高
bu	蔀 (shed)
buji	不及 (falling behind)
Cang Gong	倉公
Chang Sang	長桑
chen	辰 (7–9 am)
Chen Xiuyuan	陳修圓
Chen Zhiheng	陳治恆
Chengqi	承泣 (ST 1)
chi	尺 (foot [unit of measurement]; third position of the pulse)
chou	丑 (1–3 am)
couli	腠理 (interstices of the flesh)
Dabao	大包 (SP 21)
Dadun	大敦 (LV 1)
dazhuang	大壯 (Great Strength, one of the twelve tidal hexagrams in the *Classic of Changes*)
Dao	道 (Way)
Deng Xiaoping	鄧小平
dongzhi	冬至 (winter solstice)
Dong Zhongshu	董仲舒

Dou Cai　　　　　　　竇材
dun　　　　　　　　遯 (Retreat, one of the twelve tidal hexagrams in the *Classic of Changes*)

fang　　　　　　　　方 (formula; direction)
Fang Zhongxing　　　　方中行
Fengchi　　　　　　　風池 (GB 20)
Fengfu　　　　　　　風府 (GV 16)
Feng Menglong　　　　馮夢龍
fengshui　　　　　　風水 (*feng shui*)
fu　　　　　　　　　浮 (floating)
fu　　　　　　　　　復 (Turning Back, one of the twelve tidal hexagrams in the *Classic of Changes*)
fu　　　　　　　　　腑 (bowel; hollow organ)

Gao Baoheng　　　　　高保衡
ge　　　　　　　　　合 (unit of measurement)
gewu zhizhi　　　　　格物致知 (to investigate things to perfect knowledge)
gong　　　　　　　　工 (adept)
Gongsheng Yang Qing　公乘陽慶
gou　　　　　　　　姤 (Encountering, one of the twelve tidal hexagrams in the *Classic of Changes*)
gou　　　　　　　　鈎 (hook)
guai　　　　　　　　夬 (Eliminating, one of the twelve tidal hexagrams in the *Classic of Changes*)
guan　　　　　　　　觀 (Watching, one of the twelve tidal hexagrams in the *Classic of Changes*)
guanjie　　　　　　　關節 (joint)

hai　　　　　　　　亥 (9–11 pm)
Han Xin　　　　　　　韓信
he　　　　　　　　　合 (union)
heche　　　　　　　河車 (Water Wheel)
Hetu　　　　　　　　河圖 (River Chart)
hong　　　　　　　　洪 (flooding; bounding)
hou　　　　　　　　候 (five-day term)
Huangdi　　　　　　　黃帝 (the Yellow Emperor)
Huangfu Mi　　　　　　皇甫謐
hun　　　　　　　　魂 (soul)

ji　　　　　　　　　極 (ultimate)
Jiquan　　　　　　　　極泉 (HT 1)
jieqi　　　　　　　　節氣 (node *qi*, seasonal term, solar term)

jin	緊 (tight; tense)
Jin Yong	金庸 (Lousi Cha)
jing	精 (essence)
jing	經 (classic; channel; conformation; warp; longitude)
jingdian	經典 (classical text)
Jingming	睛明 (BL 1)
Jueyin	厥陰
Ke Xuefan	柯雪帆
kun	坤 (Responding, one of the twelve tidal hexagrams in the *Classic of Changes*)
Lake Lugu	瀘沽湖
Lei Gong	雷公
Li Bai	李白
Li Dongyuan	李東垣
Lidui	厲兌 (ST 45)
Li Shizhen	李時珍
Li Yangbo	李陽波
liang	兩 (traditional unit of weight, approximately 50 grams)
Liang Qichao	梁啟超
Liang Shuming	梁漱溟
Liao Bingzhen	廖炳真
lin	臨 (Approaching, one of the twelve tidal hexagrams in the *Classic of Changes*)
Lin Peixiang	林沛湘
Lin Yi	林億
Ling Mengchu	凌濛初
Liu Bang	劉邦
Liu Wansu	劉完素
lun	論 (treatise)
mai	脈 (pulse)
mao	毛 (hair; hair-like)
mao	卯 (5–7 am)
Mao Zedong	毛澤東
Meng Haoran	孟浩然
Pengzu	彭祖
pi	否 (Hindrance, one of the twelve tidal hexagrams in the *Classic of Changes*)
pi	痞 (glomus)
Pu Fuzhou	蒲輔周

Qi Bo	岐伯
Qimen	期門 (LV 14)
qimen dunjia	奇門遁甲 (method of divination)
qiyi	氣宜 (appropriate *qi*)
qian	乾 (Initiating, one of the twelve tidal hexagrams in the *Classic of Changes*)
Qian Xuesen	錢學森
qiao	巧 (astute)
Qin Bowei	秦伯未
qinglong	青龍 (blue-green dragon)
ribusuo	日晡所 (time period of late afternoon, 3–5 pm)
sanjiao	三焦 (triple burner)
sha	殺 (to kill)
Shanzhong	膻中 (CV 17)
Shang Binghe	尚秉和
Shanghan	傷寒 (cold damage)
Shaochong	少沖 (HT 9)
Shao Kangjie	邵康節
Shao Shi	少師
Shaoyang	少陽
Shaoyin	少陰
Shao Yu	少俞
shen	申 (3–5 pm)
shen	神 (spirit)
Shennong	神農
Shenque	神闕 (CV 8)
sheng	聖 (sage)
shi	石 (stone)
shifu	師父 (master; teacher)
shou	首 (chief)
shou sheng	受盛 (receive sacrificial offerings)
si	巳 (9–11 am)
sini	四逆 (four counterflow)
sui	遂 (succession)
Sun Simiao	孫思邈
tai	泰 (Advance, one of the twelve tidal hexagrams in the *Classic of Changes*)
taiguo	太過 (overstepping)
taiji	太極 (Supreme Ultimate)
Taijitu	太極圖 (Chart of the Supreme Ultimate)

Taiyang	太陽
Taiyin	太陰
ti	體 (substance)
Tian Bawei	田八昧 (nickname for Tian Heming 田鶴鳴)
Tianchi	天池 (PC 1)
Tiantu	天突 (CV 22)
tong	通 (passage)
Wang Bing	王冰
Wang Caigui	王財貴
Wang Donghua	王東華
Wang Hongwen	王洪文
Wang Hu	汪琥
Wang Shuhe	王叔和
Wang Zhongxuan	王仲宣
wei	未 (1–3 pm)
wei	味 (flavor)
wei	微 (subtle)
wei	緯 (woof; latitude)
weibing	未病 (not-yet disease, *qi*-stage disease)
wenbing	溫病 (warm disease)
wu	午 (11 am–1 pm)
Wu Jutong	吳鞠通
Wu Kun	吳昆
Wu Peiheng	吳佩衡
Wu Qian	吳謙
Wu Renju	吳人駒
Wu Rongzu	吳榮祖
Wu Shiji	吳師機
wuwei	無為 (non-action, non-doing, non-striving)
wuyun liuqi	五運六氣 (five movements and six *qi*; the cyclical transformation of universal *qi*)
xiazhi	夏至 (summer solstice)
xian	弦 (wiry)
xiang	象 (image)
xiangshuxue	象數學 (the study of images and numbers)
xiaoke	消渴 (dispersion-thirst)
xiaoshu	小暑 (minor heat)
xing	形 (form)
xiuxi	休息 (rest)
xu	戌 (7–9 pm)

Xu Dachun	徐大椿
xuanwu	玄武 (black warrior)
Xue Shengbai	薛生白
yang	陽
Yangming	陽明
yangsheng	養生 (nurture life/emergence)
Yang Zhenning	楊振寧
Ye Tianshi	葉天士
yin	寅 (3–5 am)
yin	陰
Yinbai	隱白 (SP 1)
yong	用 (function)
Yongquan	湧泉 (KI 1)
you	酉 (5–7 pm)
You Zaijing	尤在涇
Yu Jiayan	喻嘉言
Yu Lu	雨路
yuanqi	元氣 (prenatal *qi*)
yunqi	運氣 (abbreviation of *wuyun liuqi*; see *wuyun liuqi*)
zangfu	臟腑 (viscera-bowel)
zeifeng	賊風 (thief wind)
Zeng Guofan	曾國藩
Zeng Rongxiu	曾榮修
zhang	章 (chapter)
Zhang Congzheng	張從正
Zhang Jiebin	張介賓
Zhang Liang	張良
Zhang Rui	張銳
Zhang Xichun	張錫純
Zhang Xiju	張錫駒
Zhang Zhongjing	張仲景
zhenwu	真武 (black warrior)
zheng	證 (syndrome; pattern; sign)
Zheng Qin'an	鄭欽安
Zhengyang	正陽
zhi	至 (apex, utmost)
zhi	治 (treat; put in order; regulation)
zhijie	治節 (governing the nodes)
Zhiyin	至陰 (BL 67)
Zhongchong	中沖 (PC 9)

zhongqi	中氣 (central *qi*)
Zhong Wen	仲文
Zhou Dunyi	周敦頤
Zhou Fengwu	周鳳梧
Zhou Ruchang	周汝昌
Zhou Yan	周岩
zhu	著 (obvious)
zhuque	朱雀 (scarlet bird)
zhuzheng	主證 (primary/governing symptom)
zi	子 (11 pm–1 am)

GLOSSARY OF CHINESE TEXTS

Bencao gangmu	《本草綱目》 (Compendium of Materia Medica)
Bencao sibian lu	《本草思辨錄》 (Records of Thoughtful Differentiation of Materia Medica)
"Benshu"	本輸 (*Lingshu*, Chapter 2, "Conveyance of the Root")
"Bilun"	痺論 (*Suwen*, Chapter 43, "Treatise on Blocks")
Bian Que xinshu	《扁鵲心書》 (Bian Que's Heart Book)
Binhu maixue	《瀕湖脈學》 (Lakeside Master's Study of the Pulse)
Changsha fangge kuo	《長沙方歌括》 (Changsha Collection of Formula Verses)
Chongguang buzhu *Huangdi neijing suwen*	《重廣補注黃帝內經素問》 (Unabridged and Annotated Plain Questions of the *Yellow Emperor's Classic*)
Chunqiu	《春秋》 (Spring and Autumn Annals)
Chunqiu fanlu	《春秋繁露》 (Luxuriant Dew of the *Spring and Autumn* *Annals*)
"Cifalun"	刺法論 (*Suwen*, Chapter 72, "Treatise on the Methods of Needling")
Daxue	《大學》 (Great Learning)

Dayao	《大要》 (Great Essential)
Daodejing	《道德經》 (Classic of the Dao and Its Virtue)
Erya	《爾雅》 (Erya)
Faxian muqin	《發現母親》 (Discovering Our Mother)
Fayan	《法言》 (Laws and Teachings)
Fangjixue	《方劑學》 (Formula Studies)
"Genjie"	根結 (*Lingshu*, Chapter 5, "Clinging Root")
Gongyangzhuan	《公羊傳》 (Commentary of Gongyang)
Guangya	《廣雅》 (Guangya)
Guangyun	《廣韻》 (Extensive [Articulation of] Rhymes)
Hanshu	《漢書》 (Book of the Han)
Heji jufang	《和劑局方》 (Official Prescriptions of the Harmonious Pharmacy)
Hongloumeng	《紅樓夢》 (Dream of the Red Chamber)
Houhanshu	《後漢書》 (Book of the Later Han)
Huainanzi	《淮南子》 (Masters of Huainan)
Huangdi neijing	《黃帝內經》 (Yellow Emperor's Classic of Internal Medicine, abbreviated throughout the book as *Yellow Emperor's Classic*)
Huangdi suwen xuanminglun fang	《黃帝素問宣明論方》 (Formulas from the Discussion Illuminating the Yellow Emperor's Plain Questions)

Huanghan yixue congshu	《皇漢醫學叢書》 (Imperial Han Medical Series)
Jian	《箋》 (Commentary)
Jifeng beiji fang	《雞峰備急方》 (Emergency Prescriptions from Rooster Peak)
Jiyun	《集韻》 (Collected Rhymes)
Jiankangbao	《健康報》 (Health Report)
"Jie jingwei lun"	解精微論 (*Suwen*, Chapter 81, "Treatise on Explaining the Profound")
Jingui yaolüe	《金匱要略》 (Essentials from the Golden Cabinet)
"Jingui zhenyan lun"	金匱真言論 (*Suwen*, Chapter 4, "Treatise on True Words in the Golden Cabinet")
"Jingmai bielun"	經脈別論 (*Suwen*, Chapter 21, "Further Discourse on the Channel Vessels")
"Jiugong bafeng"	九宮八風 (*Lingshu*, Chapter 77, "Nine Mansions and Eight Winds")
Jiutangshu	《舊唐書》 (History of the Early Tang)
"Jiuzhen shieryuan"	九針十二原 (*Lingshu*, Chapter 1, "Nine Needles and Twelve Sources")
"Jutonglun"	舉痛論 (*Suwen*, Chapter 39, "Treatise on Pain")
Kangxi zidian	《康熙字典》 (Kangxi Dictionary)
Liji	《禮記》 (Record of Rites)
Lixueji	《禮學記》 (Record of the Study of Rites)
Liyue pianwen	《理瀹駢文》 (Topical Remedies in Rhyme)

Linzheng zhinan yian	《臨證指南醫案》 (Case Records as a Guide to Clinical Practice)
"Linglan midian lun"	靈蘭秘典論 (*Suwen*, Chapter 8, "Treatise on the Spiritual Orchid Secret Canon")
Lingshu	《靈樞》 (Spiritual Pivot)
"Liujie zangxiang lun"	六節臟象論 (*Suwen*, Chapter 9, "Treatise on the Six Nodes and Visceral Manifestations")
"Liuweizhi dalun"	六微旨大論 (*Suwen*, Chapter 68, "Great Treatise on the Six Subtleties")
"Liuyuan zhengji dalun"	六元正紀大論 (*Suwen*, Chapter 71, "Great Treatise on the Policies and Arrangements of the Six Principal *Qi*")
Luxinjing	《顱囟經》 (Fontanel Classic)
Lunyu	《論語》 (Analects)
Luoshu	《洛書》 (Inscription of the River Luo)
Maijue huibian	《脈訣匯辨》 (Comprehensive Differentiation of Pulse Types)
"Maiyao jingwei lun"	脈要精微論 (*Suwen*, Chapter 17, "Treatise on the Essentials of Vessels and the Subtleties of the Essence")
Meihua yishu	《梅花易數》 (Plum Flower Calculations for the Changes)
Minglao Zhongyi zhi lu	《名老中醫之路》 (The Path of Venerable Chinese Medicine Doctors)
Nanjing	《難經》 (Classic of Difficulties)
Piweilun	《脾胃論》 (Treatise on the Spleen and Stomach)
"Pingren qixiang lun"	平人氣象論 (*Suwen*, Chapter 18, "Treatise on Phenomena Reflecting the Status of *Qi* in a Normal Person")

"Relun" 熱論
 (*Suwen*, Chapter 31, "Treatise on Heat")

Renxin yu rensheng 《人心與人生》
 (The Human Mind and Human Life)

Sanguo yanyi 《三國演義》
 (Romance of the Three Kingdoms)

"Shanggu tianzhen lun" 上古天真論
 (*Suwen*, Chapter 1, "Treatise on Heavenly Truth in Remote Antiquity")

Shanghan laisu ji 《傷寒來蘇集》
 (Collected Writings on the Renewal of the Discussion of Cold Damage)

Shanghanli 《傷寒例》
 (Guide to Cold Damage)

Shanghanlun 《傷寒論》
 (Treatise on Cold Damage)

Shanghanlun jiangyi 《傷寒論講義》
 (Commentary on the *Treatise on Cold Damage*)

Shanghanlun shisijiang 《傷寒論十四講》
 (Fourteen Lectures on Cold Damage)

Shanghan zabing lun 《傷寒雜病論》
 (Treatise on Cold Damage and Miscellaneous Diseases)

Shennong bencao jing 《神農本草經》
 (Divine Farmer's Classic of Materia Medica)

"Shengqi tongtian lun" 生氣通天論
 (*Suwen*, Chapter 3, "Treatise on the Vital *Qi* Connecting to Heaven")

Shiji 《史記》
 (Records of the Grand Historian)

Shijing 《詩經》
 (Classic of Poetry)

Shiming 《釋名》
 (Explanation of Names)

Shu 《疏》
 (Explanations)

Shujing/Shu/Shangshu 《書經》/《書》/《尚書》
 (Classic of Documents)

Shuihuzhuan 《水滸傳》
 (Outlaws of the Water Margin)

"Shuire xuelun"　　　　水熱穴論
　　　　　　　　　　　(*Suwen*, Chapter 61, "Treatise on Acupoints to
　　　　　　　　　　　Treat Water and Heat")

Shunqi yiri fenwei　　《順氣一日分為四時篇》
sishi pian　　　　　　(Division of the Proper Flow of *Qi* of One Day
　　　　　　　　　　　into Four Times)

Shuogua　　　　　　　《説卦》
　　　　　　　　　　　(Explanation of the Trigrams)

Shuowen jiezi　　　　《説文解字》
　　　　　　　　　　　(Explaining Writing and Analyzing Characters)

Siku quanshu　　　　《四庫全書》
　　　　　　　　　　　(Complete Encyclopedia in Four Branches)

Siku quanshu zongmu　《四庫全書總目》
　　　　　　　　　　　(General Catalogue for the *Complete Encyclopedia
　　　　　　　　　　　in Four Branches*)

"Siqi tiaoshen dalun"　四氣調神大論
　　　　　　　　　　　(*Suwen*, Chapter 2, "Great Treatise on the Four
　　　　　　　　　　　Qi and the Tuning of the Spirit")

Suwen　　　　　　　　《素問》
　　　　　　　　　　　(Plain Questions)

Sunzi bingfa　　　　《孫子兵法》
　　　　　　　　　　　(The Art of War)

Tailu yaolu　　　　　《胎臚藥錄》
　　　　　　　　　　　(Medicinal Records of Fontanel)

"Taiyin yangming lun"　太陰陽明論
　　　　　　　　　　　(*Suwen*, Chapter 29, "Treatise on Taiyin and
　　　　　　　　　　　Yangming")

"Tongping xushi lun"　通評虛實論
　　　　　　　　　　　(*Suwen*, Chapter 28, "Treatise Thoroughly
　　　　　　　　　　　Deliberating upon Depletion and Repletion")

Tuan　　　　　　　　《彖》
　　　　　　　　　　　(Commentary on the Judgments)

Wenbing tiaobian　　《温病條辨》
　　　　　　　　　　　(Systematic Differentiation of Warm Pathogen
　　　　　　　　　　　Diseases)

"Wuchangzheng dalun"　五常政大論
　　　　　　　　　　　(*Suwen*, Chapter 70, "Great Treatise on the Five
　　　　　　　　　　　Regular Policies")

Wuyin wuwei　　　　《五音五味》
　　　　　　　　　　　(Five Sounds and Five Flavors)

"Wuyun xing dalun"　　五運行大論
　　　　　　　　　　(*Suwen*, Chapter 67, "Great Treatise on the
　　　　　　　　　　Progression of the Five Movements")

"Wuzang bielun"　　　五臟別論
　　　　　　　　　　(*Suwen*, Chapter 11, "Further Discourse on the
　　　　　　　　　　Five Viscera")

Xici　　　　　　　　《繫辭》
　　　　　　　　　　(Great Commentary)

Xiyouji　　　　　　《西遊記》
　　　　　　　　　　(Journey to the West)

Xinhua zidian　　　《新華字典》
　　　　　　　　　　(Xinhua Dictionary)

Xingming guizhi　　《性命圭旨》
　　　　　　　　　　(Principles of the Innate Disposition and the
　　　　　　　　　　Lifespan)

Yifa yuantong　　　《醫法圓通》
　　　　　　　　　　(The Unbroken Circle of Medical Methods)

Yijing/Zhouyi　　　《易經》/《周易》
　　　　　　　　　　(Classic of Changes / Changes of Zhou)

Yili zhenchuan　　　《醫理真傳》
　　　　　　　　　　(True Transmission of Medical Principles)

Yilin duoying　　　《醫林掇英》
　　　　　　　　　　(Gathering Flowers in the Forest of Medicine)

Yiyuan　　　　　　《醫原》
　　　　　　　　　　(The Source of Medicine)

Yizong jinjian　　　《醫宗金鑒》
　　　　　　　　　　(Golden Mirror of the Medical Tradition)

"Yinyang lihe lun"　　陰陽離合論
　　　　　　　　　　(*Suwen*, Chapter 6, "Treatise on the Separation
　　　　　　　　　　and Union of Yin and Yang")

Yinyang xi riyue　　《陰陽系日月》
　　　　　　　　　　(Yin and Yang as Related to the Sun and Moon)

"Yinyang yingxiang　　陰陽應象大論
dalun"　　　　　　　(*Suwen*, Chapter 5, "Great Treatise on the
　　　　　　　　　　Correspondences of Yin and Yang")

Yupian　　　　　　《玉篇》
　　　　　　　　　　(Jade Discourse)

Yunhui　　　　　　《韻會》
　　　　　　　　　　(Gathered Rhymes)

Zagua	《雜卦》 (Miscellaneous Hexagrams)
Zengyun	《增韻》 (Additional Rhymes)
Zhenduanxue	《診斷學》 (Diagnostic Techniques)
Zhenjiu jiayi jing	《針灸甲乙經》 (A–Z Classic of Acupuncture and Moxibustion)
"Zhenyao jingzhong lun"	診要經終論 (*Suwen*, Chapter 16, "Treatise on the Essentials of Diagnosis and on Exhaustion in the Channels")
Zhengyun	《正韻》 (Correct Rhymes)
Zhiai mifang	《治癌秘方》 (Secrets of Treating Cancer)
"Zhizhenyao dalun"	至真要大論 (*Suwen*, Chapter 74, "Great Treatise on the Essentials of Ultimate Truth")
Zhongguo qingnian	《中國青年》 (China Youth)
Zhongyi jichu lilun	《中醫基礎理論》 (Fundamentals of Chinese Medicine)
Zhongyi zazhi	《中醫雜誌》 (Chinese Medicine Journal)
Zhongyong	《中庸》 (Doctrine of the Mean)
Zhoubi suanjing	《周髀算經》 (Arithmetic Classic of the Gnomon and the Circular Paths of Heaven)
Zhouli	《周禮》 (Rites of Zhou)
Zhouli tianguan shu	《周禮天官書》 (Official Documents of the *Rites of Zhou*)
Zhouyi cantongqi	《周易參同契》 (The Kinship of the Three, According to the *Changes of Zhou*)
Zhouyi Shangshi xue	《周易尚氏學》 (Master Shang's Study of the *Changes of Zhou*)
Zhuangzi	《莊子》 (Zhuangzi)
Zuozhuan	《左傳》 (Commentary of Zuo)

A CHRONOLOGY OF THE DYNASTIES IN CHINESE HISTORY

Xia dynasty	2070–1600 BC
Shang dynasty	1600–1050 BC
Western Zhou dynasty	1050–770 BC
Eastern Zhou dynasty	770–250 BC
Spring and Autumn period	770–479 BC
Warring States period	476–221 BC
Qin dynasty	221–206 BC
Western Han dynasty	206 BC–AD 23
Xin dynasty	AD 9–23
Eastern Han dynasty	AD 25–220
Three Kingdoms	AD 220–280
Western Jin dynasty	AD 265–317
Eastern Jin dynasty	AD 317–420
Southern and Northern Dynasties	AD 420–589
Sui dynasty	AD 581–618
Tang dynasty	AD 618–907
Five Dynasties	AD 907–960
Northern Song dynasty	AD 960–1127
Southern Song dynasty	AD 1127–1279
Yuan dynasty	AD 1271–1368
Ming dynasty	AD 1368–1644
Qing dynasty	AD 1644–1911